FOURTH EDITION

Handbook of
Fractures

FOURTH EDITION

Handbook of
Fractures

Kenneth A. Egol, MD

Professor and Vice Chairman
Department of Orthopaedic Surgery
NYU Hospital for Joint Diseases New York University Medical Center
New York, New York

Kenneth J. Koval, MD

Professor
Department of Orthopaedics
Dartmouth Hitchcock Medical Center
Lebanon, New Hampshire

Joseph D. Zuckerman, MD

Professor and Chairman
Department of Orthopaedic Surgery
NYU Hospital for Joint Diseases
New York University Medical Center
New York, New York

Wolters Kluwer | Lippincott Williams & Wilkins
Health

Philadelphia · Baltimore · New York · London
Buenos Aires · Hong Kong · Sydney · Tokyo

Acquisitions Editor: Robert Hurley
Product Manager: Elise M. Paxson
Production Manager: Bridgett Dougherty
Senior Manufacturing Manager: Benjamin Rivera
Marketing Manager: Lisa Lawrence
Design Coordinator: Doug Smock

Printed in China

Library of Congress Cataloging-in-Publication Data
Egol, Kenneth A., 1967-
       Handbook of fractures/Kenneth A. Egol, Kenneth J. Koval, Joseph D. Zuckerman.
— 4th ed.
            p. ; cm.
       Rev. ed. of: Handbook of fractures/Kenneth J. Koval, Joseph D. Zuckerman.
       Abridgement of Rockwood and Green's fractures in adults. 7th ed. c2010.
       Includes bibliographical references and index.
       ISBN 978-1-60547-760-2 (alk. paper)
       1. Fractures--Handbooks, manuals, etc.   2. Dislocations--Handbooks, manuals, etc.
       I. Koval, Kenneth J.   II. Zuckerman, Joseph D. (Joseph David), 1952-
       III. Koval, Kenneth J. Handbook of fractures.   IV. Rockwood & Green's fractures in
       adults. V. Title.
       [DNLM: 1. Fractures, Bone—Handbooks.   2. Dislocations—Handbooks.
WE 39 E31h 2010]
       RD101.K685 2010
       617.1'5—dc22
            2009051161

To my family, Lori, Alexander, Jonathan,
and Gabrielle, and to my mentors
KJK, JDZ, and MJB.
– Kenneth A. Egol

To all those people who have believed in me
and stood by me during adversity.
– Kenneth J. Koval

To the residents and faculty of the
NYU Hospital for Joint Diseases for all
their support in the past 25 years.
– Joseph D. Zuckerman

CONTENTS

This book represents the work of many physicians who trained at the Hospital for Joint Diseases. Starting in the 1980s, the Department of Orthopaedic Surgery initiated a weekly, didactic topic-related fracture case conference. This conference consisted of a short lecture presented by a senior resident on pertinent anatomy, fracture mechanism, radiographic and clinical evaluation, and classification and treatment options, followed by a series of cases that were used to further clarify the options for fracture care. The senior resident was also responsible for preparing a handout on the fracture topic, which was distributed prior to the lecture.

Over time, it became apparent that these topic-related fracture handouts were very useful as a reference for later study and were utilized by incoming residents as an aid in the Emergency Department. This resulted in the original compilation of the "Hospital for Joint Diseases Fracture Manual," which was organized and prepared for publication "in-house," by ourselves, two senior residents Scott Alpert and Ari Ben-Yishay, and our editorial associate William Green. The "Fracture Manual" became very popular, very quickly. Its popularity led to the preparation and publication of the second edition. The third edition was designed, in part, to accompany Rockwood and Green's textbook Fractures in Adults.

This fourth edition is a complete update of the "Fracture Manual." We have tried to keep it "pocket-size" despite the ever increasing expanse of material. Most importantly, we have tried to keep the "Fracture Manual" true to its roots as a comprehensive, useful guide for the management of patients with fractures and associated injuries. We hope that the users of this "Fracture Manual" find it helpful in their daily practice of fracture care.

Kenneth A. Egol, MD
Kenneth J. Koval, MD
Joseph D. Zuckerman, MD

ACKNOWLEDGMENTS

We would like to acknowledge the following people: James Slover, MD, Timothy Rapp, MD, Ronald Moskovich, MD, Alan Strongwater, MD, and Gail Chorney, MD, for their help in preparation of this book. In addition we would like to acknowledge all of the residents and fellows, past, present, and future, at the NYU Hospital for Joint Diseases whose inquisitiveness compel us to continually update this text.

PART I

General Considerations

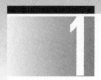

Closed Reduction, Casting, and Traction

PRINCIPLES OF CLOSED REDUCTION

- Displaced fractures, including those that will undergo internal fixation, should be reduced to minimize soft tissue trauma and provide patient comfort.
- Splints should respect the soft tissues.
  - Pad all bony prominences.
  - Allow for post injury swelling.
- Adequate analgesia and muscle relaxation are critical for success.
- Fractures are reduced using axial traction and reversal of the mechanism of injury.
- One should attempt to correct or restore length, rotation, and angulation.
- Reduction maneuvers are often specific for a particular location.
- One should try to immobilize the joint above and below the injury.
- Three-point contact and stabilization are necessary to maintain most closed reductions.

COMMON SPLINTING TECHNIQUES

- Splints may be prefabricated or custom made.
- "Bulky" Jones
  - Lower extremity splint, commonly applied for foot and ankle fractures and fractures about the knee, that uses fluffy cotton or abundant cast padding to help with post injury swelling. The splint is applied using a posterior slab and a U-shaped slab applied from medial to lateral around the malleoli. The extremity should be padded well proximal and distal to the injury.
- Sugar-tong splint
  - Upper extremity splint for distal forearm fractures that uses a U-shaped slab applied to the volar and dorsal aspects of the forearm, encircling the elbow (Fig. 1.1).
- Coaptation splint
  - Upper extremity splint for humerus fractures that uses a U-shaped slab applied to the medial and lateral aspects of the arm, encircling the elbow and overlapping the shoulder.
- Ulnar gutter splint
- Volar/dorsal hand splint

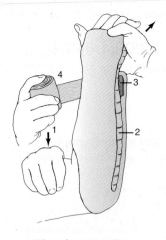

FIGURE 1.1 A sugar-tong plaster splint is wrapped around the elbow and forearm and is held using a circumferential gauze bandage. It should extend from the dorsal surface of the metacarpophalangeal joints to the volar surface of the fracture site. (From Bucholz RW, Heckman JD, Court-Brown C, eds. *Rockwood and Green's Fractures in Adults.* 6th ed. Philadelphia: Lippincott Williams & Wilkins; 2006.)

- Thumb spica splint
- Posterior slab (ankle) with or without a U-shaped splint
- Posterior slab (thigh)
- Knee immobilizer
- Cervical Collar
- Pelvic binder

Visit the University of Ottawa web site for general casting techniques and specifics on placing specific splints and casts: www.med.uottawa.ca/procedures/cast/

CASTING

- The goal is semirigid immobilization with avoidance of pressure or skin complications.
- It may be a poor choice in the treatment of acute fractures owing to swelling and soft tissue complications.
  - □ **Padding:** This is placed from distal to proximal with a 50% overlap, a minimum of two layers, and extra padding for bony prominences (fibular head, malleoli, patella, and olecranon).
  - □ **Plaster:** Cold water will maximize the molding time. Hot water may lead to burning the skin. Room temperature water is preferred.
  - □ 6-inch width for thigh
    - 4- to 6-inch width for leg
    - 4- to 6-inch width for arm
    - 2- to 4-inch width for forearm
  - □ Fiberglass
    - This is more difficult to mold but more resistant to moisture and breakdown.

- Generally, it is two to three times stronger for any given thickness.

Visit the University of Ottawa web site for general casting techniques and specifics on placing specific splints and casts: www.med.uottawa.ca/procedures/cast/

Below Knee Cast (Short Leg Cast)

- This should support the metatarsal heads.
- The ankle should be placed in neutral; apply with the knee in flexion.
- Ensure freedom of the toes.
- Build up the plantar surface for walking casts.
  - Fiberglass is preferred for durability.
- Pad the fibula head and the plantar aspect of the foot.

Above Knee Cast (Long Leg Cast)

- Apply below the knee first.
- Maintain knee flexion at 5 to 20 degrees.
- Mold the supracondylar femur for improved rotational stability.
- Apply extra padding anterior to the patella.

Short and Long Arm Casts

- The metacarpophalangeal (MCP) joints should be free.
  - Do not go past the proximal palmar crease.
- The thumb should be free to the base of the metacarpal; opposition to the fifth digit should be unobstructed.
- Even pressure should be applied to achieve the best mold.
- Avoid molding with anything but the heels of the palm, to avoid pressure points.

COMPLICATIONS OF CASTS AND SPLINTS

- Loss of reduction
- Pressure necrosis, as early as 2 hours after cast/splint application
- Tight cast or compartment syndrome
  - Univalving: 30% pressure drop
  - Bivalving: 60% pressure drop
  - Cutting of cast padding to further reduce pressure
- Thermal injury
  - Avoid plaster thicker than 10 ply
  - Avoid water hotter than 24°C
  - Unusual with fiberglass
- Cuts and burns during cast removal

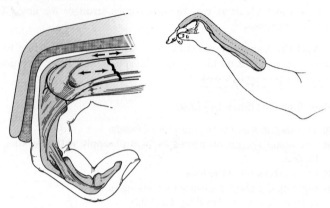

FIGURE 1.2 Position of function for the MCP joint.

- **Thrombophlebitis or pulmonary embolus:** increased with lower extremity fracture and immobilization but prophylaxis debated.
- **Joint stiffness:** Joints should be left free when possible (i.e., thumb MCP for short arm cast) and placed in position of function when not possible to leave free.

POSITIONS OF FUNCTION

- **Ankle:** neutral dorsiflexion (no equinus)
- **Hand:** MCP flexed (70 to 90 degrees), interphalangeal joints in extension (also called the intrinsic plus position) (Fig. 1.2)

TRACTION

- This allows constant controlled force for initial stabilization of long bone fractures and aids in reduction during operative procedures.
- The option for skeletal versus skin traction is case dependent.

Skin Traction

- Limited force can be applied, generally not to exceed 10 lb.
- This can cause soft tissue problems, especially in elderly patients or those with or rheumatoid-type skin.
- It is not as powerful when used during operative procedures for both length and rotational control.
- Bucks traction uses a soft dressing around the calf and foot attached to a weight off the foot of the bed.

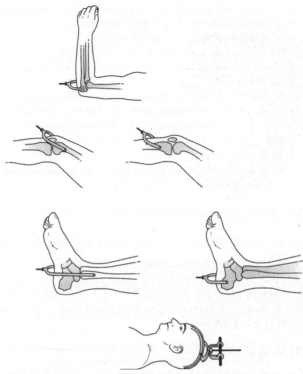

FIGURE 1.3 Skeletal traction sites. Various sites for skeletal traction are available. The techniques range from traction in the olecranon to skull traction, as illustrated here. (Modified from Connolly J. *Fractures and Dislocations: Closed Management.* Philadelphia: WB Saunders; 1995.)

□ This is an on option to provide temporary comfort in hip fractures and certain children's fractures.
□ A maximum of 7 to 10 lb of traction should be used.
□ Watch closely for skin problems, especially in elderly or rheumatoid patients.

Skeletal Traction (Fig. 1.3)

■ This is more powerful, with greater fragment control, than skin traction.
■ It permits pull up to 20% of body weight for the lower extremity.
■ It requires local anesthesia for pin insertion if the patient is awake.
　□ The anesthesia should be infiltrated down to the sensitive periosteum.

■ It is the preferred method of temporizing long bone, pelvic, and acetabular fractures until operative treatment can be performed.
■ Choice of thin wire versus Steinmann pin
  □ Thin wire is more difficult to insert with a hand drill and requires a tension traction bow. It requires use of a tension bow (Kirschner).
  □ The Steinmann pin may be either smooth or threaded.
    • A smooth pin is stronger but it can slide through the skin.
    • A threaded pin is weaker and bends more easily with increasing weights, but it will not slide and will advance more easily during insertion.
    • In general, the largest pin (5 to 6 mm) available is chosen, especially if a threaded pin is selected.

Tibial Skeletal Traction

■ The pin is placed 2 cm posterior and 1 cm distal to the tibial tubercle.
  □ It may go more distal in osteopenic bone.
■ The pin is placed from lateral to medial to direct the pin away from the common peroneal nerve.
■ The skin is released at the pin's entrance and exit points.
■ One should try to stay out of the anterior compartment.
  □ One should use a hemostat to push the muscle posteriorly.
■ A sterile dressing is applied next to the skin.

Femoral Skeletal Traction (Fig. 1.4)

■ This is the method of choice for pelvic, acetabular, and many femur fractures (especially in ligamentously injured knees).
■ The pin is placed from medial to lateral (directed away from the neurovascular bundle) at the adductor tubercle, slightly proximal to the femoral epicondyle.
  □ The location of this pin can be determined from the AP knee radiograph using the patella as a landmark.
■ One should spread through the soft tissue to bone to avoid injury to the superficial femoral artery.

Calcaneal Skeletal Traction

■ This is most commonly used with a spanning external fixation for "traveling traction," or it may be used with a Bohler-Braun frame.
■ It is used for irreducible rotational ankle fractures, some pilon fractures and extremities with multiple ipsilateral long bone fractures.

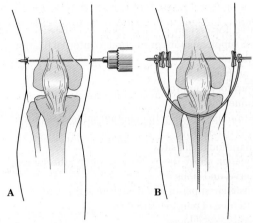

FIGURE 1.4 (A) Technique of inserting skeletal pins for femoral traction. A skeletal traction pin is inserted in the distal femur from medial to lateral. Local anesthetic is infiltrated down to the periosteum, and care is taken to avoid the neurovascular struc- tures in the posteromedial aspect of the knee. A hand drill is used to insert the 3-mm Steinmann pin, and care is taken to avoid pinching of the skin, which can be painful. **(B)** The pin is padded, and a traction bow is attached. (Modified from Connolly J. *Fractures and Dislocations: Closed Management.* Philadelphia: WB Saunders; 1995.)

- The pin is placed from medial to lateral, directed away from the neurovascular bundle, 2 to 2.5 cm posterior and inferior to the medial malleolus.

Olecranon Traction

- This is rarely used today.
- A small to medium-sized pin is placed from medial to lateral in the proximal olecranon; the bone is entered 1.5 cm from the tip of the olecranon.
- The forearm and wrist are supported with skin traction with the elbow at 90 degrees of flexion.

Gardner Wells Tongs

- This is used for cervical spine reduction and traction.
- Pins are placed one fingerbreadth above the pinna, slightly poste- rior to the external auditory meatus.
- Traction is applied starting with 5 lb and increasing in 5-lb incre- ments with serial radiographs and clinical examination.

Halo

- Indicated for certain cervical spine fractures as definitive treatment or supplementary protection to internal fixation.
- Disadvantages
  - Pin problems
  - Respiratory compromise
- Technique
  - Positioning of patient to maintain spine precautions
  - Fitting of halo ring
  - Preparation of pin sites
    - **Anterior:** above the eyebrow, avoiding the supraorbital artery, nerve, and sinus
    - **Posterior:** superior and posterior to the ear
  - Tightening of pins to 6 to 8 ft-lb
  - Retightening if loose
    - Pins only once at 24 hours after insertion
    - Frame as needed

Spanning External Fixation

- Concept of "Damage Control Orthopaedics" (DCO)
- Allows for temporary stabilization of long bones.
- Allows for transfer of patient in and out of bed.
- Does not foster an elevation of compartment pressures in affected extremities.
  - Performed in the operating room with fluoroscopy present.
  - Half pins can be placed into the ilium, femur, tibia, Calcaneus, talus, and forefoot.
  - Connected by various clamps and bars.
  - Traction applied across affected long bones and joints.

Multiple Trauma

- High-velocity trauma is the number 1 cause of death in the 18- to 44-year age group worldwide.
- Blunt trauma accounts for 80% of mortality in the <34-year age group.
- In the 1990s in the United States alone, income loss resulting from death and disability secondary to high-velocity trauma totaled 75 billion dollars annually; despite this, trauma research received <2% of the total national research budget.

The polytrauma patient is defined as follows:

- Injury severity score >18
- Hemodynamic instability
- Coagulopathy
- Closed head injury
- Pulmonary injury
- Abdominal injury

FIELD TRIAGE

Management Priorities

- Assessment and establishment of airway and ventilation
- Assessment of circulation and perfusion
- Hemorrhage control
- Patient extrication
- Shock management
- Fracture stabilization
- Patient transport

TRAUMA DEATHS

Trauma deaths tend to occur in three phases:

1. **Immediate:** This is usually the result of severe brain injury or disruption of the heart, aorta, or large vessels. It is amenable to public health measures and education, such as the use of safety helmets and passenger restraints.
2. **Early:** This occurs minutes to a few hours after injury, usually as a result of intracranial bleeding, hemopneumothorax, splenic rupture,

liver laceration, or multiple injuries with significant blood loss. These represent correctable injuries for which immediate, coordinated, definitive care at a level I trauma center can be most beneficial.

3. **Late:** This occurs days to weeks after injury and is related to sepsis, embolus, or multiple organ failure.

4. Mortality increases with increasing patient age (Fig. 2.1).

GOLDEN HOUR

- Rapid transport of the severely injured patient to a trauma center is essential for appropriate assessment and treatment.
- The patient's chance of survival diminishes rapidly after 1 hour, with a threefold increase in mortality for every 30 minutes of elapsed time without care in the severely, multiply injured patient.

THE TEAM

- The orthopaedic surgeon plays a critical role in management of the multiply injured patient.
- The trauma team is headed by the trauma general surgeon, who acts as the "captain of the ship" in directing patient care.
- The orthopaedic consult is available to assess all musculoskeletal injuries, provide initial bony stabilization, and work in concert with the trauma surgeons to treat shock and hemorrhage.
  - □ Long bone IM nailing
  - □ Pelvic external or internal fixation
  - □ Management of open wounds
  - □ Splintage
  - □ Traction
  - □ DCO

RESUSCITATION

- **Follows ABCDE:** airway, breathing, circulation, disability, exposure.

AIRWAY CONTROL

- The upper airway should be inspected to ensure patency.
- Foreign objects should be removed, and secretions suctioned.
- A nasal, endotracheal, or nasotracheal airway should be established as needed. A tracheostomy may be necessary.
- The patient should be managed as if a cervical spine injury were present. However, no patient should die from lack of an airway because of concern over a possible cervical spine injury. Gentle maneuvers, such as axial traction, are usually possible to allow for safe intubation without neurologic compromise.

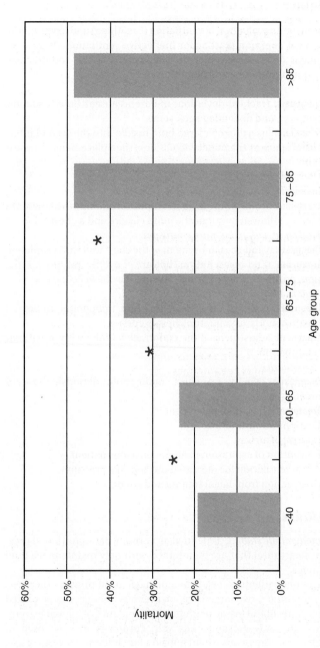

FIGURE 2.1 Mortality rate increases with increasing age.

BREATHING

- This involves evaluation of ventilation (breathing) and oxygenation.
- The most common reasons for ineffective ventilation after establishment of an airway include malposition of the endotracheal tube, pneumothorax, and hemothorax.
  - □ *Tension pneumothorax*
    Diagnosis: tracheal deviation, unilateral absent breath sounds, tympany, and distended neck veins
    Treatment: insertion of a large-bore needle into the second intercostal space at the midclavicular line, then placement of a chest tube
  - □ *Open pneumothorax*
    Diagnosis: sucking chest wound
    Treatment: occlusive dressing not taped on one side to allow air to escape, followed by surgical wound closure and a chest tube
  - □ *Flail chest with pulmonary contusion*
    Diagnosis: paradoxical movement of the chest wall with ventilation
    Treatment: fluid resuscitation (beware of overhydration), intubation, positive end-expiratory pressure may be necessary
  - □ *Endotracheal tube malposition*
    Diagnosis: malposition evident on chest radiograph, unilateral breath sounds, asymmetric chest excursion
    Treatment: adjustment of the endotracheal tube with or without reintubation
  - □ *Hemothorax*
    Diagnosis: opacity on chest radiograph, diminished/absent breath sounds
    Treatment: chest tube placement
- Indications for intubation
  - □ Control of airway
  - □ Prevention of aspiration in an unconscious patient
  - □ Hyperventilation for increased intracranial pressure
  - □ Obstruction from facial trauma and edema

CIRCULATION

- *Hemodynamic stability* is defined as normal vital signs (blood pressure, heart rate) that are maintained with only maintenance fluid volumes.
- In trauma patients, shock is hemorrhagic until proven otherwise.
- At a minimum, two large-bore intravenous lines should be placed in the antecubital fossae or groin with avoidance of injured extremities. Alternatively, saphenous vein cutdowns may be used in adults, or intraosseous (tibia) infusion for children <6 years of age.

- Serial monitoring of blood pressure and urine output is necessary, with possible central access for central venous monitoring or Swan-Ganz catheter placement for hemodynamic instability. Serial hematocrit monitoring should be undertaken until hemodynamic stability is documented.
- Peripheral blood pressure should be assessed.
- Blood pressure is necessary to palpate a peripheral pulse.

Peripheral pulse	Blood pressure
Radial	80 mm Hg
Femoral	70 mm Hg
Carotid	60 mm Hg

INITIAL MANAGEMENT OF THE PATIENT IN SHOCK

- Direct control of obvious bleeding: direct pressure control preferable to tourniquets or blind clamping of vessels.
- Large-bore venous access, Ringer lactate resuscitation, monitoring of urine output, central venous pressure, and pH.
- Blood replacement as indicated by serial hematocrit monitoring.
- Traction with Thomas splints or extremity splints to limit hemorrhage from unstable fractures.
- Consideration of angiography (with or without embolization) or immediate operative intervention for hemorrhage control.

DIFFERENTIAL DIAGNOSIS OF HYPOTENSION IN TRAUMA

Cardiogenic Shock

- Cardiac arrhythmias, myocardial damage
- Pericardial tamponade
  Diagnosis: distended neck veins, hypotension, muffled heart sounds (Beck triad)
  Treatment: pericardiocentesis through subxiphoid approach

Neurogenic Shock

- This occurs in patients with a thoracic level spinal cord injury in which sympathetic disruption results in an inability to maintain vascular tone.
- **Diagnosis:** hypotension without tachycardia or vasoconstriction. Consider in a head-injured or spinal cord–injured patient who does not respond to fluid resuscitation.
- **Treatment:** volume restoration followed by vasoactive drugs (beware of fluid overload).

Septic Shock

- Consider in patients with gas gangrene, missed open injuries, and contaminated wounds closed primarily.
- **Diagnosis:** hypotension accompanied by fever, tachycardia, cool skin, and multiorgan failure. This occurs in the early-to-late phases, but not in the acute presentation.
- **Treatment:** fluid balance, vasoactive drugs, antibiotics.

Hemorrhagic Shock

- More than 90% of patients are in acute shock after trauma.
- Consider in patients with large open wounds, active bleeding, pelvic and/or femoral fractures, and abdominal or thoracic trauma.
- **Diagnosis:** hypotension, tachycardia. In the absence of open hemorrhage, bleeding into voluminous spaces (chest, abdomen, pelvis, thigh) must be ruled out. This may require diagnostic peritoneal lavage, angiography, computed tomography (CT), MRI, or other techniques as dictated by the patient presentation.
- **Treatment:** aggressive fluid resuscitation, blood replacement, angiographic embolization, operative intervention, fracture stabilization, and other techniques as dictated by the source of hemorrhage.

CLASSIFICATION OF HEMORRHAGE

Class I: $<15\%$ loss of circulating blood volume
  Diagnosis: no change in blood pressure, pulse, or capillary refill
  Treatment: crystalloid

Class II: Fifteen percent to 30% loss of circulating blood volume
  Diagnosis: tachycardia with normal blood pressure
  Treatment: crystalloid

Class III: Thirty percent to 40% loss of circulating blood volume
  Diagnosis: tachycardia, tachypnea, and hypotension
  Treatment: rapid crystalloid replacement, then blood

Class IV: $>40\%$ loss of circulating blood volume
  Diagnosis: marked tachycardia and hypotension
  Treatment: immediate blood replacement

BLOOD REPLACEMENT

- Fully cross-matched blood is preferable; it requires approximately 1 hour for laboratory cross-match and unit preparation.
- Saline cross-matched blood may be ready in 10 minutes; it may have minor antibodies.

- Type O negative blood is used for life-threatening exsanguination.
- Warming the blood will help to prevent hypothermia.
- Monitor coagulation factors, platelets, and calcium levels.

PNEUMATIC ANTISHOCK GARMENT OR MILITARY ANTISHOCK TROUSERS

- Used to control hemorrhage associated with pelvic fractures.
- May support systolic blood pressure by increasing peripheral vascular resistance.
- May support central venous pressure by diminution of lower extremity blood pooling.
- **Advantages:** simple, rapid, reversible, immediate fracture stabilization.
- **Disadvantages:** limited access to the abdomen, pelvis, and lower extremities, exacerbation of congestive heart failure, decreased vital capacity, potential for compartment syndrome.
- Are contraindicated in patients with severe chest trauma.

INDICATIONS FOR IMMEDIATE SURGERY

Hemorrhage is secondary to

- **Liver, splenic, renal parenchymal injury:** laparotomy
- **Aortic, caval, or pulmonary vessel tears:** thoracotomy
- **Depressed skull fracture or acute intracranial hemorrhage:** craniotomy

DISABILITY (NEUROLOGIC ASSESSMENT)

- Initial survey consists of an assessment of the patient's level of consciousness, pupillary response, sensation, and motor response in all extremities, rectal tone, and sensation.
- The Glasgow coma scale (Table 2.1) assesses level of consciousness, severity of brain function, brain damage, and potential patient recovery by measuring three behavioral responses: eye opening, best verbal response, and best motor response.
- A revised trauma score results from the sum of respiratory rate, systolic blood pressure, and Glasgow coma scale and can be used to decide which patients should be sent to a trauma center (Table 2.2).

INJURY SEVERITY SCORE (ISS) (TABLE 2.3)

- This anatomic scoring system provides an overall score for patients with multiple injuries.

TABLE 2.1	Glasgow Coma Scale

Glasgow Coma Scale	Score
A Eye opening (E)	
1. Spontaneous	
2. To speech	4
3. To pain	3
4. None	2
B. Best motor response (M)	1
1. Obeys commands	
2. Localizes to stimulus	6
3. Withdraws to stimulus	5
4. Flexor posturing	4
5. Extensor posturing	3
6. None	2
C. Verbal response (V)	1
D. Oriented	
E. Confused conversation	5
F. Inappropriate words	3
G. Incomprehensible phonation	2
H. None	1

GCS = E + M + V (range, 3–15).

Note: Patients with a Glasgow coma scale of <13, a systolic blood pressure of <90, or a respiratory rate of >29 or <10/min should be sent to a trauma center. These injuries cannot be adequately evaluated by physical examination.

- It is based on the Abbreviated Injury Scale (AIS), a standardized system of classification for the severity of individual injuries from 1 (mild) to 6 (fatal).
- Each injury is assigned an AIS score and allocated to one of six body regions (head, face, chest, abdomen, extremities including pelvis, and external structures).
- The total ISS score is calculated from the sum of the squares of the three worst regional values. It is important to emphasize that only the worst injury in each body region is used.
- The ISS ranges from 1 to 75, with any region scoring 6 automatically giving a score of 75.
- The ISS limits the total number of contributing injuries to three only, one each from the three most injured regions, which may result in underscoring the degree of trauma sustained if a patient has more than one significant injury in more than three regions or multiple severe injuries in one region.
- To address some of these limitations, Osler et al. proposed a modification to the system which they termed the New Injury Severity

Revised Trauma Score: Trauma Scoring Systems		
Revised Trauma Score (RTS)	**Rate**	**Score**
A. Respiratory rate (breaths/min)	10–29	4
	>29	3
	6–9	2
	1–5	1
	0	0
B. Systolic blood pressure (mm Hg)	>89	4
	76–89	3
	50–75	2
	1–49	1
	0	0
C. Glasgow coma scale (GCS) conversion	13–15	4
	9–12	3
	6–8	2
	4–5	1
	3	0

RTS = 0.9368 GCS + 0.7326 SBP + 0.2908 RR. The RTS correlates well with the probability of survival.

Score (NISS). This is defined as the sum of squares of the AIS scores of each of a patient's three most severe injuries regardless of the body region in which they occur. Both systems have been shown to be good predictors of outcome in multiple trauma patients.

Evaluation of Multiple Trauma Patient Injury Severity Score (ISS)

Abbreviated injury scale defined body areas (external structures)
1. Soft tissue
2. Head and neck
3. Chest
4. Abdomen
5. Extremity and/or pelvis
6. Face

Severity code
1. Minor
2. Moderate
3. Severe (non-life-threatening)
4. Severe (life-threatening)
5. Critical (survival uncertain)
6. Fatal (dead on arrival)

ISS = A^2 + B^2 + C^2. A, B, and C represent individual body area severity code.

EXPOSURE

- It is important to undress the trauma patient completely and to examine the entire body for signs and symptoms of injury.

RADIOGRAPHIC EVALUATION

A radiographic trauma series consists of the following:

- Lateral cervical spine: must see all seven vertebrae and the top of T1.
  - □ Can perform swimmer's view or CT scan if needed.
  - □ In the absence of adequate cervical spine views of all vertebrae, the cervical spine cannot be "cleared" from possible injury, and a rigid cervical collar must be maintained until adequate views or a CT scan can be obtained.
  - □ Clinical clearance cannot occur if the patient has a depressed level of consciousness for any reason (e.g., ethanol intoxication).
- Anteroposterior (AP) chest.
- AP pelvis.
- CT scanning of these various regions has replaced plain films.

STABILIZATION

- The stabilization phase occurs immediately following initial resuscitation and may encompass hours to days, during which medical optimization is sought. It consists of
  1. Restoration of stable hemodynamics.
  2. Restoration of adequate oxygenation and organ perfusion.
  3. Restoration of adequate kidney function.
  4. Treatment of bleeding disorders.
- Risk of deep venous thrombosis is highest in this period and may be as high as 58% in multiply injured patients. Highest-risk injuries include spinal cord injuries, femur fractures, tibia fractures, and pelvic fractures. A high index of suspicion must be followed by duplex ultrasonography.
- Low-molecular-weight heparin, drop low dose warfarin, only low molecular weight heparin in patients without risk factors for hemorrhage has been shown to be more effective than sequential compression devices in preventing thromboses, but it is contraindicated in patients at risk for hemorrhage, especially following head trauma. Prophylaxis should be continued until adequate mobilization of the patient out of bed is achieved.
- Vena caval filters may be placed at time of angiography and are effective in patients with proximal venous thrombosis. These will only have an effect on development of embolic complications.

- Pulmonary injuries (e.g., contusion), sepsis, multiorgan failure (e.g., because of prolonged shock), massive blood replacement, and pelvic or long bone fractures may result in the adult respiratory distress syndrome (ARDS).

DECISION TO OPERATE

- Most patients are safely stabilized from a cardiopulmonary perspective within 4 to 6 hours of presentation.
- Early operative intervention is indicated for
  1. Femur or pelvic fractures, which carry high risk of pulmonary complications (e.g., fat embolus syndrome, ARDS).
  2. Active or impending compartment syndrome, most commonly associated with tibia or forearm fractures.
  3. Open fractures.
  4. Vascular disruption.
  5. Unstable cervical or thoracolumbar spine injuries.
  6. Patients with fractures of the femoral neck, talar neck, or other bones in which fracture has a high risk of osteonecrosis.
- Determination of patient medical stability
  - □ Activation of immune system results in release and suppression of mediators
    - May lead to second hit phenomena (Fig. 2.2)
  - □ Adequacy of resuscitation
    - Vital signs of resuscitation are deceptive.
    - Laboratory parameters include base deficit and lactic acidosis.
  - □ No evidence of coagulopathy
  - □ As long as homeostasis is maintained, no evidence exists that the duration of the operative procedure results in pulmonary or other organ dysfunction or worsens the prognosis of the patient.
  - □ Must be ready to change plan as patient status dictates.
  - □ Patients who are hemodynamically stable without immediate indication for surgery should receive medical optimization (i.e., cardiac risk stratification and clearance) before operative intervention.
- Decision making
  - □ Determined by general surgery, anesthesia, and orthopaedics.
  - □ Magnitude of the procedure can be tailored to the patient's condition.
  - □ Timing and extent of operative intervention based on physiologic criteria.
  - □ Early total care (ETC) is a concept that favors definitive stabilization/fixation of all orthopaedic injuries at the earliest opportunity.

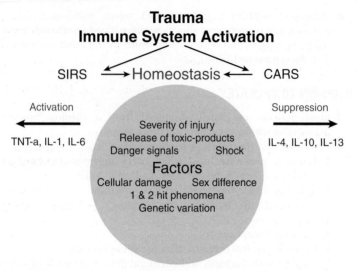

FIGURE 2.2 Factors associated with the "second hit" phenomena.

- ☐ Patients unable to undergo ETC may require damage control surgery as a temporizing and stabilizing measure.
- ■ Incomplete resuscitation
  - ☐ Based on physiologic assessment.
  - ☐ Intensive care includes monitoring, resuscitation, rewarming, and correction of coagulopathy and base deficit.
  - ☐ Once the patient is warm and oxygen delivery is normalized, reconsider further operative procedures.

CONCOMITANT INJURIES

Head Injuries

- ■ The diagnosis and initial management of head injuries take priority in the earliest phase of treatment.
- ■ Mortality rates in trauma patients are associated with severe head injury more than any other organ system.
- ■ Neurologic assessment is accomplished by the use of the Glasgow coma scale (see earlier).
- ■ Intracranial pressure monitoring may be necessary.

Evaluation

Emergency CT scan with or without intravenous contrast is indicated to characterize the injury radiographically after initial neurologic assessment.

- Cerebral contusion
  - □ **Diagnosis:** history of prolonged unconsciousness with focal neurologic signs
  - □ **Treatment:** close observation
- Epidural hemorrhage (tear of middle meningeal artery)
  - □ **Diagnosis:** loss of consciousness with intervening lucid interval, followed by severe loss of consciousness
  - □ **Treatment:** surgical decompression
- Subdural hemorrhage (tear of subdural veins)
  - □ **Diagnosis:** Neurologic signs may be slow to appear. Lucid intervals may be accompanied by progressive depressed level of consciousness.
  - □ **Treatment:** surgical decompression
- Subarachnoid hemorrhage (continuous with cerebrospinal fluid)
  - □ **Diagnosis:** signs of meningeal irritation
  - □ **Treatment:** close observation

Thoracic Injuries

- These may result from blunt (e.g., crush), penetrating (e.g., gunshot), or deceleration (e.g., motor vehicle accident) mechanisms.
- Injuries may include disruption of great vessels, aortic dissection, sternal fracture, and cardiac or pulmonary contusions, among others.
- A high index of suspicion for thoracic injuries must accompany scapular fractures.
- Emergency thoracotomy may be indicated for severe hemodynamic instability.
- Chest tube placement may be indicated for hemothorax or pneumothorax.

Evaluation

- AP chest radiograph may reveal mediastinal widening, hemothorax, pneumothorax, or musculoskeletal injuries.
- CT with intravenous contrast is indicated with suspected thoracic injuries and may demonstrate thoracic vertebral injuries.

Abdominal Injuries

These may accompany blunt or penetrating trauma.

Evaluation

- CT scan with oral and intravenous contrast may be used to diagnose intra-abdominal or intrapelvic injury. Pelvic fractures, lumbosacral fractures, or hip disorders may be observed.

- Diagnostic peritoneal lavage remains the gold standard for immediate diagnosis of operable intra-abdominal injury. Usually it is reserved for situations in which the patient is too unstable for the CT scanner.
- Positive peritoneal lavage
  Gross blood, bile, or fecal material
  >100,000 red blood cells per milliliter
  >500 white blood cells per milliliter
- Ultrasound (FAST) has been increasingly utilized to evaluate fluid present in the abdominal and chest cavities.

Genitourinary Injuries

Fifteen percent of abdominal trauma results in genitourinary injury.

Evaluation

- If genitourinary injury is suspected (e.g., blood seen at the urethral meatus), a retrograde urethrogram should be performed before indwelling bladder catheter insertion. Urethral injury may necessitate placement of a suprapubic catheter. If a pelvic fracture is present, communication with the urologist is mandatory.
- If hematuria is present, a voiding urethrogram, cystogram, and intravenous pyelogram are indicated.

3 Open Fractures

- An *open fracture* refers to osseous disruption in which a break in the skin and underlying soft tissue communicates directly with the fracture and its hematoma. The term *compound fracture* refers to the same injury, but is archaic.
- One-third of patients with open fractures are multiply injured.
- Any wound occurring on the same limb segment as a fracture must be suspected to be a consequence of an open fracture until proven otherwise.
- Soft tissue injuries in an open fracture may have three important consequences:
  1. Contamination of the wound and fracture by exposure to the external environment.
  2. Crushing, stripping, and devascularization that results in soft tissue compromise and increased susceptibility to infection.
  3. Destruction or loss of the soft tissue envelope may affect the method of fracture immobilization, compromise the contribution of the overlying soft tissues to fracture healing (e.g., contribution of osteoprogenitor cells), and result in loss of function from muscle, tendon, nerve, vascular, ligament, or skin damage.

MECHANISM OF INJURY

- Open fractures result from the application of a violent force. The applied kinetic energy ($0.5 \, mv^2$) is dissipated by the soft tissue and osseous structures (Table 3.1).

TABLE 3.1   Energy Transmitted by Injury Mechanism

Injury	Energy (ft-lb)
Fall from curb	100
Skiing injury	300–500
High-velocity gunshot wound (single missile)	2,000
20-mph bumper injury (assumes bumper strikes fixed target)	100,000

From Bucholz RW, Heckman JD, Court-Brown C, et al., eds. *Rockwood and Green's Fractures in Adults*, 6th ed. Philadelphia: Lippincott Williams & Wilkins, 2006.

■ The amount of bony displacement and comminution is suggestive of the degree of soft tissue injury and is proportional to the applied force.

CLINICAL EVALUATION

1. **Patient assessment involves ABCDE:** airway, breathing, circulation, disability, and exposure.
2. Initiate resuscitation and address life-threatening injuries.
3. Evaluate injuries to the head, chest, abdomen, pelvis, and spine.
4. Identify all injuries to the extremities.
5. Assess the neurovascular status of injured limb(s).
6. **Assess skin and soft tissue damage:** Exploration of the wound in the emergency setting is not indicated if operative intervention is planned because it risks further contamination with limited capacity to provide useful information and may precipitate further hemorrhage.
   □ Obvious foreign bodies that are easily accessible may be removed in the emergency room under sterile conditions.
   □ Irrigation of wounds with sterile normal saline may be performed in the emergency room if a significant surgical delay is expected.
   □ Sterile injection of joints with saline may be undertaken to determine egress from wound sites to evaluate possible continuity.
7. Identify skeletal injury; obtain necessary radiographs.

COMPARTMENT SYNDROME

■ An open fracture does not preclude the development of compartment syndrome, particularly with severe blunt trauma or crush injuries.
■ Severe pain, decreased sensation, pain to passive stretch of fingers or toes, and a tense extremity are all clues to the diagnosis. A strong suspicion or an unconscious patient in the appropriate clinical setting warrants monitoring of compartment pressures.
■ Compartment pressures >30 mm Hg raise concern and within 30 mm Hg of the diastolic blood pressure (ΔP) indicate compartment syndrome; immediate fasciotomies should be performed.
■ Distal pulses may remain present long after muscle and nerve ischemia and damage are irreversible.

VASCULAR INJURY

■ Ankle Brachial Indices (ABIs) should be obtained if signs of vascular compromise exist.

    □ Obtained by measuring diastolic pressure at the ankle and arm.
    □ Normal ratio is >0.9.
- An angiogram should be obtained if a vascular injury is suspected.
- Indications for angiogram include the following:
  - □ Knee dislocation with ABI <0.9
  - □ Cool, pale foot with poor distal capillary refill
  - □ High-energy injury in an area of compromise (e.g., trifurcation of the popliteal artery)
  - □ Documented ABI <0.9 associated with a lower extremity injury (note: preexisting peripheral vascular disease may result in abnormal ABIs; comparison with the contralateral extremity may reveal underlying vascular disease)

RADIOGRAPHIC EVALUATION

- Extremity radiographs are obtained as indicated by clinical setting, injury pattern, and patient complaints. Every attempt should be made to obtain at least two views of the extremity at 90 degrees to one another. It is important to include the joint above and below an apparent limb injury.
- Additional studies may include a CT if there is intra-articular involvement.

CLASSIFICATION

Gustilo and Anderson (Open Fractures) (Tables 3.2 and 3.3)

- This was originally designed to classify soft tissue injuries associated with open tibial shaft fractures and was later extended to all open fractures. While description includes size of skin wound, the subcutaneous soft tissue injury that is directly related to the energy imparted to the extremity is of more significance. For this reason, final typing of the wound is reserved until after operative debridement.
- It is useful for communicative purposes however, despite variability in interobserver reproducibility.

Type I: Clean skin opening of <1 cm, usually from inside to outside; minimal muscle contusion; simple transverse or short oblique fractures

Type II: Laceration >1 cm long, with extensive soft tissue damage; minimal-to-moderate crushing component; simple transverse or short oblique fractures with minimal comminution

Type III: Extensive soft tissue damage, including muscles, skin, and neurovascular structures; often a high-energy injury with a severe crushing component

TABLE 3.2 | Classification of Open Fractures

Type	Wound	Level of Contamination	Soft Tissue Injury	Bone Injury
I	<1 cm long	Clean	Minimal	Simple, minimal comminution
II	>1 cm long	Moderate	Moderate, some muscle damage	Moderate comminution
III[a]				
A	Usually >10 cm long	High	Severe with crushing	Usually comminuted; soft tissue coverage of bone possible
B	Usually >10 cm long	High	Very severe loss of coverage; usually requires soft tissue reconstructive surgery	Bone coverage poor; variable, may be moderate-to-severe comminution
C	Usually >10 cm long	High	Very severe loss of coverage plus vascular injury requiring repair; may require soft tissue reconstructive surgery	Bone coverage poor; variable, may be moderate-to-severe comminution

[a] Segmental fractures, farmyard injuries, fractures occurring in a highly contaminated environment, shotgun wounds, or high-velocity gunshot wounds automatically result in classification as type III open fractures.

From Bucholz RW, Heckman JD, Court-Brown C, et al., eds. *Rockwood and Green's Fractures in Adults*. 6th ed. Philadelphia: Lippincott Williams & Wilkins, 2006.

	Factors that Modify Open Fracture Classification Regardless of Initial Skin Defect

Contamination
A. Exposure to soil
B. Exposure to water (pools, lakes/streams)
C. Exposure to fecal matter (barnyard)
D. Exposure to oral flora (bite)
E. Gross contamination on inspection
F. Delay in treatment >12 hours

Signs of high-energy mechanism
A. Segmental fracture
B. Bone loss
C. Compartment syndrome
D. Crush mechanism
E. Extensive degloving of subcutaneous fat and skin
F. Requires flap coverage (any size defect)

From Bucholz RW, Heckman JD, Court-Brown C, et al., eds. *Rockwood and Green's Fractures in Adults.* 6th ed. Philadelphia: Lippincott Williams & Wilkins, 2006.

IIIA: Extensive soft tissue laceration, adequate bone coverage; segmental fractures, gunshot injuries, minimal periosteal stripping

IIIB: Extensive soft tissue injury with periosteal stripping and bone exposure requiring soft tissue flap closure; usually associated with massive contamination

IIIC: Vascular injury requiring repair

Tscherne Classification of Open Fractures

■ This takes into account wound size, level of contamination, and fracture mechanism.

Grade I: Small puncture wound without associated contusion, negligible bacterial contamination, low-energy mechanism of fracture

Grade II: Small laceration, skin and soft tissue contusions, moderate bacterial contamination, variable mechanisms of injury

Grade III: Large laceration with heavy bacterial contamination, extensive soft tissue damage, with frequent associated arterial or neural injury

Grade IV: Incomplete or complete amputation with variable prognosis based on location and nature of injury (e.g., cleanly amputated middle phalanx vs. crushed leg at the proximal femoral level)

Tscherne Classification of Closed Fractures

■ This classifies soft tissue injury in closed fractures and takes into account indirect versus direct injury mechanisms.

Grade 0:   Injury from indirect forces with negligible soft tissue damage

Grade I: Closed fracture caused by low-to-moderate energy mechanisms, with superficial abrasions or contusions of soft tissues overlying the fracture

Grade II: Closed fracture with significant muscle contusion, with possible deep, contaminated skin abrasions associated with moderate-to-severe energy mechanisms and skeletal injury; high risk for compartment syndrome

Grade III: Extensive crushing of soft tissues, with subcutaneous degloving or avulsion, and arterial disruption or established compartment syndrome

TREATMENT

Emergency Room Management

After initial trauma survey and resuscitation for life-threatening injuries (see Chapter 2):

1. Perform a careful clinical and radiographic evaluation as outlined earlier.
2. Wound hemorrhage should be addressed with direct pressure rather than limb tourniquets or blind clamping.
3. Initiate parenteral antibiosis (see later).
4. Assess skin and soft tissue damage; place a moist sterile dressing on the wound.
5. Perform provisional reduction of fracture and place in a splint, brace, or traction.
6. **Operative intervention:** Open fractures constitute orthopaedic urgencies. The optimal timing of surgical intervention is unclear from the literature. The only intervention that has been shown to diminish the incidence of infection in these cases is the early administration of intravenous antibiotics. There is growing evidence that open fractures in the absence of a non-limb threatening (vascular compromise, compartment syndrome) can be delayed up until 24 hours. The patient should undergo formal wound exploration, irrigation, and debridement before definitive fracture fixation, with the understanding that the wound may require multiple debridements.

Important

- Do not irrigate, debride, or probe the wound in the emergency room if immediate operative intervention is planned: This may further contaminate the tissues and force debris deeper into the wound. If a significant surgical delay (>24 hours) is anticipated, gentle irrigation with normal saline may be performed. Only obvious foreign bodies that are easily accessible should be removed.
- Bone fragments should not be removed in the emergency room, no matter how seemingly nonviable they may be.

Antibiotic Coverage for Open Fractures

Type I, II:	First-generation cephalosporin
Type III:	Add an aminoglycoside
Farm injuries:	Add penicillin and an aminoglycoside

Tetanus prophylaxis should also be given in the emergency room (see later). The current dose of toxoid is 0.5 mL regardless of age; for immune globulin, the dose is 75 U for patients <5 years of age, 125 U for those 5 to 10 years old, and 250 U for those >10 years old. Both shots are administered intramuscularly, each from a different syringe and into a different site.

Requirements for Tetanus Prophylaxis

Immunization history	dT	TIG	dT	TIG
Incomplete (<3 doses) or not known	+	−	+	+
Complete/>10 years since last dose	+	−	+	−
Complete/<10 years since last dose	−	−	−a	−

Key: +, prophylaxis required; −, prophylaxis not required; dT, diphtheria and tetanus toxoids; TIG, tetanus immune globulin; a, required if >5 years since last dose.

Operative Treatment

Irrigation and Debridement

Adequate irrigation and debridement are the most important steps in open fracture treatment:

- The wound should be extended proximally and distally in line with the extremity to examine the zone of injury.
- The clinical utility of intraoperative cultures has been highly debated and remains controversial.
- Meticulous debridement should be performed, starting with the skin subcutaneous fat and muscle (Table 3.4).

TABLE 3.4	Factors of Muscle Viability
Color	Normally beefy red; rarely, carbon monoxide exposure can be deceiving
Consistency	Normally firm, not easily disrupted
Capacity to bleed	Can be deceiving because arterioles in necrotic muscle can bleed Typically reliable
Contractility	Responsive to forceps pinch or low cautery setting Typically reliable

From Bucholz RW, Heckman JD, Court-Brown C, et al., eds. *Rockwood and Green's Fractures in Adults.* 6th ed. Philadelphia: Lippincott Williams & Wilkins, 2006.

- ☐ Large skin flaps should not be developed because this further devitalizes tissues that receive vascular contributions from vessels arising vertically from fascial attachments.
- ☐ A traumatic skin flap with a base-to-length ratio of 1:2 will frequently have a devitalized tip, particularly if it is distally based.
- ☐ Tendons, unless severely damaged or contaminated, should be preserved.
- ☐ Osseous fragments devoid of soft tissue may be discarded.
- ■ Extension into adjacent joints mandates exploration, irrigation, and debridement.
- ■ The fracture surfaces should be exposed fully by recreation of the injury mechanism.
- ■ Lavage irrigation, with or without antibiotic solution (acts as a surfactant), should be performed. Some authors favor pulsatile lavage. There is growing evidence that low flow, high volume irrigation may produce less damage to the surrounding tissues with the same effect. The addition of antibiotic to the solution has not been shown to be efficacious.
- ■ Meticulous hemostasis should be maintained, because blood loss may already be significant and the generation of clot may contribute to dead space and nonviable tissue.
- ■ Fasciotomy should be considered if concern for compartment syndrome exists, especially in the obtunded patient.
- ■ Historically, it has been advocated that traumatic wounds should not be closed. One should close the surgically extended part of the wound only. More recently, most centers have been closing the traumatic open wound over a drain or vacuum-assisted closure (VAC) system (Fig. 3.1) after debridement with close observation for signs or symptoms of sepsis.

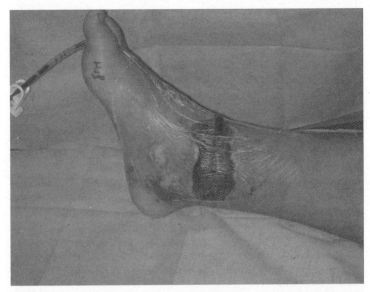

FIGURE 3.1 Example of a VAC dressing sponge utilized for an open medial ankle wound.

■ The wound, if left open, should be dressed with saline-soaked gauze, synthetic dressing, a VAC sponge, or an antibiotic bead pouch.

■ Serial debridement(s) should be performed every 24 to 48 hours as necessary until there is no evidence of necrotic soft tissue or bone. Definitive delayed primary or secondary wound closure should follow.

Foreign Bodies

Foreign bodies, both organic and inorganic ones, must be sought and removed because they can lead to significant morbidity if they are left in the wound. (Note: Gunshot injuries are discussed separately.)

■ Wood may become blood soaked and difficult to differentiate from muscle.

■ Cloth and leather are usually found between tissue planes and may be remote from the site of injury.

■ Road tar and oil may require special attention. Emulsifants such as Bisacodyl may be helpful during debridement to remove.

■ The foreign material itself usually incites an inflammatory response, whereas intrinsic crevices may harbor pathogenic organisms or spores.

Fracture Stabilization

In open fractures with extensive soft tissue injury, fracture stabilization (internal or external fixation, IM nails) provides protection from additional soft tissue injury, maximum access for wound management, and maximum limb and patient mobilization (see individual chapters for specific fracture management).

Soft Tissue Coverage and Bone Grafting

- Wound coverage is performed once there is no further evidence of necrosis.
- The type of coverage—delayed primary closure, split-thickness skin graft, rotational or free muscle flaps—is dependent on the severity and location of the soft tissue injury.
- Bone grafting can be performed when the wound is clean, closed, and dry. The timing of bone grafting after free flap coverage is controversial. Some advocate bone grafting at the time of coverage; others wait until the flap has healed (normally 6 weeks).

Limb Salvage

Choice of limb salvage versus amputation in Gustilo Grade III injuries is controversial. Immediate or early amputation may be indicated if:

1. The limb is nonviable: irreparable vascular injury, warm ischemia time >8 hours, or severe crush with minimal remaining viable tissue.
2. Even after revascularization the limb remains so severely damaged that function will be less satisfactory than that afforded by a prosthesis.
3. The severely damaged limb may constitute a threat to the patient's life, especially in patients with severe, debilitating, chronic disease.
4. The severity of the injury would demand multiple operative procedures and prolonged reconstruction time that is incompatible with the personal, sociologic, and economic consequences the patient is willing to withstand.
5. The patient presents with an injury severity score (ISS; see Chapter 2) of >20 in whom salvage of a marginal extremity may result in a high metabolic cost or large necrotic/inflammatory load that could precipitate pulmonary or multiple organ failure.

Many of the predictive scores such as the mangled extremity severity score (MESS) have been shown to be poor predictors of successful limb salvage (LEAP Study).

COMPLICATIONS

- **Infection:** Open fractures may result in cellulitis or osteomyelitis, despite aggressive, serial debridements, copious lavage, appropriate antibiosis, and meticulous wound care. Certain anatomic areas may be more prone to infection than others. The tibia with its one-third subcutaneous nature will be affected by the soft tissue stripping at the fracture site more so than a forearm injury with greater soft tissue coverage. Gross contamination at the time of injury is causative, although retained foreign bodies, amount of soft tissue compromise (wound type), nutritional status, and multisystem injury are risk factors for infection.
- **Missed compartment syndrome:** This devastating complication results in severe loss of function, most commonly in the forearm, foot, and leg. It may be avoided by a high index of suspicion with serial neurovascular examinations accompanied by compartment pressure monitoring, prompt recognition of impending compartment syndrome, and fascial release at the time of surgery.

4 Gunshot Wounds

BALLISTICS

- **Low velocity (>2,000 ft/sec):** This includes all handguns.
- **High velocity (>2,000 ft/sec):** This includes all military rifles and most hunting rifles.
- Shotgun wounding potential is dependent on
  1. Chote (shot pattern)
  2. Load (size of the individual pellet)
  3. Distance from the target

ENERGY

- The kinetic energy (KE) of any moving object is directly proportional to its mass (m) and the square of its velocity (v^2), and is defined by the equation: $KE = 1/2 \, (mv^2)$.
- The energy delivered by a missile to a target is dependent on
  1. The energy of the missile on impact (striking energy)
  2. The energy of the missile on exiting the tissue (exit energy)
  3. The behavior of the missile while traversing the target: tumbling, deformation, fragmentation

TISSUE PARAMETERS

- The wounding potential of a bullet depends on the missile parameters, including caliber, mass, velocity, range, composition, and design, as well as those of the target tissue.
- The degree of injury created by the missile is generally dependent on the specific gravity of the traversed tissue: higher specific gravity = greater tissue damage.
- A missile projectile achieves a high kinetic energy because of its relatively high velocity. The impact area is relatively small, resulting in a small area of entry with a momentary vacuum created by the soft tissue shock wave. This can draw adjacent material, such as clothing and skin, into the wound.
- The direct passage of the missile through the target tissue becomes the permanent cavity. The permanent cavity is small, and its tissues are subjected to crush (Fig. 4.1).
- The temporary cavity (cone of cavitation) is the result of a stretch-type injury from the dissipation of imparted kinetic energy

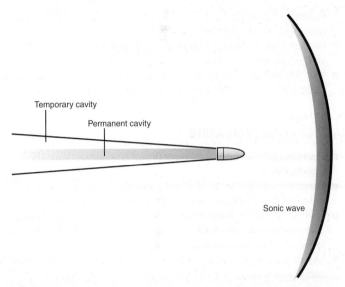

FIGURE 4.1 The two areas of tissue injury: the permanent cavity and the temporary cavity. The permanent cavity is caused by localized areas of cell necrosis proportional to the size of the projectile as it travels through. Temporary cavitization causes a transient lateral displacement of tissue. The shock wave, although measurable, has not been found to cause injury in tissue. (From Bucholz RW, Heckman JD, Court-Brown C, et al., eds. *Rockwood and Green's Fractures in Adults.* 6th ed. Philadelphia: Lippincott Williams & Wilkins; 2006.)

(i.e., shock wave). It is large, and its size distinguishes high-energy from low-energy wounds.

■ Gases are compressible, whereas liquids are not; therefore, penetrating missile injuries to the chest may produce destructive patterns only along the direct path of impact as a result of air-filled structures, whereas similar injuries to fluid-filled structures (e.g., liver, muscle) produce considerable displacement of the incompressible liquid with shock-wave dissipation, resulting in significant momentary cavities. This may lead to regions of destruction apparently distant to the immediate path of the missile with resultant soft tissue compromise.

CLINICAL EVALUATION

■ Following initial trauma survey and management (see Chapter 2), specific evaluation of the gunshot injury will vary based on the location of injury and patient presentation. Careful neurovascular examination must be undertaken to rule out the possibility of disruption to vascular or neural elements.

- Entrance wounds are characterized by a reddish zone of abraded skin—"the abrasion ring" Radiographic Evaluation.
- Exit wounds are larger in size than entrance wounds and more irregular in shape (e.g., stellate, slit-like, or crescent).

RADIOGRAPHIC EVALUATION

- Standard AP and lateral radiographs of the injured sites should be obtained.
- Fractures caused by low-velocity missiles tend to have multiple nondisplaced fracture lines that can potentially displace.
- Specific attention must be paid to retained missile fragments, degree of fracture comminution, and the presence of other potential foreign bodies (e.g., gravel).
- Missile fragments can often be found distant to the site of missile entry or exit.

TREATMENT OF ORTHOPAEDIC GUNSHOT INJURIES

Low-Velocity Wounds

- Steps in treatment include
  1. Administration of antibiotics (first-generation cephalosporin), tetanus toxoid, and antitoxin.
  2. Irrigation and debridement of the entrance and exit skin edges. Furthermore, one must understand that nonvital tissue and detritus may have been introduced to the fracture site. If so, operative debridement in the operating room may be required.
  3. Indications for operative debridement:
     - Retention in the subarachnoid space
     - Articular involvement (intra-articular bone or missile fragments)
     - Vascular disruption
     - Gross contamination
     - Massive hematoma
     - Severe tissue damage
     - Compartment syndrome
     - Gastrointestinal contamination
  4. **Fracture treatment:** Unstable fracture patterns are treated surgically, while stable patterns may be treated functionally following debridement.

High-Velocity and Shotgun Wounds

- These should be treated as high-energy injuries with significant soft tissue damage.
- Steps in treatment include
  1. Administration of antibiotics (first-generation cephalosporin), tetanus toxoid, and antitoxin
  2. Extensive and often multiple operative debridements
  3. Fracture stabilization
  4. Delayed wound closure with possible skin grafts or flaps for extensive soft tissue loss

Important: Gunshot wounds that pass through the abdomen and exit through the soft tissues with bowel contamination deserve special attention. These require debridement of the intra-abdominal and extra-abdominal missile paths, along with administration of broad-spectrum antibiotics covering gram-negative and anaerobic pathogens.

COMPLICATIONS

- **Retained missile fragments:** These are generally tolerated well by the patient and do not warrant a specific indication for surgery or a hunt for fragments at the time of surgery unless they cause symptoms (pain, loss of function), are superficial in location especially on the palms or soles, are involved in an infected wound, or are intra-articular in location. Occasionally, the patient will develop a draining sinus through which fragments will be expressed.
- **Infection:** Studies have demonstrated that gunshot injuries are not necessarily "sterile injuries" as was once thought. This is secondary to skin flora, clothing, and other foreign bodies that are drawn into the wound at the time of injury. In addition, missiles that pass through the mouth or abdomen are seeded with pathogens that are then dispersed along the missile path. Meticulous debridement and copious irrigation will minimize the possibility of wound infection, abscess formation, and osteomyelitis.
- **Neurovascular disruption:** The incidence of damage to neurovascular structures is much higher in high-velocity injuries (military weapons, hunting rifles), owing to the energy dissipation through tissues created by the shock wave. Temporary cavitation may produce traction or avulsion injuries to structures remote from the immediate path of the missile. These may result in injuries ranging from neuropraxia and thrombosis to frank disruption of neural and vascular structures.

■ **Lead poisoning:** Synovial or cerebrospinal fluid is caustic to lead components of bullet missiles, resulting in lead breakdown products that may produce severe synovitis and low-grade lead poisoning. Intra-articular or subarachnoid retention of missiles or missile fragments is thus an indication for exploration and removal.

5 Pathologic Fractures

DEFINITION

- A pathologic fracture is one that occurs when the normal integrity and strength of bone have been compromised by invasive disease or destructive processes.
- Causes include neoplasm (primary tumor or metastatic disease), necrosis, metabolic disease, disuse, infection, osteoporosis, or iatrogenic causes (e.g., surgical defect).
- Fractures more common in benign tumors (vs. malignant tumors).
  - □ Most are asymptomatic before fracture.
  - □ Antecedent nocturnal symptoms are rare.
  - □ Most common in children:
    - Humerus
    - Femur
    - Unicameral bone cyst, non-ossifying fibroma, fibrous dysplasia, eosinophilic granuloma are common predisposing conditions
- Primary malignant tumors
  - □ These are relatively rare.
  - □ Osteosarcoma, Ewing sarcoma, chondrosarcoma, malignant fibrous histiocytoma, fibrosarcoma are examples.
  - □ They may occur later in patients with radiation induced osteonecrosis (Ewing sarcoma, lymphoma).
  - □ Suspect a primary tumor in younger patients with aggressive-appearing lesions:
    - Poorly defined margins (wide zone of transition)
    - Matrix production
    - Periosteal reaction
  - □ Patients usually have antecedent pain before fracture, especially night pain.
  - □ Pathologic fracture complicates but does not mitigate against limb salvage.
  - □ Local recurrence is higher.
- Patients with fractures and underlying suspicious lesions or history should be referred for evaluation and possibly biopsy.
- Always obtain a biopsy of a solitary destructive bone lesion, even in patients with a history of primary carcinoma, before proceeding with definitive fixation.

MECHANISM OF INJURY

- Pathologic fractures may occur as a result of minimal trauma or even during normal activities.
- Alternatively, pathologic fractures may occur during high-energy trauma involving a region that is predisposed to fracture.

CLINICAL EVALUATION

- **History:** Suspicion of pathologic fracture should be raised in patients presenting with fracture involving
  □ Normal activity or minimal trauma
  □ Excessive pain at the site of fracture prior to injury
  □ Patients with a known primary malignant disease or metabolic disease
  □ A history of multiple fractures
  □ Risk factors such as smoking or environmental exposure to carcinogens
- **Physical examination:** In addition to the standard physical examination performed for the specific fracture encountered, attention should be directed to evaluation of a possible soft tissue mass at fracture site or evidence of primary disease such as lymphadenopathy, thyroid nodules, breast masses, prostate nodules, rectal lesions, as well as examination of other painful regions to rule out impending fractures.

LABORATORY EVALUATION (TABLE 5.1)

- Complete blood cell count (CBC) with differential, red blood cell indices, and peripheral smear
- Erythrocyte sedimentation rate (ESR)
- **Chemistry panel:** electrolytes, with calcium, phosphate, albumin, globulin, alkaline phosphatase
- Urinalysis
- Stool guaiac
- Serum and urine protein electrophoresis (SPEP, UPEP) to rule out possible myeloma
- Twenty-four-hour urine hydroxyproline to rule out Paget disease
- **Specific tests:** thyroid function tests (TFTs), carcinoembryonic antigen (CEA), parathyroid hormone (PTH), prostate-specific antigen (PSA)

RADIOGRAPHIC EVALUATION

- **Plain radiographs:** As with all fractures, include the joint above and below the fracture. It is difficult to measure size accurately,

TABLE 5.1	Disorders producing osteopenia

	Laboratory Value			
Disorder	Serum Calcium	Serum Phosphorus	Serum Alkaline Phosphatase	Urine
Osteoporosis	Normal	Normal	Normal	Normal Ca
Osteomalacia	Normal	Normal	Normal	Low Ca
Hyperparathyroidism	Normal to high	Normal to low	Normal	High Ca
Renal osteodystrophy	Low	High	High	
Paget disease	Normal	Normal	Very high	Hydroxyproline
Myeloma[a]	Normal	Normal	Normal	Protein

[a] Abnormal serum or urine immunoelectrophoresis.
From Bucholz RW, Heckman JD, Court-Brown C, et al., eds. *Rockwood and Green's Fractures in Adults.* 6th ed. Philadelphia: Lippincott Williams & Wilkins, 2006.

particularly with permeative lesions; >30% of bone must be lost before it is detectable by plain radiography.

- **Chest radiograph:** to rule out primary lung tumor or metastases in all cases.
- **Bone scan:** This is the most sensitive indicator of skeletal disease. It gives information on the presence of multiple lesions, correlates "hot" areas with plain x-rays, and may be "cold" with myeloma.
- **CT:** This is a more sensitive test for lesions that destroy <30% bone. It also shows soft tissue extension of a lesion.
- **MRI:** More useful for primary bone tumor. Shows the bony extent of the lesion, bone marrow changes, periosteal reaction, and soft tissue extension. Spine MRI is also useful to evaluate for spinal canal compromise.
- **PET scan:** More sensitive than bone scan in finding metastatic lesions. Especially helpful in primary lung carcinoma.
- Other useful tests in evaluating a patient with suspected pathologic fracture of unknown origin include the following (Table 5.2):
  □ Upper/lower gastrointestinal series
  □ Endoscopy
  □ Mammography
  □ Computed tomography of the chest, abdomen, and pelvis

Despite an elaborate workup, the primary disease process will not be identified in 15% of patients with suspected metastatic disease.

	Search for Primary Source in Patient with Suspected Metastatic Bone Lesion

1. History, especially of thyroid, breast, or prostate nodule
2. Review of systems, especially gastrointestinal symptoms, weight loss, flank pain, hematuria
3. Physical examination, especially lymph nodes, thyroid, breast, abdomen, prostate, testicles, and rectum
4. Total-body technetium-99m bone scan
5. Laboratory: complete blood count, erythrocyte sedimentation rate, calcium, phosphate, urinalysis, prostate-specific antigen, immunoelectrophoresis, and alkaline phosphatase
6. Biopsy: frozen section before prophylactic fixation

From Bucholz RW, Heckman JD, eds. *Rockwood and Green's Fractures in Adults.* 5th ed. Baltimore: Lippincott Williams & Wilkins, 2002:561.

CLASSIFICATION

Springfield

This is based on the pattern of bone invasion.

Systemic

- **Osteoporosis:** This is the most common cause of pathologic fractures in the elderly population.
- **Metabolic bone disease:** Osteomalacia, hyperparathyroidism, and renal osteodystrophy may be present.
- **Paget disease:** This is present in 5% to 15% of the elderly population. Pathologic fracture is the most common orthopaedic complication, seen in 10% to 30% of patients and often the first manifestation of unrecognized Paget disease.

Localized

- This accounts for the majority of pathologic fractures and includes
  - □ Primary malignancy of bone.
  - □ Hematopoietic disorders: myeloma, lymphoma, leukemia.
  - □ Metastatic disease:
    - Most pathologic fractures (80%) from metastatic disease arise from lesions of the breast, lung, thyroid, kidney, prostate.
    - Most common locations include the spine, ribs, pelvis, femur, humerus.

Classification by Pathologic Process

Systemic Skeletal Disease

- Bones are weak and predisposed to fracture. Healing and callus formation are normal.

- Correctable disorders include osteomalacia, disuse osteoporosis, hyperparathyroidism, renal osteodystrophy, and steroid-induced osteoporosis.
- Noncorrectable disorders include osteogenesis imperfecta, polyostotic fibrous dysplasia, osteopetrosis, postmenopausal osteoporosis, Paget disease, rheumatoid arthritis, and Gaucher disease.

Local Disease

- Benign primary bone tumors
  □ Nonossifying fibroma, unicameral bone cyst, aneurysmal bone cyst, enchondroma, chondromyxoid fibroma, giant cell tumor, osteoblastoma, chondroblastoma, eosinophilic granuloma
- Malignant primary bone tumors
  □ Ewing sarcoma, multiple myeloma, non-Hodgkin lymphoma, osteosarcoma, chondrosarcoma, fibrosarcoma, malignant fibrous histiocytoma
- Carcinoma metastasized to bone

Miscellaneous

- Irradiated bone
- Congenital pseudarthrosis
- Localized structural defects

TREATMENT

Initial Treatment

- **Standard fracture care:** reduction and immobilization
- Evaluation of underlying pathologic process
- Optimization of medical condition

Nonoperative Treatment

- In general, fractures through primary benign lesions of bone will heal without surgical management.
- Healing time is slower than in normal bone, particularly after radiation therapy and chemotherapy.
- Contrary to popular belief, the fracture will not stimulate involution of the lesion.

Operative Treatment

- Goals of surgical intervention are
  □ Prevention of disuse osteopenia

- ☐ Mechanical support for weakened or fractured bone to permit the patient to perform daily activities
- ☐ Pain relief
- ☐ Decreased length and cost of hospitalization
- Internal fixation, with or without cement augmentation, is the standard of care for most pathologic fractures, particularly long bones. Internal fixation will eventually fail if the bone does not unite.
- Resection and prosthetic reconstruction may be considered for impending pathologic fractures in periarticular locations or for failed attempts of internal fixation
- Loss of fixation is the most common complication in the treatment of pathologic fractures, owing to poor bone quality.
- Contraindications to surgical management of pathologic fractures are
  - ☐ General condition of the patient inadequate to tolerate anesthesia and the surgical procedure
  - ☐ Mental obtundation or decreased level of consciousness that precludes the need for local measures to relieve pain
  - ☐ Life expectancy of <1 month (controversial)
- Adequate patient management requires multidisciplinary care by oncologists, internal medicine physicians, and radiation therapists.
  - ☐ Radiation and chemotherapy are useful adjunctive therapies in the treatment of pathologic fractures, as well as potential mainstays of therapy in cases of metastatic disease.
    - These treatments are used to decrease the size of the lesion, stop lesion progression, and alleviate symptoms.
    - They delay soft tissue healing and should not be administered until 10 to 21 days postoperatively.
    - Renal cell carcinoma is more resistant to radiation and chemotherapy.
  - ☐ For renal cell and thyroid carcinomas, preoperative local embolization should be performed.
- Goals of surgery in treating patients with pathologic fractures are
  - ☐ Pain relief
  - ☐ Restoration of function
  - ☐ Facilitation of nursing care
- Pathologic fracture survival
  - ☐ Seventy-five percent of patients with a pathologic fracture will be alive after 1 year.
  - ☐ The average survival is $\sim$21 months and varies according to primary diagnosis (e.g. shorter for lung carcinoma).
- Pathologic fracture treatment includes

- ☐ Biopsy, especially for solitary lesions before proceeding with definitive surgery
- ☐ Nails versus plates versus arthroplasty
  - Interlocked cephalomedullary nails to stabilize the entire bone (e.g. cephalomedullary nails for femoral lesions)
  - Arthroplasty for periarticular fractures, especially around the hip
- ☐ Cement augmentation, which is often necessary
- ☐ Radiation and chemotherapy
- ☐ Aggressive rehabilitation

Adjuvant Therapy: Radiation Therapy and Chemotherapy

- ■ Role in treatment of pathologic fractures:
  - ☐ Palliate symptoms
  - ☐ Diminish lesion size
  - ☐ Prevent advancement of lesion

Metastases of Unknown Origin

- ■ Three percent to 4% of all carcinomas have no known primary site.
- ■ Ten percent to 15% of these patients have bone metastases.

Management of Specific Pathologic Fractures

Femur Fractures

- ■ The proximal femur is involved in >50% of long bone pathologic fractures resulting from high weight-bearing stresses.
- ■ Pathologic fractures of the femoral neck generally do not unite regardless of the degree of displacement; these require proximal femoral replacement. If the acetabulum is not involved, a hemiarthroplasty may be indicated; however, with acetabular involvement, total hip replacement is required.
- ■ Pathologic femoral shaft fractures may be managed with intramedullary nailing.
- ■ Indications for prophylactic fixation (Harrington) are
  - ☐ Cortical bone destruction ≥50%
  - ☐ Proximal femoral lesion ≥2.5 cm
  - ☐ Pathologic avulsion of the lesser trochanter
  - ☐ Persistent pain following irradiation
- ■ Mirel's scoring system for prophylactic fixation (*Clin Orthop* 1989) is useful (Table 5.3).

TABLE 5.3	Mirel's Criteria for Risk of Fracture		
	Number Assigned		
Variable	**1**	**2**	**3**
Site	Upper arm	Lower extremity	Peritrochanteric
Pain	Mild	Moderate	Severe
Lesion[a]	Blastic	Mixed	Lytic
Size	<1/3 diameter of the bone	1/3–2/3 diameter of the bone	>2/3 diameter of the bone

Each patient's situation is assessed a number (1, 2, or 3) to each aspect of his or her presentation (site, pain, lesion, and size) and then the numbers are added to obtain a total number to indicate the patient's risk for fracture. Mirel's data suggest that those patients whose total number is 7 or less can be irradiated and observed, but those with a number of 8 or more should have prophylactic internal fixation.
[a] By radiography.
From Bucholz RW, Heckman JD, Court-Brown C, et al., eds. *Rockwood and Green's Fractures in Adults.* 6th ed. Philadelphia: Lippincott Williams & Wilkins, 2006.

■ Advantages of prophylactic fixation compared to fixation after fracture occurs are as follows:
  □ Decreased morbidity
  □ Shorter hospital stay
  □ Easier rehabilitation
  □ Pain relief
  □ Faster and less complicated surgery
  □ Decreased surgical blood loss

Humerus Fractures

■ The humeral shaft is frequently involved with metastatic disease, thus increasing the possibility of humeral shaft fracture.
■ Prophylactic fixation of impending pathologic fractures is not recommended on a routine basis.
■ Operative stabilization of pathologic fractures of the humerus may be performed to alleviate pain, to reduce the need for nursing care, and to optimize patient independence.

Spine Fractures

■ If painful, but no neurologic loss, or loss of height, can treat with radiation therapy.

- For fractures caused by osteoporosis, myeloma, metastatic carcinoma, and percutaneous cement placement in the vertebral body can be used. There is concern for leakage of cement into the canal and adjacent veins.
- For neurological loss, spinal decompression and fusion with internal fixation can be done anteriorly or posteriorly.

Periprosthetic Fractures

TOTAL HIP ARTHROPLASTY

Femoral Shaft Fractures

Epidemiology

- **Intraoperative:** There is a 0.8% to 2.3% incidence overall, including cemented and uncemented components.
- **Postoperative:** There is a 0.1% incidence.
- They occur more frequently with noncemented components, with an incidence of 2.6% to 4% to as high as 21% for noncemented revisions.
- Mortality associated with age >70 and male sex (men 2.1% vs. 1.2% in women).

Risk Factors

- **Osteopenia:** Osteoporosis or bone loss secondary to osteolysis.
- Rheumatoid arthritis.
- THA following failed open reduction and internal fixation (ORIF).
- Stress risers secondary to cortical defects.
- Revision surgery.
- **Inadequate implant site preparation:** Large implant with inadequate reaming or broaching may be responsible.
- **Pericapsular pathology:** A scarred capsule with inadequate release may result in intraoperative fracture.
- **Loose components:** Loose femoral components are responsible for up to 33% of periprosthetic femur fractures.

Surgical Considerations (to Avoid Periprosthetic Fracture during Revision Surgery)

- Use longer-stem prosthesis, spanning twice the bone diameter beyond the defect.
- Consider bone grafting the defect.
- Strut allograft or plate support.
- Place cortical windows in an anterolateral location on the femur in line with the neutral bending axis.
- Leave cortical windows <30% of the bone diameter.
- Choose the correct starting point for reaming and broaching.

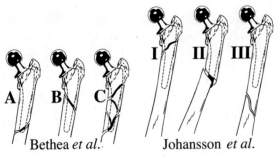

FIGURE 6.1 Classification scheme proposed by Johansson.

Classification

Johansson (Fig. 6.1)

Type I: Fracture proximal to the prosthetic tip with the stem remaining in the medullary canal

Type II: Fracture extending beyond the distal stem with dislodgement of the stem from the distal canal

Type III: Fracture entirely distal to the tip of the prosthesis

Cooke and Newman (Modification of Bethea et al.)

Type I: Explosion type with comminution around the stem; prosthesis always loose and fracture inherently unstable

Type II: Oblique fracture around the stem; fracture pattern stable, but prosthetic loosening usually present

Type III: Transverse fracture at the distal tip of the stem; fracture unstable, but prosthetic fixation usually unaffected

Type IV: Fracture entirely distal to the prosthesis; fracture unstable, but prosthetic fixation usually unaffected

American Academy of Orthopaedic Surgeons Classification (Fig. 6.2).

This divides the femur into three separate regions:

Level I: Proximal femur distally to the lower extent of the lesser trochanter

Level II: 10 cm of the femur distal to level I

Level III: Covers remainder of femur distal to level II

Type I: Fracture proximal to the intertrochanteric line that usually occurs during dislocation of the hip

Type II: Vertical or spiral split that does not extend past the lower extent of the lesser trochanter

Type III: Vertical or spiral split that extends past the lower extent of the lesser trochanter but not beyond level II, usually

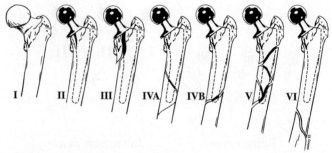

FIGURE 6.2 American Academy of Orthopaedic Surgeons classification of fractures associated with hip arthroplasty. (Modified from Petty W, ed. *Total Joint Replacement.* Philadelphia: WB Saunders; 1991:291–314.)

at the junction of the middle and distal thirds of the femoral stem

Type IV: Fractures that traverse or lie within the area of the femoral stem in level III, with type IVA being a spiral fracture around the tip and type IVB being a simple transverse or short oblique fracture

Type V: Severely comminuted fractures around the stem in level III

Type VI: Fractures distal to the stem tip, also in level III

Vancouver Classification (Fig. 6.3)

Type A: Fracture in the trochanteric region

AG: Greater trochanter region

AL: Lesser trochanteric region

Type B: Around or just distal to the stem

B1: Stable prosthesis

B2: Unstable prosthesis

B3: Unstable prosthesis plus inadequate bone stock

Type C: Well below the stem

Treatment Principles

■ Treatment depends on
  □ Location of the fracture.
  □ Stability of the prosthesis.
    • A loose stem should be revised.
  □ Bone stock.
  □ Age and medical condition of the patient.
  □ Accurate reduction and secure fixation.

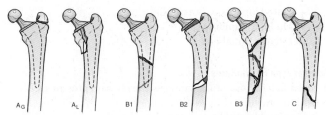

FIGURE 6.3 Vancouver classification scheme for periprosthetic fractures about total hip arthroplasties. (Modified from Duncan CP, Masri BA. Fractures of the femur after hip replacement. In: Jackson D, ed. *Instructional Course Lectures 44*. Rosemont, IL: American Academy of Orthopaedic Surgeons; 1995:293–304.)

- Options include
  - □ **Nonoperative treatment:** limited weight bearing, brace, cast, or traction.
  - □ ORIF (with plate and screws or cable and/or strut allograft).
  - □ Revision plus ORIF.

Vancouver Type A Fractures
- These are usually stable and minimally displaced.
- ORIF is used to maintain abductor function with wide displacement.
- Revision of acetabular component is indicated with severe polyethylene wear.

Vancouver Type B1 Fractures
- These are usually treated with internal fixation.
- Options for fixation include
  - □ Wires or cables
  - □ Plate and screws and/or cables
  - □ Cortical onlay allograft
  - □ Combination
- Long-term results depend on
  - □ Implant alignment
  - □ Preservation of the periosteal blood supply
  - □ Adequacy of stress riser augmentation
- Routine bone graft is used with ORIF.

Vancouver Type B2 Fractures
- Revision arthroplasty and ORIF are used.
- Choice of implant includes
  - □ **Uncemented prosthesis:**
    - • Extensive coated long-stem curved prosthesis

- Fluted long-stem prosthesis
- Modular implants
  □ Cemented prosthesis

Vancouver Type B3 Fractures
- No sufficient bone stock supports the revision prosthesis.
- Options include
  □ Proximal femoral reconstruction
    - Composite allograft
    - Scaffold technique
  □ Proximal femoral replacement
- Treatment depends on
  □ The age of the patient
  □ The severity of the bone defect
  □ The functional class of the patient

Vancouver Type C Fractures
- Treat independently of the arthroplasty.
- Use a plate and screws and/or cables with or without a strut allograft.
- Do not create any new stress riser.

Acetabular Fractures

- Nondisplaced fractures should be observed and treated with crutches and limited weight bearing. There is a high incidence of late loosening of the acetabular component, requiring revision.
- Associated intraoperatively with significant underreaming prior to press fit cup.
- Late fracture is associated with osteolysis or stress shielding.
- Must assess for pelvic discontinuity.
- Displaced fractures should be treated by ORIF, and the component should be revised.

TOTAL KNEE ARTHROPLASTY

Supracondylar Femur Fractures

Epidemiology

- The postoperative incidence is 0.6% to 2.8% in primaries and up to 6.3% in revisions.
- They generally occur within 10 years after surgery, usually secondary to relatively minor trauma.

Risk Factors

Supracondylar fractures after total knee replacement are multifactorial in origin, and risk factors include

- Osteoporosis
- Preexisting neurologic disease
- Knee stiffness/arthrofibrosis
- Notching of the anterior cortex:
  - □ **Biomechanical analysis:** 3 mm of anterior notching reduces torsional strength by 29%.
  - □ There is a high correlation between notching and supracondylar fractures in patients with rheumatoid arthritis and significant osteopenia.
  - □ In the absence of significant osteopenia, there is no correlation between notching and supracondylar fractures.
  - □ If notching >3 mm is noted intraoperatively, stemmed implant may be considered to avoid.

Classification

Neer, with Modification by Merkel
Type I: Minimally displaced supracondylar fracture
Type II: Displaced supracondylar fracture
Type III: Comminuted supracondylar fracture
Type IV: Fracture at the tip of the prosthetic femoral stem of fracture of the diaphysis above the prosthesis
Type V: Any fracture of the tibia

Periprosthetic Femur Fractures about Total Knees (Lewis and Rorabeck)
This classification takes into account both fracture displacement and prosthesis stability (Fig. 6.4).
Type I: The fracture is nondisplaced, and the bone-prosthesis interface remains intact.
Type II: The interface remains intact, but the fracture is displaced.
Type III: The patient has a loose or failing prosthesis in the presence of either a displaced or a nondisplaced fracture.

Treatment

Principles
- Anatomic and mechanical alignments are critical.
- Nondisplaced fractures may be treated nonoperatively.
- ORIF is indicated if the alignment is unacceptable by closed means and if bone stock is adequate for fixation devices.
- Immediate prosthetic revision is indicated in selected cases.

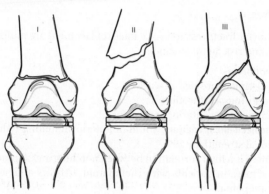

FIGURE 6.4 Classification scheme for periprosthetic fracture of the knee. (Modified from Lewis PL, Rorabeck CH. Periprosthetic fractures. In: Engh GA, Rorabeck CH, eds. *Revision Total Knee Arthroplasty.* Baltimore: Williams & Wilkins; 1997:275–295.)

Nonoperative Treatment

■ Long leg casting or cast bracing for 4 to 8 weeks may be used to treat minimally displaced fractures.

Operative Treatment

■ Displaced periprosthetic fractures around a total knee replacement are almost always managed with ORIF because of the difficulties in maintaining acceptable alignment after displacement.
  □ A blade plate, dynamic condylar screw, dynamic compression plate, condylar buttress plate, locked plate, or retrograde intramedullary nailing may be used for operative stabilization. (NB: nonunion rates are higher with use of IM nail.)
  □ Primary revision with a stemmed component may be considered if there is involvement of the bone-implant interface and if prosthesis is loose.
  □ Bone loss may be addressed with autologous grafting.
  □ Cases of severe bone loss, especially in the metaphyseal region, may be addressed with distal femoral replacement with a specialized prosthesis designed for oncology management.
■ Fractures around the diaphysis or the tip of a femoral component may be treated with cortical strut grafts and cerclage wiring, dynamic compression plate, locked plate, or a combination of techniques.
■ Acceptable alignment guidelines:
  □ Angulation <5 to 10 degrees in either plane
  □ <5-mm translation

□ <10-degree rotation
□ <1-cm shortening

Tibial Fractures

Risk Factors

- Significant trauma (shaft fractures)
- Tibial component malalignment associated with increased medial plateau stress fractures
- Revision surgery with press-fit stems to bypass a defect
- Loose components and osteolysis
- More common with increase in unicompartmental knee replacement
- Pin site placement

Classification

Periprosthetic Tibial Fractures (Felix et al.)

- **Classification is based on three factors:** location of the fracture, stability of the implant, and whether the fracture occurred intraoperatively or postoperatively (Fig. 6.5).

Type I: Occur in the tibial plateau
Type II: Adjacent to the stem
Type III: Distal to the prosthesis
Type IV: Involve the tubercle

- The stability of the implant is then used to classify the fractures further:
  □ Subtype A is a well-fixed implant.
  □ Subtype B is loose.
  □ Subtype C fractures are intraoperative.

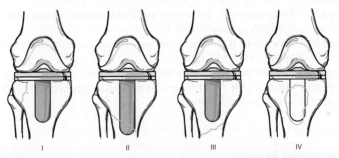

FIGURE 6.5 Classification of periprosthetic tibial fractures. (Modified from Felix NA, Stuart MJ, Hansen AD. Periprosthetic fractures of the tibia associated with total knee arthroplasty. *Clin Orthop.* 1997;345:113–124.)

Treatment

Nonoperative Treatment
- Closed reduction and cast immobilization may be performed for most tibial shaft fractures after alignment is restored.
- Early conversion to a cast brace to preserve knee range of motion is advised.

Operative Treatment
- Periprosthetic tibial fractures not involving the plateau require ORIF if closed reduction and cast immobilization are unsuccessful.
- Type I fractures involving the tibial plateau typically involve the bone-implant interface, necessitating revision of the tibial component.

Patella Fractures

Epidemiology

- The postoperative incidence is 0.3% to 5.4% (reported as high as 21%).

Risk Factors

- Large, central peg component
- Excessive resection of the patella during prosthetic implantation
- Lateral release, with devascularization of the patella
- Malalignment
- Thermal necrosis (secondary to methylmethacrylate)
- Excessive femoral component flexion

Classification

Goldberg

Type I:	Fractures not involving cement/implant composite or quadriceps mechanism
Type II:	Fractures involving cement/implant composite and/or quadriceps mechanism
Type IIIA:	Inferior pole fractures with patellar ligament disruption
Type IIIB:	Inferior pole fractures without patellar ligament disruption
Type IV:	Fracture-dislocations

Treatment

Nonoperative Treatment
- Fractures without component loosening, extensor mechanism rupture, or malalignment of the implant (type I or IIIB) may be

treated nonoperatively (these situations compose the majority of clinical cases).

■ The patient may be placed in a knee immobilizer for 4 to 6 weeks, with partial weight bearing on crutches.

Operative Treatment

■ Indicated for patients with disruption of the extensor mechanism, patellar dislocation, or prosthetic loosening.

■ Treatment options include

  □ ORIF with revision of the prosthetic patella. This is indicated for type II, IIIA, and IV fractures.

  □ **Fragment excision:** This may be undertaken for small fragments that do not compromise implant stability or patellar tracking.

  □ **Patellectomy:** This may be necessary in cases of extensive comminution or devascularization with osteonecrosis.

  □ Surgical considerations include adequate medial arthrotomy, adequate lateral release, preservation of the superior lateral geniculate artery, and preservation of the patellar fat pad.

TOTAL SHOULDER ARTHROPLASTY

Epidemiology

■ Periprosthetic fractures of the shoulder complicate approximately 1.6% to 2.3% of cases.

Risk Factors

■ Excessive reaming of the proximal humerus
■ Overimpaction of the humeral component
■ Excessive torque placed on the humerus during implant insertion

Classification

University of Texas San Antonio Classification of Periprosthetic Shoulder Fractures (Fig. 6.6)

Type I: Fractures occurring proximal to the tip of the humeral prosthesis

Type II: Fractures occurring in the proximal portion of the humerus with distal extension beyond the tip of the humeral prosthesis

Type III: Fractures occurring entirely distal to the tip of the humeral prosthesis

Type IV: Fractures occurring adjacent to the glenoid prosthesis

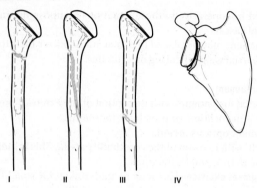

FIGURE 6.6 Classification of periprosthetic shoulder fractures. Type I: fractures occurring proximal to the tip of the prosthesis. Type II: fractures occurring in the proximal portion of the humerus with distal extension beyond the tip of the prosthesis. Type III: fractures occurring entirely distal to the tip of the prosthesis. Type IV: fractures occurring adjacent to the glenoid prosthesis. (From Bucholz RW, Heckman JD, eds. *Rockwood and Green's Fractures in Adults.* 5th ed. Baltimore: Lippincott Williams & Wilkins; 2002:587.)

Treatment

- **Controversial:** Some advocate nonoperative treatment with surgical intervention indicated for compromise of prosthetic fixation and intraoperative fractures. Others advocate aggressive operative stabilization of all periprosthetic fractures of the shoulder.

Nonoperative Treatment

- Closed treatment involves fracture brace, isometric exercises, and early range-of-motion exercises until radiographic evidence of healing.

Operative Treatment

- Primary goals include fracture union, prosthesis stability, and maintenance of motion.
- ORIF may be performed with cerclage wiring and possible bone grafting.
- Revision to a long-stem prosthesis may be required for cases with gross implant loosening.
- Options for postoperative immobilization range from sling immobilization for comfort until range-of-motion exercises can be

instituted, to shoulder spica casting for 6 weeks in cases of tenuous fixation.

TOTAL ELBOW ARTHROPLASTY

Epidemiology

- The overall prevalence of periprosthetic fractures of the elbow is approximately 13%.
- Most fractures are preceded by prosthetic loosening and thinning of the cortices. These occur more commonly in the humerus than in the ulna.

Risk Factors

- Osteoporosis
- Paucity of bone between the medial and lateral columns of the distal humerus
- Abnormal humeral bowing in the sagittal plane
- Size and angulation of the humeral and ulnar medullary canals
- Excessive reaming to accommodate the prostheses
- Revision elbow surgery

Classification (Fig. 6.7)

Type I: Fracture of the humerus proximal to the humeral component
Type II: Fracture of the humerus or ulna in any location along the length of the prosthesis
Type III: Fracture of the ulna distal to the ulnar component
Type IV: Fracture of the implant

Treatment

Nonoperative Treatment

- Nondisplaced periprosthetic fractures that do not compromise implant stability may be initially addressed with splinting at 90 degrees and early isometric exercises.
- The splint may then be changed to a fracture brace for 3 to 6 weeks.

Operative Treatment

- Displaced type I or II fractures may be managed with ORIF with cerclage wire fixation, or with plates and screws. Alternatively, revision to a long-stem humeral component may be performed, with the component extending at least two diameters proximal to the tip of the implant. Supplemental bone grafting may be used as necessary.

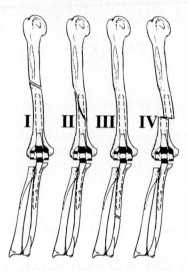

FIGURE 6.7 Classification of periprosthetic elbow fractures. Type I: fractures of the humerus proximal to the humeral component. Type II: fractures of the humerus or ulna in any location along the length of the prosthesis (including those fractures that extend proximal and distal to the humeral and ulnar components, respectively). Type III: fracture of the ulna distal of the ulnar component. Type IV: fracture of the implant. (From Bucholz RW, Heckman JD, eds. *Rockwood and Green's Fractures in Adults*. 5th ed. Baltimore: Lippincott Williams & Wilkins; 2002:601.)

- Type III fractures are usually amenable to cerclage wiring.
- If stable fixation of implant components cannot be obtained, consideration should be given to more constrained prostheses.
- Type IV fractures require component revision.
- Displaced olecranon fractures should be fixed with a tension band and cement.

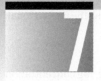

Orthopaedic Analgesia

PHARMACOLOGY: CLASSES OF DRUGS

- Local anesthetics
- Vasoconstrictors
- Opioids
- Sedatives (benzodiazepines)
- Others

LOCAL ANESTHETICS

- Basic function
  - □ These drugs act by blocking voltage-gated sodium channels in axons, preventing action potential.
- Local effect
  - □ Block is most effective in smaller, myelinated fibers that fire at high frequency.
  - □ Pain and temperature fibers are much more sensitive than pressure fibers, which are more sensitive than motor and proprioceptive fibers.
- Toxicity
  - □ Central nervous system (CNS)
    - Results from intravenous absorption or injection and high plasma levels.
    - They block inhibitory pathways, leading to unopposed excitatory components.
    - *Signs and* symptoms include dizziness, *tongue numbness*, nystagmus, and seizures (tonic-clonic).
  - □ Cardiovascular-depressive effects
    - Weaker contraction and arteriolar dilatation occur.
    - High doses can result in ventricular fibrillation, which is difficult to treat. Twenty percent intralipid is now being used as an agent to reverse significant cardiac toxicity.
  - □ Neurotoxicity
    - In high concentrations, they can directly damage peripheral nerve fibers.
- **Lidocaine:** rapid, potent, high penetration
  - □ Short acting

☐ **Most widely used local anesthetic:** local anesthesia, regional, spinal, epidural
- **Bupivacaine:** slower, potent
  - ☐ Longer lasting than lidocaine
  - ☐ Can separate motor and sensory block by altering concentration
  - ☐ Increased cardiac toxicity possibly
- Ropivicaine
  - ☐ "Safer" version of bupivicaine with same analgesic characteristics considered to be associated with a lower incidence of significant cardiac toxicity
- Maximal dose of commonly used local anesthetics
  - ☐ **Lidocaine:** 5 mg/kg (7 mg/kg if combined with epinephrine)
    - Calculation example:
      Percent concentration $\times$ 10 = mg/mL of drug
      1% lidocaine = 10 mg/mL of lidocaine
    - 30-kg child, 1% lidocaine without epinephrine
      10 mg/mL of lidocaine
      5 mg/kg $\times$ 30 kg = 150 mg allowed
      150 mg/10 mg/mL = 15 mL of 1% lidocaine
  - ☐ **Bupivacaine:** 1.5 mg/kg (3 mg/kg with epinephrine)

VASOCONSTRICTORS

- Allow for longer-lasting blockade (decreased blood flow, less drug leaves area).
- They may also decrease local blood loss.
- Epinephrine
  - ☐ Most widely used, diluted to 1/200,000
  - ☐ Should *not* be used for a digital block, Bier block, or ankle block
  - ☐ **Mnemonic for areas *not* to use epinephrine:** nose, hose (penis), fingers, toes
- Phenylephrine is occasionally used in spinal anesthesia.

OPIOIDS

- They are derived from the seed of the opium poppy, *Papaver somniferum.*
- Morphine and codeine are directly from the plant; others are synthesized.
- They act by binding to specific opioid receptors in the CNS (μ, δ, κ).
  - ☐ Th μ receptor is the one most responsible for the analgesic effect.
  - ☐ The action is both presynaptic and postsynaptic.

- Central action/pain modulation
  - □ When activated, the μ receptor inhibits γ-aminobutyric acid (GABA)-ergic neurons that would otherwise inhibit pain inhibitory neurons.
  - □ They may also affect neurons in the thalamus and midbrain, to modulate pain stimuli.
- CNS effects
  - □ Analgesia, euphoria, sedation, respiratory depression, cough suppression, miosis, nausea
- Peripheral effects
  - □ **Cardiovascular:** bradycardia
  - □ **Gastrointestinal:** decreased motility, constipation, constriction of biliary tree
  - □ **Genitourinary:** decreased renal function and increased sphincter tone
- Morphine
  - □ Naturally occurring, oldest member of this drug class
  - □ Dosing for adults
    - Loading dose of 0.05 to 0.10 mg/kg intravenously (IV) followed by 0.8 to 10.0 mg/hour IV titrated to pain
  - □ **Onset:** 5 minutes
  - □ **Relatively long lasting:** 3 to 4 hours
  - □ Better for continuous dull pain rather than sharp/severe pain
  - □ Used for postoperative PCA 1-mg increments with a lockout of 6 to 10 min. Basal rates tend to increase episodes of hypoxia
- Meperidine (Demerol)
  - □ Most common emergency department narcotic
  - □ One-tenth as potent as morphine
  - □ Dosing for adults
    - Fifteen to 35 mg/hour slow IV infusion or 50 to 150 mg subcutaneously/intramuscularly every 3 to 4 hours as needed
  - □ **Poorly titrated:** 5- to 10-minute onset and 2- to 3-hour duration
  - □ Potential for CNS stimulation
  - □ Less commonly used for pain than in the past
  - □ Concern about bad interactions with MAO inhibitors
- Fentanyl
  - □ 100$\times$ more potent and 7,000$\times$ more lipophilic than morphine
  - □ **Rapid uptake:** 30 to 60 seconds with peak analgesia in 2 to 3 minutes
  - □ **Duration:** 20 to 30 minutes
  - □ **Dose:** 1 μg/kg slowly, with sedation often at 3 to 4 μg/kg
  - □ **Risks:** "tight chest syndrome," bradycardia, respiratory depression
- Naloxone, naltrexone (Narcan)
  - □ Opioid antagonist

- ☐ Strong affinity for μ receptor
- ☐ Binds to receptor, but does not activate it, rapidly reversing the opioid effect within 1 to 3 minutes
- ☐ **Usual dose:** 0.1 to 0.4 mg IV (0.01 mg/kg in children)
- ☐ Shorter half-life than most agonists, so multiple doses may be necessary

SEDATIVES

- ■ Benzodiazepines
  - ☐ In general, they produce anxiolysis and sedation and encourage sleep.
  - ☐ They are metabolized in the liver and excreted in the urine.
  - ☐ Mechanism
    - • They act centrally, bind to, and activate the GABA-A receptor.
    - • GABA is major inhibitory neurotransmitter in the CNS.
    - • The GABA receptor is the chloride channel.
    - • When activated, they hyperpolarize the membrane, making it less excitable.
  - ☐ Effects
    - • Sedation, hypnosis, anesthesia, amnesia (anterograde), anti-convulsant effects, muscle relaxation, respiratory depression (especially in pulmonary patients)
    - • Often increased when combined with opioids
- ■ Midazolam
  - ☐ **Peak effect:** 2 to 3 minutes
  - ☐ Water soluble, hepatic metabolization
  - ☐ Easily titrated with doses every 5 to 7 minutes
  - ☐ 1 to 2 mg per dose (0.1 mg/kg/dose in children)
- ■ Flumazenil
  - ☐ Blocks the effect of benzodiazepines at the GABA receptor level.
  - ☐ It has a much shorter half-life than most benzodiazepines that are used clinically.
  - ☐ The dose is 0.1 to 0.2 mg IV (0.02 mg/kg in children).
  - ☐ Use with caution because it may precipitate seizures.
- ■ Ketamine
  - ☐ Dissociative anesthetic
  - ☐ Catatonic, amnestic, without loss of consciousness or loss of protective reflexes
  - ☐ Blockade of glutamic acid at the N-methyl-D-aspartate receptor subtype
  - ☐ May stimulate cardiovascular system and increase blood flow
  - ☐ **Dose:** 1 mg/kg IV
  - ☐ **Rapid onset:** 1 to 3 minutes

  □ **Duration:** 15 to 20 minutes
  □ **Occasional hallucinations on emergence:** can be avoided with a small dose of midazolam
  □ **May increase salivation:** atropine, 0.01 mg/kg, given before ketamine
 ■ Propofol
  □ Isopropylphenol compound
  □ Rapid onset, short duration (half-life 30 minutes but lipid soluble so clinical duration is less)
  □ Minimal gastrointestinal side effects or nausea
  □ **Provides general anesthesia:** sedation, hypnosis, without analgesia or amnesia
  □ **Complications:** respiratory depression, hypotension, pain at injection site
  □ Need for anesthesia/emergency department assistance with airway
  □ **Dose:** 0.5 to 1.0 mg/kg for induction of sedation
  □ **Highly titratable:** 25 to 100 μg/kg/minute infusion after initial bolus

NITROUS OXIDE

 ■ Inhaled agent
 ■ Given in varying 50/50 to 70/30 mixture with oxygen
 ■ Flow controlled by patient holding the mask
 ■ Provides analgesia and anxiolysis, some sedation
 ■ *Rapid onset and offset*
 ■ **Short duration:** resolves within 5 minutes of removing mask
 ■ Often used as an adjunct with other forms of anesthesia, or for short procedures
 ■ Very safe for brief procedures

REGIONAL BLOCKS AND CONSCIOUS SEDATION

Hematoma block, regional blocks, Bier block (if proper equipment and training available), and conscious sedation can all be effectively used by orthopaedists for fracture reduction and select procedures.

Hematoma Block

 ■ This replaces the fracture hematoma with local anesthetic.
 ■ It provides analgesia for closed reductions.
 ■ It provides postreduction analgesia.
 ■ Technique
  □ Sterile preparation of the fracture site is indicated.

□ Enter the fracture hematoma with a large-bore needle, aspirating hematoma fluid.

□ Replace the hematoma with 10 to 15 mL of 1% lidocaine without epinephrine.

   • Bupivacaine may be added to help with postreduction pain. *Give in safe dose such as 10 mL of 0.25%.*

□ Wait 5 to 7 minutes, then perform the reduction maneuver.

■ Risks

   □ Systemic toxicity

   • Potential risk of the local anesthetic's entering the bloodstream directly via the bone's blood supply.

   • Infection

      Theoretically converting a closed fracture to an open one. Single case report in orthopaedic literature.

Regional Blocks

■ They provide anesthesia to a certain area of the body, without general whole-body effects.

■ They are useful in fracture-dislocation reduction, as well as minor and major surgical procedures on the extremities.

■ They are also beneficial for postprocedure analgesia.

■ Local anesthetic is injected around the peripheral *nerves or plexi*.

■ Length of block depends on the choice of anesthetic, as well as the use of epinephrine.

Digital Block

■ Indications include finger fracture, laceration, nailbed injury, and finger/nailbed infection.

■ *Do not use epinephrine.*

■ Technique (Fig. 7.1)

   □ Pronate the hand (skin on the dorsum is less sensitive).

   □ Use two injection sites, at each side of the metacarpophalangeal.

   □ Use about 2 mL per nerve (8 mL total).

Wrist Block (Fig. 7.2)

■ Median nerve

   □ Indications include multiple finger fractures and finger/nailbed lacerations.

   □ Technique

   • Supinate the forearm.

   • The needle is placed between the palmaris longus and the flexor carpi radialis, 2 cm proximal to the wrist flexion crease.

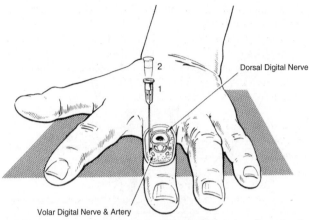

2

1

Dorsal Digital Nerve

Volar Digital Nerve & Artery

FIGURE 7.1 Surgical anatomy for the Digital Block Technique (From Consins MJ, Bridenbaugh PO, eds. *Neural Blockade*. 3rd ed. Philadelphia: Lippincott-Raven; 1998.)

- If paresthesia is elicited, inject 3 to 5 mL at this site.
- If no paresthesia occurs, then inject 5 mL in fan-shaped fashion.
■ Ulnar nerve
  □ **Indications:** ulnar-sided lacerations, reductions of boxer's fracture (if anesthesia is required)
  □ **Technique:** supinated hand, 6 cm proximal to wrist crease, just radial to flexor carpi ulnaris, 8 to 10 mL (more distal block will miss the dorsal branch, which can be blocked by a wheal ulnar to the flexor carpi ulnaris)
■ Radial nerve
  □ Indications include thumb and dorsum of hand lacerations.
  □ Technique
    - Field block is performed on the pronated hand at the level of the snuff box.
    - This is superficial to the extensor palmaris longus tendon.
    - Start at the snuff box and continue over the entire dorsum of the hand.
    - A dose of 5 to 8 mL is required.

Elbow Block

■ Indications include procedures of the hand and wrist.
■ **Four nerves are involved:** median, ulnar, radial, and lateral antebrachial cutaneous.
■ Median nerve

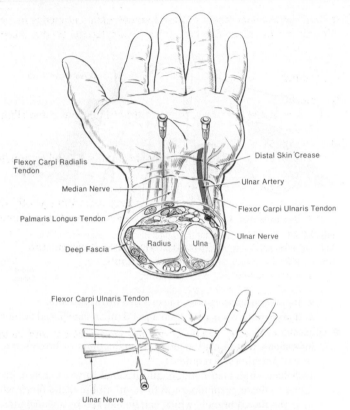

FIGURE 7.2 Surgical anatomy for the Wrist Block Technique (From Consins MJ, Bridenbaugh PO, eds. *Neural Blockade.* 3rd ed. Philadelphia: Lippincott-Raven; 1998.)

- □ Draw a line between the medial and lateral condyles of the humerus.
- □ The skin wheal is just medial to the brachial artery.
- □ Advance the needle until paresthesia is obtained.
- □ Inject 3 to 5 mL of lidocaine.
- ■ Ulnar nerve
  - □ The elbow is flexed.
  - □ Inject 1 cm proximal to the line that connects the medial epicondyle and the olecranon.
  - □ Use 3 to 5 mL of lidocaine.
  - □ Inject very superficially.
  - □ *Too much fluid can cause "compartment syndrome."*

■ Radial/musculocutaneous (lateral antebrachial cutaneous nerve)
   □ At the intercondylar line, inject 2 cm lateral to the biceps tendon.

Axillary Block

■ Indications
   □ These include hand and forearm procedures and some elbow procedures.
■ Technique (Fig. 7.3)
   □ The patient is supine with the shoulder abducted and externally rotated.
   □ Palpate the axillary artery in the distal axilla.
   □ Some advocate going through the artery, depositing two-thirds of the total anesthetic (20 to 30 mL) behind the artery and one-third superficial to it.
   □ Others suggest going on either side of the palpable artery.
   □ Think of the four nerves in four quadrants:
      • **Musculocutaneous:** 9 to 12 o'clock
      • **Median:** 12 to 3 o'clock
      • **Ulnar:** 3 to 6 o'clock
      • **Radial:** 6 to 9 o'clock
   □ *Other techniques include ultrasound guided blocks and nerve stimulation techniques.*

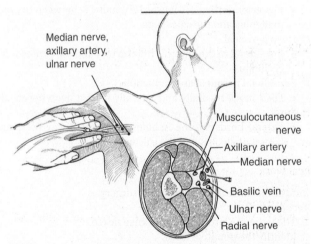

FIGURE 7.3 Surgical anatomy for the Axillary Block Technique (From Doyle JR, *Hand and Wrist.* Philadelphia: Lippincott Williams & Wilkins; 2006.)

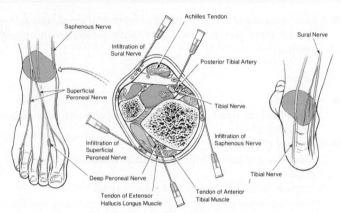

FIGURE 7.4 Surgical anatomy for the Ankle Block Technique (From Consins MJ, Bridenbaugh PO, eds. *Neural Blockade*. 3rd ed. Philadelphia: Lippincott-Raven; 1998.)

Ankle Block

- Indications include any foot and ankle procedure.
- **The block must include all five nerves:** tibial, superficial and deep peroneal, saphenous and sural nerves (Fig. 7.4).
  □ Tibial
    - Posterior to the posttibial artery, halfway between the medial malleolus and the calcaneus
  □ Deep peroneal
    - Just lateral to the anterior tibial artery and the extensor hallucis longus
  □ Superficial peroneal and saphenous
    - Field block medially and laterally from a deep peroneal site
  □ Sural
    - Lateral border of the Achilles tendon, halfway between the lateral malleolus and the calcaneus

Popliteal Block

- Indications include foot and ankle surgery.
- Technique
  □ The patient is prone, with the knee flexed.
  □ Identify the popliteal fossa.
  □ Inject 7 cm superior to the skin crease, 1 cm lateral to the midline, lateral to the artery.
  □ Advance in an anterosuperior direction.

- Add a field block of the saphenous distal to the medial tibial plateau for a more complete block.
- Ultrasound guided and nerve stimulation techniques can be used for this block.

Bier Block (Fig. 7.5)

- It is also known as regional IV anesthesia.
- This was developed by August Bier in 1908.
- Indications include hand/wrist procedures and fracture reductions.
- Technique
  - Start the IV infusion in the hand. *Place IV catheter. Do not run IV fluid.*
  - Place double tourniquets around the upper arm.
  - Exsanguinate the upper extremity.
  - Inflate the more proximal tourniquet.
  - Inject lidocaine without epinephrine (1.5 mg/kg dilute solution or 3 mg/kg, ~50 mL 0.5%) and without any preservative.
  - The tourniquet must stay inflated for 25 to 30 minutes. *If the patient has tourniquet pain, the distal tourniquet may be inflated followed by deflation of the proximal tourniquet.*
- Risks
  - Tourniquet pain
  - Length of block most often limited by the ability to tolerate the tourniquet
  - Systemic toxicity
  - **Theoretic risks:** severe cardiovascular and CNS side effects with early release of the tourniquet and a large intravascular bolus of lidocaine

MODERATE SEDATION

- Alteration in consciousness
  - Decreased anxiety
  - Pain relief
- Patient able to maintain patent airway and have intact protective airway reflexes
- Patient able to respond to verbal or physical stimuli
- Sedation a continuum
  - Awake/light sedation
  - Anxiolysis, patient essentially responding normally
  - Conscious sedation
    - Response requiring verbal or physical stimuli, airway maintained

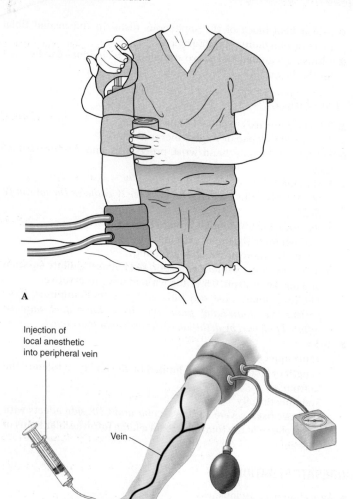

Injection of
local anesthetic
into peripheral vein

Vein

A

B

FIGURE 7.5 (**A** and **B**) Intravenous regional blockade (Bier block). (From Bucholz RW, Heckman JD, eds. *Rockwood and Green's Fractures in Adults.* 5th ed. Baltimore: Lippincott Williams & Wilkins; 2002:102.)

- □ Deep sedation
  - Repeated or painful stimuli necessary for response, airway patency questionable
- □ General anesthesia
  - Unarousable, airway not protected
- ■ When to use it?
  - □ Any time a potentially painful procedure needs to be performed in the outpatient setting
  - □ For procedures not requiring general anesthesia and that are reasonably short in duration
  - □ When appropriate monitoring equipment is available
  - □ *When patient is appropriately NPO*
- ■ Contraindications
  - □ Clinically unstable patient requiring other more urgent procedures
  - □ Refusal by a competent patient
  - □ **Relative contraindication:** long-lasting procedures, likely to require general anesthetic for success
- ■ Appropriate equipment
  - □ IV access
  - □ Pulse oximetry
  - □ Electrocardiographic monitor
  - □ Blood pressure cuff
  - □ Airway management equipment
  - □ Supplemental oxygen
  - □ Reversal medications (naloxone, flumazenil)
- ■ Technique
  - □ This typically involves combining an opioid (morphine or fentanyl) for analgesia and a benzodiazepine (midazolam) for sedation, relaxation, and amnesia.
  - □ Titrate dosing to achieve appropriate level of sedation while minimizing the risk of adverse outcome.
  - □ The patient should at all times be responsive to physical or verbal stimuli (therefore should have protective airway reflexes intact).
  - □ Remember that these patients have likely already had large doses of opioids for pain control.
  - □ Be aware of "dose stacking," giving additional doses of narcotics before waiting to see the effects of the prior doses.
- ■ Risks
  - □ Respiratory depression/hypoventilation
  - □ Risk of respiratory depression potentiated by a combination of opioids and benzodiazepines

□ Moderated by appropriate dosing, monitoring, and presence of reversal agents
□ Aspiration
□ Theoretic risk in nonfasted, sedated patients
□ No reported incidences of aspiration during emergency department conscious sedation in the current literature
■ Disposition
□ Vital signs, mental status, motor function returning to baseline
□ Pain control with oral analgesics
□ Adequate oral intake
□ Responsible adult present to monitor for continued effects of sedatives

PART II

Axial Skeleton Fractures

8 General Spine

EPIDEMIOLOGY

- There are approximately 11,000 new spinal cord injuries requiring treatment each year.
- Injury to the vertebral column occurs much less frequently than injury to the appendicular skeleton, and vertebral column fractures account for approximately 6% of all fractures.
- Fifteen percent to 20% of vertebral fractures can occur at multiple noncontiguous levels.
- Motor vehicle accidents account for >50% of all traumatic spinal cord injuries.
- In patients with a spinal cord injury, the overall mortality during the initial hospitalization is 17%.
- Approximately 2% to 6% of trauma patients sustain a cervical spine fracture.
- The ratio of male to female patients sustaining vertebral fractures is 4:1.
- The lifetime direct medical cost of spinal cord injury is estimated to be between $630,000 and $970,000 per injured person, with an aggregate annual cost estimated at $7.74 billion for the United States alone.

ANATOMY

- The spinal cord occupies approximately 35% of the canal at the level of the atlas (C1) and 50% of the canal in the lower cervical spine and thoracolumbar segments. The remainder of the canal is filled with epidural fat, cerebrospinal fluid, and dura mater.
- The *conus medullaris* represents the caudal termination of the spinal cord. It contains the sacral and coccygeal myelomeres and lies dorsal to the L1 body and L1–2 intervertebral disc.
- The *cauda equina* (literally translated means "horse's tail") represents the motor and sensory roots of the lumbosacral myelomeres. These roots are less likely to be injured because they have more room in the canal and are not tethered to the same degree as the spinal cord. Furthermore, the motor nerve roots are composed of lower motor neurons, which are more resilient to injury than the upper motor neurons of the brain and spinal cord.

■ A *reflex arc* is a simple sensorimotor pathway that can function without using either ascending or descending white matter long-tract axons. A spinal cord level that is anatomically and physiologically intact may demonstrate a functional reflex arc at that level despite dysfunction of the spinal cord cephalad to that level.

MECHANISM OF INJURY

A long-standing and fundamental problem of classifying spinal injury based on presumed mechanism of injury is that the same mechanism of injury can result in morphologically different patterns of injury; similar morphologic patterns of injury can also be the result of different injury mechanisms, and the patterns of head deflection do not predict spinal injury patterns. Several characteristics of the injury force that determine the extent of neural tissue damage have been identified. These include the rate of force application, the degree of neural tissue compression, and the duration of neural tissue compression.

Primary Injury

Primary injury refers to physical tissue disruption caused by mechanical forces.

■ **Contusion:** This sudden, brief compression by a displaced structure affects central tissues primarily and accounts for the majority of primary injuries; thus, it is responsible for the majority of neurologic deficits. Contusion injuries are potentially reversible, although irreversible neuronal death occurs along with vascular injury and intramedullary hemorrhage.

■ **Compression:** Injury results from decreased size of the spinal canal; it may occur with translation or angulation of the spinal column, as in burst injuries or epidural hematomas. Injury occurs by
    □ Mechanical deformation interrupting axonal flow
    □ Interruption of spinal vascularity resulting in ischemia of neurologic structures

■ **Stretch:** Injury results in longitudinal traction, as in the case of a flexion-distraction injury. Injury occurs as a result of capillary and axonal collapse secondary to tensile distortion.

■ **Laceration:** This is caused by penetrating foreign bodies, missile fragments, or displaced bone.

Secondary Injury

Secondary injury refers to additional neural tissue damage resulting from the biologic response initiated by physical tissue disruption.

Local tissue elements undergo structural and chemical changes. These changes, in turn, elicit systemic responses. Changes in local blood flow, tissue edema, metabolite concentrations, and concentrations of chemical mediators lead to propagation of interdependent reactions. This pathophysiologic response, referred to as secondary injury, can propagate tissue destruction and functional loss.

CLINICAL EVALUATION

- **Assess the patient:** Airway, breathing, circulation, disability, and exposure (ABCDE). Avoid the head-tilt–chin-lift maneuver, hypoxia, and hypotension.
- **Initiate resuscitation:** Address life-threatening injuries.
- Evaluate the patient's level of consciousness.
- Evaluate injuries to the head, chest, abdomen, pelvis, and spine. The spine should be protected at all times during the management of a multiply injured patient. The ideal position is with the whole spine immobilized in a neutral position on a firm surface. This may be achieved manually or with a combination of semirigid cervical collars, side head supports, and strapping. Strapping should be applied to the shoulders and pelvis as well as the head to prevent the neck becoming the center of rotation of the body.

    Take extreme care when logrolling the patient to assess the spinal column, as there is significant risk of injuring the spinal cord if there is instability. Examine the skin for bruising and abrasions, and palpate spinous processes for tenderness and diastasis. The patient should be placed on a scoop stretcher or long spine board with the head and neck supported.

    □ Calenoff found a 5% incidence of multiple noncontiguous vertebral injuries. Half of the secondary lesions were initially missed, with a mean delay of 53 days in diagnosis; 40% of secondary lesions occurred above the primary lesion and 60% below. The region T2 through T7 accounted for 47% of primary lesions in this population but only 16% of reported spinal injuries in general.

    □ **Injuries of the vertebral column tend to cluster at the junctional areas:** the craniocervical junction (occiput to C2), the cervicothoracic junction (C7–T1), and the thoracolumbar junction (T11–L2). These areas represent regions of stress concentration, where a rigid segment of the spine meets a more flexible segment. Also contributing to stress concentration in these regions are changes at these levels in the movement constraints of vertebrae.

    □ Among these injuries, the most serious and most frequently missed is craniocervical dissociation.

    □ In trauma patients, thoracic and lumbar fractures are concentrated at the thoracolumbar junction, with 60% of thoracic and lumbar fractures occurring between T11 and L2 vertebral levels.

☐ Three common patterns of noncontiguous spinal injuries are as follows.

Pattern A: Primary injury at C5–7, with secondary injuries at T12 or in the lumbar spine

Pattern B: Primary injury at T2–4, with secondary injuries in the cervical spine

Pattern C: Primary injury at Tl2–L2, with a secondary injury at L4–5

■ Assess injuries to the extremities.

■ Complete the neurologic examination to evaluate reflexes, sensation (touch, pain), and motor function (Fig. 8.1 and Tables 8.1 and 8.2).

■ Perform a rectal examination to test for perianal sensation, resting tone, and the bulbocavernosus reflex.

Spinal Shock

■ Spinal shock is defined as spinal cord dysfunction based on physiologic rather than structural disruption. Resolution of spinal shock may be recognized when reflex arcs caudal to the level of injury begin to function again, usually within 24 hours of injury.

■ Spinal shock should be distinguished from neurogenic shock, which refers to hypotension associated with loss of peripheral vascular resistance in spinal cord injury.

Neurogenic Shock

■ Neurogenic shock (Table 8.3) refers to flaccid paralysis, areflexia, and lack of sensation to physiologic spinal cord "shutdown" in response to injury.

■ It is most common in cervical and upper thoracic injuries.

■ It almost always resolves within 24 to 48 hours.

■ The bulbocavernosus reflex (S3–4) is the first to return (Table 8.4).

■ Neurogenic shock occurs secondary to sympathetic outflow disruption (T1–L2) with resultant unopposed vagal (parasympathetic) tone.

■ Initial tachycardia and hypertension immediately after injury are followed by hypotension accompanied by bradycardia and venous pooling.

■ Hypotension from neurogenic shock may be differentiated from cardiogenic, septic, and hypovolemic shock by the presence of associated bradycardia, as opposed to tachycardia.

■ Treatment is based on administration of isotonic fluids, with careful assessment of fluid status (beware of overhydration).

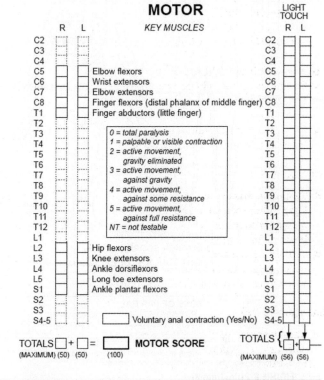

FIGURE 8.1 Neurologic examination recommended by the American Spinal Injury Association (ASIA). **(A)** Motor score and **(B)** Sensory score. (From Bucholz RW, Heckman JD, Court-Brown C, et al., eds. *Rockwood and Green's Fractures in Adults.* 6th ed. Philadelphia: Lippincott Williams & Wilkins; 2006.)

■ Recognizing neurogenic shock as distinct from hemorrhagic shock is critical for safe initial resuscitation of a trauma patient. Treatment of neurogenic shock is pharmacologic intervention to augment peripheral vascular tone. This vascular tone may be essential for

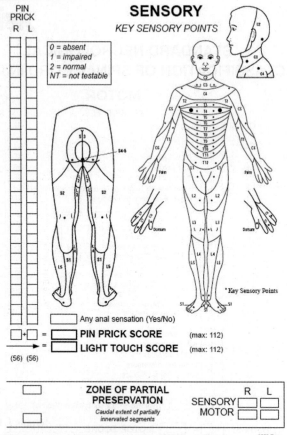

B

FIGURE 8.1 (Continued)

effective resuscitation. Fluid overload from excessive fluid volume administration, typical in treatment of hemorrhagic shock, can result in pulmonary edema in the setting of neurogenic shock.

Bulbocavernosus Reflex

- The bulbocavernosus reflex refers to contraction of the anal sphincter in response to stimulation of the trigone of the bladder with either a squeeze on the glans penis, a tap on the mons pubis, or a pull on a urethral catheter.
- The absence of this reflex indicates spinal shock.

Elements of ASIA Neurologic Assessment

Examination	Method	Testing Locations	Grading
Required elements of ASIA neurologic impairment assessment			
Pinprick (sharp/dull)	Discriminate sharp and dull ends of a standard safety pin	28 dermatomes specified by designated bony prominences	0, 1, 2, NT
Light touch	Identify contact with a cotton swab tip		0, 1 (absent, present)
Deep anal sensation	Digital rectal examination	Pressure on rectal wall	
Key muscles	Patient is in supine position	10 key muscles	0, 1, 2, 3, 4, 5*, NT
Optional elements of ASIA neurologic impairment assessment			
Joint movement appreciation (proprioception)	Support proximal portion and move distal portion by gripping medial and lateral edges	Wrist Thumb interphalangeal joint Small finger proximal interphalangeal joint Knee Ankle Great toe interphalangeal joint	0, 1, 2, NT
Deep pressure sensation	Apply pressure with thumb or index finger	Wrist radial styloid Thumb nail bed Small finger nail bed Ankle medial malleolus Great toe nail bed Small toe nail bed	0, 1 (absent, present)
Diaphragm	Observe under fluoroscopy	Movement over two or more interspaces	0, 1 (absent, present)
Deltoids	Shoulder abduction	C5–6 ± 4	0, 1, 2, 3, 4, 5, 5*, NT
Abdominal muscles	Observe movement of umbilicus (Beevor sign: umbilicus moves up in T9 through T11 lesions)	T6 through T12	0, 1, 2, 3, 4, 5, 5*, NT

(continued)

TABLE 8.1 (Continued)

Examination	Method	Testing Locations		Grading
Hip adductors	Palpate adductor longus	L2–3		0, 1, 2, 3, 4, 5, 5*, NT
Hamstrings	Knee flexion	Plurisegmental		0, 1, 2, 3, 4, 5, 5*, NT

Motor Grades Score	Description	Sensory Grades Score		Description
0	No visible or palpable contraction	0		Absent → unable to distinguish
1	Any visible or palpable contraction	1		Impaired → able to distinguish but intensity is abnormal
2	Full range of motion of joint with gravity eliminated	2		Normal
3	Full range of motion of joint against gravity	NT		Not testable
4	Full range of motion of joint against some resistance			
5*	Able to exert sufficient resistance to be normal according to examiner's judgment			
5	Normal according to examiner's judgment if inhibiting factors are not present			
NT	Not testable			

ASIA, American Spinal Injury Association.
From ASIA. *Standards for Neurological Classification of Spinal Injury.* Chicago: American Spinal Injury Association; 1996, with permission.

TABLE 8.2	Definitions of Terms Describing Spinal Cord Injury
Impairment	Loss of motor and sensory function
Disability	Loss in daily life functioning
Tetraplegia	Loss of motor and/or sensory function in the cervical segments
Paraplegia	Loss of motor and/or sensory function in the thoracic, lumbar, or sacral segments
Dermatome	Area of skin innervated by sensory axons within each segmental nerve
Myotome	Collection of muscle fibers by the motor axons within each segmental nerve
Neurologic level	The most caudal segment with normal sensory and motor function on both sides
Sensory level	The most caudal segment with normal sensory function on both sides
Motor level	The most caudal segment with normal motor function on both sides
Skeletal level	Radiographic level of greatest vertebral damage
Sensory score	Numeric summary value of sensory impairment
Motor score	Numeric summary value of motor impairment
Incomplete injury	Partial preservation of sensory and/or motor function below the neurologic level *and* sensory and/or motor preservation of the lowest sacral segment
Complete injury	Absence of sensory and motor function in the lowest sacral segment
Zone of partial preservation	Dermatomes and myotomes caudal to the neurologic level that remain partially innervated Only used in complete injuries

From ASIA. *Standards for Neurological Classification of Spinal Injury.* Chicago: American Spinal Injury Association; 1996, with permission.

- The return of the bulbocavernosus reflex heralds the end of spinal shock and generally occurs within 24 hours of the initial injury.
- The presence of a complete lesion after spinal shock has resolved portends a virtually nonexistent chance of neurologic recovery.
- The bulbocavernosus reflex is not prognostic for lesions involving the conus medullaris or the cauda equina.

RADIOGRAPHIC EVALUATION

- The lateral cervical spine radiograph is routine in the standard evaluation of trauma patients. Patients complaining of neck pain should undergo complete radiographic evaluation of the cervical spine, including anteroposterior and odontoid views.
- Lateral radiographic examination of the entire spine is recommended in patients with spine fractures when complete clinical

TABLE 8.3	Neurogenic and Hypovolemic Shock

Neurogenic Shock	Hypovolemic Shock
As the result of loss of sympathetic outflow	**As the result of hemorrhage**
Hypotension	Hypotension
Bradycardia	Tachycardia
Warm extremities	Cold extremities
Normal urine output	Low urine output

From Bucholz RW, Heckman JD, Court-Brown C, et al., eds. *Rockwood and Green's Fractures in Adults.* 6th ed. Philadelphia: Lippincott Williams & Wilkins; 2006;
Grundy D, Swain A, Russell J. ABC of spinal cord injury: early management and complications–II. *Br Med J.* 1986;292:123–125;
Piepmeier JM, Lehmann KB, Lane JG. Cardiovascular instability following acute cervical spinal cord trauma. *Cent Nerv Syst Trauma.* 1985;2:153–160; and Zipnick RI, Scalea TM, Trooskin SZ, et al. Hemodynamic responses to penetrating spinal cord injuries. *J Trauma.* 1993;35:578–582; discussion 582–583, with permission.

assessment is impaired by neurologic injury or other associated injuries.

- Despite using all the radiographic techniques available, uncertainty about cervical spinal clearance may remain. Continued protection of the neck and serial studies may ultimately demonstrate occult injuries.
- Magnetic resonance imaging may aid in assessing spinal cord or root injury as well as the degree of canal compromise.

CLASSIFICATION

The functional consequences of spinal cord injury are usually described by terms that refer to the severity and pattern of neurologic dysfunction: complete spinal cord injury, incomplete injury, and transient spinal cord dysfunction describe different grades of severity of neurologic injury. Names for different types of spinal cord injury syndromes, such as anterior cord syndrome, central cord syndrome, and Brown-Séquard syndrome, refer to patterns of neurologic dysfunction observed during clinical evaluation.

GRADING OF NEUROLOGIC INJURY

Spinal Cord Injury: Complete

- No sensation or voluntary motor function is noted caudal to the level of injury in the presence of an intact bulbocavernosus reflex. (The sacral levels are commonly quoted as being S2, S3, and S4.)
- Reflex returns below the level of the cord injury.

TABLE

8.4

Spinal Cord and Conus Medullaris Reflexes

Reflex	Location of Lesion	Stimulus	Normal Response	Abnormal Response
Babinski	Upper motor neuron	Stroking the plantar aspect of foot proximal lateral to distal medial	Toes plantarflex	Toes extend and splay
Oppenheim	Upper motor neuron	Rubbing the tibial crest proximal to distal	Toes plantarflex	Toes extend and splay
Cremasteric	T12–L1	Stroking the medial thigh proximal to distal	Upward motion of the scrotum	No motion of the scrotum
Anal wink	S2–S4	Stroking skin around anus	Anal sphincter contracts	No anal sphincter contraction
Bulbocavernosus	S3–S4	Squeezing the penis in males, applying pressure to clitoris in females, or tugging the bladder catheter in either	Anal sphincter contracts	No anal sphincter contraction

From Bucholz RW, Heckman JD, Court-Brown C, et al., eds. *Rockwood and Green's Fractures in Adults.* 6th ed. Philadelphia: Lippincott Williams & Wilkins; 2006.

- The level of injury is named by the last spinal level of partial neurologic function.
- One can expect up to one to two levels of additional root return, although the prognosis for recovery is extremely poor.

Spinal Cord Injury: Incomplete

- Some neurologic function persists caudal to the level of injury after the return of the bulbocavernosus reflex.
- As a rule, the greater the function distal to the lesion and the faster the recovery, the better is the prognosis.
- Sacral sparing is represented by perianal sensation, voluntary rectal motor function, and great toe flexor activity; it indicates at least partial continuity of white matter long tracts (corticospinal and spinothalamic) with implied continuity between the cerebral cortex and lower sacral motor neurons. It indicates incomplete cord injury, with the potential for a greater return of cord function following resolution of spinal shock.

PATTERNS OF INCOMPLETE SPINAL CORD INJURY (TABLE 8.5)

Brown-Séquard Syndrome

- This is a hemicord injury with ipsilateral muscle paralysis, loss of proprioception and light touch sensation, and contralateral hypesthesia to pain and temperature.
- The prognosis is good, with over 90% of patients regaining bowel and bladder function and ambulatory capacity.

Central Cord Syndrome

- This is most common and is frequently associated with an extension injury to an osteoarthritic spine in a middle-aged person.
- It presents with flaccid paralysis of the upper extremities (more involved) and spastic paralysis of the lower extremities (less involved), with the presence of sacral sparing.
- Radiographs frequently demonstrate no fracture or dislocation because the lesion is created by a pincer effect between anterior osteophytes and posterior infolding of the ligamentum flavum.
- The prognosis is fair, with 50% to 60% of patients regaining motor and sensory function to the lower extremities, although permanent central gray matter destruction results in poor hand function.

TABLE
8.5

Descriptions of Incomplete Cord Injury Patterns

Syndrome	Lesion	Clinical Presentation
Bell cruciate paralysis	Long-tract injury at the level of decussation in brainstem	Variable cranial nerve involvement, greater upper extremity weakness than lower, greater proximal weakness than distal
Anterior cord	Anterior gray matter, descending corticospinal motor tract, and spinothalamic tract injury with preservation of dorsal columns	Variable motor and pain and temperature sensory loss with preservation of proprioception and deep pressure sensation
Central cord	Incomplete cervical white matter injury	Sacral sparing and greater weakness in the upper limbs than the lower limbs
Brown-Séquard	Injury to one lateral half of cord and preservation of contralateral half	Ipsilateral motor and proprioception loss and contralateral pain and temperature sensory loss
Conus medullaris	Injury to the sacral cord (conus) and lumbar nerve roots within the spinal canal	Areflexic bladder, bowel, and lower limbs; may have preserved bulbocavernosus and micturition reflexes
Cauda equina	Injury to the lumbosacral nerve roots within the spinal canal	Areflexic bladder, bowel, and lower limbs
Root injury	Avulsion or compression injury to single or multiple nerve roots (brachial plexus avulsion)	Dermatomal sensory loss, myotomal motor loss, and absent deep tendon reflexes

From ASIA. *Standards for Neurological Classification of Spinal Injury.* Chicago: American Spinal Injury Association; 1996, with permission.

Anterior Cord Syndrome

- This is common and involves motor and pain/temperature loss (corticospinal and spinothalamic tracts) with preserved light touch and proprioception (dorsal columns).
- The prognosis is good if recovery is evident and progressive within 24 hours of injury. Absence of sacral sensation to temperature or pinprick after 24 hours portends a poor outcome, with functional recovery in 10% of patients according to one series.

Posterior Cord Syndrome

- This is rare and involves loss sensation of deep pressure, deep pain, and proprioception with full voluntary power, pain, and temperature sensation.

Conus Medullaris Syndrome

- This is seen in T12–L1 injuries and involves a loss of voluntary bowel and bladder control (S2–4 parasympathetic control) with preserved lumbar root function.
- It may be complete or incomplete; the bulbocavernosus reflex may be permanently lost.
- It is uncommon as a pure lesion and more common with an associated lumbar root lesion (mixed conus–cauda lesion).

NERVE ROOT LESIONS

- Isolated root lesions may occur at any level and may accompany spinal cord injury.
- This may be partial or complete and results in radicular pain, sensory dysfunction, weakness, hyporeflexia, or areflexia.

CAUDA EQUINA SYNDROME

- This is caused by multilevel lumbosacral root compression within the lumbar spinal canal.
- Clinical manifestations include saddle anesthesia, bilateral radicular pain, numbness, weakness, hyporeflexia or areflexia, and loss of voluntary bowel or bladder function.

GRADING SYSTEMS FOR SPINAL CORD INJURY

Frankel Classification

Grade A:　　Absent motor and sensory function
Grade B:　　Absent motor function; sensation present

Grade C: Motor function present, but not useful (2/5 or 3/5); sensation present
Grade D: Motor function present and useful (4/5); sensation present
Grade E: Normal motor (5/5) and sensory function

American Spinal Injury Association (ASIA) Impairment Scale

Grade A: **Complete:** No motor or sensory function is preserved in sacral segments S4–5.
Grade B: **Incomplete:** Sensory but not motor function is preserved below the neurologic level and extends through the sacral segment S4–5.
Grade C: **Incomplete:** Motor function is preserved below the neurologic level; most key muscles below the neurologic level have a muscle grade <3.
Grade D: **Incomplete:** Motor function is preserved below the neurologic level; most key muscles below the neurologic level have a muscle grade >3.
Grade E: **Normal:** Motor and sensory function is normal.

ASIA Neurologic Assessment

According to ASIA definitions, the neurologic injury level is the most caudal segment of the spinal cord with normal motor and sensory function on both sides: right and left sensation and right and left motor function. For functional scoring, 10 key muscle segments corresponding to innervation by C5, C6, C7, C8, T1, L2, L3, L4, L5, and S1 are each given a functional score of 0 to 5 out of 5. For sensory scoring, both right and left sides are graded for a total of 100 points. For the 28 sensory dermatomes on each side of the body, sensory levels are scored on a zero- to two-point scale, yielding a maximum possible pinprick score of 112 points for a patient with normal sensation.

TREATMENT

Note: Specific fractures of the cervical and thoracolumbar spines will be covered in their respective chapters.

Immobilization

1. A rigid cervical collar is indicated until the patient is cleared radiographically and clinically. A patient with a depressed level of consciousness (e.g., from ethanol intoxication) cannot be cleared clinically.

2. A special backboard with a head cutout must be used for children to accommodate their proportionally larger head size and prominent occiput.

3. The patient should be removed from the backboard (by logrolling) as soon as possible to minimize pressure sore formation.

Medical Management of Acute Spinal Cord Injury

- Intravenous methylprednisolone
  - □ May improve recovery of neurologic injury
  - □ Is currently considered the "standard of care" for spinal cord injury if it is administered within 8 hours of injury; it improves motor recovery among patients with complete and partial cord injuries
  - □ Has a loading dose of 30 mg/kg
    - 5.4 mg/kg/hour over the next 24 hours if started within 3 hours of spinal cord injury
    - 5.4 mg/kg/hour over the next 48 hours if started within 8 hours of spinal cord injury
  - □ Has no benefit, similar to other steroids, if started more than 8 hours after injury
  - □ Is not indicated for pure root lesions
- Experimental pharmacologic agents include
  - □ Naloxone (opiate receptor antagonist).
  - □ Thyrotropin-releasing hormone.
  - □ **G$_{M1}$ gangliosides:** A membrane glycolipid that, when administered within 72 hours of injury, resulted in a significant increase in motor scores. Administer 100 mg/day for up to 32 days after injury. It is not recommended for simultaneous use with methylprednisolone.

COMPLICATIONS

- **Gastrointestinal:** Ileus, regurgitation and aspiration, and hemorrhagic gastritis are common early complications, occurring as early as the second day after injury. Gastritis is thought to be the result of sympathetic outflow disruption with subsequent unopposed vagal tone resulting in increased gastric activity. Passage of a nasogastric tube and administration of histamine (H_2) receptor antagonists should be used as prophylaxis against these potential complications.
- **Urologic:** Urinary tract infections are recurrent problems in the long-term management of paralyzed patients. An indwelling urinary catheter should remain in the patient during the acute, initial

management only to monitor urinary output, which is generally low with neurogenic shock because of venous pooling and a low-flow state. Following this, sterile intermittent catheterization should be undertaken to minimize potential infectious sequelae.

■ **Pulmonary:** Acute quadriplegic patients are able to inspire only using their diaphragm because their abdominal and intercostal muscles are paralyzed. Vital capacity ranges from 20% to 25% of normal, and the patient is unable forcibly to expire, cough, or clear pulmonary secretions. Management of fluid balance is essential in the patient in neurogenic shock because volume overload rapidly results in pulmonary edema with resolution of shock. Positive pressure or mechanical ventilation may be necessary for adequate pulmonary function. Without aggressive pulmonary toilet, pooling of secretions, atelectasis, and pneumonia are common and are associated with high morbidity and mortality.

■ **Skin:** Problems associated with pressure ulceration are common in spinal cord–injured patients owing to anesthesia of the skin. Turning the patient every 2 hours, careful inspection and padding of bony prominences, and aggressive treatment of developing decubitus ulcers are essential to prevent long-term sequelae of pressure ulceration.

CLEARING THE SPINE

■ A cleared spine in a patient implies that diligent spine evaluation is complete and the patient does not have a spinal injury requiring treatment.

■ The necessary elements for a complete spine evaluation are
   1. History to assess for high-risk events and high-risk factors
   2. Physical examination to check for physical signs of spinal injury or neurologic deficit
   3. Imaging studies based on an initial evaluation

■ **Patients with a diagnosed cervical spine fracture have at least one of the following four characteristics:** midline neck tenderness, evidence of intoxication, abnormal level of alertness, or several painful injuries elsewhere.

■ Therefore, criteria for *clinical* clearance are
   1. No posterior midline tenderness
   2. Full pain-free active range of motion
   3. No focal neurologic deficit
   4. Normal level of alertness
   5. No evidence of intoxication
   6. No distracting injury

- Radiographs are not necessary for patients who are alert, are not intoxicated, have isolated blunt trauma, and have no neck tenderness on physical examination.
- The process of clearing the thoracolumbar spine is similar to that for clearing the cervical spine. Only anteroposterior and lateral view radiographs are necessary. Patients with clear mental status, no back pain, and no other major injuries do not need radiographs of the entire spine to exclude a spinal fracture.

9 Cervical Spine

EPIDEMIOLOGY

- Cervical spine injuries usually occur secondary to high-energy mechanisms, including motor vehicle accident (45%) and falls from a height (20%).
- Less commonly, cervical spine injuries occur during athletic participation (15%), most notably during American football and diving events, and as a result of acts of violence (15%).
- Neurologic injury occurs in 40% of patients with cervical spine fractures.
- Spinal cord damage is more frequently associated with lower rather than upper cervical spine fractures and dislocations.
- Approximately 2% to 6% of trauma patients sustain a cervical spine fracture.
- More than half of spinal cord injuries involve the cervical region.
- Twenty percent of trauma patients who present with a focal neurologic deficit will have an associated cervical spine fracture.
- Spinal cord damage is more frequently associated with lower rather than upper cervical spine fractures and dislocations.

ANATOMY

- The *atlas* is the first cervical vertebra, which has no body. Its two large lateral masses provide the only two weight-bearing articulations between the skull and the vertebral column.
  - ☐ The tectoral membrane and the alar ligaments are the key to providing normal craniocervical stability.
  - ☐ The anterior tubercle is held adjacent to the odontoid process of C2 by the *transverse ligament of the atlas* (Gray's Anatomy).
  - ☐ About 50% of total neck flexion and extension occurs between the occiput and C2, 25° at occiput-C1, and 20° at C1–2.
  - ☐ The vertebral artery emerges from the foramen transversarium and passes between C1 and the occiput, traversing a depression on the superior aspect of the C1 ring. Fractures are common in this location.
- The *axis* is the second cervical vertebra, whose body is the largest of the cervical vertebrae as it incorporates the odontoid process (dens).

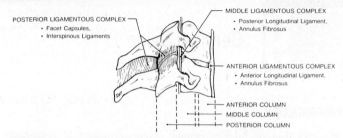

FIGURE 9.1 The components of the cervical three-column spine. The ligamentous complexes resist distractive forces. The bony structures counteract compression. (From Rockwood CA Jr, Green DP, Bucholz RW, Heckman JD, eds. *Rockwood and Green's Fractures in Adults.* Vol 2. 4th ed, Philadelphia: Lippincott-Raven; 1996:1489.)

- □ Transverse ligament of the atlas (horizontal band of the cruciform ligament) provides primary support for the atlantoaxial joint.
- □ The alar ligaments are secondary stabilizers of the atlantoaxial joint.
- □ The facet joint capsules at occiput-C1 and C1–C2 provide little support.
- □ Fifty percent of total neck rotation occurs at the C1–C2 junction.
- ■ C3–C7 can be conceptualized as a three-column system (Denis) (Fig. 9.1):
  - □ **Anterior column:** The anterior vertebral body and intervertebral disc resist compressive loads, while the anterior longitudinal ligament and annulus fibrosis are the most important checkreins to distractive forces (extension).
  - □ **Middle column:** The posterior vertebral body and uncovertebral joints resist compression, while the posterior longitudinal ligament and annulus fibrosis limit distraction.
  - □ **Posterior column:** The facet joints and lateral masses resist compressive forces, while the facet joint capsules, interspinous ligaments, and supraspinous ligaments counteract distractive forces.
  - □ The vertebral artery enters the foramen transversarium of C6 and ascends through the foramina transversarium to C1. Injuries to the vertebral arteries are uncommon because of the redundancy of the vessel.

MECHANISM OF INJURY

- ■ Motor vehicle accidents (primarily in young patients), falls (primarily in older patients), diving accidents, and blunt trauma account for the majority of cervical spine injuries.

■ Forced flexion or extension resulting from unrestrained deceleration forces, with or without distraction or axial compression, is the mechanism for most cervical spine injuries.

CLINICAL EVALUATION

1. **Patient assessment is indicated:** airway, breathing, circulation, disability, and exposure (ABCDE).
   Airway patency is the first priority.
   Breathing or adequate ventilation is the next priority.
   Circulation or recognition of the shock state is the next priority.
   Disability refers to doing a brief neurologic examination.
   Exposure is the final part of the initial examination. Completely undress the patient, and maintain body temperature.
2. **Initiate resuscitation:** Address life-threatening injuries. Maintain rigid cervical immobilization.
3. Tracheal intubation and central line placement are often performed in the emergency setting. During intubation, manipulation of the neck can potentially displace unstable cervical fractures or dislocations. Manual in-line stabilization should be maintained throughout the intubation process. Alternatively, mask ventilation can be continued until fiberoptic or nasotracheal intubation can be safely performed. If an unstable spine is highly suspected, a cricothyroidotomy may be the safest alternative for airway control.
4. **Evaluate the level of consciousness and neurologic impairment:** Glasgow Coma Scale (see Chapter 2).
5. Assess head, neck, chest, abdominal, pelvic, extremity injury.
6. **Ascertain the patient's history:** mechanism of injury, witnessed head trauma, movement of extremities/level of consciousness immediately following trauma, etc.
7. Physical examination
   □ Neck pain
   □ Lacerations and contusions on scalp, face, or neck
8. Neurologic examination
   □ Cranial nerves
   □ Complete sensory and motor examination
   □ Upper and lower extremity reflexes
   □ **Rectal examination:** perianal sensation, rectal tone
   □ Bulbocavernosus reflex (see Chapter 8)

RADIOGRAPHIC EVALUATION

■ **Lateral cervical spine radiograph:** This will detect 85% of cervical spine injuries. One must visualize the atlantooccipital junction, all seven cervical vertebrae, and the cervicothoracic junction (as inferior as the superior aspect of T1). This may necessitate downward traction on both upper extremities or a swimmer's view (upper extremity proximal to the x-ray beam abducted 180 degrees, axial traction on the contralateral upper extremity, and the beam directed 60 degrees caudad). Patients complaining of neck pain should undergo complete radiographic evaluation of the cervical spine, including anteroposterior (AP) and odontoid views. On the lateral cervical spine radiograph, one may appreciate:

1. Acute kyphosis or loss of lordosis
2. **Continuity of radiographic "lines":** anterior vertebral line, posterior vertebral line, facet joint line, or spinous process line
3. Widening or narrowing of disc spaces
4. Increased distance between spinous processes or facet joints
5. Prevertebral soft tissue swelling, which depends on the level in question, or an abnormal contour of the tissues:
   - **At C1:** >10 mm
   - **At C3, C4:** >7 mm
   - **At C5, C6, C7:** >20 mm
6. Radiographic markers of cervical spine instability, including the following:
   - Compression fractures with >25% loss of height
   - Angular displacements >11 degrees between adjacent vertebrae (as measured by Cobb angle)
   - Translation >3.5 mm
   - Intervertebral disc space separation >1.7 mm (Figs. 9.2 and 9.3)

■ Computed tomography (CT) and/or magnetic resonance imaging (MRI) may be valuable to assess the upper cervical spine or the cervicothoracic junction, especially if it is inadequately visualized by plain radiography.

■ The proposed advantages of CT over a lateral cervical film as an initial screening tool are that it is more sensitive for detecting fractures and more consistently enables assessment of the occipitocervical and cervicothoracic junctions. A potential disadvantage of CT as an initial radiographic assessment is that subtle malalignment, facet joint gapping, or intervertebral distraction is difficult to assess using axial images alone.

■ The most useful applications of MRI are in detecting traumatic disc herniation, epidural hematoma, spinal cord edema or compression, and posterior ligamentous disruption. An additional application of MRI is the ability to visualize vascular structures. MR arteriograms can be used to assess the patency of the vertebral arteries.

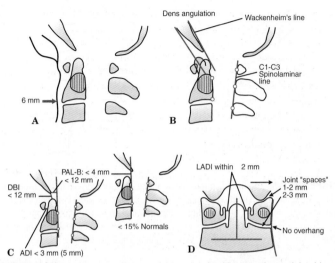

FIGURE 9.2 (A) Prevertebral soft tissue shadow. In a healthy recumbent adult without an endotracheal tube, the prevertebral soft tissue shadow should not exceed 6 mm. **(B)** Bony screening lines and dens angulation. The anterior cortex of the odontoid should parallel the posterior cortex of the anterior ring of the atlas. Any kyphotic or lordotic deviation should be viewed with suspicion for an odontoid fracture or transverse ligament of the atlas disruption. Wackenheim line is drawn as a continuation from the clivus caudally. The tip of the odontoid should be within 1 to 2 mm of this line. The C1–C3 spinolaminar line's reference points are drawn from the anterior cortex of the laminae of the atlas, axis, and C3 segments, which should fall within 2 mm of one another. Greater deviation should raise suspicion of atlantoaxial translation or disruption of the neural arches of either segment. **(C)** Ligamentous injury reference lines (lateral x-rays). The atlas-dens interval (ADI) should be <3 mm in an adult (5 mm in a child). The space available for the cord is measured as the distance from the posterior cortex of the odontoid tip to the anterior cortex of the posterior arch of the atlas and should amount to more than 13 mm. The dens-basion interval (DBI) is the distance between the odontoid tip and the distal end of the basion. It should be <12 mm in adults. The posterior axis line (PAL-B) should not be more than 4 mm anterior and should be <12 mm posterior to the basion. **(D)** Bony screening lines (anteroposterior imaging). The left and right lateral atlas-dens intervals (LADIs) should be symmetric to one another (with 2-mm deviation). The bony components of the atlantooccipital joints should be symmetric and should not be spaced more than 2 mm apart on anteroposterior images. (Courtesy of Fred Mann, MD, Professor of Radiology, University of Washington, Seattle.)

- Stress flexion/extension radiographs rarely if ever should be performed if instability is suspected; they should be performed in the awake and alert patient only. In a patient with neck pain, they are best delayed until spasm has subsided, which can mask instability.

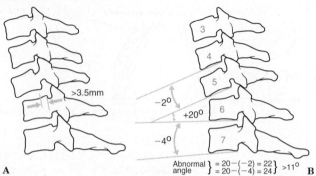

FIGURE 9.3 Radiographic indications of instability. Greater than 3.5 mm of translation **(A)** or 11 degrees of angulation **(B)** and widening of the separation between spinous processes are indications of instability on the lateral plain film. (Adapted from Bucholz RW. Lower cervical spine injuries. In: Browner BD, Jupiter JB, Levine AM, et al., eds. *Skeletal Trauma*. Vol 1. Philadelphia: WB Saunders; 1992:707.)

The atlantodens interval (ADI) should be <3 mm in adults and <5 mm in children.

■ Traction x-rays are taken during reductions only.

CLASSIFICATION

OTA Classification of Cervical Spine Injuries

See Fracture and Dislocation Classification Compendium at http://www.ota.org/compendium/compendium.html.

INJURIES TO THE OCCIPUT-C1–C2 COMPLEX

■ As with other transitional regions of the spine, the craniocervical junction is highly susceptible to injury. This region's vulnerability to injury is particularly high because of the large lever-arm induced cranially by the skull and the relative freedom of movement of the craniocervical junction, which relies disproportionately on ligamentous structures rather than on intrinsic bony stability.

Occipital Condyle Fractures

■ These are frequently associated with C1 fractures as well as cranial nerve palsies.

■ The mechanism of injury involves compression and lateral bending; this causes either compression fracture of the condyle as it presses against the superior facet of C1 or avulsion of the alar ligament with extremes of atlantooccipital rotation.

■ CT is frequently necessary for diagnosis.

CLASSIFICATION (FIG. 9.4)

Type I: Impaction of condyle; usually stable
Type II: Shear injury associated with basilar or skull fractures; potentially unstable
Type III: Condylar avulsion; unstable

■ Treatment includes rigid cervical collar immobilization for 8 weeks for stable injuries and halo immobilization or occipital-cervical fusion for unstable injuries.

■ Craniocervical dissociation should be considered with any occipital condyle fracture.

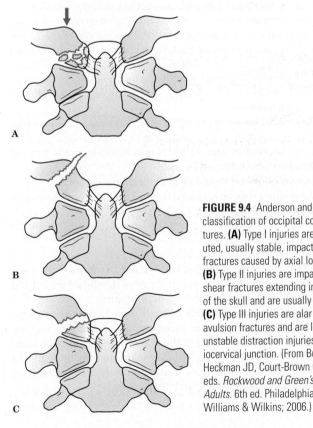

FIGURE 9.4 Anderson and Montesano classification of occipital condyle fractures. **(A)** Type I injuries are comminuted, usually stable, impaction fractures caused by axial loading. **(B)** Type II injuries are impaction or shear fractures extending into the base of the skull and are usually stable. **(C)** Type III injuries are alar ligament avulsion fractures and are likely to be unstable distraction injuries of the craniocervical junction. (From Bucholz RW, Heckman JD, Court-Brown C, et al., eds. *Rockwood and Green's Fractures in Adults.* 6th ed. Philadelphia: Lippincott Williams & Wilkins; 2006.)

Occipitoatlantal Dislocation (Craniovertebral Dissociation)

- This is almost always fatal, with postmortem studies showing it to be the leading cause of death in motor vehicle accidents; rare survivors have severe neurologic deficits ranging from complete C1 flaccid quadriplegia to mixed incomplete syndromes such as Brown-Séquard.
- This is twice as common in children, owing to the inclination of the condyles.
- It is associated with submental lacerations, mandibular fractures, and posterior pharyngeal wall lacerations.
- It is associated with injury to the cranial nerves (the abducens and hypoglossal nerves are most commonly affected by craniocervical injuries), the first three cervical nerves, and the vertebral arteries.
- The cervicomedullary syndromes, which include cruciate paralysis as described by Bell and hemiplegia cruciata initially described by Wallenberg, represent the more unusual forms of incomplete spinal cord injury and are a result of the specific anatomy of the spinal tracts at the junction of the brainstem and spinal cord. Cruciate paralysis can be similar to a central cord syndrome, although it normally affects proximal more than distal upper extremity function. Hemiplegia cruciata is associated with ipsilateral arm and contralateral leg weakness.
- Mechanism is a high-energy injury resulting from a combination of hyperextension, distraction, and rotation at the craniocervical junction.
- The diagnosis is often missed, but it may be made on the basis of the lateral cervical spine radiograph:
  - The tip of odontoid should be in line with the basion.
  - The odontoid–basion distance is 4 to 5 mm in adults and up to 10 mm in children.
  - Translation of the odontoid on the basion is never >1 mm in flexion/extension views.
  - Powers ratio (BC/OA) should be <1 (Fig. 9.5).
  - In adults, widening of the prevertebral soft tissue mass in the upper neck is an important warning sign of significant underlying trauma and may be the only sign of this injury.
  - Fine-cut CT scans with slices no more than 2 mm wide are helpful to understand articular incongruities or complex fracture patterns more clearly. MRI of the craniovertebral junction is indicated for patients with spinal cord injury and can be helpful to assess upper cervical spine ligamentous injuries as well as subarachnoid and prevertebral hemorrhage.

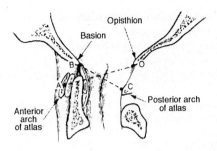

FIGURE 9.5 Powers ratio. (From Browner BD, Jupiter JB, Levine AM, et al., eds. *Skeletal Trauma.* Vol 1. Philadelphia: WB Saunders; 1992:668.)

- Classification based on the position of the occiput in relation to C1 is as follows:

Type I: Occipital condyles anterior to the atlas; most common

Type II: Condyles longitudinally dissociated from atlas without translation; result of pure distraction

Type III: Occipital condyles posterior to the atlas

- The Harborview classification attempts to quantify stability of craniocervical junction. Surgical stabilization is reserved for type II and III injuries.

Type I: Stable with displacement <2 mm

Type II: Unstable with displacement <2 mm

Type III: Gross instability with displacement >2 mm

- Immediate treatment includes halo-vest application with strict avoidance of traction. Reduction maneuvers are controversial and should ideally be undertaken with fluoroscopic visualization.
- Long-term stabilization involves fusion between the occiput and the upper cervical spine.

Atlas Fractures

- These are rarely associated with neurologic injury.
- Instability invariably equates to the presence of transverse alar ligament insufficiency, which can be diagnosed either by direct means, such as by identifying bony avulsion on CT scan or ligament rupture on MRI, or indirectly by identifying widening of the lateral masses.
- Fifty percent of these injuries are associated with other cervical spine fractures, especially odontoid fractures and spondylolisthesis of the axis.

- Cranial nerve lesions of VI to XII and neurapraxia of the suboccipital and greater occipital nerves may be associated.
- Vertebral artery injuries may cause symptoms of basilar insufficiency such as vertigo, blurred vision, and nystagmus.
- Patients may present with neck pain and a subjective feeling of "instability."
- The mechanism of injury is axial compression with elements of hyperextension and asymmetric loading of condyles causing variable fracture patterns.
- Classification (Levine) (Fig. 9.6)
  1. Isolated bony apophysis fracture
  2. Isolated posterior arch fracture

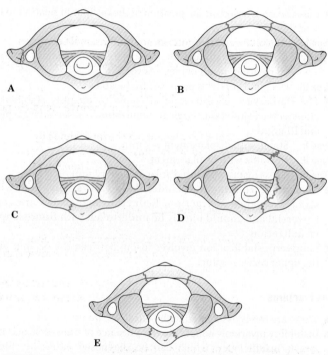

FIGURE 9.6 Classification of atlas fractures (according to Levine). **(A)** Isolated bony apophysis fracture. **(B)** Isolated posterior arch fracture. **(C)** Isolated anterior arch fracture. Comminuted, or lateral mass, fracture **(D)** and burst fracture **(E)**, three or more fragments. (From Bucholz RW, Heckman JD, Court-Brown C, et al., eds. *Rockwood and Green's Fractures in Adults*. 6th ed. Philadelphia: Lippincott Williams & Wilkins; 2006.)

   3. Isolated anterior arch fracture
   4. Comminuted lateral mass fracture
   5. Burst fracture, also known as the Jefferson fracture
- Treatment
   □ Initial treatment includes halo traction/immobilization.
   □ Stable fractures (posterior arch or nondisplaced fractures involving the anterior and posterior portions of the ring) may be treated with a rigid cervical orthosis.
   □ Less stable configurations (asymmetric lateral mass fracture with "floating" lateral mass, burst fractures) may require prolonged halo immobilization.
   □ C1–C2 fusion may be necessary to alleviate chronic instability and/or pain.

Transverse Ligament Rupture (Traumatic C1–C2 Instability)

- This rare, usually fatal, injury is seen mostly in older age groups (50s to 60s).
- The mechanism of injury is forced flexion.
- The clinical picture ranges from severe neck pain to complete neurologic compromise.
- Rupture of the transverse ligament may be determined by
   1. Visualizing the avulsed lateral mass fragment on CT scan.
   2. Atlantoaxial offset >6.9 mm on an odontoid radiograph.
   3. ADI >3 mm in adults. An ADI >5 mm in adults also implies rupture of the alar ligaments.
   4. Direct visualization of the rupture on MRI.
- Treatment
   □ Initial treatment includes halo traction/immobilization.
   □ In the cases of avulsion, halo immobilization is continued until osseous healing is documented.
   □ C1–C2 fusion is indicated for tears of the transverse ligament without bony avulsion, chronic instability, or pain (Fig. 9.7).

Atlantoaxial Rotary Subluxation and Dislocation

- In this rare injury, patients present with confusing complaints of neck pain, occipital neuralgia, and, occasionally, symptoms of vertebrobasilar insufficiency. In chronic cases, the patient may present with torticollis.
- It is infrequently associated with neurologic injury.

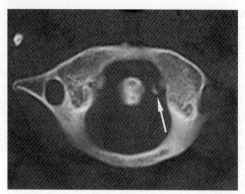

FIGURE 9.7 Axial CT image demonstrating transverse ligament rupture with atlantoaxial subluxation. (Reproduced with permission from Bucholz RW, Heckman JD, Court-Brown C, et al., eds. *Rockwood and Green's Fractures in Adults.* 6th ed. Philadelphia: Lippincott Williams & Wilkins; 2006.)

- The mechanism of injury is flexion/extension with a rotational component, although in some cases it can occur spontaneously with no reported history of trauma.
- Odontoid radiographs may show asymmetry of C1 lateral masses with unilateral facet joint narrowing or overlap (wink sign). The C2 spinous process may be rotated from the midline on an AP view.
- The subluxation may be documented on dynamic CT scans; failure of C1 to reposition on a dynamic CT scan indicates fixed deformity.
- Classification (Fielding)

Type I: Odontoid as a pivot point; no neurologic injury; ADI <3 mm; transverse ligament intact (47%)

Type II: Opposite facet as a pivot; ADI <5 mm; transverse ligament insufficient (30%)

Type III: Both joints anteriorly subluxed; ADI >5 mm; transverse and alar ligaments incompetent

Type IV: Rare; both joints posteriorly subluxed

Type V: **Levine and Edwards:** frank dislocation; extremely rare

- Treatment
  - □ Cervical halter traction in the supine position and active range-of-motion exercises for 24 to 48 hours initially are followed by ambulatory orthotic immobilization with active range-of-motion exercises until free motion returns.
  - □ Rarely, fixed rotation with continued symptoms and lack of motion indicates a C1–C2 posterior fusion.

Fractures of the Odontoid Process (Dens)

- A high association exists with other cervical spine fractures.
- There is a 5% to 10% incidence of neurologic involvement with presentation ranging from Brown-Séquard syndrome to hemiparesis, cruciate paralysis, and quadriparesis.
- Vascular supply arrives through the apex of the odontoid and through its base with a watershed area in the neck of the odontoid.
- High-energy mechanisms of injury include motor vehicle accident or falls with avulsion of the apex of the dens by the alar ligament or lateral/oblique forces that cause fracture through the body and base of the dens.
- Classification (Anderson and D'Alonzo) (Fig. 9.8)

Type I: Oblique avulsion fracture of the apex (5%)

Type II: Fracture at the junction of the body and the neck; high nonunion rate, which can lead to myelopathy (60%)

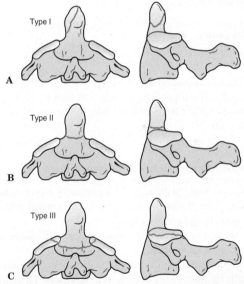

FIGURE 9.8 The odontoid fracture classification of Anderson and D'Alonzo. **(A)** Type I fractures of the odontoid tip represent alar ligament avulsions. **(B)** Type II fractures occur at the odontoid waist, above the C2 lateral masses. **(C)** Type III fractures extend below the odontoid waist to involve the body and lateral masses of C2. Hadley has added the type IIA fracture with segmental comminution at the base of the odontoid (not shown). (From Bucholz RW, Heckman JD, Court-Brown C, et al., eds. *Rockwood and Green's Fractures in Adults.* 6th ed. Philadelphia: Lippincott Williams & Wilkins; 2006.)

Type IIA: Highly unstable comminuted injury extending from the waist of the odontoid into the body of the axis

Type III: Fracture extending into the cancellous body of C2 and possibly involving the lateral facets (30%)

■ Treatment

Type I: If it is an isolated injury, stability of the fracture pattern allows for immobilization in a cervical orthosis.

Type II: This is controversial, because the lack of periosteum and cancellous bone and the presence in watershed area result in a high incidence of nonunion (36%). Risk factors include age >50 years, >5 mm displacement, and posterior displacement. It may require screw fixation of the odontoid or C1–C2 posterior fusion for adequate treatment. Nonoperative treatment is halo immobilization.

Type III: There is a high likelihood of union with halo immobilization owing to the cancellous bed of the fracture site.

C2 Lateral Mass Fractures

■ Patients often present with neck pain, limited range of motion, and no neurologic injury.

■ The mechanisms of injury are axial compression and lateral bending.

■ CT is helpful for diagnosis.

■ A depression fracture of the C2 articular surface is common.

■ Treatment ranges from collar immobilization to late fusion for chronic pain.

Traumatic Spondylolisthesis of C2 (Hangman's Fracture)

■ This is associated with a 30% incidence of concomitant cervical spine fractures. It may be associated with cranial nerve, vertebral artery, and craniofacial injuries.

■ The incidence of spinal cord injury is low with types I and II and high with type III injuries.

■ The mechanism of injury includes motor vehicle accidents and falls with flexion, extension, and axial loads. This may be associated with varying degrees of intervertebral disc disruption. Hanging mechanisms involve hyperextension and distraction injury, in which the patient may experience bilateral pedicle fractures and complete disruption of disc and ligaments between C2 and C3.

■ Classification (Levine and Edwards; Effendi) (Fig. 9.9)

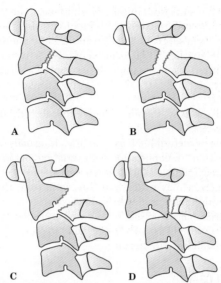

FIGURE 9.9 Classification of traumatic spondylolisthesis of the axis (hangman's fracture) (according to Effendi, modified by Levine). **(A)** Type I, nondisplaced fracture of the pars interarticularis. **(B)** Type II, displaced fracture of the pars interarticularis. **(C)** Type IIA, displaced fracture of the pars interarticularis with disruption of the C2–C3 discoligamentous complex. **(D)** Type III, dislocation of C2–C3 facets joints with fractured pars interarticularis. (From Bucholz RW, Heckman JD, Court-Brown C, et al., eds. *Rockwood and Green's Fractures in Adults.* 6th ed. Philadelphia: Lippincott Williams & Wilkins; 2006.)

Type I: Nondisplaced, no angulation; translation <3 mm; C2–C3 disc intact (29%); relatively stable

Type Ia: Atypical unstable lateral bending fractures that are obli-quely displaced and usually involve only one pars interarticularis, extending anterior to the pars and into the body on the con-tralateral side

Type II: Significant angulation at C2–C3; translation >3 mm; most common injury pattern; unstable; C2–C3 disc disrupted (56%); subclassified into flexion, extension, and olisthetic types

Type IIA: Avulsion of entire C2–C3 intervertebral disc in flexion with injury to posterior longitudinal ligament, leaving the anterior longitudinal ligament intact; results in severe angulaion; no translation; unstable; probably caused by flexion-distraction injury (6%); traction contraindicated

Type III: Rare; results from initial anterior facet dislocation of C2 on C3 followed by extension injury fracturing the neural arch; results in severe angulation and translation with unilateral or bilateral facet dislocation of C2–C3; unstable (9%); type III injuries most commonly associated with spinal cord injury

■ Treatment

Type I: This usually requires rigid cervical orthosis for up to 6 weeks.

Type II: This is determined by stability; it usually requires halo traction/immobilization with serial radiographic confirmation of reduction for at least 6 weeks.

Type IIA: Traction may exacerbate the condition; therefore, only immobilization may be indicated.

Type III: Initial halo traction is followed by open reduction and posterior fusion of C2–C3, with fracture fixation and/or possible anterior fusion.

INJURIES TO C3–C7

■ Vertebral bodies have a superior cortical surface that is concave in the coronal plane and convex in the sagittal plane, allowing for flexion, extension, and lateral tilt by the gliding motion of the facets.

■ The uncinate process projects superiorly from the lateral aspect of the vertebral body. With degenerative changes, these may articulate with the superior vertebra, resulting in an uncovertebral joint (of Luschka).

■ The mechanism of injury includes motor vehicle accidents, falls, diving accidents, and blunt trauma.

■ Radiographic evaluation consists of AP, lateral, and odontoid views of the cervical spine, as described earlier in the section on radiographic evaluation of cervical spine instability.

  □ If cervical spine instability is suspected, flexion/extension views may be obtained in a willing, conscious, and cooperative patient without neurologic compromise. A "stretch" test (Panjabi and White) may be performed with longitudinal cervical traction. An abnormal test is indicated by a >1.7-mm interspace separation or a >7.5-degree change between vertebrae.

  □ CT scans with reconstructions may be obtained to characterize fracture pattern and degree of canal compromise more clearly.

  □ MRI may be undertaken to delineate spinal cord, disc, and canal abnormalities further.

☐ The amount of normal cervical motion at each level has been extensively described, and this knowledge can be important in assessing spinal stability after treatment. Flexion-extension motion is greatest at the C4–5 and C5–6 segments, averaging about 20 degrees. Axial rotation ranges from 2 to 7 degrees at each of the subaxial motion segments; the majority (45% to 50%) of rotation occurs at the C1–C2 articulation. Lateral flexion is 10 to 11 degrees per level in the upper segments (C2–5). Lateral motion decreases caudally, with only 2 degrees observed at the cervicothoracic junction.

Classification (Allen-Ferguson) (Fig. 9.10)

1. Compressive flexion (shear mechanism resulting in "teardrop" fractures)

Stage I: Blunting of anterior body; posterior elements intact

Stage II: "Beaking" of the anterior body; loss of anterior vertebral height

Stage III: Fracture line passing from anterior body through the inferior subchondral plate

Stage IV: Inferoposterior margin displaced <3 mm into the neural canal

Stage V: "Teardrop" fracture; inferoposterior margin >3 mm into the neural canal; failure of the posterior ligaments and the posterior longitudinal ligament

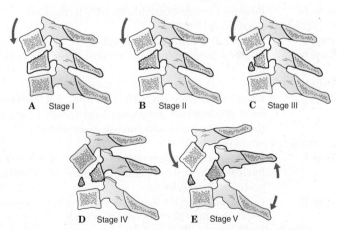

FIGURE 9.10 (A–E) The five stages of compression flexion injuries. (From Bucholz RW, Heckman JD, Court-Brown C, et al., eds. *Rockwood and Green's Fractures in Adults.* 6th ed. Philadelphia: Lippincott Williams & Wilkins; 2006.)

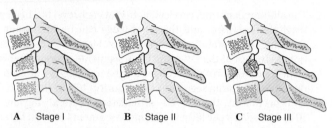

A Stage I   **B** Stage II   **C** Stage III

FIGURE 9.11 (A–C) The three stages of vertical compression injuries. (From Bucholz RW, Heckman JD, Court-Brown C, et al., eds. *Rockwood and Green's Fractures in Adults.* 6th ed. Philadelphia: Lippincott Williams & Wilkins; 2006.)

2. Vertical compression (burst fractures) (Fig. 9.11)

Stage I: Fracture through the superior or inferior endplate with no displacement

Stage II: Fracture through both endplates with minimal displacement

Stage III: Burst fracture; displacement of fragments peripherally and into the neural canal

3. Distractive flexion (dislocations) (Fig. 9.12)

Stage I: Failure of the posterior ligaments, divergence of the spinous processes, and facet subluxation

Stage II: Unilateral facet dislocation; translation always <50%

Stage III: Bilateral facet dislocation; translation of 50% and "perched" facets

Stage IV: Bilateral facet dislocation with 100% translation

4. Compressive extension (Fig. 9.13)

Stage I: Unilateral vertebral arch fracture

Stage II: Bilateral laminar fracture without other tissue failure

Stages III, IV: Theoretic continuum between stages II and V

Stage V: Bilateral vertebral arch fracture with full vertebral body displacement anteriorly; ligamentous failure at the posterosuperior and anteroinferior margins

5. Distractive extension (Fig. 9.14)

Stage I: Failure of anterior ligamentous complex or transverse fracture of the body; widening of the disc space and no posterior displacement

Stage II: Failure of posterior ligament complex and superior displacement of the body into the canal

6. Lateral flexion (Fig. 9.15)

Stage I: Asymmetric, unilateral compression fracture of the vertebral body plus a vertebral arch fracture on the ipsilateral side without displacement

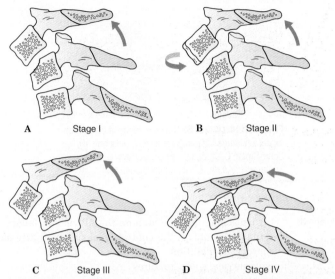

FIGURE 9.12 (A–D) The four stages of distraction flexion injuries. (From Bucholz RW, Heckman JD, Court-Brown C, et al., eds. *Rockwood and Green's Fractures in Adults*. 6th ed. Philadelphia: Lippincott Williams & Wilkins; 2006.)

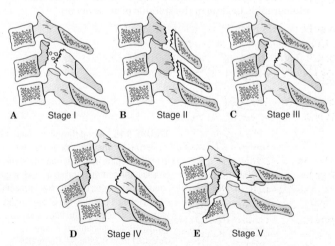

FIGURE 9.13 (A–E) The five stages of compression extension injuries. (From Bucholz RW, Heckman JD, Court-Brown C, et al., eds. *Rockwood and Green's Fractures in Adults*. 6th ed. Philadelphia: Lippincott Williams & Wilkins; 2006.)

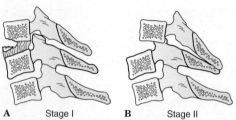

A   Stage I   **B**   Stage II

FIGURE 9.14 (A and B) The two stages of distraction extension injuries. (From Bucholz RW, Heckman JD, Court-Brown C, et al., eds. *Rockwood and Green's Fractures in Adults.* 6th ed. Philadelphia: Lippincott Williams & Wilkins; 2006.)

Stage II: Displacement of the arch on the AP view or failure of the ligaments on the contralateral side with articular process separation

7. Miscellaneous cervical spine fractures
   - □ **"Clay shoveler's" fracture:** This is an avulsion of the spinous processes of the lower cervical and upper thoracic vertebrae. Historically, this resulted from muscular avulsion during shoveling in unyielding clay with force transmission through the contracted shoulder girdle. Treatment includes restricted motion and symptomatic treatment until clinical improvement or radiographic healing of the spinous process occurs.

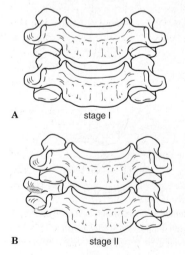

A   stage I

B   stage II

FIGURE 9.15 Lateral flexion injuries. Blunt trauma from the side places the ipsilateral spine in distraction while compressing the contralateral spine. **(A)** Stage I injury, asymmetric centrum fracture with a unilateral arch fracture. **(B)** Stage II injury, with displacement of the body and contralateral ligamentous failure. (Adapted from Rizzolo SJ, Cotler JM. Unstable cervical spine injuries: specific treatment approaches. *J Am Acad Orthop Surg.* 1993;1:57–66.)

- ☐ **Sentinel fracture:** This fracture occurs through the lamina on either side of the spinous process. A loose posterior element may impinge on the cord. Symptomatic treatment only is indicated unless spinal cord compromise exists.

- ☐ **Ankylosing spondylitis:** This may result in calcification and ossification of the ligamentous structures of the spine, producing "chalk stick" fractures after trivial injuries. These fractures are notoriously unstable because they tend to occur through brittle ligamentous structures. Attempts at reduction, or even repositioning the patient, may result in catastrophic spinal cord injury as the injury involves all three spinal columns. Treatment includes traction with minimal weight in neutral or the presenting position of the neck, with aggressive immobilization with either halo vest or open stabilization.

- ☐ **Gunshot injuries:** Missile impact against bony elements may cause high-velocity fragmentation frequently associated with gross instability and complete spinal cord injury. Surgical extraction of missile fragments is rarely indicated in the absence of canal compromise. Missiles that traverse the esophagus or pharynx should be removed, with aggressive exposure and debridement of the missile tract. These injuries carry high incidences of abscess formation, osteomyelitis, and mediastinitis.

TREATMENT: GENERAL CERVICAL SPINE

Initial Treatment

- ■ Immobilization with a cervical orthosis (for stable fractures) or skull traction (for unstable injuries) should be maintained in the emergency setting before CT for evaluation of spinal and other system injuries. Skull or skeletal traction may be applied using Gardner-Wells tongs or preferably by application of a halo-crown, which can be used for traction and subsequently attached to a vest assembly (halo-vest).

- ■ Vasopressor support is indicated for suspected neurogenic shock and emergency assessment for potential intracranial trauma.

- ■ Patients with neurologic injuries should be considered for intravenous methylprednisolone per the NASCIS II and III protocol (30 mg/kg loading dose and then 5.4 mg/kg for 24 hours if started within 3 hours, for 48 hours if started within 8 hours. Steroids have no benefit if they are started more than 8 hours after injury).

- ■ The majority of cervical spine fractures can be treated nonoperatively. The most common method of nonoperative treatment is immobilization in a cervical orthosis. In reality, orthoses decrease motion rather than effect true immobilization. Motion at the occipital-cervical junction is slightly increased by most cervical collars.

- ☐ **Soft cervical orthosis:** This produces no significant immobilization and is a supportive treatment for minor injuries.
- ☐ **Rigid cervical orthosis (Philadelphia collar):** This is effective in controlling flexion and extension; however, it provides little rotational or lateral bending stability.
- ☐ **Poster braces:** These are effective in controlling midcervical flexion, with fair control in other planes of motion.
- ☐ **Cervicothoracic orthoses:** These are effective in flexion and extension and rotational control, with limited control of lateral bending.
- ☐ **Halo device:** This provides the most rigid immobilization (of external devices) in all planes.
- ☐ For traction, Gardner-Wells tongs are applied one finger's width above the pinna of the ear in line with the external auditory canal. Slight anterior displacement will apply an extension force, whereas posterior displacement will apply a flexion force, useful when reducing facet dislocations (Fig. 9.16).

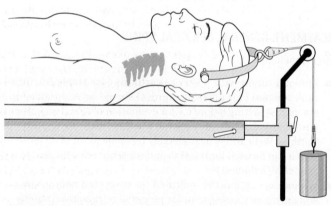

FIGURE 9.16 Closed reduction technique. Diagram of cranial tong technique for maintaining alignment and stability of the spine. Weight is increased gradually with a maximum of 45 to 50 lb (10 lb for the head and 5 lb for each successive interspace). Patients with an unrevealing examination may require a magnetic resonance imaging scan before reduction to rule out a space-occupying lesion in the vertebral canal. Failure of reduction may also necessitate such a scan. (Adapted from Bucholz RW. Lower cervical spine injuries. In: Browner BD, Jupiter JB, Levine AM, et al., eds. *Skeletal Trauma*. Vol 1. Philadelphia: WB Saunders; 1992:638.)

☐ Numerous complications are associated with the use of cervical collars. Skin breakdown at bony prominences, in particular, the occiput, mandible, and sternum, can occur. Up to 38% of patients with severe closed head injuries can develop skin complications with prolonged use.

■ **Patients with neural deficits from burst-type injuries:** Traction is used to stabilize and indirectly decompress the canal via ligamentotaxis.

■ **Patients with unilateral or bilateral facet dislocations and complete neural deficits:** Gardner-Wells tong traction and reduction by sequentially increasing the amount of traction are indicated.

■ Traction is contraindicated in distractive cervical spine injuries and type IIA spondylolisthesis injuries of C2.

■ Patients with incomplete neural deficits or who are neurologically intact with unilateral and bilateral facet dislocations require MRI before reduction via traction to evaluate for a herniated disc, especially if a patient is not awake and alert and able to cooperate with serial examinations during reduction maneuvers.

■ A halo has been recommended for patients with isolated occipital condyle fractures, unstable atlas ring fractures, odontoid fractures, and displaced neural arch fractures of the axis.

■ The halo vest relies on a firm fit of the vest around the torso and is poorly tolerated by elderly patients and patients with pulmonary compromise or thoracic deformities, such as those with ankylosing spondylitis.

■ The halo ring should be applied 1 cm above the ears. Anterior pin sites should be placed below the equator of the skull above the supraorbital ridge, anterior to the temporalis muscle, and over the lateral two-thirds of the orbit. Posterior sites are variable and are placed to maintain horizontal orientation of the halo. Pin pressure should be 6 to 8 lb in the adult and should be retightened at 24 hours. Pin care is optional.

■ Prolonged recumbence carries an increased morbidity and mortality risk, and consideration should be given to the use of a RotoRest bed and mechanical as well as pharmacologic thromboprophylaxis.

■ Because of the normally wide spinal canal diameter, decompression of neural elements in upper cervical spine fractures is not commonly required for traumatic conditions.

■ The optimal time to perform surgery, particularly in patients with neurologic deficits, remains unclear. The two most commonly proposed benefits of earlier versus later surgery are improved rates of neurologic recovery and improved ability to mobilize the patient without concern of spinal displacement. To date, little human clinical evidence supports the view that early surgical decompression and stabilization improve neurologic recovery rates. However, clinical series have demonstrated that surgery performed as soon as 8 hours after injury does not appear to increase the rate of complications or lead to neurologic decline.

Stabilization of the Upper Cervical Spine (Occiput-C2)

- The mainstay of operative treatment of upper cervical fractures and dislocations remains fusion with instrumentation, most commonly performed from the posterior approach. In order of frequency, the most common upper cervical fusion procedures are atlantoaxial fusion, occipitocervical fusion, and, least commonly, C1–C3 fusion.
- Fusion of the occiput-C2 limits 50% of flexion and extension.
- Fusion of C1–C2 limits 50% of rotation.

Anterior Approach

There are three main indications for anterior upper cervical spine exposure in trauma.

1. Screw fixation of a type II odontoid fracture
2. Anterior interbody fusion and plating of the C2–C3 interspace for a type IIA or III hangman's fracture
3. Anterior arthrodesis of the atlantoaxial articulations as a rare salvage procedure for failed posterior atlantoaxial fusion attempts

Posterior Approach

Most upper cervical fractures are treated through a posterior approach.

- Modified Brooks or Gallie arthrodesis uses sublaminar wires and a bone graft between the arches of C1 and C2.
  - □ Flexion control is obtained via the wires, extension via the bone blocks, and rotation via friction between the bone blocks and the posterior arches.
- Transarticular screws (Magerl) are effective, especially if the posterior elements of C1 and C2 are fractured.
- Lateral mass screw fixation of C1 and (pedicle) screw fixation of C2 with rods between C1 and C2 (Harms fixation) also provides effective posterior fixation.

Osteosynthesis

- The two indications for direct fracture repair in the upper cervical spine involve the treatment of type II odontoid fractures or type II traumatic spondylolistheses of C2 with interfragmentary screw fixation.

- This is not indicated for fixation of anteriorly displaced odontoid fractures.

Stabilization of the Lower Cervical Spine (C3–C7)

- Fifty percent of flexion/extension and 50% of rotation are evenly divided between each of the facet articulations.
- Fusion of each level reduces motion by a proportionate amount.
- **Posterior decompression and fusion:**
  - ☐ The posterior approach to the cervical spine is a midline, extensile approach that can be used to access as many spinal levels as necessary, with a variety of instrumentation techniques in use.
  - ☐ In the majority of acute, traumatic, subaxial spinal injuries, posterior decompression via laminectomy is not necessary. Canal compromise is most frequently caused by dislocation, translation, or retropulsed vertebral body fragments. In rare cases of anteriorly displaced posterior arch fragments, laminectomy would be indicated to directly remove the offending compressive elements. This is not true, however, in cases of acute spinal cord injury associated with multilevel spondylotic stenosis or ossification of the posterior longitudinal ligament, in which a posterior decompressive procedure may be considered the procedure of choice if cervical lordosis has been maintained.
  - ☐ Open reduction of dislocated facet joints is typically performed using a posterior approach.
- Bilateral lateral mass plating
  - ☐ This can be utilized for a variety of fractures including facet fractures, facet dislocations, and "teardrop" (compressive flexion stage V) fractures.
  - ☐ Single-level fusions are sufficient for dislocations, although multilevel fusions may be required for more unstable patterns.
  - ☐ This can stop fusion at levels with fractured spinous processes or laminae, thus avoiding the fusion of extra levels with consequent loss of motion.
- Anterior decompression and fusion
  - ☐ These are used for vertebral body burst fractures with spinal cord injury and persistent anterior cord compression.
  - ☐ The anterior approach to the subaxial spine utilizes the interval plane between the sternocleidomastoid (lateral) and anterior strap (medial) muscles. Deeper, the interval of dissection is

between the carotid sheath laterally and the trachea/esophagus medially.

☐ MRI, myelography, and CT are valuable in preoperative assessment of bony and soft tissue impingement on the spinal cord.

☐ A simple discectomy or corpectomy in which osseous fragments are removed from the canal and a tricortical iliac or fibular graft placed between the vertebral bodies by a variety of techniques can be performed.

☐ In the presence of a herniated cervical disc associated with dislocated facet joints, one may elect to perform an anterior discectomy and decompression before facet reduction.

☐ Anterior plating or halo vest immobilization adds stability during healing.

COMPLICATIONS

Complications of spinal cord injury are covered in Chapter 8.

10 Thoracolumbar Spine

EPIDEMIOLOGY

- Neurologic injury complicates 15% to 20% of fracture at the thoracolumbar level.
- Sixty-five percent of thoracolumbar fractures occur as a result of motor vehicle trauma or fall from a height, with the remainder caused by athletic participation and assault.
- Most isolated thoracic and lumbar spine fractures are related to osteoporosis and involve minimal or no trauma.
- Osteoporosis accounts for approximately 750,000 vertebral fractures annually in the United States, and far outnumbers the 15,000 trauma-related thoracic and lumbar spine fractures.
- Thoracolumbar trauma occurs most frequently in male patients between 15 and 29 years of age.
- Ninety percent of vertebral fractures occur in the thoracolumbar spine.
- Neurologic injury occurs in approximately 25% of thoracic and lumbar fractures.
- Sixty percent of thoracolumbar fractures occur between T11 and L2 vertebral levels.

ANATOMY

See Chapter 8 for a general definition of terms.

- The thoracolumbar spine consists of 12 thoracic vertebrae and 5 lumbar vertebrae.
- The thoracic level is kyphotic, and the lumbar region is lordotic. The thoracolumbar region, as a transition zone, is especially prone to injury.
- The thoracic spine is much stiffer than the lumbar spine in flexion-extension and lateral bending, reflecting the restraining effect of the rib cage as well as the thinner intervertebral discs of the thoracic spine.
- Rotation is greater in the thoracic spine, achieving a maximum at T8–T9. The reason is the orientation of the lumbar facets, which limit the rotation arc to approximately 10 degrees for the lumbar spine versus 75 degrees for the thoracic spine.

- The conus medullaris ends at the L1–L2 level. The cauda equina, which comprises the motor and sensory roots of the lumbosacral myelomeres (Fig. 10.1), lies caudal to the conus.
- The corticospinal tracts demonstrate polarity, with cervical fibers distributed centrally and sacral fibers peripherally.
- The ratio of the spinal canal dimensions to the spinal cord dimensions is smallest in the T2–T10 region, which makes this area prone to neurologic injury after trauma.
- Neurologic deficits secondary to skeletal injury from the first through the tenth thoracic levels are frequently complete deficits, primarily related to spinal cord injury with varying levels of root injury. The proportion of root injury increases with more caudal injuries, with skeletal injuries caudal to L1 causing exclusively root (lower motor neuron) injury.
- The region between T2 and T10 is a circulatory watershed area, deriving its proximal blood supply from antegrade vessels in the upper thoracic spine and distally from retrograde flow from the purported artery of Adamkiewicz, which can be variably located between T9 and L2.
- Most thoracic and lumbar injuries occur within the region between T11 and L1, commonly referred to as the thoracolumbar junction. This increased susceptibility can be explained by a variety of factors. The thoracolumbar junction is a transition zone between the relatively stiff thoracic spine and the more mobile lumbar spine.

MECHANISM OF INJURY

- These generally represent high-energy injuries, typically from motor vehicle accident or falls from a height.
- They may represent a combination of flexion, extension, compression, distraction, torsion, and shear.

CLINICAL EVALUATION

1. **Patient assessment:** This involves airway, breathing, circulation, disability, and exposure (ABCDE). Please see also Chapter 9.
2. **Initiate resuscitation:** Address life-threatening injuries. Maintain spine immobilization. Watch for neurogenic shock (hypotension and bradycardia).
3. **Evaluate the level of consciousness and neurologic impairment:** Glasgow Coma Scale.
4. Assess head, neck, chest, abdominal, pelvic, extremity injury.

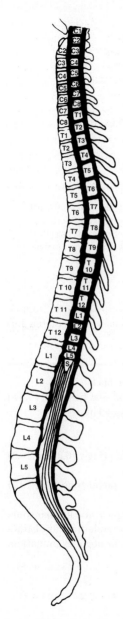

FIGURE 10.1 The relationship between myelomeres (spinal cord segments) and the vertebral bodies. (From Benson DR, Keenen TL. Evaluation and treatment of trauma to the vertebral column. *Instr Course Lect.* 1990;39:577.)

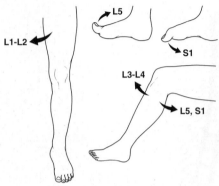

FIGURE 10.2 A screening examination of the lower extremities assesses the motor function of the lumbar and first sacral nerve roots: hip adductors, L1–L2; knee extension, L3–L4; knee flexion, L5–S1; great toe extension, L5; and great toe flexion, S1. (From Benson DR, Keenen TL. Evaluation and treatment of trauma to the vertebral column. *Instr Course Lect*. 1990;39:583.)

5. **Ascertain the history:** mechanism of injury, witnessed head trauma, movement of extremities/level of consciousness immediately following trauma, etc.
6. Physical examination
   - Back pain and tenderness
   - Lacerations, abrasions, and contusions on back
   - Abdominal and/or chest ecchymosis from seat belt injury (also suggestive of liver, spleen, or other abdominal injury)
7. Neurologic examination
   - Cranial nerves
   - Complete motor and sensory examination (Figs. 10.2 and 10.3)
   - Upper and lower extremity reflexes
   - Rectal examination: perianal sensation, rectal tone (Fig. 10.4)
   - Bulbocavernosus reflex (Fig. 10.5)
8. In the alert and cooperative patient, the thoracic and lumbar spine can be "cleared" with the absence of pain or tenderness or distraction mechanism of injury and a normal neurologic examination. Otherwise, imaging is required.

RADIOGRAPHIC EVALUATION

- Anteroposterior (AP) and lateral views of the thoracic and lumbar spine are obtained.

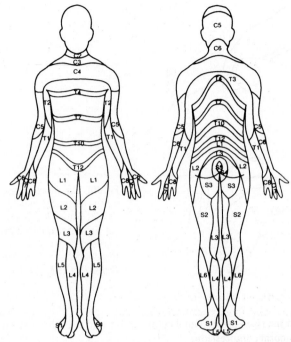

FIGURE 10.3 A pain and temperature dermatome chart. These sensory modalities are mediated by the lateral spinothalamic tract. Note that C4 includes the upper chest just superior to T2. The rest of the cervical and T1 roots are located in the upper extremities. There is overlap in the territories subserved by each sensory root and variation among individuals. (From Benson DR, Keenen TL. Evaluation and treatment of trauma to the vertebral column. *Instr Course Lect.* 1990;39:584.)

- Abnormal widening of the interpedicular distance signifies lateral displacement of vertebral body fragments, typical of burst fractures.
- Vertebral body height loss can be measured by comparing the height of the injured level with adjacent uninjured vertebrae.
- Quantification of sagittal plane alignment can be performed using the Cobb method.
- Chest and abdominal radiographs obtained during the initial trauma survey are not adequate for assessing vertebral column injury.
- Computed tomography (CT) and/or magnetic resonance imaging of the injured area may be obtained to characterize the fracture

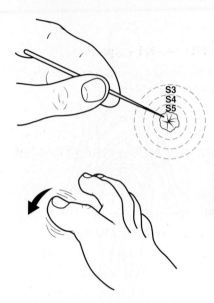

FIGURE 10.4 Sacral sparing may include the triad of perianal sensation, rectal tone, and great toe flexion. (From Benson DR, Keenen TL. Evaluation and treatment of trauma to the vertebral column. *Instr Course Lect.* 1990;39:580.)

further, to assess for canal compromise, and to evaluate the degree of neural compression.

■ CT scans provide finer detail of the bony involvement in thoracolumbar injuries, and MRI can be used to evaluate for soft tissue injury to the cord, intervertebral discs or for posterior ligamentous disruption.

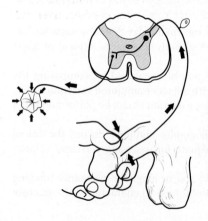

FIGURE 10.5 The bulbocavernosus reflex arc is mediated by the conus medullaris and the lower three sacral roots. Stimulation of the glans penis, glans clitoris, or gentle traction on a Foley catheter to stimulate the bladder will evoke contraction of the rectal sphincter. (From Benson DR, Keenen TL. Evaluation and treatment of trauma to the vertebral column. *Instr Course Lect.* 1990;39:578.)

CLASSIFICATION

OTA Classification of Thoracic and Lumbar Spine Injuries

See Fracture and Dislocation Classification Compendium at http://www.ota.org/compendium/compendium.html.

McAfee et al.

Classification is based on the failure mode of the middle osteoligamentous complex (posterior longitudinal ligament, posterior half of vertebral body, and posterior annulus fibrosus).

- Axial compression
- Axial distraction
- Translation within the transverse plane

This led to the following six injury patterns in this classification:

1. Wedge-compression fracture
2. Stable burst fracture
3. Unstable burst fracture
4. Chance fracture
5. Flexion-distraction injury
6. Translational injuries

McCormack et al.

- This is a "load-sharing classification."
- A point value is assigned to the degree of vertebral body comminution, fracture fragment apposition, and kyphosis. Based on their primary outcome of hardware failure, McCormack et al. concluded that injuries with scores >6 points would be better treated with the addition of anterior column reconstruction to posterior stabilization. A recent study demonstrated very high interobserver and intraobserver reliability of this classification system.

Denis

Minor Spinal Injuries

Articular process fractures (1%)
Transverse process fractures (14%)
Spinous process fractures (2%)
Pars interarticularis fractures (1%)

Major Spinal Injuries

Compression fractures (48%)
Burst fractures (14%)

Fracture-dislocations (16%)
Seat belt–type injuries (5%)

- Compression fractures
  - These can be anterior (89%) or lateral (11%).
  - They are rarely associated with neurologic compromise.
  - They are generally stable injuries, although they are considered unstable if associated with loss of >50% vertebral body height, angulation >20 to 30 degrees, or multiple adjacent compression fractures.
  - The middle column remains intact; it may act as a hinge with a posterior column distraction injury (seen with compression in 40% to 50%).
  - Four subtypes are described based on endplate involvement (Fig. 10.6):

  Type A: Fracture of both endplates (16%)
  Type B: Fracture of superior endplate (62%)
  Type C: Fracture of inferior endplate (6%)
  Type D: Both endplates intact (15%)

  - Treatment includes an extension orthosis (Jewett brace or thoracolumbar spinal orthosis) with early ambulation for most fractures, which are stable. Reduction of the wedge kyphosis under conscious sedation and application of an extension body cast (Böhler) remains an option. Unstable fractures (>50% height loss or 20 to 30 degrees of kyphosis in nonosteoporotic bone

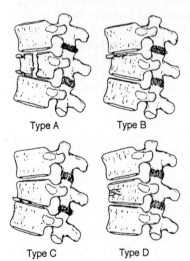

Type A   Type B

Type C   Type D

FIGURE 10.6 Compression fractures. (From Browner BD, Jupiter JD, Levine MA, eds. *Skeletal Trauma*. Philadelphia: WB Saunders; 1992:746.)

strongly suggests the possibility of posterior ligament complex disruption, which places the patient at risk of increasing kyphotic deformity or neurologic deficit) may require hyperextension casting or open reduction and internal fixation. Posterior ligamentous injury may be inferred by observing widening of the interspinous distance. MRI is sensitive to presence of posterior interspinous ligament and soft tissue injury. Upper thoracic fractures are not amenable to casting or bracing and require surgical management to prevent significant kyphosis.

- Burst fractures
  - □ No direct relationship exists between the percentage of canal compromise and the degree of neurologic injury.
  - □ The mechanism is compression failure of the anterior and middle columns under an axial load.
  - □ An association exists between lumbar burst fractures, longitudinal laminar fractures, and neurologic injury.
  - □ These injuries result in loss of posterior vertebral body height and splaying of pedicles on radiographic evaluation.
  - □ Five types are recognized (Fig. 10.7):

  Type A: Fracture of both endplates (24%)
  Type B: Fracture of the superior endplate (49%)
  Type C: Fracture of inferior endplate (7%)
  Type D: Burst rotation (15%)
  Type E: Burst lateral flexion (5%)

  - □ Treatment may consist of hyperextension casting if no neurologic compromise exists and the fracture pattern is stable (see compression fractures, earlier).
  - □ Early stabilization is advocated to restore sagittal and coronal plane alignment in cases with
    - Neurologic deficits
    - Loss of vertebral body height >50%
    - Angulation >20 to 30 degrees
    - Canal compromise of >50%
    - Scoliosis >10 degrees
  - □ Anterior, posterior, and combined approaches have been used.
  - □ Posterior surgery relies on indirect decompression via ligamentotaxis and avoids the morbidity of anterior exposure in patients who have concomitant pulmonary or abdominal injuries; it also has shorter operative times and decreased blood loss. Anterior approaches allow for direct decompression. Posterior instrumentation alone cannot directly reconstitute anterior column support and is therefore somewhat weaker in compression than anterior instrumentation. This has led to a higher incidence of

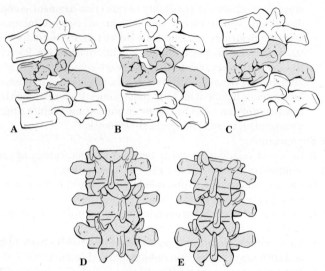

FIGURE 10.7 (A–E) Denis classification of burst fractures. Type A involves fractures of both endplates, type B involves fractures of the superior endplate, and type C involves fractures of the inferior endplate. Type D is a combination of a type A fracture with rotation. Type E fractures exhibit lateral translation. (From Bucholz RW, Heckman JD, Court-Brown C, et al., eds. *Rockwood and Green's Fractures in Adults.* 6th ed. Philadelphia: Lippincott Williams & Wilkins; 2006.)

progressive kyphosis and instrumentation failure when treating highly comminuted fractures.
- Instrumentation should provide distraction and extension moments.
- Harrington rods distract posteriorly, which tends to produce kyphosis, and are thus contraindicated for use in the lower lumbar spine.
- Laminectomies should not be done without instrument stabilization.
■ Flexion-distraction injuries (Chance fractures, seat belt–type injuries)
- Patients are usually neurologically intact.
- Up to 50% may have associated abdominal injuries.
- Flexion-distraction injury results in compression failure of the anterior column and tension failure of the posterior and middle columns.
- Injuries rarely occur through bone alone and are most commonly the result of osseous and ligamentous failure (Fig. 10.8).

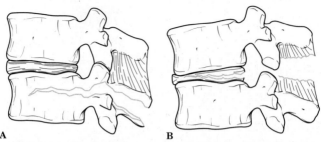

A   B

FIGURE 10.8 Flexion-distraction injuries. The bony Chance fracture **(A)** is often associated with lap seat belt use. This fracture was originally described by Bohler years before Chance. A flexion-distraction injury can occur entirely through soft tissue **(B)**. (From Bucholz RW, Heckman JD, eds. *Rockwood and Green's Fractures in Adults.* 5th ed. Baltimore: Lippincott Williams & Wilkins; 2002.)

- ☐ One may see increased interspinous distance on the AP and lateral views.
- ☐ Four types are recognized:

Type A: One-level bony injury (47%)

Type B: One-level ligamentous injury (11%)

Type C: Two-level injury through bony middle column (26%)

Type D: Two-level injury through ligamentous middle column (16%)

- ☐ Treatment consists of hyperextension casting for type A injuries.
- ☐ For injuries with compromise of the middle and posterior columns with ligamentous disruption (types B, C, D), posterior spinal fusion with compression should be performed.
- ☐ The primary goal of surgery for flexion-distraction injuries is not to reverse neurologic deficit but to restore alignment and stability to enable early patient mobilization and to prevent secondary displacement.
- ☐ Unless a herniated disc is noted on a preoperative MRI and warrants anterior discectomy, posterior reduction and compressive stabilization of the involved segment are usually adequate.
- ■ Fracture-dislocations
  - ☐ All three columns fail under compression, tension, rotation, or shear, with translational deformity.
  - ☐ Three types, with different mechanisms (Denis), are known as follows:

Type A: **Flexion-rotation:** posterior and middle column fail in tension and rotation; anterior column fails in compression and rotation; 75% with neurologic deficits, 52% of these being complete lesions (Fig. 10.9)

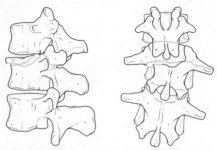

FIGURE 10.9 A flexion-rotation type of fracture-dislocation. (From Bucholz RW, Heckman JD, eds. *Rockwood and Green's Fractures in Adults*. 5th ed. Baltimore: Lippincott Williams & Wilkins; 2002.)

Type B: **Shear:** shear failure of all three columns, most commonly in the posteroanterior direction; all cases with complete neurologic deficit (Fig. 10.10)

Type C: **Flexion-distraction:** tension failure of posterior and middle columns, with anterior tear of annulus fibrosus and stripping of the anterior longitudinal ligament; 75% with neurologic deficits (all incomplete) (Fig. 10.11)

☐ Generally, these are highly unstable injuries that require surgical stabilization.

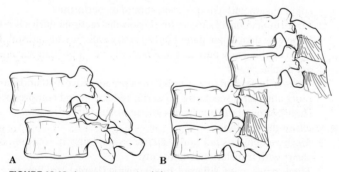

FIGURE 10.10 A posteroanterior **(A)** shear-type fracture-dislocation. An anteroposterior **(B)** shear-type fracture-dislocation. This nomenclature is based on the direction of the shear force that would produce the injury when applied to the superior vertebra. (From Bucholz RW, Heckman JD, eds. *Rockwood and Green's Fractures in Adults*. 5th ed. Baltimore: Lippincott Williams & Wilkins; 2002.)

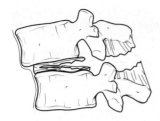

FIGURE 10.11 A flexion-distraction type of dislocation. (From Bucholz RW, Heckman JD, eds. *Rockwood and Green's Fractures in Adults.* 5th ed. Baltimore: Lippincott Williams & Wilkins; 2002.)

- ☐ Posterior surgery is usually most useful for achieving reduction and stability in these injuries.
- ☐ The characteristic deformity of fracture-dislocations is translational malalignment of the involved vertebrae. Realigning the spine is often difficult and is best performed by direct manipulation of the vertebra with bone clamps or elevators. Gradual distraction may be needed to reduce dislocations with no associated fracture.
- ☐ Patients whose fractures are stabilized within 3 days of injury have a lower incidence of pneumonia and a shorter hospital stay than those with fractures stabilized more than 3 days after injury.
- ☐ Patients without neurologic deficit do not typically need urgent surgery. Surgery can be performed when the patient has been adequately stabilized medically. A similar approach should be employed in patients that have complete neurologic injuries when there is little chance for significant recovery.

SPINAL STABILITY

A spinal injury is considered unstable if normal physiologic loads cause further neurologic damage, chronic pain, and unacceptable deformity.

White and Punjabi

Defined scoring criteria have been developed for the assessment of clinical instability of spine fractures (Tables 10.1 and 10.2).

Denis

The three-column model of spinal stability (Fig. 10.12 and Table 10.3) is as follows:

1. **Anterior column:** anterior longitudinal ligament, anterior half of the vertebral body, and anterior annulus

TABLE 10.1 Thoracic and Thoracolumbar Spine Stability Scale	
Element	**Point Value**
Anterior elements unable to function	2
Posterior elements unable to function	2
Disruptions of costovertebral articulations	1
Radiographic criteria	4
Sagittal displacement >2.5 mm (2 pts)	
Relative sagittal plane angulation >5 degrees (2 pts)	
Spinal cord or cauda equina damage	2
Dangerous loading anticipated	1

Instability: total of ≥5 points
From White A, Punjabi M. *Clinical Biomechanics of the Spine*. Philadelphia: JB Lippincott; 1990:335.

2. **Middle column:** posterior half of vertebral body, posterior annulus, and posterior longitudinal ligament
3. **Posterior column:** posterior neural arches (pedicles, facets, and laminae) and posterior ligamentous complex (supraspinous ligament, interspinous ligament, ligamentum flavum, and facet capsules)

TABLE 10.2 Lumbar Spine Stability Scale	
Element	**Point Value**
Anterior elements unable to function	2
Posterior elements unable to function	2
Radiographic criteria	4
Flexion/extension x-rays	
Sagittal plane translation >4.5 mm or 15% (2 pts)	
Sagittal plane rotation (2 pts)	
>15 degrees at L1–2, L2–3, and L3–4	
>20 degrees at L4–5	
>25 degrees at L5–S1	
OR	
Resting x-rays	
Sagittal plane displacement >4.5 mm or 15% (2 pts)	
Relative sagittal plane angulation >22 degrees (2 pts)	
Spinal cord or cauda equina damage	2
Cauda equina damage	3
Dangerous loading anticipated	1

Instability: total of ≥5 points
From White A, Punjabi M. *Clinical Biomechanics of the Spine*. Philadelphia: JB Lippincott; 1990:335.

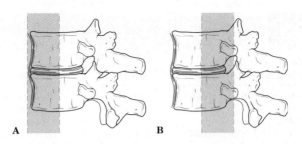

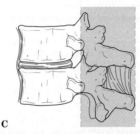

FIGURE 10.12 The three columns of the spine, as proposed by Francis Denis. The anterior column **(A)** consists of the anterior longitudinal ligament, anterior part of the vertebral body, and the anterior portion of the annulus fibrosis. The middle column **(B)** consists of the posterior longitudinal ligament, posterior part of the vertebral body, and posterior portion of the annulus. The posterior column **(C)** consists of the bony and ligamentous posterior elements. (Modified from Denis F. The three-column spine and its significance in the classification of acute thoracolumbar spine injuries. *Spine.* 1983;8:817–831.)

☐ Instability exists with disruption of any two of the three columns.
☐ **Thoracolumbar stability usually follows the middle column:** if it is intact, then the injury is usually stable.

Three degrees of instability are recognized:

First degree (mechanical instability): potential for late kyphosis

- Severe compression fractures
- Seat belt–type injuries

Second degree (neurologic instability): potential for late neurologic injury

- Burst fractures without neurologic deficit

Third degree (mechanical and neurologic instability):

- Fracture-dislocations
- Severe burst fractures with neurologic deficit

| | | **TABLE 10.3** | Basic Types of Spinal Fractures and Columns Involved in Each |

	Column Involvement		
Type of Fracture	**Anterior**	**Middle**	**Posterior**
Compression	Compression	None	None or distraction (in severe fractures)
Burst	Compression	Compression	None or distraction
Seat belt	None or compression	Distraction	Distraction
Fracture-dislocation	Compression and/or anterior rotation, shear	Distraction and/or rotation, shear	Distraction and/or rotation, shear

From Denis F. The three-column spine and its significance in the classification of acute thoracolumbar spinal injuries. *Spine* 1983;8:817–831.

McAfee

This author noted that burst fractures can be unstable, with early progression of neurologic deficits and spinal deformity as well as late onset of neurologic deficits and mechanical back pain.

- ■ **Factors indicative of instability in burst fractures:**
  - □ 50% canal compromise
  - □ >15 to 25 degrees of kyphosis
  - □ >40% loss of anterior body height

GUNSHOT WOUNDS

- ■ In general, fractures associated with low-velocity gunshot wounds are stable fractures. This is the case with most handgun injuries. They are associated with a low infection rate and can be prophylactically treated with 48 hours of a broad-spectrum antibiotic. Transintestinal gunshot wounds require special attention. In these cases, the bullet passes through the colon, intestine, or stomach before passing through the spine. These injuries carry a significantly higher rate of infection. Broad-spectrum antibiotics should be continued for 7 to 14 days. High-energy wounds, as caused by a rifle or military assault weapon, require open debridement and stabilization.
- ■ Neural injury is often secondary to a blast effect in which the energy of the bullet is absorbed and transmitted to the soft tissues. Because of this unique mechanism, decompression is rarely indicated. One exception is when a bullet fragment is found in the

spinal canal between the level of T12 and L5 in the presence of a neurologic deficit. Rarely, delayed bullet extraction may be indicated for lead toxicity or late neurologic deficits owing to migration of a bullet fragment. Steroids after gunshot wounds to the spine are not recommended, because they have demonstrated no neurologic benefit and appear to be associated with a higher rate of nonspinal complications.

PROGNOSIS AND NEUROLOGIC RECOVERY

Bradford and McBride

■ The authors modified the Frankel grading system of neurologic injury for thoracolumbar injuries, dividing Frankel D types (impaired but functional motor function) based on degree of motor function as well as bowel and bladder function:

Type A: Complete motor and sensory loss

Type B: Preserved sensation, no voluntary motor

Type C: Preserved motor, nonfunctional

Type D1: Low-functional motor (3+/5+) and/or bowel or bladder paralysis

Type D2: Midfunctional motor (3+ to 4+/5+) and/or neurogenic bowel or bladder dysfunction

Type D3: High-functional motor (4+/5+) and normal voluntary bowel or bladder function

Type E: Complete motor and sensory function normal

■ In patients with thoracolumbar spine fractures and incomplete neurologic injuries, greater neurologic improvement (including return of sphincter control) was found in those treated by anterior spinal decompression versus posterior or lateral spinal decompression.

Dall and Stauffer

■ They prospectively examined neurologic injury and recovery patterns for T12–L1 burst fractures with partial paralysis and >30% initial canal compromise.

■ Conclusions

☐ Severity of neurologic injury did not correlate with fracture pattern or amount of CT-measured canal compromise.

☐ Neurologic recovery did not correlate with the treatment method or amount of canal decompression.

☐ Neurologic recovery did correlate with the initial fracture pattern (four types):

Type I: <15 degrees of kyphosis; maximal canal compromise at level of ligamentum flavum

Type II: <15 degrees of kyphosis; maximal compromise at the bony posterior arch

Type III: >15 degrees of kyphosis; maximal compromise at the bony arch

Type IV: >15 degrees of kyphosis; maximal compromise at the level of the ligamentum flavum

- **Type I or Type II:** Significant neurologic recovery occurred in >90%, regardless of the severity of the initial paralysis or treatment method.
- **Type III:** Significant neurologic recovery occurred in <50%.
- **Type IV:** The response was variable.

Camissa et al.

- They associated dural tears in 37% of burst fractures with associated laminar fractures; all patients had neurologic deficits.
- They concluded that the presence of a preoperative neurologic deficit in a patient who had a burst fracture and an associated laminar fracture was a sensitive (100%) and specific (74%) predictor of dural laceration, as well as a predictor of risk for associated entrapment of neural elements.

Keenen et al.

- They reported an 8% incidence of dural tears in all surgically treated spine fractures, 25% in lumbar burst fractures.
- In patients with burst fractures and a dural tear, 86% had neurologic deficits versus 42% in those with burst fractures without a dural tear.

COMPLICATIONS

Complications of spinal cord injury are covered in Chapter 8.

PART III

Upper Extremity Fractures and Dislocations

11 Clavicle Fractures

EPIDEMIOLOGY

- Clavicle fractures account for 2.6% to 12% of all fractures and for 44% to 66% of fractures about the shoulder.
- Middle third fractures account for 80% of all clavicle fractures, whereas fractures of the lateral and medial third of the clavicle account for 15% and 5%, respectively.

ANATOMY

- The clavicle is the first bone to ossify (fifth week of gestation) and the last ossification center (sternal end) to fuse, at 22 to 25 years of age.
- The clavicle is S-shaped, with the medial end convex forward and the lateral end concave forward.
- It is widest at its medial end and thins laterally.
- The medial and lateral ends have flat expanses that are linked by a tubular middle, which has sparse medullary bone.
- The clavicle functions as a strut, bracing the shoulder from the trunk and allowing the shoulder to function at optimal strength.
- The medial one-third protects the brachial plexus, the subclavian and axillary vessels, and the superior lung. It is strongest in axial load.
- The junction between the two cross-sectional configurations occurs in the middle third and constitutes a vulnerable area to fracture, especially with axial loading. Moreover, the middle third lacks reinforcement by muscles or ligaments distal to the subclavius insertion, resulting in additional vulnerability.
- The distal clavicle contains the coracoclavicular ligaments.
  - □ The two components are the trapezoid and conoid ligaments.
  - □ They provide vertical stability to the acromioclavicular (AC) joint.
  - □ They are stronger than the AC ligaments.

MECHANISM OF INJURY

- Falls onto the affected shoulder account for most (87%) of clavicular fractures, with direct impact accounting for only 7% and falls onto an outstretched hand accounting for 6%.

- Although rare, clavicle fractures can occur secondary to muscle contractions during seizures or atraumatically from pathologic mechanisms or as stress fractures.

CLINICAL EVALUATION

- Patients usually present with splinting of the affected extremity, with the arm adducted across the chest and supported by the contralateral hand to unload the injured shoulder.
- A careful neurovascular examination is necessary to assess the integrity of neural and vascular elements lying posterior to the clavicle.
- The proximal fracture end is usually prominent and may tent the skin. Assessment of skin integrity is essential to rule out open fracture.
- The chest should be auscultated for symmetric breath sounds. Tachypnea may be present as a result of pain with inspiratory effort; this should not be confused with diminished breath sounds, which may be present from an ipsilateral pneumothorax caused by an apical lung injury.

ASSOCIATED INJURIES

- Up to 9% of patients with clavicle fractures have additional fractures, most commonly rib fractures.
- Most brachial plexus injuries are associated with proximal third clavicle fractures (traction injury).

RADIOGRAPHIC EVALUATION

- Standard anteroposterior radiographs are generally sufficient to confirm the presence of a clavicle fracture and the degree of fracture displacement.
- A 30-degree cephalad tilt view provides an image without the overlap of the thoracic anatomy.
- An apical oblique view can be helpful in diagnosing minimally displaced fractures, especially in children. This view is taken with the involved shoulder angled 45 degrees toward the x-ray source, which is angled 20 degrees cephalad.
- A chest x-ray allows for side to side comparison, including normal length.
- Computed tomography may be useful, especially in proximal third fractures, to differentiate sternoclavicular dislocation from epiphyseal injury, or distal third fractures, to identify articular involvement.

CLASSIFICATION

Descriptive

Clavicle fractures may be classified according to anatomic description, including location, displacement, angulation, pattern (e.g., greenstick, oblique, transverse), and comminution.

Allman

- **Group I:** fracture of the middle third (80%). This is the most common fracture in both children and adults; proximal and distal segments are secured by ligamentous and muscular attachments.
- **Group II:** fracture of the distal third (15%). This is subclassified according to the location of the coracoclavicular ligaments relative to the fracture:

Type I: **Minimal displacement:** interligamentous fracture between the conoid and trapezoid or between the coracoclavicular and AC ligaments; ligaments still intact (Fig. 11.1)

Type II: **Displaced secondary to a fracture medial to the coracoclavicular ligaments:** higher incidence of nonunion

IIA: Conoid and trapezoid attached to the distal segment (Fig. 11.2)

IIB: Conoid torn, trapezoid attached to the distal segment (Fig. 11.3)

Type III: **Fracture of the articular surface of the AC joint with no ligamentous injury:** may be confused with first-degree AC joint separation (Fig. 11.4)

30% chance of displaced distal clavicle fx

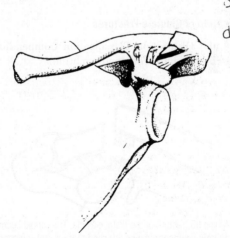

FIGURE 11.1 A type I fracture of the distal clavicle (group II). The intact ligaments hold the fragments in place. (From Rockwood CA Jr, Green DP, Bucholz RW, Heckman JD, eds. *Rockwood and Green's Fractures in Adults.* Vol 1. 4th ed, Philadelphia: Lippincott–Raven; 1996:1117.)

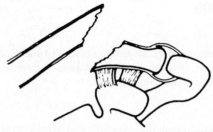

FIGURE 11.2 A type IIA distal clavicle fracture. In type IIA, both conoid and trapezoid ligaments are on the distal segment, whereas the proximal segment without ligamentous attachments is displaced. (From Rockwood CA Jr, Green DP, Bucholz RW, Heckman JD, eds. *Rockwood and Green's Fractures in Adults.* Vol 1. 4th ed, Philadelphia: Lippincott–Raven; 1996:1118.)

- **Group III:** fracture of the proximal third (5%). Minimal displacement results if the costoclavicular ligaments remain intact. It may represent epiphyseal injury in children and teenagers. Subgroups include

Type I: Minimal displacement
Type II: Displaced
Type III: Intraarticular
Type IV: Epiphyseal separation
Type V: Comminuted

OTA Classification of Clavicle Fractures

See Fracture and Dislocation Classification Compendium at http://www.ota.org/compendium/compendium.html.

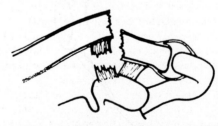

FIGURE 11.3 A type IIB fracture of the distal clavicle. The conoid ligament is ruptured, whereas the trapezoid ligament remains attached to the distal segment. The proximal fragment is displaced. (From Rockwood CA Jr, Green DP, Bucholz RW, Heckman JD, eds. *Rockwood and Green's Fractures in Adults.* Vol 1. 4th ed, Philadelphia: Lippincott–Raven; 1996:1118.)

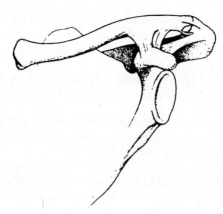

FIGURE 11.4 A type III distal clavicle fracture, involving only the articular surface of the acromioclavicular joint. No ligamentous disruption or displacement occurs. These fractures present as late degenerative changes of the joint. (From Rockwood CA Jr, Green DP, Bucholz RW, Heckman JD, eds. *Rockwood and Green's Fractures in Adults.* Vol 1 4th ed, Philadelphia: Lippincott–Raven; 1996:1119.)

TREATMENT

Nonoperative

- Most minimally displaced clavicle fractures can be successfully treated nonoperatively with some form of immobilization.
- Comfort and pain relief are the main goals. A sling has been shown to give the same results as a figure-of-eight bandage, providing more comfort and fewer skin problems.
- The goals of the various methods of immobilization are as follows:
  □ Support the shoulder girdle, raising the lateral fragment in an upward, outward, and backward direction (sling).
  □ Depress the medial fragment (figure of eight).
  □ Maintain some degree of fracture reduction (both).
  □ Allow for the patient to use the ipsilateral hand and elbow.
- Regardless of the method of immobilization utilized, some degree of shortening and deformity usually result.
- In general, immobilization is used for 4 to 6 weeks.
- During the period of immobilization, active range of motion of the elbow, wrist, and hand should be performed.

Operative

- The surgical indications for midshaft clavicle fractures are controversial and have been changing recently.

- The accepted indications for operative treatment of acute clavicle fractures are open fracture, associated neurovascular compromise, and skin tenting with the potential for progression to open fracture.
- Controversy exists over management of midshaft clavicle fractures with substantial displacement ("z-deformity") and shortening (>1 to 2 cm).
  □ Although most displaced midshaft fractures will unite, studies have reported shoulder dysfunction and patient dissatisfaction with the resulting cosmetic deformity.
  □ There is also more recent evidence that functional outcome may be improved in some of these patients with surgical treatment. Furthermore, the presence of a malunion may portend inferior function.
- Controversy also exists over management of type II distal clavicle fractures.
  □ Some authors have indicated that all type II fractures require operative management.
  □ Others report that if the bone ends are in contact, healing can be expected even if there is some degree of displacement. In this situation, nonoperative management consists of sling immobilization and progressive range of shoulder motion.
- Operative fixation may be accomplished via the use of
  □ **Plate fixation:** This is placed either on the superior or on the anteroinferior aspect of the clavicle.
    • Plate and screw fixation requires a more extensive exposure than intramedullary devices but has the advantage of more secure fixation.
    • Plate and screw fixation may be prominent, particularly if placed on the superior aspect of the clavicle. Anteroinferior plating may preclude this finding.
  □ **Intramedullary fixation (Hagie pin, Rockwood pin):** This is placed in antegrade fashion through the lateral fragment and then in retrograde fashion into the medial fragment.
    • Use of intramedullary fixation requires frequent radiographic follow-up to monitor the possibility of hardware migration and a second procedure for hardware removal.
    • Intramedullary pins are prone to skin erosion at the hardware insertion site laterally. These implants have been reported to be associated with complications in up to 50% of cases.
  □ Operative treatment of type II distal clavicle fractures consists of reducing the medial fragment to the lateral fragment. This is accomplished by using either coracoclavicular fixation (Mersilene tape, sutures, wires, or screws) or fixation across the AC joint,

through the lateral fragment and into the medial fragment (lateral clavicle plates).

COMPLICATIONS

- **Neurovascular compromise:** This is uncommon and can result from either the initial injury or secondary to compression of adjacent structures by callus and/or residual deformity. Subclavian vessels are at risk with superior plating.
- **Malunion:** This may cause a bony prominence and may be associated with poorer DASH scores at one year.
- **Nonunion:** The incidence of nonunion following clavicle fractures ranges from 0.1% to 13.0%, with 85% of all nonunions occurring in the middle third.
  - □ Factors implicated in the development of nonunions of the clavicle include (1) severity of initial trauma (open wound), (2) extent of displacement of fracture fragments, (3) soft tissue interposition, (4) refracture, (5) inadequate period of immobilization, and (6) primary open reduction and internal fixation.
- **Posttraumatic arthritis:** This may occur after intraarticular injuries to the sternoclavicular or AC joint.

12 Acromioclavicular and Sternoclavicular Joint Injuries

ACROMIOCLAVICULAR (AC) JOINT INJURY

Epidemiology

- Most common in the second decade of life, associated with contact athletic activities.
- Acromioclavicular dislocations represent 9% to 10% of acute traumatic injuries to the shoulder girdle.
- More common in males (5 to 10:1).

Anatomy (Fig. 12.1)

- The AC joint is a diarthrodial joint, with fibrocartilage-covered articular surfaces, located between the lateral end of the clavicle and the medial acromion.
- Inclination of the plane of the joint may be vertical or inclined medially 50 degrees.
- The AC ligaments (anterior, posterior, superior, inferior) strengthen the thin capsule. Fibers of the deltoid and trapezius muscles blend with the superior AC ligament to strengthen the joint.
- The AC joint has minimal mobility through a meniscoid, intraarticular disc that demonstrates an age-dependent degeneration until it is essentially nonfunctional beyond the fourth decade.

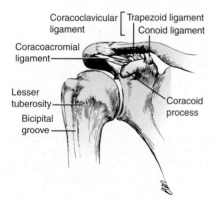

FIGURE 12.1. Normal anatomy of the acromioclavicular joint. (From Bucholz RW, Heckman JD, Court-Brown C, et al., eds. *Rockwood and Green's Fractures in Adults.* 6th ed. Philadelphia: Lippincott Williams & Wilkins; 2006.)

- The horizontal stability of the AC joint is conferred by the AC ligaments, whereas the vertical stability is maintained by the coracoclavicular ligaments (conoid-medial, trapezoid-lateral).
- The average coracoclavicular distance is 1.1 to 1.3 cm.

Mechanism of Injury

- **Direct:** This is the most common mechanism, resulting from a fall onto the shoulder with the arm adducted, driving the acromion medial and inferior.
- **Indirect:** This is caused by a fall onto an outstretched hand with force transmission through the humeral head and into the AC articulation (Fig. 12.2).

Associated Fractures and Injuries

- **Fractures:** clavicle, acromion process, and coracoid process
- Pneumothorax or pulmonary contusion with type VI AC separations

Clinical Evaluation

- The patient should be examined while in the standing or sitting position with the upper extremity in a dependent position, thus stressing the AC joint and emphasizing deformity.

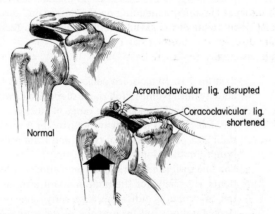

FIGURE 12.2. An indirect force applied up through the upper extremity (e.g., a fall on the outstretched hand) may superiorly displace the acromion from the clavicle, thus producing injury to the acromioclavicular ligaments. However, stress is not placed on the coracoclavicular ligaments. (From Bucholz RW, Heckman JD, Court-Brown C, et al., eds. *Rockwood and Green's Fractures in Adults*. 6th ed. Philadelphia: Lippincott Williams & Wilkins; 2006.)

- The characteristic anatomic feature is a downward sag of the shoulder and arm.
- A standard shoulder examination should be performed, including assessment of neurovascular status and possible associated upper extremity injuries. Inspection may reveal an apparent step-off deformity of the injured AC joint, with possible tenting of the skin overlying the distal clavicle. Range of shoulder motion may be limited by pain. Tenderness may be elicited over the AC joint.

Radiographic Evaluation

- A standard trauma series of the shoulder (anteroposterior [AP], scapular-Y, and axillary views) is usually sufficient for the recognition of AC injury. The Zanca view is taken with the x-ray beam in 10 to 15 degrees of cephalic tilt. This view allows better visualization of the distal clavicle.
- Ligamentous injury to the coracoclavicular joints may be assessed via stress radiographs, in which weights (10 to 15 lb) are strapped to the wrists, and an AP radiograph is taken of both shoulders to compare coracoclavicular distances (difficult to do in the acute setting and had little clinical application).

Classification

- This injury is classified depending on the degree and direction of displacement of the distal clavicle (Table 12.1 and Fig. 12.3).

Treatment

Type I: Rest for 7 to 10 days, ice packs, sling. Refrain from full activity until painless, full range of motion (2 weeks).

Type II: Sling for 1 to 2 weeks, gentle range of motion as soon as possible. Refrain from heavy activity for 6 weeks. More than 50% of patients with type I and II injuries remain symptomatic at long-term follow-up.

Type III: For inactive, nonlaboring, or recreational athletic patients, especially for the nondominant arm, nonoperative treatment is indicated: sling, early range of motion, strengthening, and acceptance of deformity. Younger, more active patients with more severe degrees of displacement and laborers who use their upper extremity above the horizontal plane may benefit from operative stabilization. Repair is generally avoided in contact athletes because of the risk of reinjury.

TABLE

12.1   Classification of Acromioclavicular (AC) Joint Injury

Type	Anatomy	Clinical Examination	Radiographic Examination
I	Sprain of the AC ligament	AC joint tenderness, minimal pain with arm motion, no pain in coracoclavicular interspace	No abnormality
II	AC ligament tear with joint disruption, coracoclavicular ligaments sprained	Distal clavicle slightly superior to acromion and mobile to palpation; tenderness in the coracoclavicular space	Slight elevation of the distal end of the clavicle; AC joint widening. Stress films show coracoclavicular space unchanged from normal shoulder.
III	AC and coracoclavicular ligaments torn with AC joint dislocation. The deltoid and trapezius muscles are usually detached from the distal clavicle.	The upper extremity and distal fragment are depressed and the distal end of the proximal fragment may tent the skin. The AC joint is tender, and coracoclavicular widening is evident.	Radiographs demonstrate the distal clavicle superior to the medial border of the acromion; stress views reveal a widened coracoclavicular interspace 25% to 100% greater than the normal side.
IV	Distal clavicle displaced posteriorly into or through the trapezius. The deltoid and trapezius muscles are detached from the distal clavicle.	There is more pain than in type III; the distal clavicle is displaced posteriorly away from the acromion.	Axillary radiograph or computed tomography scan demonstrates posterior displacement of the distal clavicle.
V	Distal clavicle grossly and severely displaced superiorly (>100%). The deltoid and trapezius muscles are detached from the distal clavicle.	Typically associated with tenting of the skin	Radiographs demonstrate the coracoclavicular interspace to be 100% to 300% greater than the normal side.
VI	The AC joint is dislocated, with the clavicle displaced inferior to the acromion or the coracoid; the coracoclavicular interspace is decreased compared with normal. The deltoid and trapezius muscles are detached from the distal clavicle.	The shoulder has a flat appearance with a prominent acromion; associated clavicle and upper rib fractures and brachial plexus injuries result from high-energy trauma.	One of two types of inferior dislocation: subacromial or subcoracoid

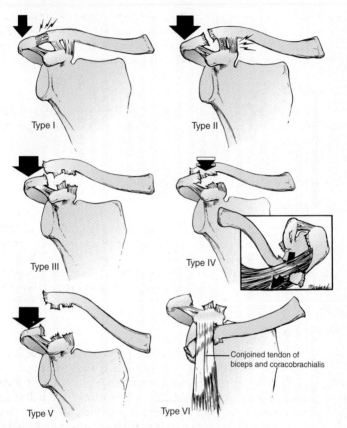

FIGURE 12.3. Classification of ligamentous injuries to the acromioclavicular (AC) joint. **Top left:** In the type I injury, a mild force applied to the point of the shoulder does not disrupt either the AC or the coracoclavicular ligaments. **Top right:** A moderate to heavy force applied to the point of the shoulder will disrupt the AC ligaments, but the coracoclavicular ligaments remain intact (type II). **Center left:** When a severe force is applied to the point of the shoulder, both the AC and the coracoclavicular ligaments are disrupted (type III). **Center right:** In a type IV injury, not only are the ligaments disrupted, but also the distal end of the clavicle is displaced posteriorly into or through the trapezius muscle. **Bottom left:** A violent force applied to the point of the shoulder not only ruptures the AC and coracoclavicular ligaments but also disrupts the muscle attachments and creates a major separation between the clavicle and the acromion (type V). **Bottom right:** This is an inferior dislocation of the distal clavicle in which the clavicle is inferior to the coracoid process and posterior to the biceps and coracobrachialis tendons. The AC and coracoclavicular ligaments are also disrupted (type VI). (From Bucholz RW, Heckman JD, Court-Brown C, et al., eds. *Rockwood and Green's Fractures in Adults.* 6th ed. Philadelphia: Lippincott Williams & Wilkins; 2006.)

Types IV–VI: These are generally treated with open reduction, and surgical repair or reconstruction of the coracoclavicular ligaments is performed for vertical stability, although no level-one evidence for this treatment exists.

Complications

- **Coracoclavicular ossification:** not associated with increased disability
- **Distal clavicle osteolysis:** associated with chronic dull ache and weakness
- AC arthritis

STERNOCLAVICULAR (SC) JOINT INJURY

Epidemiology

- Injuries to the SC joint are rare; Cave et al. reported that of 1,603 shoulder girdle dislocations, only 3% were SC, with 85% glenohumeral and 12% AC dislocations.
- Approximately 80% of dislocations of the SC joint are caused by either motor vehicle accidents (47%) or sports-related injuries (31%).

Anatomy (Fig. 12.4)

- The SC joint is a diarthrodial joint, representing the only true articulation between the upper extremity and the axial skeleton.
- The articular surface of the clavicle is much larger than that of the sternum; both are covered with fibrocartilage. Less than half of the medial clavicle articulates with the sternum; thus, the SC joint has the distinction of having the least amount of bony stability of the major joints of the body.
- Joint integrity is derived from the saddle-like configuration of the joint (convex vertically and concave anteroposteriorly), as well as from surrounding ligaments:
  - The intraarticular disc ligament is a checkrein against medial displacement of the clavicle.
  - The extraarticular costoclavicular ligament resists rotation and medial-lateral displacement.
  - The interclavicular ligament helps to maintain shoulder poise.
- Range of motion is 35 degrees of superior elevation, 35 degrees of combined AP motion, and 50 degrees of rotation around its long axis.
- The medial clavicle physis is the last physis to close. It ossifies at 20 years and fuses with the shaft at 25 to 30 years. Therefore, many supposed SC joint dislocations may actually be physeal injuries.

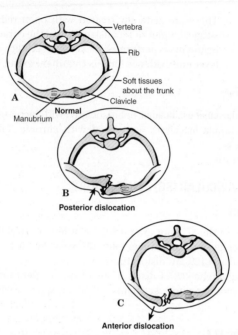

FIGURE 12.4. Cross sections through the thorax at the level of the sternoclavicular joint. **(A)** Normal anatomic relations. **(B)** Posterior dislocation of the sternoclavicular joint. **(C)** Anterior dislocation of the sternoclavicular joint. (From Bucholz RW, Heckman JD, Court-Brown C, et al., eds. *Rockwood and Green's Fractures in Adults.* 6th ed. Philadelphia: Lippincott Williams & Wilkins; 2006.)

Mechanism of Injury (Fig. 12.5)

- **Direct:** Force applied to the anteromedial aspect of the clavicle forces the clavicle posteriorly into the mediastinum to produce posterior dislocation. This may occur when an athlete is in the supine position and another athlete falls on him or her, when an individual is run over by a vehicle, or when an individual is pinned against a wall by a vehicle.

- **Indirect:** Force can be applied indirectly to the SC joint from the anterolateral (producing anterior SC dislocation) or posterolateral (producing posterior SC dislocation) aspects of the shoulder. This is most commonly seen in football "pileups," in which an athlete is lying obliquely on his shoulder and force is applied with the individual unable to change position.

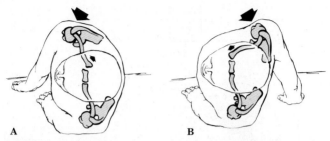

A   B

FIGURE 12.5. Mechanisms that produce anterior or posterior dislocations of the sternoclavicular joint. **(A)** If the patient is lying on the ground and compression force is applied to the posterolateral aspect of the shoulder, the medial end of the clavicle will be displaced posteriorly. **(B)** When the lateral compression force is directed from the anterior position, the medial end of the clavicle is dislocated anteriorly. (From Bucholz RW, Heckman JD, Court-Brown C, et al., eds. *Rockwood and Green's Fractures in Adults.* 6th ed. Philadelphia: Lippincott Williams & Wilkins; 2006.)

Clinical Evaluation

■ The patient typically presents supporting the affected extremity across the trunk with the contralateral, uninjured arm. The patient's head may be tilted toward the side of injury to decrease stress across the joint, and the patient may be unwilling to place the affected scapula flat on the examination table.

■ Swelling, tenderness, and painful range of shoulder motion are usually present, with a variable change of the medial clavicular prominence, depending on the degree and direction of injury.

■ Neurovascular status must be assessed, because the brachial plexus and major vascular structures are in the immediate vicinity of the medial clavicle.

■ With posterior dislocations, venous engorgement of the ipsilateral extremity, shortness of breath, painful inspiration, difficulty swallowing, and a choking sensation may be present. The chest must be auscultated to ensure bilaterally symmetric breath sounds.

Radiographic Evaluation

■ AP chest radiographs typically demonstrate asymmetry of the clavicles that should prompt further radiographic evaluation. This view should be scrutinized for the presence of pneumothorax if the patient presents with breathing complaints.

■ **Hobbs view:** In this 90-degree cephalocaudal lateral view, the patient leans over the plate, and the radiographic beam is angled behind the neck (Fig. 12.6).

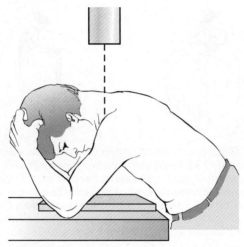

FIGURE 12.6. Hobbs view: positioning of the patient for x-ray evaluation of the sternoclavicular joint, as recommended by Hobbs. (Modified from Hobbs DW. Sternoclavicular joint: a new axial radiographic view. *Radiology.* 1968;90:801–802; in Bucholz RW, Heckman JD, Court-Brown C, et al., eds. *Rockwood and Green's Fractures in Adults.* 6th ed. Philadelphia: Lippincott Williams & Wilkins; 2006.)

- **Serendipity view:** This 40-degree cephalic tilt view is aimed at the manubrium. With an anterior dislocation, the medial clavicle lies above the interclavicular line; with a posterior dislocation, the medial clavicle lies below this line (Fig. 12.7).
- **Computed tomography (CT) scan:** This is the best technique to evaluate injuries to the SC joint. CT is able to distinguish fractures of the medial clavicle from dislocation as well as delineate minor subluxations that would otherwise go unrecognized.

Classification

Anatomic

- **Anterior dislocation:** more common
- Posterior dislocation

Etiologic

- Sprain or subluxation
  - □ **Mild:** joint stable, ligamentous integrity maintained

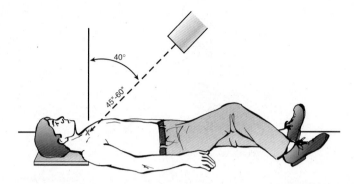

FIGURE 12.7. Serendipity view: positioning of the patient to take the "serendipity" view of the sternoclavicular joints. The x-ray tube is tilted 40 degrees from the vertical position and is aimed directly at the manubrium. The nongrid cassette should be large enough to receive the projected images of the medial halves of both clavicles. In children, the tube distance from the patient should be 45 inches; in thicker-chested adults, the distance should be 60 inches. (From Bucholz RW, Heckman JD, Court-Brown C, et al., eds. *Rockwood and Green's Fractures in Adults.* 6th ed. Philadelphia: Lippincott Williams & Wilkins; 2006.)

  ☐ **Moderate:** subluxation, with partial ligamentous disruption
  ☐ **Severe:** unstable joint, with complete ligamentous compromise
  ■ **Acute dislocation:** complete ligamentous disruption with frank translation of the medial clavicle
  ■ **Recurrent dislocation:** rare
  ■ Unreduced dislocation
  ■ **Atraumatic:** may occur with spontaneous dislocation, developmental (congenital) dislocation, osteoarthritis, condensing osteitis of the medial clavicle, SC hyperostosis, or infection

Treatment

  ■ **Mild sprain:** Ice is indicated for the first 24 hours with sling immobilization for 3 to 4 days and a gradual return to normal activities as tolerated.
  ■ **Moderate sprain or subluxation:** Ice is indicated for the first 24 hours with a clavicle strap, sling and swathe, or figure-of-eight bandage for 1 week, then sling immobilization for 4 to 6 weeks.
  ■ Severe sprain or dislocation (Fig. 12.8)
    ☐ **Anterior:** As for nonoperative treatment, it is controversial whether one should attempt closed reduction because it is usually unstable; a sling is used for comfort. Closed reduction may

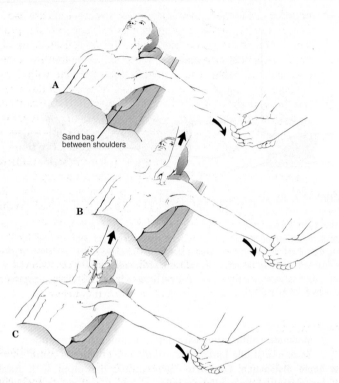

Sand bag
between shoulders

FIGURE 12.8. Technique for closed reduction of the sternoclavicular joint. **(A)** The patient is positioned supine with a sandbag placed between the two shoulders. Traction is then applied to the arm against countertraction in an abducted and slightly extended position. In anterior dislocations, direct pressure over the medial end of the clavicle may reduce the joint. **(B)** In posterior dislocations, in addition to the traction it may be necessary to manipulate the medial end of the clavicle with the fingers to dislodge the clavicle from behind the manubrium. **(C)** In stubborn posterior dislocations, it may be necessary to prepare the medial end of the clavicle in sterile fashion and to use a towel clip to grasp around the medial clavicle to lift it back into position. (From Bucholz RW, Heckman JD, Court-Brown C, et al., eds. *Rockwood and Green's Fractures in Adults*. 6th ed. Philadelphia: Lippincott Williams & Wilkins; 2006.)

be accomplished using general anesthesia, or narcotics and muscle relaxants for the stoic patient. The patient is placed supine with a roll between the scapulae. Direct, posteriorly directed pressure usually results in reduction. Postreduction care consists of a clavicle strap, sling and swathe, or figure-of-eight bandage for 4 to 6 weeks. Some advocate a bulky anterior dressing with elastic tape to maintain reduction.

- ☐ **Posterior:** A careful history and physical examination are necessary to rule out associated pulmonary or neurovascular problems. Prompt closed or open reduction is indicated, usually under general anesthesia. Closed reduction is often successful and remains stable. The patient is placed supine with a roll between the scapulae. Closed reduction may be obtained with traction with the arm in abduction and extension. Anteriorly directed traction on the clavicle with a towel clip may be required. A clavicle strap, sling and swathe, or figure-of-eight bandage is used for immobilization for 4 to 6 weeks. A general or thoracic surgeon should be available in the event that the major underlying neurovascular structures are inadvertently damaged.

- ■ **Medial physeal injury:** Closed reduction is usually successful, with postreduction care consisting of a clavicle strap, sling and swathe, or figure-of-eight bandage immobilization for 4 to 6 weeks.

- ■ Operative management of SC dislocation may include fixation of the medial clavicle to the sternum using fascia lata, subclavius tendon, or suture, osteotomy of the medial clavicle, or resection of the medial clavicle. The use of Kirschner wires or Steinmann pins is discouraged, because migration of hardware may occur.

Complications

- ■ Poor cosmesis is the most common complication with patients complaining of an enlarged medial prominence.

- ■ Complications are more common with posterior dislocations and reflect the proximity of the medial clavicle to mediastinal and neurovascular structures. The complication rate has been reported to be as high as 25% with posterior dislocation. Complications include the following:
  - ☐ Pneumothorax
  - ☐ Laceration of the superior vena cava
  - ☐ Venous congestion in the neck
  - ☐ Esophageal rupture
  - ☐ Subclavian artery compression
  - ☐ Carotid artery compression
  - ☐ Voice changes

13 Scapula Fractures

EPIDEMIOLOGY

- This relatively uncommon injury represents only 3% to 5% of all shoulder fractures and 0.5% to 1% of all fractures.
- The mean age of patients with fracture of the scapula is 35 to 45 years.

ANATOMY

- This flat, triangular bone links the upper extremity to the axial skeleton.
- Protection from impact is provided by the large surrounding muscle mass as well as the mobility of the scapula on the chest wall, further aiding in force dissipation.

MECHANISM OF INJURY

- Significant high-energy trauma is usually required to fracture the scapula, as is evidenced by the common cause of injury—motor vehicle accident in approximately 50% of cases and motorcycle accident in 11% to 25%.
- Indirect injury occurs through axial loading on the outstretched arm (scapular neck, glenoid, intra-articular fracture).
- Direct trauma occurs from a blow or fall (scapula body fracture) or through direct trauma to the point of the shoulder (acromion, coracoid fracture).
- Shoulder dislocation may cause a glenoid fracture.
- Muscles or ligaments may cause an avulsion fracture.

ASSOCIATED INJURIES

- The presence of a scapula fracture should raise suspicion of associated injuries, because 35% to 98% of scapula fractures occur in the presence of comorbid injuries including
  - **Ipsilateral upper torso injuries:** fractured ribs, clavicle, sternum, shoulder trauma
  - **Pneumothorax:** seen in 11% to 55% of scapula fractures
  - **Pulmonary contusion:** present in 11% to 54% of scapula fractures

- ☐ **Injuries to neurovascular structures:** brachial plexus injuries, vascular avulsions
- ☐ **Spine injuries:** 20% lower cervical spine, 76% thoracic spine, 4% lumbar spine

CLINICAL EVALUATION

- ■ A full trauma evaluation is indicated, with attention to airway, breathing, circulation, disability, and exposure.
- ■ The patient typically presents with the upper extremity supported by the contralateral hand in an adducted and immobile position, with painful range of motion, especially shoulder abduction.
- ■ A careful examination for associated injures should be performed, with a thorough neurovascular assessment.
- ■ Compartment syndrome overlying the scapula is uncommon, but it must be ruled out in the presence of pain out of proportion to the apparent injury. *Comolli sign* is triangular swelling of the posterior thorax overlying the scapula and is suggestive of hematoma resulting in increased compartment pressures.

RADIOGRAPHIC EVALUATION

- ■ May first be picked up on a chest x-ray. Initial radiographs should include a trauma series of the shoulder, consisting of a true antero-posterior view, an axillary view, and a scapular-Y view (true scapular lateral); these generally are able to demonstrate most glenoid, scapular neck, body, and acromion fractures.
  - ☐ The axillary view may be used to delineate acromial and glenoid rim fractures further.
  - ☐ An acromial fracture should not be confused with an *os acromiale*, which is a rounded, unfused apophysis and is present in approximately 3% of the population. When present, it is bilateral in 60% of cases.
  - ☐ *Glenoid hypoplasia,* or *scapular neck dysplasia,* is an unusual abnormality that may resemble glenoid impaction and may be associated with humeral head or acromial abnormalities. It has a benign course and is usually noted incidentally.
- ■ A 45-degree cephalic tilt (Stryker notch) radiograph is helpful to identify coracoid fractures.
- ■ Computed tomography may be useful for further characterizing intra-articular glenoid fractures.
- ■ Because of the high incidence of associated injuries, especially to thoracic structures, a chest radiograph is an essential part of the evaluation.

CLASSIFICATION

Anatomic Classification (Zdravkovic and Damholt) (Fig. 13.1)

Type I:	Scapula body
Type II:	Apophyseal fractures, including the acromion and coracoid
Type III:	Fractures of the superolateral angle, including the scapular neck and glenoid

Ideberg Classification of Intra-articular Glenoid Fractures (Fig. 13.2)

Type I:	Avulsion fracture of the anterior margin
Type IIA:	Transverse fracture through the glenoid fossa exiting inferiorly
Type IIB:	Oblique fracture through the glenoid fossa exiting inferiorly
Type III:	Oblique fracture through the glenoid exiting superiorly and often associated with an acromioclavicular joint injury
Type IV:	Transverse fracture exiting through the medial border of the scapula
Type V:	Combination of a type II and type IV pattern
Type VI:	Comminuted glenoid fracture

Classification of Acromial Fractures (Kuhn et al.) (Fig. 13.3)

Type I:	Minimally displaced
Type II:	Displaced but does not reduce the subacromial space
Type III:	Displaced with narrowing of the subacromial space

Classification of Coracoid Fractures (Ogawa et al.) (Fig. 13.4)

Type I:	Proximal to the coracoclavicular ligament
Type II:	Distal to the coracoclavicular ligament

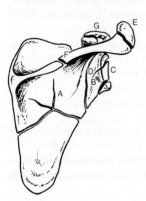

FIGURE 13.1 Anatomic classification. (*A*) scapula body; (*B,C*) glenoid; (*D*) scapula neck; (*E*) acromion; (*F*) scapula spine; (*G*) coracoid.

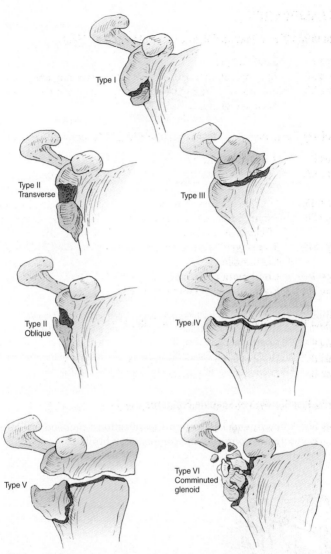

FIGURE 13.2 Ideberg classification of glenoid fractures into five types, with the comminuted type VI of Goss added. The classification is historical, because decision making is based on displacement of the articular component. (From Bucholz RW, Heckman JD, Court-Brown C, et al., eds. *Rockwood and Green's Fractures in Adults*. 6th ed. Philadelphia: Lippincott Williams & Wilkins; 2006.)

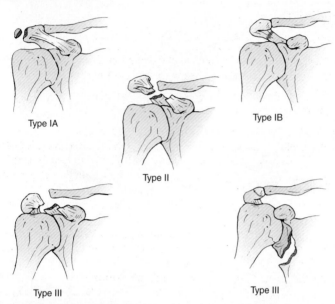

FIGURE 13.3 Type I acromion fractures are nondisplaced and include type IA (avulsion) and type IB (complete fracture). Type II fractures are displaced, but they do not reduce the subacromial space. Type III fractures cause a reduction in subacromial space. (Modified from Kuhn JE, Blasier RB, Carpenter JE. Fractures of the acromion process: a proposed classification system. *J Orthop Trauma.* 1994;8:6–13.)

OTA Classification of Scapula Fractures

■ See Fracture and Dislocation Classification Compendium http://www.ota.org/compendium/compendium.html.

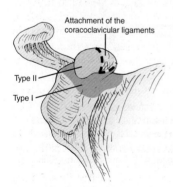

FIGURE 13.4 Classification of coracoid fractures: type I is proximal to the coracoclavicular ligament attachment and type II is distal. (Modified from Ogawa K, Yoshida A, Takahashi M, Ui M. Fractures of the coracoid process. *J Bone Joint Surg Br.* 1979;79:17–19.)

TREATMENT

Nonoperative

Most scapula fractures (extra-articular) are amenable to nonoperative treatment, consisting of sling use and early range of shoulder motion.

Operative

- Surgical indications are controversial, but include
  - □ Displaced intra-articular glenoid fractures involving greater than 25% of the articular surface, with or without subluxation.
  - □ Scapular neck fractures with greater than 40-degree angulation or 1-cm medial translation.
  - □ Scapular neck fractures with an associated displaced clavicle fracture.
  - □ Fractures of the acromion that impinge on the subacromial space.
  - □ Fractures of the coracoid process that result in a functional acromioclavicular separation.
  - □ Comminuted fractures of the scapular spine.
- Specific treatment options include
  - □ **_Glenoid fractures_ (Ideberg classification):**

Type I: Fractures involving greater than one-fourth of the glenoid fossa that result in instability may be amenable to open reduction and internal fixation with screw fixation using an anterior or posterior approach.

Type II: Inferior subluxation of the humeral head may result, necessitating open reduction, especially when associated with a greater than 5-mm articular step-off. An anterior approach typically provides adequate exposure.

Type III: Reduction is often difficult and may require superior exposure for superior to inferior screw placement, partial-thickness clavicle removal, or distal clavicle resection in addition to anterior exposure for reduction. Additional stabilization of the superior suspensory shoulder complex (SSSC) may be necessary.

Type IV: Open reduction should be considered for displaced fractures, especially those in which the superior fragment of the glenoid displaces laterally.

Type V: Operative management does not necessarily result in improved functional results as compared with nonoperative treatment with early motion, but it should be considered for articular step-off greater than 5 mm.

□ **Scapular body fractures:** Operative fixation is rarely indicated, with nonoperative measures generally effective. Open reduction may be considered when neurovascular compromise is present and exploration is required.

□ **Glenoid neck fractures:** These generally may be treated symptomatically, with early range-of-motion exercises. If the injury is accompanied by a displaced clavicle fracture, an unstable segment may exist, including the glenoid, acromion, and lateral clavicle. Internal fixation of the clavicular fracture generally results in adequate stabilization for healing of the glenoid fracture.

□ **Acromion fractures:** Os acromiale must first be ruled out, as well as concomitant rotator cuff injuries. Displaced acromion fractures may be stabilized by dorsal tension banding, if displacement causes subacromial impingement.

□ **Coracoid fractures:** Complete third-degree acromioclavicular separation accompanied by a significantly displaced coracoid fracture is an indication for open reduction and internal fixation of both injuries.

□ **Floating shoulder:** This consists of double disruptions of the superior shoulder suspensory complex (SSSC).

■ The SSSC is a bone-soft tissue ring that includes the glenoid process, coracoid process, coracoclavicular ligaments, distal clavicle, acromioclavicular joint, and acromial process (Fig. 13.5).

■ The superior strut is the middle third clavicle.

■ The inferior strut is the lateral scapular body and spine.

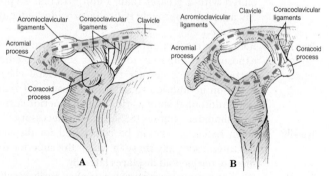

FIGURE 13.5 Superior shoulder suspensory complex anatomy. **(A)** Anteroposterior view. **(B)** True lateral view. (Modified from Goss TP. Double disruption of the superior shoulder suspensory complex. *J Orthop Trauma.* 1993;7:99–106.)

- Traumatic disruption of two or more components of the SSSC usually secondary to high-energy injury is frequently described as a floating shoulder.
- Historically, operative management has been recommended because of potential instability and displacement of the glenoid. This may lead to shortening, loss of range of shoulder motion, and potential weakness.
- Recent series of nonoperative treatment of floating shoulders have reported good results.

COMPLICATIONS

- **Associated injuries:** These account for most serious complications, because of the high-energy nature of these injuries. Increased mortality is associated with concomitant first rib fracture.
- **Malunion:** Fractures of the scapula body generally unite with nonoperative treatment; when malunion occurs, it is generally well tolerated but may result in painful scapulothoracic crepitus.
- **Nonunion:** This is extremely rare, but when present and symptomatic it may require open reduction and internal fixation.
- **Suprascapular nerve injury:** This may occur in association with scapula body, neck, or coracoid fractures that involve the suprascapular notch (Fig. 13.6).

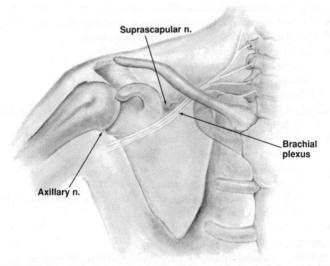

FIGURE 13.6 Schematic diagram showing the positions of the brachial plexus relative to the scapula. (From Bucholz RW, Heckman JD, Court-Brown C, et al., eds. *Rockwood and Green's Fractures in Adults.* 6th ed. Philadelphia: Lippincott Williams & Wilkins; 2006.)

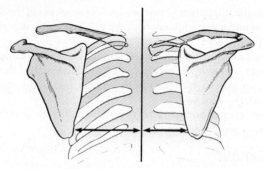

FIGURE 13.7 Diagram of scapulothoracic dissociation, demonstrating lateral displacement of the scapula on the injured side **(left)** compared with the normal side **(right)** on a nonrotated chest radiograph. (From Bucholz RW, Heckman JD, Court-Brown C, et al., eds. *Rockwood and Green's Fractures in Adults.* 6th ed. Philadelphia: Lippincott Williams & Wilkins; 2006.)

Scapulothoracic Dissociation

- This injury is a traumatic disruption of the scapula from the posterior chest wall.
- This rare, life-threatening injury is essentially a subcutaneous forequarter amputation.
- The mechanism is a violent traction and rotation force, usually as a result of a motor vehicle or motorcycle accident.
- Neurovascular injury is common:
  - □ **Complete brachial plexopathy:** 80%
  - □ **Partial plexopathy:** 15%
  - □ **Subclavian or axillary artery:** 88%
- It can be associated with fracture or dislocation about the shoulder or without obvious bone injury.
- Diagnosis includes
  - □ Massive swelling of shoulder region
  - □ A pulseless arm
  - □ A complete or partial neurologic deficit
  - □ Lateral displacement of the scapula on a nonrotated chest radiograph, which is diagnostic (Fig. 13.7)
- Classification

Type I: Musculoskeletal injury alone
Type IIA: Musculoskeletal injury with vascular disruption
Type IIB: Musculoskeletal injury with neurologic impairment
Type III: Musculoskeletal injury with both neurologic and vascular injury

- Initial treatment
  - ☐ Patients are often polytraumatized.
  - ☐ Advanced trauma life support protocols should be followed.
  - ☐ Angiography of the limb with vascular repair and exploration of brachial plexus are performed as indicated.
  - ☐ Stabilization of associated bone or joint injuries is indicated.
- Later treatment
  - ☐ Neurologic
    - At 3 weeks, electromyography is indicated.
    - At 6 weeks, cervical myelography or magnetic resonance imaging is performed.
    - Shoulder arthrodesis and/or above elbow amputation may be necessary if the limb is flail.
    - Nerve root avulsions and complete deficits have a poor prognosis.
    - Partial plexus injuries have good prognosis, and functional use of the extremity is often regained.
    - MRI—"empty sleeve sign"
  - ☐ Osseous
    - If initial exploration of the brachial plexus reveals a severe injury, primary above elbow amputation should be considered.
    - If cervical myelography reveals three or more pseudo-meningoceles, the prognosis is similarly poor.
- This injury is associated with a poor outcome including flail extremity in 52%, early amputation in 21%, and death in 10%.

Intrathoracic Dislocation of the Scapula

- This is extremely rare.
- The inferior angle of the scapula is locked in the intercostal space.
- Chest computed tomography may be needed to confirm the diagnosis.
- Treatment consists of closed reduction and immobilization with a sling and swathe for 2 weeks, followed by progressive functional use of the shoulder and arm.

14

Glenohumeral Dislocation

EPIDEMIOLOGY

- The shoulder is the most commonly dislocated major joint of the body, accounting for up to 45% of dislocations.
- Most shoulder dislocations are anterior; this occurs between eight and nine times more frequently than posterior dislocation, the second most common direction of dislocation.
- The incidence of glenohumeral dislocation is 17 per 100,000 population per year.
- Incidence peaks were found in the age-group 21 to 30 years among men and in the age-group 61 to 80 years among women.
- Recurrence rate in all ages was 50%, but rose to almost 89% in the 14 to 20 year age-group.
- Inferior (luxatio erecta) and superior shoulder dislocations are rare.

ANATOMY (FIG. 14.1)

- Glenohumeral stability depends on various passive and active mechanisms, including
  - □ **Passive:**
    1. Joint conformity.
    2. Vacuum effect of limited joint volume.
    3. Adhesion and cohesion owing to the presence of synovial fluid.
    4. **Scapular inclination:** for >90% of shoulders, the critical angle of scapular inclination is between 0 and 30 degrees, below

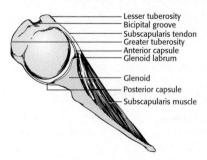

Lesser tuberosity
Bicipital groove
Subscapularis tendon
Greater tuberosity
Anterior capsule
Glenoid labrum

Glenoid
Posterior capsule
Subscapularis muscle

FIGURE 14.1 Views of the shoulder bony anatomy. (From Bucholz RW, Heckman JD, Court-Brown C, et al., eds. *Rockwood and Green's Fractures in Adults.* 6th ed. Philadelphia: Lippincott Williams & Wilkins; 2006.)

which the glenohumeral joint is considered unstable and prone to inferior dislocation.

5. Ligamentous and capsular restraints (Fig. 14.2).
   - **Joint capsule:** Redundancy prevents significant restraint, except at terminal ranges of motion. The anteroinferior capsule limits anterior subluxation of the abducted shoulder. The posterior capsule and teres minor limit internal rotation. The anterior capsule and lower subscapularis restrain abduction and external rotation.
   - **Superior glenohumeral ligament:** This is the primary restraint to inferior translation of the adducted shoulder.
   - **Middle glenohumeral ligament:** This is variable, poorly defined, or absent in 30%. It limits external rotation at 45 degrees of abduction.
   - **Inferior glenohumeral ligament:** This consists of three bands, the superior of which is of primary importance to prevent anterior dislocation of the shoulder. It limits external rotation at 45 to 90 degrees of abduction.
6. Glenoid labrum.
7. **Bony restraints:** acromion, coracoid, glenoid fossa.

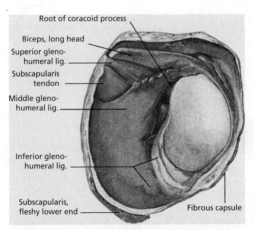

FIGURE 14.2 Anterior glenohumeral ligaments. This drawing shows the anterosuperior, anteromedial, and anteroinferior glenohumeral ligaments. The anteromedial and anteroinferior glenohumeral ligaments are often avulsed from the glenoid or glenoid labrum in traumatic anterior instability. (From *Grant's Atlas of Anatomy.* 4th ed. Baltimore: Williams & Wilkins; 1956.)

□ **Active:**
  1. Biceps, long head.
  2. Rotator cuff.

■ Coordinated shoulder motion involves
  1. Glenohumeral motion.
  2. Scapulothoracic motion.
  3. Clavicular and sternoclavicular motion.
  4. Acromioclavicular motion.

■ **Pathoanatomy of shoulder dislocations:**
  □ Stretching or tearing of the capsule.
  □ Usually off the glenoid, but occasionally off the humeral avulsion of the glenohumeral ligaments (HAGL lesion).
  □ Labral damage.
  □ A "Bankart" lesion refers to avulsion of anteroinferior labrum off the glenoid rim. It may be associated with a glenoid rim fracture ("bony Bankart").

■ **Hill-Sachs lesion:** A posterolateral head defect is caused by an impression fracture on the glenoid rim; this is seen in 27% of acute anterior dislocations and 74% of recurrent anterior dislocations (Fig. 14.3).

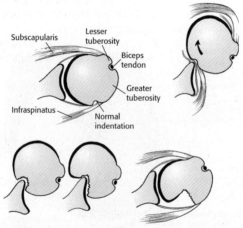

FIGURE 14.3 Hill-Sachs lesion associated with anterior shoulder dislocation. On dislocation, the posterior aspect of the humeral head engages the anterior glenoid rim. The glenoid rim then initiates an impression fracture that can enlarge. (From Bucholz RW, Heckman JD, Court-Brown C, et al., eds. *Rockwood and Green's Fractures in Adults.* 6th ed. Philadelphia: Lippincott Williams & Wilkins; 2006.)

- **Shoulder dislocation with associated rotator cuff tear:**
  - ☐ This is common in older patients.
    - • **>40 years of age:** 35% to 40%
    - • **>60 years of age:** may be as high as 80%
  - ☐ Beware of inability to lift the arm in an older patient following a dislocation.

ANTERIOR GLENOHUMERAL DISLOCATION

Incidence

- Anterior dislocations represent 90% of shoulder dislocations.

Mechanism of Injury

Anterior glenohumeral dislocation may occur as a result of trauma, secondary to either direct or indirect forces.

- Indirect trauma to the upper extremity with the shoulder in abduction, extension, and external rotation is the most common mechanism.
- Direct, impaction forces to the posterior shoulder may produce an anterior dislocation.
- Convulsive mechanisms and electrical shock typically produce posterior shoulder dislocations, but they may also result in an anterior dislocation.
- Recurrent instability related to congenital or acquired laxity or volitional mechanisms may result in anterior dislocation with minimal trauma.

Clinical Evaluation

- It is helpful to determine the nature of the trauma, the chronicity of the dislocation, pattern of recurrence with inciting events, and the presence of laxity or a history of instability in the contralateral shoulder.
- The patient typically presents with the injured shoulder held in slight abduction and external rotation. The acutely dislocated shoulder is painful, with muscular spasm.
- Examination typically reveals squaring of the shoulder owing to a relative prominence of the acromion, a relative hollow beneath the acromion posteriorly, and a palpable mass anteriorly.
- A careful neurovascular examination is important, with attention to axillary nerve integrity. Deltoid muscle testing is usually not possible, but sensation over the deltoid may be assessed. Deltoid atony may be present and should not be confused with axillary nerve injury. Musculocutaneous nerve integrity can be assessed

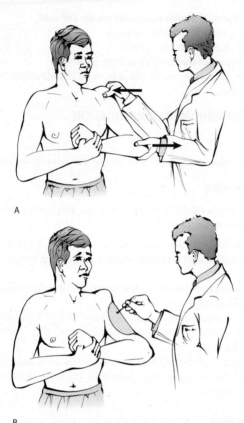

A

B

FIGURE 14.4 Technique for testing axillary nerve function. With the arm adducted and stabilized by the examiner, the patient is asked to abduct the arm. The motor component **(A)** of the axillary nerve is documented by observing or palpating deltoid muscle contraction. The sensory component **(B)** of the axillary nerve is documented by testing the sensation to the lateral aspect of the upper arm. (From Bucholz RW, Heckman JD, Court-Brown C, et al., eds. *Rockwood and Green's Fractures in Adults*. 6th ed. Philadelphia: Lippincott Williams & Wilkins; 2006.)

by the presence of sensation on the anterolateral forearm (Fig. 14.4).

■ Patients may present after spontaneous reduction or reduction in the field. If the patient is not in acute pain, examination may reveal

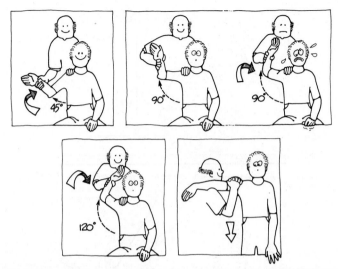

FIGURE 14.5 Evaluation of the injured shoulder in varying degrees of abduction. Top left: External rotation force is applied to the arm in 45 degrees of abduction. Top right: The shoulder is abducted 90 degrees. Next, the external rotation force with some extension is applied, which produces pain, usually posteriorly, and marked apprehension in the patient. This position most commonly produces pain and severe apprehension. Bottom left: The external rotation and extension force is applied to the arm in 120 degrees of abduction. This causes apprehension in some patients but not as marked with the arm in 90 degrees of abduction. Bottom right: The Feagin test. With the patient's elbow resting on the top of the physician's shoulder, a downward force on the proximal humerus in some instances produces apprehension. (From Bucholz RW, Heckman JD, eds. *Rockwood and Green's Fractures in Adults.* 5th ed. Baltimore: Lippincott Williams & Wilkins; 2001.)

a positive *apprehension test,* in which passive placement of the shoulder in the provocative position (abduction, extension, and external rotation) reproduces the patient's sense of instability and pain (Fig. 14.5).

Radiographic Evaluation

- **Trauma series of the affected shoulder:** Anteroposterior (AP), scapular-Y, and axillary views are taken in the plane of the scapula (Figs. 14.6 and 14.7).
- **Velpeau axillary:** If a standard axillary cannot be obtained because of pain, the patient may be left in a sling and leaned obliquely backward 45 degrees over the cassette. The beam is directed caudally,

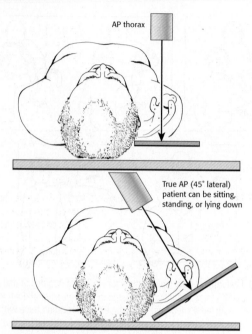

FIGURE 14.6 Technique for obtaining anteroposterior (AP) **(upper panel)** and true AP **(lower panel)** x-rays of the shoulder. In an AP view, the x-ray actually represents an oblique view of the shoulder joint. In a true AP view, the x-ray beam is parallel to the joint so overlap between the humeral head and the glenoid surface is minimal. (From Bucholz RW, Heckman JD, Court-Brown C, et al., eds. *Rockwood and Green's Fractures in Adults.* 6th ed. Philadelphia: Lippincott Williams & Wilkins; 2006.)

orthogonal to the cassette, resulting in an axillary view with magnification (Fig. 14.8).

■ Special views:

  □ **West Point axillary:** This is taken with patient prone with the beam directed cephalad to the axilla 25 degrees from the horizontal and 25 degrees medial. It provides a tangential view of the anteroinferior glenoid rim (Fig. 14.9).

  □ **Hill-Sachs view:** This AP radiograph is taken with the shoulder in maximal internal rotation to visualize a posterolateral defect.

  □ **Stryker notch view:** The patient is supine with the ipsilateral palm on the crown of the head and the elbow pointing straight

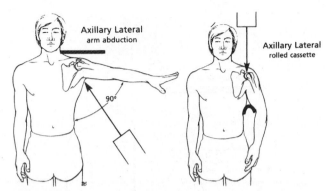

FIGURE 14.7 **(A)** The axillary lateral x-ray view. Ideally, the arm is abducted 70 to 90 degrees and the beam is directed superiorly up to the x-ray cassette. **(B)** When the patient cannot fully abduct the arm, a curved cassette can be placed in the axilla and the beam can be directed inferiorly through the glenohumeral joint onto the cassette. (From Rockwood CA, Szalay EA, Curtis RJ, et al., X-ray evaluation of shoulder problems. In: Rockwood CA, Matsen FA III, eds. *The Shoulder.* Philadelphia: WB Saunders; 1990:119–225.)

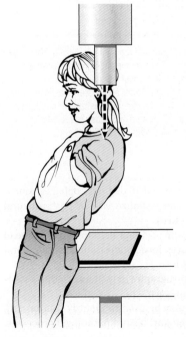

FIGURE 14.8 Positioning of the patient for the Velpeau axillary lateral view x-ray. (Modified from Bloom MH, Obata WG. Diagnosis of posterior dislocation of the shoulder with use of Velpeau axillary and angle-up roentgenographic views. *J Bone Joint Surg Am.* 1967;49:943–949.)

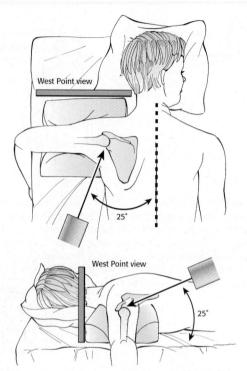

FIGURE 14.9 West Point view for the identification of a glenoid rim lesion. This x-ray is taken with the patient in the prone position. The beam is angled approximately 25 degrees **(A)** to provide a tangential view of the glenoid. In addition, the beam is angled 25 degrees downward **(B)** to highlight the anterior and posterior aspects of the glenoid. In this fashion, the entire glenoid rim can be clearly visualized. (From Bucholz RW, Heckman JD, Court-Brown C, et al., eds. *Rockwood and Green's Fractures in Adults.* 6th ed. Philadelphia: Lippincott Williams & Wilkins; 2006.)

upward. The x-ray beam is directed 10 degrees cephalad, aimed at the coracoid. This view can visualize 90% of posterolateral humeral head defects (Fig. 14.10).

   □ Computed tomography may be useful in defining humeral head or glenoid impression fractures, loose bodies, and anterior labral bony injuries (bony Bankart lesion).
   ■ Single- or double-contrast arthrography may be utilized to evaluate rotator cuff pathologic processes.
   ■ Magnetic resonance imaging may be used to identify rotator cuff, capsular, and glenoid labral (Bankart lesion) pathologic processes.

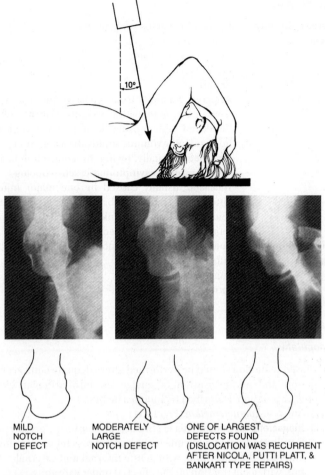

MILD
NOTCH
DEFECT

MODERATELY
LARGE
NOTCH DEFECT

ONE OF LARGEST
DEFECTS FOUND
(DISLOCATION WAS RECURRENT
AFTER NICOLA, PUTTI PLATT, &
BANKART TYPE REPAIRS)

FIGURE 14.10 (A) The position of the patient for the Stryker notch view. The patient is supine with the cassette posterior to the shoulder. The humerus is flexed approximately 120 degrees so the hand can be placed on top of the patient's head. Note that the angle of the x-ray tube is 10 degrees superior. **(B)** Defects in the posterolateral aspect of the humeral head are seen in three different patients with recurring anterior dislocations of the shoulder. (Modified from Hall RH, Isaac F, Booth CR. Dislocation of the shoulder with special reference to accompanying small fractures. *J Bone Joint Surg.* 1959;41:489–494.)

Classification

Degree of stability: Dislocation versus subluxation

Chronology: Congenital

Acute versus chronic

Locked (fixed)

Recurrent

Acquired: generally from repeated minor injuries (swimming, gymnastics, weights); labrum often intact but with capsular laxity; increased glenohumeral joint volume; subluxation common

Force: **Atraumatic:** usually owing to congenital laxity; noninjury; often asymptomatic; self-reducing

Traumatic: usually caused by one major injury; anterior or inferior labrum may be detached (Bankart lesion); unidirectional; generally requires assistance for reduction

Patient contribution: Voluntary versus involuntary

Direction: Subcoracoid

Subglenoid

Intrathoracic

Treatment

Nonoperative

- Closed reduction should be performed after adequate clinical evaluation and administration of analgesics, intra-articular block and/or sedation. Described techniques include
  - □ *Traction-countertraction* (Fig. 14.11)
  - □ **Hippocratic technique:** This is effective with only one person performing reduction, with one foot placed across the axillary folds and onto the chest wall, with gentle internal and external rotation with axial traction on the affected upper extremity.
  - □ **Stimson technique:** After administration of analgesics and/or sedatives, the patient is placed prone on the stretcher with the affected upper extremity hanging free. Gentle, manual traction or 5 lb of weight is applied to the wrist, with reduction effected over 15 to 20 minutes (Fig. 14.12).
  - □ **Milch technique:** With the patient supine and the upper extremity abducted and externally rotated, thumb pressure is applied by the physician to push the humeral head into place.
  - □ **Kocher maneuver:** The humeral head is levered on the anterior glenoid to effect reduction; this is not recommended because of increased risk of fracture.

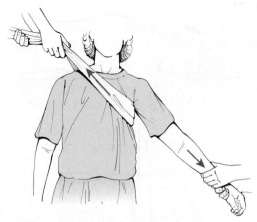

FIGURE 14.11 Closed reduction of the left shoulder with traction against countertraction. (From Bucholz RW, Heckman JD, Court-Brown C, et al., eds. *Rockwood and Green's Fractures in Adults.* 6th ed. Philadelphia: Lippincott Williams & Wilkins; 2006.)

- Postreduction care includes immobilization for 2 to 5 weeks. A shorter period of immobilization may be used for patients older than 40 years of age because stiffness of the ipsilateral hand, wrist, elbow, and shoulder tends to complicate treatment. Younger patients with a history of recurrent dislocation may require longer periods of immobilization.
- In comparison to a simple sling, immobilization in a Velpeau dressing does not appear to alter the subsequent development of recurrent instability.
- Therapy should be instituted following immobilization, including increasing degrees of shoulder external rotation, flexion, and abduction as time progresses, accompanied by full, active range of motion to the hand, wrist, and elbow.
- Irreducible acute anterior dislocation (rare) is usually the result of interposed soft tissue and requires open reduction.

Operative

- Indications for surgery include
  - Soft tissue interposition
  - Displaced greater tuberosity fracture that remains >5 mm superiorly displaced following joint reduction

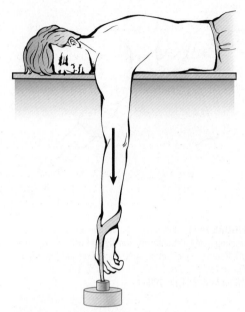

FIGURE 14.12 The Stimson technique for closed shoulder reduction. With the patient in prone position, a weight is hung from the wrist to distract the shoulder joint. Eventually, with sufficient fatigue in the shoulder musculature, the joint can be easily reduced. (From Bucholz RW, Heckman JD, Court-Brown C, et al., eds. *Rockwood and Green's Fractures in Adults.* 6th ed. Philadelphia: Lippincott Williams & Wilkins; 2006.)

- ☐ Glenoid rim fracture >5 mm in size
- ☐ Selective repair in the acute period (e.g., in young athletes)
- Surgical options for stabilization include arthroscopic ligamentous repair of the anterior labrum. Procedures such as capsular shift, capsulorrhaphy, muscle or tendon transfers, and bony transfers are reserved for refractory cases.
- Postoperative management typically includes the use of a shoulder immobilizer for up to 3 weeks in patients <30 years, 2 weeks for patients 30 to 40 years, and 1 to 2 weeks for patients >50 years of age, depending on the type of surgical stabilization. Patients are allowed to remove the immobilizer two to four times per day for shoulder, wrist, and hand range-of-motion exercises. Therapy is aimed at active and passive range of motion and regaining upper extremity strength.

Complications

- **Recurrent anterior dislocation:** related to ligament and capsular changes.
  - ☐ The most common complication after dislocation is recurrent dislocation
  - ☐ **Incidence:**
    - **Age 20 years:** 80% to 92% (lower in nonathletes)
    - **Age 30 years:** 60%
    - **Age 40 years:** 10% to 15%
  - ☐ Most recurrences occur within the first 2 years and tend to occur in men.
  - ☐ Prognosis is most affected by age at the time of initial dislocation.
  - ☐ Incidence is unrelated to the type or length of immobilization.
  - ☐ Patient activity has been identified as an independent factor for developing recurrent instability.
- **Osseous lesions:**
  - ☐ Hill-Sachs lesion
  - ☐ Glenoid lip fracture ("bony Bankart lesion")
  - ☐ Greater tuberosity fracture
  - ☐ Fracture of acromion or coracoid
  - ☐ Posttraumatic degenerative changes
- **Soft tissue injuries:**
  - ☐ Rotator cuff tear (older patients)
  - ☐ Capsular or subscapularis tendon tears
- **Vascular injuries:** These typically occur in elderly patients with atherosclerosis and usually involve the axillary artery. They may occur at the time of open or closed reduction.
- **Nerve injuries:** These involve most commonly the musculocutaneous and axillary nerves, usually in elderly individuals; neurapraxia almost always recovers, but if it persists beyond 3 months, it requires further evaluation with possible exploration.

POSTERIOR GLENOHUMERAL DISLOCATION

Incidence

- These injuries represent 10% of shoulder dislocations and 2% of shoulder injuries.
- They are often unrecognized by primary care and emergency physicians, with 60% to 80% missed on initial examination.

Mechanism of Injury

- **Indirect trauma:** This is the most common mechanism.
  - ☐ The shoulder typically is in the position of adduction, flexion, and internal rotation.

- ☐ Electric shock or convulsive mechanisms may produce posterior dislocations owing to the greater muscular force of the internal rotators (latissimus dorsi, pectoralis major, and subscapularis muscles) compared with the external rotators of the shoulder (infraspinatus and teres minor muscles).
- ■ **Direct trauma:** This results from force application to the anterior shoulder, resulting in posterior translation of the humeral head.

Clinical Evaluation

- ■ Clinically, a posterior glenohumeral dislocation does not present with striking deformity; the injured upper extremity is typically held in the traditional sling position of shoulder internal rotation and adduction. These injuries may be missed if a complete radiographic series is not obtained.
- ■ A careful neurovascular examination is important to rule out axillary nerve injury, although it is much less common than with anterior glenohumeral dislocation.
- ■ On examination, limited external rotation (often <0 degrees) and limited anterior forward elevation (often <90 degrees) may be appreciated.
- ■ A palpable mass posterior to the shoulder, flattening of the anterior shoulder, and coracoid prominence may be observed.

Radiographic Evaluation

- ■ **Trauma series of the affected shoulder:** AP, scapular-Y, and axillary views. A Velpeau axillary view (see earlier) may be obtained if the patient is unable to position the shoulder for a standard axillary view.
- ■ On a standard AP view of the shoulder, signs suggestive of a posterior glenohumeral dislocation include
  - ☐ Absence of the normal elliptic overlap of the humeral head on the glenoid.
  - ☐ **Vacant glenoid sign:** The glenoid appears partially vacant (space between anterior rim and humeral head >6 mm).
  - ☐ **Trough sign:** impaction fracture of the anterior humeral head caused by the posterior rim of glenoid (reverse Hill-Sachs lesion). This is reported to be present in 75% of cases.
  - ☐ **Loss of profile of neck of humerus:** The humerus is in full internal rotation.
  - ☐ Void in the superior/inferior glenoid fossa, owing to inferosuperior displacement of the dislocated humeral head.

- Glenohumeral dislocations are most readily recognized on the axillary view; this view may also demonstrate the reverse Hill-Sachs defect.
- Computed tomography scans are valuable in assessing the percentage of the humeral head involved with an impaction fracture.

Classification

Etiologic Classification

Traumatic: Sprain, subluxation, dislocation, recurrent, fixed (unreduced)

Atraumatic: Voluntary, congenital, acquired (due to repeated microtrauma)

Anatomic Classification

Subacromial (98%): Articular surface directed posteriorly with no gross displacement of the humeral head as in anterior dislocation; lesser tuberosity typically occupies glenoid fossa; often associated with an impaction fracture on the anterior humeral head

Subglenoid (very rare): Humeral head posterior and inferior to the glenoid

Subspinous (very rare): Humeral head medial to the acromion and inferior to the spine of the scapula

Treatment

Nonoperative

- Closed reduction requires full muscle relaxation, sedation, and analgesia.
  - □ The pain from an acute, traumatic posterior glenohumeral dislocation is usually greater than that with an anterior dislocation and may require general anesthesia for reduction.
  - □ With the patient supine, traction should be applied to the adducted arm in the line of deformity with gentle lifting of the humeral head into the glenoid fossa.
  - □ The shoulder should not be forced into external rotation, because this may result in a humeral head fracture if an impaction fracture is locked on the posterior glenoid rim.
  - □ If prereduction radiographs demonstrate an impaction fracture locked on the glenoid rim, axial traction should be accompanied by lateral traction on the upper arm to unlock the humeral head.

- Postreduction care should consist of a sling and swathe if the shoulder is stable. If the shoulder subluxes or redislocates in the sling and swathe, a shoulder spica should be placed with the amount of external rotation determined by the position of stability. Immobilization is continued for 3 to 6 weeks, depending on the age of the patient and the stability of the shoulder.
  - □ With a large anteromedial head defect, better stability may be achieved with immobilization in external rotation.
  - □ External rotation and deltoid isometric exercises may be performed during the period of immobilization.
  - □ After discontinuation of immobilization, an aggressive internal and external rotator strengthening program is instituted.

Operative

- Indications for surgery include
  - □ Major displacement of an associated lesser tuberosity fracture
  - □ A large posterior glenoid fragment
  - □ Irreducible dislocation or an impaction fracture on the posterior glenoid preventing reduction
  - □ Open dislocation
  - □ An anteromedial humeral impaction fracture (reverse Hill-Sachs lesion)
  - □ **Twenty to 40% humeral head involvement:** transfer the lesser tuberosity with attached subscapularis into the defect (modified McLaughlin procedure)
  - □ **Greater than 40% humeral head involvement:** hemiarthroplasty with neutral version of the prosthesis
- Surgical options include open reduction, infraspinatus muscle/tendon plication (reverse Putti-Platt procedure), long head of the biceps tendon transfer to the posterior glenoid margin (Boyd-Sisk procedure), humeral and glenoid osteotomies, and capsulorraphy.
- Voluntary dislocators should be treated nonoperatively, with counseling and strengthening exercises.

Complications

- **Fractures:** These include fractures of the posterior glenoid rim, humeral shaft, lesser and greater tuberosities, and humeral head.
- **Recurrent dislocation:** The incidence is increased with atraumatic posterior glenohumeral dislocations, large anteromedial humeral head defects resulting from impaction fractures on the glenoid rim, and large posterior glenoid rim fractures. They may require surgical stabilization to prevent recurrence.

- **Neurovascular injury:** This is much less common in posterior versus anterior dislocation, but it may include injury to the axillary nerve as it exits the quadrangular space or to the nerve to the infraspinatus (branch of the suprascapular nerve) as it traverses the spinoglenoid notch.
- **Anterior subluxation:** This may result from "overtightening" posterior structures, forcing the humeral head anteriorly. It may cause limited flexion, adduction, and internal rotation.

INFERIOR GLENOHUMERAL DISLOCATION (LUXATIO ERECTA)

- This very rare injury is more common in elderly individuals.

Mechanism of Injury (Fig. 14.13)

- It results from a hyperabduction force causing impingement of the neck of the humerus on the acromion, which levers the humeral head out inferiorly.
- The superior aspect of articular surface is directed inferiorly and is not in contact with the inferior glenoid rim. The humeral shaft is directed superiorly.
- Rotator cuff avulsion and tear, pectoralis injury, proximal humeral fracture, and injury to the axillary artery or brachial plexus are common.

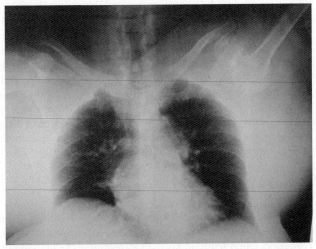

FIGURE 14.13 Locked inferior dislocation of the glenohumeral joint, also known as *luxatio erectae.*

Clinical Evaluation

- Patients typically present in a characteristic "salute" fashion, with the humerus locked in 110 to 160 degrees of abduction and forward elevation. Pain is usually severe.
- The humeral head is typically palpable on the lateral chest wall and axilla.
- A careful neurovascular examination is essential, because neurovascular compromise almost always complicates these dislocations.

Radiographic Evaluation

- **Shoulder trauma series:** AP, scapular-Y, and axillary views are taken.
- The AP radiograph is typically diagnostic, with inferior dislocation of the humeral head and superior direction of the humeral shaft along the glenoid margin.
- The radiograph must be carefully scrutinized for associated fractures, which are common and may be clinically not detected because of a diffusely painful shoulder.

Treatment

Nonoperative

- Reduction may be accomplished by the use of traction–countertraction maneuvers.
- Axial traction should be performed in line with the humeral position (superolaterally), with a gradual decrease in shoulder abduction. Countertraction should be applied with a sheet around the patient, in line with, but opposite to the traction vector.
- The arm should be immobilized in a sling for 3 to 6 weeks, depending on the age of the patient. Older individuals may be immobilized for shorter periods to minimize shoulder stiffness.

Operative

- Occasionally, the dislocated humeral head "buttonholes" through the inferior capsule and soft tissue envelope, preventing closed reduction. Open reduction is then indicated with enlarging of the capsular defect and repair of the damaged structures.

Complications

- **Neurovascular compromise:** This complicates nearly all cases of infe-rior glenohumeral dislocation, but it usually recovers following reduction.

SUPERIOR GLENOHUMERAL DISLOCATION

- This very rare injury is less common than inferior glenohumeral dislocation.

Mechanism of Injury

- Extreme anterior and superior directed force applied to the ad-ducted upper extremity, such as a fall from a height onto the upper extremity, forces the humeral head superiorly from the glenoid fossa.
- It is associated with fractures of the acromion, clavicle, coracoid, and humeral tuberosities, as well as injury to the acromioclavicu-lar joint.
- Typically it is accompanied by soft tissue injury to the rotator cuff, glenohumeral capsule, biceps tendon, and surrounding musculature.

Clinical Evaluation

- The patient typically presents with a foreshortened upper extrem-ity held in adduction.
- Clinical examination typically reveals a palpable humeral head above the level of the acromion.
- Neurovascular injuries are common and must be ruled out.

Radiographic Evaluation

- **Trauma series of the affected shoulder:** AP, scapular-Y, and axillary views are obtained.
- The AP radiograph is typically diagnostic, with dislocation of the humeral head superior to the acromion process.
- The radiograph must be carefully scrutinized for associated frac-tures, which are common and may be clinically not detected because of a diffusely painful shoulder.

Treatment

- Closed reduction should be attempted with the use of analgesics and sedatives.

- Axial traction with countertraction may be applied in an inferior direction, with lateral traction applied to the upper arm to facilitate reduction.
- As with inferior dislocations, soft tissue injury and associated fractures are common; irreducible dislocations may require open reduction.

Complications

- Neurovascular complications are usually present and typically represent traction injuries that resolve with reduction.

15

Proximal Humerus Fractures

EPIDEMIOLOGY

- Proximal humerus fractures comprise 4% to 5% of all fractures and represent the most common humerus fracture (45%).
- The increased incidence in the older population is related to osteoporosis.
  - Three hundred thousand per year (more common than hip fracture).
  - Eighty-five percent are nondisplaced.
- The 2:1 female-to-male ratio is likely related to issues of bone density as well.

ANATOMY

- The shoulder has the greatest range of motion of any articulation in the body; this is due to the shallow glenoid fossa that is only 25% of the size of the humeral head and the fact that the major contributor to stability is not bone, but a soft tissue envelope composed of muscle, capsule, and ligaments.
- The proximal humerus is retroverted 35 to 40 degrees relative to the epicondylar axis.
- The four osseous segments (Neer) (Fig. 15.1) are
  1. The humeral head
  2. The lesser tuberosity
  3. The greater tuberosity
  4. The humeral shaft
- **Deforming muscular forces on the osseous segments (Fig. 15.1):**
  1. The greater tuberosity is displaced superiorly and posteriorly by the supraspinatus and external rotators.
  2. The lesser tuberosity is displaced medially by the pull of the subscapularis.
  3. The humeral shaft is displaced medially by the pectoralis major.
  4. The deltoid insertion causes abduction of the proximal fragment.
- **Neurovascular supply:**
  1. The major blood supply is from the anterior and posterior humeral circumflex arteries.

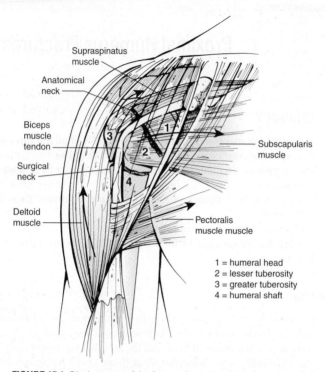

FIGURE 15.1 Displacement of the fracture fragments depends on the pull of the muscles of the rotator cuff and the pectoralis major. (From Bucholz RW, Heckman JD, Court-Brown C, et al., eds. *Rockwood and Green's Fractures in Adults.* 6th ed. Philadelphia: Lippincott Williams & Wilkins; 2006.)

2. The arcuate artery is a continuation of the ascending branch of the anterior humeral circumflex. It enters the bicipital groove and supplies most of the humeral head. Small contributions to the humeral head blood supply arise from the posterior humeral circumflex, reaching the humeral head via tendo-osseous anastomoses through the rotator cuff. Fractures of the anatomic neck are uncommon, but they tend to have a poor prognosis because of the precarious vascular supply to the humeral head.

3. The axillary nerve courses just anteroinferior to the glenohumeral joint, traversing the quadrangular space. It is at particular risk for traction injury owing to its relative rigid fixation at the posterior cord and deltoid, as well as its proximity to the inferior capsule where it is susceptible to injury during anterior dislocation and anterior fracture-dislocation.

MECHANISM OF INJURY

- Most common is a fall onto an outstretched upper extremity from a standing height, typically in an older, osteoporotic woman.
- Younger patients typically present with proximal humeral fractures following high-energy trauma, such as a motor vehicle accident. These usually represent more severe fractures and dislocations, with significant associated soft tissue disruption and multiple injuries.
- Less common mechanisms include
  1. Excessive shoulder abduction in an individual with osteoporosis, in which the greater tuberosity prevents further rotation
  2. Direct trauma, usually associated with greater tuberosity fractures
  3. Electrical shock or seizure
  4. **Pathologic processes:** malignant or benign processes in the proximal humerus

CLINICAL EVALUATION

- Patients typically present with the upper extremity held closely to the chest by the contralateral hand, with pain, swelling, tenderness, painful range of motion, and variable crepitus.
- Ecchymosis about the proximal humerus may not be apparent immediately after injury. Chest wall and flank ecchymosis may be present and should be differentiated from thoracic injury.
- A careful neurovascular examination is essential, with particular attention to axillary nerve function. This may be assessed by the presence of sensation on the lateral aspect of the proximal arm overlying the deltoid. Motor testing is usually not possible at this stage because of pain. Inferior translation of the distal fragment may result from deltoid atony and is not a true glenohumeral dislocation; this usually resolves by 4 weeks after fracture, but if it persists, it may represent a true axillary nerve injury.

RADIOGRAPHIC EVALUATION

- Refer back to Figs 14.6–14.8. Those are the Standard shoulder views.

CLASSIFICATION

Neer (Fig. 15.2)

- **Four parts:** These are the greater and lesser tuberosities, humeral shaft, and humeral head.

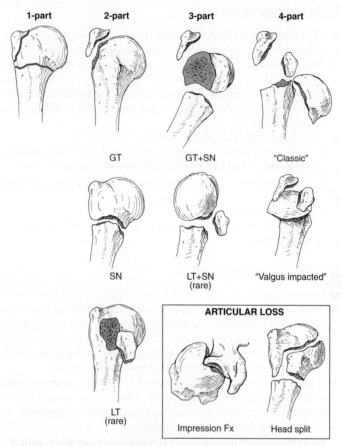

FIGURE 15.2 The Neer classification of proximal humerus fractures. (Reprinted with permission from Neer CS. Displaced proximal humeral fractures: I. Classification and evaluation. *J Bone Joint Surg Am.* 1970;52:1077–1089.)

- A part is defined as displaced if >1 cm of fracture displacement or >45 degrees of angulation.
- Fracture types include
  - **One-part fractures:** no displaced fragments regardless of number of fracture lines
  - **Two-part fractures (any of the following):**
    - Anatomic neck

- Surgical neck
- Greater tuberosity
- Lesser tuberosity
□ **Three-part fractures:**
  - Surgical neck with greater tuberosity
  - Surgical neck with lesser tuberosity
□ Four-part fractures
□ Fracture-dislocation
□ Articular surface fracture

OTA Classification of Proximal Humerus Fractures

See Fracture and Dislocation Classification Compendium at http://www.ota.org/compendium/compendium.html.

TREATMENT

- Minimally displaced fractures (one-part)
  □ Up to 85% of proximal humerus fractures are minimally displaced or nondisplaced.
  □ Sling immobilization or swathe for comfort.
  □ Frequent radiographic follow-up is important to detect loss of fracture reduction.
  □ Early shoulder motion may be instituted at 7 to 10 days if the patient has a stable or impacted fracture.
  □ Pendulum exercises are instructed initially followed by passive range-of-motion exercises.
  □ Six weeks post injury, active range-of-motion exercises are usually started.
  □ Resistive exercises are started anywhere from 6 to 12 weeks.
  □ Return to near full range of motion and function is the expected outcome by one year.
- Two-part fractures
  □ **Anatomic neck fractures:** These are rare and difficult to treat by closed reduction. They require open reduction and internal fixation (ORIF) (younger patients) or prosthesis (e.g., shoulder hemiarthroplasty) and have been historically associated with a high incidence of osteonecrosis.
  □ Surgical neck fractures
    - If the fracture is reducible and the patient has good-quality bone, one can consider fixation with percutaneously inserted terminally threaded pins or cannulated screws.

Problems associated with multiple pin fixation include nerve injury (axillary), pin loosening, pin migration, and inability to move the arm.

- Irreducible fractures (usually interposed soft tissue) and fractures in osteopenic bone require ORIF with anyone of a variety of implants.

□ **Greater tuberosity fractures:** If they are displaced more than 5 to 10 mm (5 mm for superior translation), they require ORIF with or without rotator cuff repair; otherwise, they may develop nonunion and subacromial impingement. A greater tuberosity fracture associated with anterior dislocation may reduce on reduction of the glenohumeral joint and be treated nonoperatively. Isolated greater tuberosity fractures can be approached through a superior deltoid split.

□ **Lesser tuberosity fractures:** They may be treated closed unless displaced fragment blocks internal rotation; one must rule out associated posterior dislocation.

■ Three-part fractures

□ These are unstable due to opposing muscle forces; as a result, closed reduction and maintenance of reduction are often difficult.

□ Displaced fractures require operative fixation, except in severely debilitated patients or those who cannot tolerate surgery.

□ Younger individuals should have an attempt at ORIF; preservation of the vascular supply is of paramount importance with minimization of soft tissue devascularization.

□ The delto-pectoral approach is the workhorse of the shoulder and allows for an extensile approach to the proximal humerus. ORIF or arthroplasty is well performed through this approach (Fig. 15.3).

□ The advance of locking plate technology has led to enhanced fixation in osteoporotic bone and thus improved outcomes in the more recent literature. Older patients may benefit from primary prosthetic replacement (hemiarthroplasty).

■ Four-part fractures

□ Incidence of osteonecrosis ranges from 4% to 35%.

□ ORIF may be attempted in patients if the humeral head is located within the glenoid fossa and there appears to be soft tissue continuity. Fixation is best achieved with locking plate and screw fixation, suture, and/or wire fixation.

□ Primary prosthetic replacement of the humeral head (hemiarthroplasty) is a secondary option in the elderly.

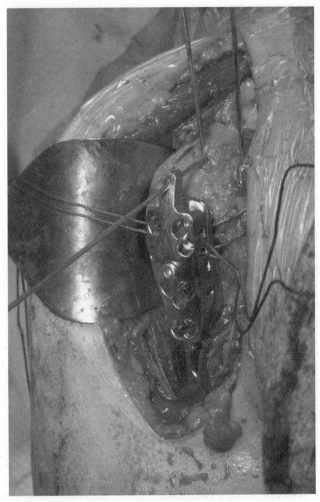

FIGURE 15.3 Right shoulder delto-pectoral approach demonstrating access to the proximal humers. Locking plate applied with rotator cuff sutures passed for enhanced fixation.

- • Hemiarthroplasty is associated with predictable pain relief, but unpredictable results from the standpoint of function.
- ☐ Four-part valgus-impacted proximal humerus fractures represent variants that are associated with lower rate of osteonecrosis and have excellent results with ORIF (Fig. 15.3).

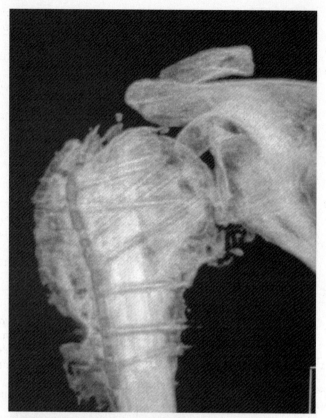

FIGURE 15.4 3D CT Scan depicting heterotopic ossification following fracture dislocation of the shoulder.

■ Fracture-dislocations
  □ **Two-part fracture-dislocations:** These may be treated closed after shoulder reduction unless the fracture fragments remain displaced.
  □ **Three- and four-part fracture-dislocations:** ORIF is used in younger individuals and hemiarthroplasty in the elderly, depending on the length of dislocation. The brachial plexus and axillary artery are in proximity to the humeral head fragment with anterior fracture-dislocations.
  □ Recurrent dislocation is rare following fracture union.

- □ Hemiarthroplasty for anatomic neck fracture-dislocation is recommended because of the high incidence of osteonecrosis.
- □ These injuries may be associated with increased incidence of myositis ossificans with repeated attempts at closed reduction.
- ■ Articular surface fractures (Hill-Sachs, reverse Hill-Sachs)
  - □ These are most often associated with posterior dislocations.
  - □ Patients with >40% of humeral head involvement may require hemiarthroplasty; ORIF should initially be considered in patients <40 years of age, if possible.

COMPLICATIONS

- ■ **Vascular injury:** This is infrequent (5% to 6%); the axillary artery is the most common site (proximal to anterior circumflex artery). The incidence is increased in older individuals with atherosclerosis because of the loss of vessel wall elasticity. There is a rich collateral circulation about the shoulder, which could mask vascular injury.
- ■ Neural injury
  - □ **Brachial plexus injury:** This is infrequent (6%).
  - □ **Axillary nerve injury:** This is particularly vulnerable with anterior fracture-dislocation because the nerve courses on the inferior capsule and is prone to traction injury or laceration. Complete axillary nerve injuries that do not improve within 2 to 3 months may require electromyographic evaluation and exploration.
- ■ **Chest injury:** Intrathoracic dislocation may occur with surgical neck fracture-dislocations; pneumothorax and hemothorax must be ruled out in the appropriate clinical setting.
- ■ **Myositis ossificans:** This is uncommon and is associated with chronic unreduced fracture-dislocations and repeated attempts at closed reduction. It may also be related to timing of surgery and deltoid split approaches (Fig. 15.4).
- ■ **Shoulder stiffness:** It may be minimized with an aggressive, supervised physical therapy regimen and may require open lysis of adhesions for recalcitrant cases.
- ■ **Osteonecrosis:** This may complicate 3% to 14% of three-part proximal humeral fractures, 4% to 34% of four-part fractures, and a high rate of anatomic neck fractures.
- ■ **Nonunion:** This occurs particularly in displaced two-part surgical neck fractures with soft tissue interposition. Other causes include excessive traction, severe fracture displacement, systemic disease,

poor bone quality, inadequate fixation, and infection. It may be addressed with ORIF with or without bone graft or prosthetic replacement.

■ **Malunion:** This occurs after inadequate closed reduction or failed ORIF and may result in impingement of the greater tuberosity on the acromion, with subsequent restriction of shoulder motion.

16 Humeral Shaft Fractures

EPIDEMIOLOGY

- A common injury, representing 3% to 5% of all fractures.
- Incidence is 14.5 per 100,000 per year.
- Two percent to 10% are open fractures.
- Sixty percent involve middle third of the diaphysis, 30% involve proximal third of diaphysis, and 10% involve distal third of diaphysis.
- Bimodal age distribution with a peak in the third decade is seen in males and peak in the seventh decade is seen in females.

ANATOMY

- The humeral shaft extends from the pectoralis major insertion to the supracondylar ridge. In this interval, the cross-sectional shape changes from cylindric to narrow in the anteroposterior direction.
- The vascular supply to the humeral diaphysis arises from perforating branches of the brachial artery, with the main nutrient artery entering the medial humerus distal to the midshaft (Fig. 16.1).
- The musculotendinous attachments of the humerus result in characteristic fracture displacements (Table 16.1).

MECHANISM OF INJURY

- **Direct (most common):** Direct trauma to the arm from a blow or motor vehicle accident results in transverse or comminuted fractures.
- **Indirect:** A fall on an outstretched arm or rotational injury results in spiral or oblique fractures, especially in elderly patients. Uncommonly, throwing injuries with extreme muscular contraction have been reported to cause humeral shaft fractures.
- **Fracture pattern depends on the type of force applied:**
  - □ **Compressive:** proximal or distal humeral fractures
  - □ **Bending:** transverse fractures of the humeral shaft
  - □ **Torsional:** spiral fractures of the humeral shaft
  - □ **Torsional and bending:** oblique fracture, often accompanied by a butterfly fragment

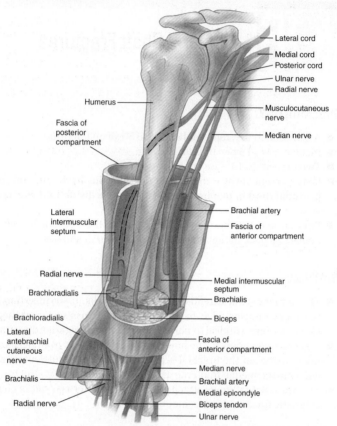

FIGURE 16.1 The neurovascular anatomy of the upper arm. (From Bucholz RW, Heckman JD, Court-Brown C, et al., eds. *Rockwood and Green's Fractures in Adults*. 6th ed. Philadelphia: Lippincott Williams & Wilkins; 2006.)

TABLE 16.1   Position of Fracture Fragments

Fracture Location	Proximal Fragment	Distal Fragment
Above pectoralis major insertion	Abducted, rotated externally by rotator cuff	Medial, proximal by deltoid and pectoralis major
Between pectoralis major and deltoid tuberosity	Medial by pectoralis, teres major, and latissimus dorsi	Lateral, proximal by deltoid
Distal to deltoid tuberosity	Abducted by deltoid	Medial, proximal by biceps and triceps

CLINICAL EVALUATION

■ Patients with humeral shaft fractures typically present with pain, swelling, deformity, and shortening of the affected arm.

■ A careful neurovascular examination is essential, with particular attention to radial nerve function. In cases of extreme swelling, serial neurovascular examinations are indicated with possible measurement of compartment pressures.

■ Physical examination frequently reveals gross instability with crepitus on gentle manipulation.

■ Soft tissue abrasions and minor lacerations must be differentiated from open fractures.

■ Intra-articular extensions of open fractures may be determined by intra-articular injection of saline distant from the wound site and noting extravasation of fluid from the wound.

RADIOGRAPHIC EVALUATION

■ AP and lateral radiographs of the humerus should be obtained, including the shoulder and elbow joints on each view. To obtain views at 90 degrees from each other, the patient, NOT the arm, should be rotated (transthoracic lateral), as manipulation of the injured extremity will typically result in distal fragment rotation only.

■ Traction radiographs may aid in fracture definition in cases of severely displaced or comminuted fracture patterns.

■ Computed tomography, bone scans, and MRI are rarely indicated except in cases in which pathologic fracture is suspected.

CLASSIFICATION

Descriptive

■ Open versus closed
■ **Location:** proximal third, middle third, distal third
■ **Degree:** nondisplaced, displaced
■ **Direction and character:** transverse, oblique, spiral, segmental, comminuted
■ Intrinsic condition of bone
■ Articular extension

OTA Classification

■ See Fracture and Dislocation Classification Compendium at http:// www.ota.org/ compendium/compendium.html.

TREATMENT

- The goal is to establish union with an acceptable humeral alignment and to restore the patient to preinjury level of function.
- Both patient and fracture characteristics, including patient age and functional level, presence of associated injuries, soft tissue status, and fracture pattern, need to be considered when selecting an appropriate treatment option.

NONOPERATIVE

- Nonoperative treatment requirements are
  - □ An understanding by the treating physician of the postural and muscular forces that must be controlled
  - □ Dedication to close patient supervision and follow-up
  - □ A cooperative and preferably upright and mobile patient
  - □ An acceptable reduction
- Most humeral shaft fractures (>90%) will heal with nonsurgical management.
- Twenty degrees of anterior angulation, 30 degrees of varus angulation, and up to 3 cm of bayonet apposition are acceptable and will not compromise function or appearance.
- **Hanging cast:** This utilizes dependency traction by the weight of the cast and arm to effect fracture reduction.
  - □ Indications include displaced midshaft humeral fractures with shortening, particularly spiral or oblique patterns. Transverse or short oblique fractures represent relative contraindications because of the potential for distraction and healing complications.
  - □ The patient must remain upright or semiupright at all times with the cast in a dependent position for effectiveness.
  - □ It may be exchanged for functional bracing following early callus formation.
  - □ More than 95% union is reported.
- **Coaptation splint:** This utilizes dependency traction and hydrostatic pressure to effect fracture reduction, but with greater stabilization and less distraction than a hanging arm cast. The forearm is suspended in a collar and cuff.
  - □ It is indicated for the acute treatment of humeral shaft fractures with minimal shortening and for short oblique or transverse fracture patterns that may displace with a hanging arm cast.
  - □ Disadvantages include irritation of the patient's axilla and the potential for splint slippage.
  - □ It is frequently exchanged for functional bracing 1 to 2 weeks after injury.

- **Thoracobrachial immobilization (Velpeau dressing):** This is used in elderly patients or children who are unable to tolerate other methods of treatment and in whom comfort is the primary concern.
  - □ It is indicated for minimally displaced or nondisplaced fractures that do not require reduction.
  - □ Passive shoulder pendulum exercises may be performed within 1 to 2 weeks after injury.
  - □ It may be exchanged for functional bracing 1 to 2 weeks after injury.
- **Shoulder spica cast:** This has limited application, because operative management is typically performed for the same indications.
  - □ It is indicated when the fracture pattern necessitates significant abduction and external rotation of the upper extremity.
  - □ Disadvantages include difficulty of cast application, cast weight and bulkiness, skin irritation, patient discomfort, and inconvenient upper extremity position.
- **Functional bracing:** This utilizes hydrostatic soft tissue compression to effect and maintain fracture alignment while allowing motion of adjacent joints.
  - □ It is typically applied 1 to 2 weeks after injury, after the patient has been placed in a hanging arm cast or coaptation splint and swelling has subsided.
  - □ It consists of an anterior and posterior (or medial-lateral) shell held together with Velcro straps.
  - □ Success depends on an upright patient and brace tightening daily.
  - □ Contraindications include massive soft tissue injury, an unreliable patient, and an inability to obtain or maintain acceptable fracture reduction.
  - □ A collar and cuff may be used to support the forearm, but sling application may result in varus angulation.
  - □ The functional brace is worn for a minimum of 8 weeks after fracture or until radiographic evidence of union.

Operative

- Indications for operative treatment are
  - □ Multiple trauma
  - □ Inadequate closed reduction or unacceptable malunion
  - □ Pathologic fracture
  - □ Associated vascular injury
  - □ "Floating elbow"
  - □ Segmental fracture
  - □ Intra-articular extension

- □ Bilateral humeral fractures
- □ Open fracture
- □ Neurologic loss following penetrating trauma
- □ Radial nerve palsy after fracture manipulation (controversial)
- □ Nonunion
- ■ Surgical approaches to the humeral shaft include
  1. **Anterolateral approach:** preferred for proximal third humeral shaft fractures; radial nerve identified in the interval between the brachialis and brachioradialis and traced proximally. The brachialis muscle is split to afford access to the shaft. This can be extended proximally to the shoulder or distally to the elbow.
  2. **Anterior approach:** muscular interval between the biceps and brachialis muscles.
  3. **Posterior approach:** provides excellent exposure to most of the humerus, but cannot be extended proximally to the shoulder; muscular interval between the lateral and long heads of the triceps. The medial head is split. The radial nerve must be identified in the spiral groove usually at the mid portion of the arm.

Surgical Techniques

Open Reduction and Plate Fixation

- ■ This is associated with the best functional results. It allows direct fracture reduction and stable fixation of the humeral shaft without violation of the rotator cuff.
- ■ Radiographs of the uninjured, contralateral humerus may be used for preoperative templating.
- ■ A 4.5-mm dynamic compression plate (large fragment) with fixation of six to eight cortices proximal and distal to the fracture is typically used (Fig. 16.2).
- ■ Lag screws should be utilized wherever possible.
- ■ One should preserve soft tissue attachments to butterfly fragments.

Intramedullary Fixation

- ■ Indications include
  - □ Segmental fractures in which plate placement would require considerable soft tissue dissection
  - □ Humerus fractures in extremely osteopenic bone
  - □ Pathologic humerus fractures
- ■ It is associated with a high incidence of shoulder pain following antegrade humeral nailing.
- ■ **Two types of intramedullary nails are available for use in the humeral shaft:** flexible nails and interlocked nails.

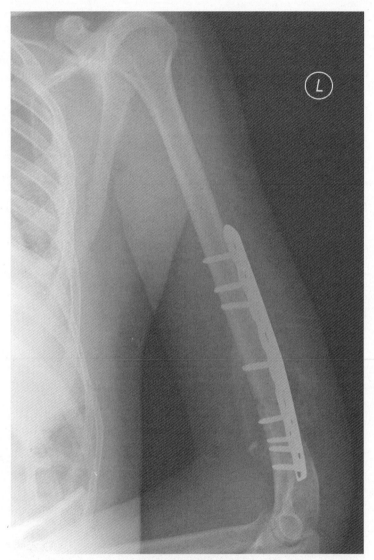

FIGURE 16.2 Plate and screw fixation of a distal third humeral shaft fracture.

■ Flexible nails
  □ **Rationale:** Fill the canal with multiple nails to achieve an interference fit.
  □ These nails have relatively poor stability.

- ☐ Use should be reserved for humeral shaft fractures with transverse patterns or minimal comminution.
- ■ Interlocked nails
  - ☐ These nails have proximal and distal interlocking capabilities and are able to provide rotational and axial fracture stability (Fig. 16.3).

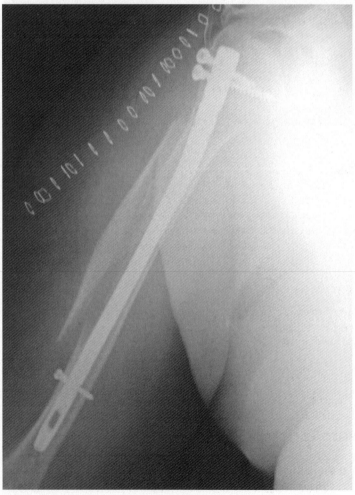

FIGURE 16.3 IM nail fixation of a humeral shaft fracture.

- ☐ With antegrade nailing, the axillary nerve is at risk for injury during proximal locking screw insertion. Screws protruding beyond the medial cortex may potentially impinge on the axillary nerve during internal rotation. Anterior to posterior screws are avoided because of the potential for injury to the main trunk of the axillary nerve.
- ☐ Distal locking usually consists of a single screw in the anteroposterior plane. Distal locking screw can be inserted anterior to posterior or posterior to anterior via an open technique to minimize the risk of neurovascular injury. Lateral to medial screws risk injury to lateral antebrachial cutaneous nerve and the radial nerve.
- ■ Either type of nails can be inserted through antegrade or retrograde techniques.
- ■ If antegrade technique is elected, most methods attempt to avoid the rotator cuff to minimize postoperative shoulder problems.
- ■ The proximal aspect of the nail should be countersunk to prevent subacromial impingement.

External Fixation (Fig. 16.4)
- ■ Indications include
  - ☐ Infected nonunions
  - ☐ Burn patients with fractures
  - ☐ Open fractures with extensive soft tissue loss
- ■ Complications include pin tract infection, neurovascular injury, and nonunion.

Postoperative Rehabilitation

Range-of-motion exercises for the hand and wrist should be started immediately after surgery; shoulder and elbow range of motion should be instituted as pain subsides.

COMPLICATIONS
- ■ Radial nerve injury occurs in up to 18% of cases.
  - ☐ It is most common with middle third fractures, although best known for its association with Holstein-Lewis type distal third fracture, which may entrap or lacerate the nerve as it passes through the intermuscular septum.
  - ☐ Most injuries are neurapraxias or axonotmesis; function will return within 3 to 4 months; laceration is more common in penetrating trauma.

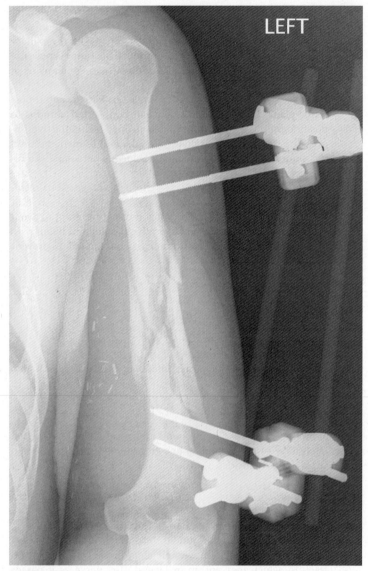

FIGURE 16.4 External fixation of a humeral shaft fracture sustained secondary to gunshot wound. Vascular repair followed this temporary bony stabilization.

□ With secondary palsies that occur during fracture reduction, it has not been clearly established that surgery will improve the ultimate recovery rate compared with nonsurgical management.

□ Delayed surgical exploration should be done after 3 to 4 months if there is no evidence of recovery by electromyography or nerve conduction velocity studies.

□ **Advantages of late over early nerve exploration:**
- Enough time will have passed for recovery from neurapraxia or neurotmesis.
- Precise evaluation of a nerve lesion is possible.
- The associated fracture may have united.
- The results of secondary nerve repair are as good as those of primary repair.

■ **Vascular injury:** This is uncommon but may be associated with fractures of the humeral shaft lacerating or impaling the brachial artery or with penetrating trauma.

□ The brachial artery has the greatest risk for injury in the proximal and distal third of arm.

□ It constitutes an orthopaedic emergency; arteriography is controversial because it may prolong time to definitive treatment for an ischemic limb.

□ Arterial inflow should be established within 6 hours.

□ At surgery, the vessel should be explored and repaired and the fracture should be stabilized.

□ If limb viability is not in jeopardy, bone repair may precede vascular repair.

□ External fixation should be considered an option.

■ Nonunion occurs in up to 15% of cases.

□ Risk factors include fracture at the proximal or distal third of the humerus, transverse fracture pattern, fracture distraction, soft tissue interposition, and inadequate immobilization.

□ It may necessitate open reduction and internal fixation with bone grafting.

■ **Malunion:** This may be functionally inconsequential; arm musculature and shoulder, elbow, and trunk range of motion can compensate for angular, rotational, and shortening deformities.

17 Distal Humerus

EPIDEMIOLOGY

- Fractures of the adult distal humerus are relatively uncommon, comprising approximately 2% of all fractures and one-third of all humerus fractures.
- Distal humerus fractures have a bimodal age distribution, with peak incidences occurring in males between the ages of 12 to 19 years and in females aged 80 years and older.
- In contrast, >60% of distal humerus fractures in the elderly occur from low-energy injuries, such as a fall from standing height.
- The incidence of distal humerus fractures in adults as being 5.7 per 100,000 per year.
- Intercondylar fractures of the distal humerus are the most common fracture pattern.
- Extension-type supracondylar fractures of the distal humerus account for >80% of all supracondylar fractures in adults.

ANATOMY

- The distal humerus may be conceptualized as medial and lateral "columns," each of which is roughly triangular and is composed of an *epicondyle*, or the nonarticulating terminal of the supracondylar ridge, and a *condyle*, which is the articulating unit of the distal humerus (Fig. 17.1).
- The articulating surface of the capitellum and trochlea projects distally and anteriorly at an angle of 40 to 45 degrees. The centers of the arcs of rotation of the articular surfaces of each condyle lie on the same horizontal axis; thus, malalignment of the relationships of the condyles to each other changes their arc of rotation, thus limiting flexion and extension (Fig. 17.2).
- The trochlear axis compared with the longitudinal axis is 4 to 8 degrees of valgus.
- The trochlear axis is 3 to 8 degrees externally rotated.
- The intramedullary canal ends 2 to 3 cm above the olecranon fossa.

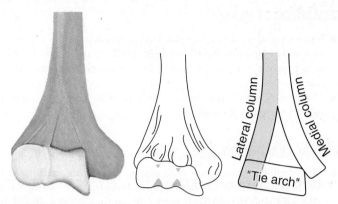

FIGURE 17.1 The distal most part of the lateral column is the capitellum, and the distal most part of the medial column is the nonarticular medial epicondyle. The trochlea is the medial most part of the articular segment and is intermediate in position between the medial epicondyle and capitellum. The articular segment functions architecturally as a "tie arch."

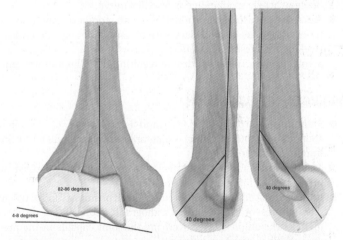

FIGURE 17.2 The joint surface to shaft axis is 4 to 8 degrees of valgus—the A-carrying angle **(A)**. The articular segment juts forward from the line of the shaft at 40 degrees and functions architecturally as the tie arch at the point of maximum column divergence distally. The medial epicondyle is on the projected axis of the shaft, whereas the lateral epicondyle is projected slightly forward from the axis **(B,C)**.

MECHANISM OF INJURY

- Most low-energy distal humeral fractures result from a simple fall in middle-aged and elderly women in which the elbow is either struck directly or axially loaded in a fall onto the outstretched hand.
- Motor vehicle and sporting accidents are more common causes of injury in younger individuals.

CLINICAL EVALUATION

- Signs and symptoms vary with degree of swelling and displacement; considerable swelling frequently occurs, rendering landmarks difficult to palpate. However, the normal relationship of the olecranon, medial, and lateral condyles should be maintained, roughly delineating an equilateral triangle.
- Crepitus with range of motion and gross instability may be present; although this is highly suggestive of fracture, no attempt should be made to elicit it because neurovascular compromise may result.
- A careful neurovascular evaluation is essential because the sharp, fractured end of the proximal fragment may impale or contuse the brachial artery, median nerve, or radial nerve.
- Serial neurovascular examinations with compartment pressure monitoring may be necessary with massive swelling; cubital fossa swelling may result in vascular impairment or the development of a volar compartment syndrome resulting in Volkmann ischemia.

RADIOGRAPHIC EVALUATION

- Standard anteroposterior (AP) and lateral views of the elbow should be obtained. Oblique radiographs may be helpful for further fracture definition.
- Traction radiographs may better delineate the fracture pattern and may be useful for preoperative planning.
- In nondisplaced fractures, an anterior or posterior "fat pad sign" may be present on the lateral radiograph, representing displacement of the adipose layer overlying the joint capsule in the presence of effusion or hemarthrosis.
- Minimally displaced fractures may result in a decrease in the normal condylar shaft angle of 40 degrees seen on the lateral radiograph.
- Because intercondylar fractures are much more common than supracondylar fractures in adults, the AP (or oblique) radiograph should be scrutinized for evidence of a vertical split in the intercondylar region of the distal humerus.

- Computed tomography may be utilized to delineate fracture fragments further.

CLASSIFICATION

Descriptive

- Supracondylar fractures
  - □ Extension-type
  - □ Flexion-type
- Transcondylar fractures
- Intercondylar fractures
- Condylar fractures
- Capitellum fractures
- Trochlea fractures
- Lateral epicondylar fractures
- Medial epicondylar fractures
- Fractures of the supracondylar process

OTA Classification of Fractures of the Distal Humerus

See Fracture and Dislocation Classification Compendium at http://www.ota.org/ compendium/compendium.html.

GENERAL TREATMENT PRINCIPLES

- Anatomic articular reduction
- Stable internal fixation of the articular surface
- Restoration of articular axial alignment
- Stable internal fixation of the articular segment to the metaphysis and diaphysis
- Early range of elbow motion

SPECIFIC FRACTURE TYPES

Extra-articular Supracondylar Fracture

- This results from a fall onto an outstretched hand with or without an abduction or adduction force.
- The majority are extension patterns with a minority being flexion types.

Treatment

Nonoperative

- This is indicated for nondisplaced or minimally displaced fractures, as well as for severely comminuted fractures in elderly patients with limited functional ability.

- Posterior long arm splint is placed in at least 90 degrees of elbow flexion if swelling and neurovascular status permit, with the forearm in neutral.
- Posterior splint immobilization is continued for 1 to 2 weeks, after which range-of-motion exercises are initiated in a hinged brace. The splint or brace may be discontinued after approximately 6 weeks, when radiographic evidence of healing is present.
- Frequent radiographic evaluation is necessary to detect loss of fracture reduction.

Operative
- Indications
  - ☐ Significantly displaced fractures
  - ☐ Vascular injury
  - ☐ Open fracture
  - ☐ Inability to maintain acceptable reduction
- **Open reduction and internal fixation:** Plate fixation is used on each column, either in parallel, set at 90 degrees or 180 degrees from one another. Plate fixation is the procedure of choice, because this allows for early range of elbow motion. Extra-articular fractures may be approached posteriorly by elevating up either side of the triceps or through a triceps-split approach.
- Total elbow replacement may be considered, but it is rarely indicated in elderly patients who otherwise are active with good preinjury function in whom a severely comminuted fracture of the distal humerus is deemed unreconstructable. The medial, triceps-sparing approach should be utilized, rather than an olecranon osteotomy, for exposure of the elbow joint.
- Range-of-motion exercises should be initiated as soon as the patient is able to tolerate therapy.

Complications

- **Volkmann ischemic contracture (rare):** This may result from unrecognized compartment syndrome with subsequent neurovascular compromise. A high index of suspicion accompanied by aggressive elevation and serial neurovascular examinations with or without compartment pressure monitoring must be maintained.
- **Loss of elbow range of motion:** generally the rule following any fracture about the elbow. Loss of extension due to callus formation in the olecranon fossa. Loss of flexion due to capsular contracture and/or H.O.
- Heterotopic bone formation may occur.

Transcondylar Fractures

- These occur primarily in elderly patients with osteopenic bone.

Mechanism of Injury

- Mechanisms that produce supracondylar fractures may also result in transcondylar fractures: a fall onto an outstretched hand with or without an abduction or adduction component or a force applied to a flexed elbow.

Treatment

Nonoperative

- This is indicated for nondisplaced or minimally displaced fractures or in elderly patients who are debilitated and functioning poorly.
- Range-of-motion exercises should be initiated as soon as the patient is able to tolerate therapy.

Operative

- Operative treatment should be undertaken for open fractures, unstable fractures, or displaced fractures.
- Open reduction and plate fixation are the preferred treatment. Precontoured locked plates should be utilized in order to enhance fixation in this usually osteopenic fracture pattern.
- Total elbow arthroplasty (semiconstrained) may be considered in the elderly patient with good preinjury functional status if fixation cannot be obtained.

Intercondylar Fractures

- This is the most common distal humeral fracture.
- Comminution is common.
- Fracture fragments are often displaced by unopposed muscle pull at the medial (flexor mass) and lateral (extensor mass) epicondyles, which rotate the articular surfaces.

Mechanism of Injury

- Force is directed against the posterior aspect of an elbow flexed >90 degrees, thus driving the ulna into the trochlea.

Riseborough and Radin

Type I:	Nondisplaced
Type II:	Slight displacement with no rotation between the condylar fragments

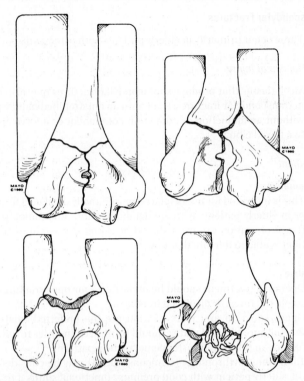

FIGURE 17.3 Riseborough and Radin classification. **(A)** Type I undisplaced condylar fracture of the elbow. **(B)** Type II displaced but not rotated T-condylar fracture. **(C)** Type III displaced and rotated T-condylar fracture. **(D)** Type IV displaced, rotated, and comminuted condylar fracture. (From Bryan RS. Fractures about the elbow in adults. *AAOS Instr Course Lect.* 1981;30:200–223.)

Type III: Displacement with rotation
Type IV: Severe comminution of the articular surface (Fig. 17.3)

Classification

OTA Classification
See Fracture and Dislocation Classification Compendium at http://www.ota.org/compendium/compendium.html.

Treatment

■ Treatment must be individualized according to patient age, bone quality, and degree of comminution.

Nonoperative
- This is indicated for nondisplaced fractures, elderly patients with displaced fractures and severe osteopenia and comminution, or patients with significant comorbid conditions precluding operative management. Nonoperative options for displaced fractures include
  - ☐ **Cast immobilization:** This has few advocates; it represents the "worst of both worlds"—inadequate fracture reduction and prolonged immobilization.
  - ☐ **"Bag of bones":** The arm is placed in a collar and cuff with as much flexion as possible after initial reduction is attempted; gravity traction helps effect reduction. The idea is to obtain a painless "pseudarthrosis," which allows for motion.

Operative
- Open reduction and internal fixation
  - ☐ The indication is a displaced reconstructible fracture.
  - ☐ Goals of fixation are to restore articular congruity and to secure the supracondylar component.
  - ☐ Methods of fixation
    - Interfragmentary screws
    - **Dual plate fixation:** one plate medially and another plate placed posterolaterally, 90 degrees from the medial plate or two plates on either column, 180 degrees from one another
- **Total elbow arthroplasty (cemented, semiconstrained):** This may be considered in markedly comminuted fractures and with fractures in osteoporotic bone.
- Surgical exposures
  - ☐ Tongue of triceps (Campbell's)
    - Does not allow full exposure of joint.
    - Deters early active motion for fear of triceps rupture.
  - ☐ **Olecranon osteotomy:** intra-articular; a chevron is best for rotational stability. It requires identification and mobilization of the ulnar nerve.
  - ☐ A triceps-sparing extensile posterior approach (Bryan and Morrey) may be used. It requires identification and mobilization of the ulnar nerve.
- **Postoperative care:** Early range of motion of the elbow is essential unless fixation is tenuous.

Complications

- **Posttraumatic arthritis:** This results from articular injury at time of trauma as well as a failure to restore articular congruity.

- **Failure of fixation:** Postoperative collapse of fixation is related to the degree of comminution, the stability of fixation, and protection of the construct during the postoperative course.
- **Loss of motion (extension):** This is increased with prolonged periods of immobilization. Range-of-motion exercises should be instituted as soon as the patient is able to tolerate therapy, unless fixation is tenuous.
- Heterotopic bone.
- **Neurologic injury:** (Up to 15%) The ulnar nerve is most commonly injured during surgical exposure.
- **Nonunion of osteotomy:** 5% to 15%.
- Infection.

Condylar Fractures

- These are rare in adults and are much more common in the pediatric age group.
- Less than 5% of all distal humerus fractures are condylar; lateral fractures are more common than medial.
- **Medial condyle fractures:** These include the trochlea and medial epicondyle and are less common than medial epicondylar fractures.
- **Lateral condyle fractures:** These include the capitellum and lateral epicondyle.

Mechanism of Injury

- Abduction or adduction of the forearm with elbow extension

Classification

Milch

Two types are designated for medial and lateral condylar fractures; the key is the lateral trochlear ridge (Fig. 17.4):

Type I: Lateral trochlear ridge left intact
Type II: Lateral trochlear ridge part of the condylar fragment (medial or lateral)
- These are less stable.
- They may allow for radioulnar translocation if capsuloligamentous disruption occurs on the contralateral side.

Jupiter

This is low or high, based on proximal extension of fracture line to supracondylar region.

OTA Classification

See Fracture and Dislocation Classification Compendium at http://www.ota.org/ compendium/compendium.html.

- **Low:** equivalent to Milch type I fracture
- **High:** equivalent to Milch type II fracture

Treatment

- Anatomic restoration of articular congruity is essential to maintain the normal elbow arc of motion and to minimize the risk of posttraumatic arthritis.

Nonoperative

- Indicated for nondisplaced or minimally displaced fractures or for patients with displaced fractures who are not considered candidates for operative treatment.
- It consists of posterior splinting with the elbow flexed to 90 degrees and the forearm in supination or pronation for lateral or medial condylar fractures, respectively.

Operative

- Indicated for open or displaced fractures.
- Consists of screw fixation with or without collateral ligament repair if necessary, with attention to restoration of the rotational axes.
- Prognosis depends on
  - □ The degree of comminution
  - □ The accuracy of reduction
  - □ The stability of internal fixation
- Range-of-motion exercises should be instituted as soon as the patient can tolerate therapy.

Complications

- **Lateral condyle fractures:** Improper reduction or failure of fixation may result in cubitus valgus and tardy ulnar nerve palsy requiring nerve transposition.
- **Medial condyle fractures:** Residual incongruity is more problematic owing to involvement of the trochlear groove. These may result in
  - □ Posttraumatic arthritis, especially with fractures involving the trochlear groove
  - □ Ulnar nerve symptoms with excess callus formation or malunion
  - □ Cubitus varus with inadequate reduction or failure of fixation

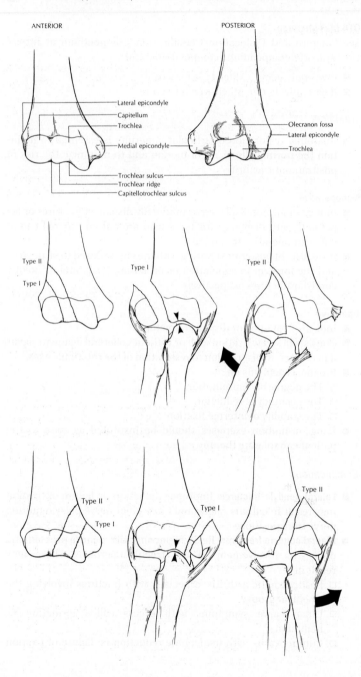

Capitellum Fractures

■ These represent <1% of all elbow fractures.
■ They occur in the coronal plane, parallel to the anterior humerus.
■ Little or no soft tissue attachments result in a free articular fragment that may displace.
■ Anterior displacement of the articular fragment into the coronoid or radial fossae may result in a block to flexion.

Mechanism of Injury

■ A fall onto an outstretched hand with the elbow in varying degrees of flexion; force is transmitted through the radial head to the capitellum. Fracture occurs secondary to shear.
■ These are occasionally associated with radial head fractures.

Classification

OTA Classification
See Fracture and Dislocation Classification Compendium at http://www.ota.org/ compendium/compendium.html.

Additional Classification (Fig. 17.5)
Type I: **Hahn-Steinthal fragment:** large osseous component of capitellum, sometimes with trochlear involvement

---

FIGURE 17.4 Classification of condylar fractures according to Milch and the location of the common fracture lines seen in type I and II fractures of the lateral **(B)** and medial **(C)** condyles. **(A)** Anterior view of the anatomy of the distal articular surface of the humerus. The capitellotrochlear sulcus divides the capitellar and trochlear articular surfaces. The lateral trochlear ridge is the key to analyzing humeral condyle fractures. In type I fractures, the lateral trochlear ridge remains with the intact condyle, providing medial to lateral elbow stability. In type II fractures, the lateral trochlear ridge is a part of the fractured condyle, which may allow the radius and ulna to translocate in a medial-to-lateral direction with respect to the long axis of the humerus. **(B)** Fractures of the lateral condyle. In type I fractures, the lateral trochlear ridge remains intact, therefore preventing dislocation of the radius and ulna. In type II fractures, the lateral trochlear ridge is a part of the fractured lateral condyle. With capsuloligamentous disruption medially, the radius and ulna may dislocate. **(C)** Fractures of the medial condyle. In type I fractures, the lateral trochlear ridge remains intact to provide medial to lateral stability of the radius and ulna. In type II fractures, the lateral trochlear ridge is a part of the fractures medial condyle. With lateral capsuloligamentous disruption, the radius and ulna may dislocate medially on the humerus. (From Rockwood CA Jr, Green DP, Bucholz RW, Heckman JD, eds. *Rockwood and Green's Fractures in Adults.* Vol 1. 4th ed. Philadelphia: Lippincott–Raven; 1996:954.)

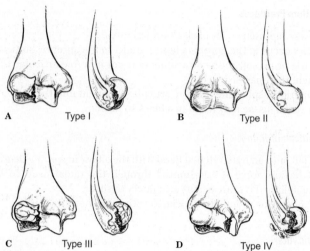

FIGURE 17.5 (A) Type I (Hahn-Steinthal fragment) large osseous component of capitellum, sometimes with trochlear involvement. **(B)** Type II (Kocher-Lorenz fragment) articular cartilage with minimal subchondral bone attached—"uncapping of the condyle." **(C)** Type III: Markedly comminuted (Morrey). **(D)** Type IV: Extension into the trochlea (McKee). (From Ruchelsman DE, Tejwani NC, Kwon YW, et al., Coronal plane partial articular fractures of the distal humerus: current concepts in management. *J Am Acad Orthop Surg* 2008;16:716–728, with permission.)

Type II:	**Kocher-Lorenz fragment:** articular cartilage with minimal subchondral bone attached: "uncapping of the condyle"
Type III:	Markedly comminuted (Morrey)
Type IV:	Extension into the trochlea (McKee)

Treatment

Nonoperative
- This is primarily used for nondisplaced fractures.
- It consists of immobilization in a posterior splint for 3 weeks followed by range of elbow motion.

Operative
- The goal is anatomic restoration.
- Open reduction and internal fixation
    - This technique is indicated for displaced type I fractures.
    - Via a posterolateral or posterior approach, screws may be placed from a posterior to anterior direction; alternatively, headless screws may be placed from anterior to posterior.
    - Fixation should be stable enough to allow early range of elbow motion.

- Excision
  - □ This is rarely indicated for severely comminuted type I fractures and most type II fractures. Care must be taken in the elderly as these are often type IV fractures, which if excised will lead to elbow instability.
  - □ This may be the recommended treatment in chronic missed fractures with limited range of elbow motion.

Complications

- **Osteonecrosis:** This is relatively uncommon.
- **Posttraumatic arthritis:** The risk is increased with failure to restore articular congruity and excision of the articular fragment.
- **Cubitus valgus:** This may result after excision of articular fragment or with an associated lateral condylar or radial head fracture. It is associated with tardy ulnar nerve palsy.
- **Loss of motion (flexion):** This is associated with retained chondral or osseous fragments that may become entrapped in the coronoid or radial fossae.

Trochlea Fractures (Laugier's Fracture)

- Extremely rare.
- It is associated with elbow dislocation.

Mechanism of Injury

- Tangential shearing force resulting from elbow dislocation.

Treatment

- Nondisplaced fractures may be managed with posterior splinting for 3 weeks followed by range-of-motion exercises.
- Displaced fractures should receive open reduction and internal fixation with Kirschner wire or screw fixation.
- Fragments not amenable to internal fixation should be excised.

Complications

- Posttraumatic arthritis may result with retained osseous fragments within the elbow joint or incongruity of the articular surface.
- Restricted range of motion may result from malunion of the trochlear fragment.

Lateral Epicondylar Fractures

- Extremely rare

Mechanism of Injury

- Direct trauma is the mechanism in adults.
- Prepubescent patients may experience avulsion fractures.

Treatment

- Symptomatic immobilization is followed by early range of elbow motion.

Complications

- Nonunion may result in continued symptoms of pain exacerbated by wrist or elbow motion.

Medial Epicondylar Fractures

- These are more common than lateral epicondylar fractures owing to the relative prominence of the epicondyle on the medial side of the elbow.

Mechanism of Injury

- In children and adolescents, the medial epicondyle may be avulsed during a posterior elbow dislocation.
- In adults, it is most commonly the result of direct trauma, although it can occur as an isolated fracture or associated with elbow dislocation.

Treatment

- Nondisplaced or minimally displaced fractures may be managed by short-term immobilization for 10 to 14 days in a posterior splint with the forearm pronated and the wrist and elbow flexed.
- Operative indications
  - □ Relative indications include displaced fragments in the presence of ulnar nerve symptoms, elbow instability to valgus stress, wrist flexor weakness, and symptomatic nonunion of the displaced fragment.
  - □ **Open reduction and internal fixation versus excision:** Excision is indicated for fragments not amenable to internal fixation or that are incarcerated within the joint space and are irreducible.

Complications

- **Posttraumatic arthritis:** This may result from osseous fragments retained within the joint space.

■ **Weakness of the flexor mass:** This may result from nonunion of the fragment or malunion with severe distal displacement.

Fractures of the Supracondylar Process

■ The supracondylar process is a congenital osseous or cartilaginous projection that arises from the anteromedial surface of the distal humerus.

■ The ligament of Struthers is a fibrous arch connecting the supracondylar process with the medial epicondyle, from which fibers of the pronator teres or the coracobrachialis may arise.

■ Through this arch traverse the median nerve and the brachial artery.

■ Fractures are rare, with a reported incidence between 0.6% and 2.7%, but they may result in pain and median nerve or brachial artery compression.

Mechanism of Injury

■ Direct trauma to the anterior aspect of the distal humerus.

Treatment

■ Most of these fractures are amenable to nonoperative treatment with symptomatic immobilization in a posterior elbow splint in relative flexion until pain free, followed by range-of-motion and strengthening exercises.

■ Median nerve or brachial artery compression may require surgical exploration and release.

Complications

■ **Myositis ossificans:** The risk is increased with surgical exploration.

■ **Recurrent spur formation:** This may result in recurrent symptoms of neurovascular compression, necessitating surgical exploration and release, with excision of the periosteum and attached muscle fibers to prevent recurrence.

18 Elbow Dislocation

EPIDEMIOLOGY

- Accounts for 11% to 28% of injuries to the elbow.
- Posterior dislocation is most common.
- The annual incidence of elbow dislocations is 6 to 8 cases per 100,000 population per year.
- Posterior dislocations of the elbow are the predominant type and account for 80% to 90% of all elbow dislocations.
- Simple dislocations are purely ligamentous.
- Complex dislocations are those that occur with an associated fracture and represent just under 50% of elbow dislocations.
- Highest incidence in the 10- to 20-year old age group associated with sports injuries; recurrent dislocation is uncommon.

ANATOMY

- The elbow is a "modified hinge" joint with a high degree of intrinsic stability owing to joint congruity, opposing tension of triceps and flexors, and ligamentous constraints.
- The three separate articulations are
  □ Ulnotroclear (hinge)
  □ Radiocapitellar (rotation)
  □ Proximal radioulnar (rotation)
- Stability (Fig. 18.1)
  □ **Anterior-posterior:** trochlea-olecranon fossa (extension); coronoid fossa, radiocapitellar joint, biceps-triceps-brachialis (flexion).
  □ **Valgus:** The medial collateral ligament (MCL) complex: the anterior bundle is the primary stabilizer in flexion and extension, and the anterior capsule and radiocapitellar joint function in extension.
  □ **Varus:** The lateral ulnar collateral ligament is static, and the anconeus muscle is dynamic.
  □ Function of the MCL
    • It is the primary medial stabilizer, especially the anterior band.
    • Full extension provides 30% of valgus stability.
    • Ninety degrees of flexion provides >50% of valgus stability.

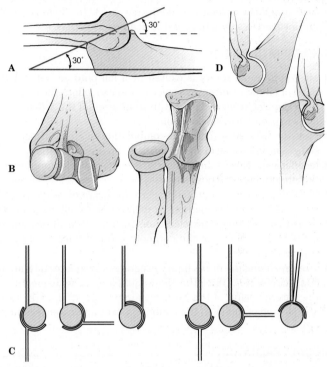

FIGURE 18.1 The elbow is an inherently stable joint. **(A)** The trochlear notch of the ulna provides a nearly 180-degree capture of the trochlea, which tilts posteriorly approximately 30 degrees. **(B)** The ridge in the center of the trochlear notch interdigitates with a groove on the trochlea, further enhancing stability. **(C)** Flexion of the elbow is enhanced by the anterior translation of the trochlea with respect to the humeral shaft as well as the coronoid and radial fossae on the anterior surface of the humerus that accept the coronoid process and radial head, respectively. **(D)** Posteriorly, the olecranon fossa enhances extension by accommodating the olecranon process. (From Bucholz RW, Heckman JD, Court-Brown C, et al., eds. *Rockwood and Green's Fractures in Adults.* 6th ed. Philadelphia: Lippincott Williams & Wilkins; 2006.)

- Resection of anterior band will cause gross instability except in extension.
  - ☐ Lateral ligaments
    - These prevent posterior subluxation and rotation of the ulna away from the humerus with the forearm supination (posterolateral rotatory instability).
- ■ **Normal range of motion:** 0 to 150 degrees flexion, 85 degrees supination, and 80 degrees pronation

■ **Functional range of motion:** a 100-degree arc, 30 to 130 degrees flexion, 50 degrees supination, and 50 degrees pronation

MECHANISM OF INJURY

■ Most commonly, injury is caused by a fall onto an outstretched hand or elbow, resulting in a levering force to unlock the olecranon from the trochlea combined with translation of the articular surfaces to produce the dislocation.

■ **Posterior dislocation:** This is a combination of elbow hyperextension, valgus stress, arm abduction, and forearm supination.

■ **Anterior dislocation:** A direct force strikes the posterior forearm with the elbow in a flexed position.

■ Most elbow dislocations and fracture-dislocations result in injury to all the capsuloligamentous stabilizers of the elbow joint. The exceptions include trans-olecranon fracture-dislocations and injuries with fractures of the coronoid involving nearly the entire coronoid process.

■ The capsuloligamentous injury progresses from lateral to medial (Hori circle) (Fig. 18.2); the elbow can completely dislocate with the anterior band of the MCL remaining intact. There is a variable degree of injury to the common flexor and extensor musculature.

CLINICAL EVALUATION

■ Patients typically guard the injured upper extremity, which shows variable gross instability and swelling.

■ A careful neurovascular examination is essential and should be performed before radiography or manipulation.

■ Following manipulation or reduction, repeat neurovascular examination should be performed to assess neurovascular status.

■ Serial neurovascular examinations should be performed when massive antecubital swelling exists or when the patient is felt to be at risk for compartment syndrome.

■ Angiography may be necessary to evaluate vascular compromise.
  □ Following reduction, if arterial flow is not re-established and the hand remains poorly perfused, the patient should be prepared for arterial reconstruction with saphenous vein grafting.
  □ Angiography should be performed in the operating room and should never delay operative intervention when vascular compromise is present.
  □ The radial pulse may be present with brachial artery compromise as a result of collateral circulation.
  □ The absence of a radial pulse in the presence of a warm, well-perfused hand likely represents arterial spasm.

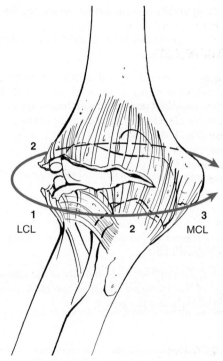

FIGURE 18.2 The capsuloligamentous structures of the elbow are injured in a lateral to medial progression during dislocation of the elbow. The elbow can dislocate with the anterior band of the medial collateral ligament (MCL) remaining intact. (From Bucholz RW, Heckman JD, Court-Brown C, et al., eds. *Rockwood and Green's Fractures in Adults.* 6th ed. Philadelphia: Lippincott Williams & Wilkins; 2006.)

ASSOCIATED INJURIES

■ Associated fractures most often involve the radial head and/or coronoid process of the ulna. Shear fractures of the capitellum and/or trochlea are less common.

■ Acute neurovascular injuries are uncommon; the ulnar nerve and anterior interosseous branches of the median nerve are most commonly involved.

■ The brachial artery may be injured, particularly with an open dislocation.

RADIOGRAPHIC EVALUATION

■ Standard anteroposterior and lateral radiographs of the elbow should be obtained.

- Radiographs should be scrutinized for associated fractures about the elbow.
- CT scans may help identify bony fracture fragments not discernable on plain radiographs.

CLASSIFICATION

- Simple versus complex (associated with fracture)
- According to the direction of displacement of the ulna relative to the humerus (Fig. 18.3):
  - □ Posterior
  - □ Posterolateral
  - □ Posteromedial
  - □ Lateral
  - □ Medial
  - □ Anterior

TREATMENT PRINCIPLES

- Restoration of the inherent bony stability of the elbow is the goal.
- Restoration of the trochlear notch of the ulna, particularly the coronoid process, is also the goal.

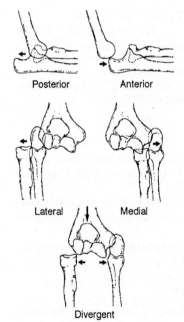

Posterior   Anterior

Lateral   Medial

Divergent

FIGURE 18.3 Elbow dislocations. (From Browner BD, Jupiter JB, Levine AM, eds. *Skeletal Trauma.* Philadelphia: WB Saunders; 1992:1142, with permission.)

- Radiocapitellar contact is very important to the stability of the injured elbow.
- The lateral collateral ligament is more important than the MCL in the setting of most cases of traumatic elbow instability.
- The trochlear notch (coronoid and olecranon), radial head, and lateral collateral ligament should be repaired or reconstructed, but the MCL rarely needs to be repaired.
- MCL will usually heal properly with active motion, and its repair is not necessary for stability.
- Postreduction stability testing should allow for extension of the elbow to –30 degrees of extension before subluxation or dislocation.

FRACTURE-DISLOCATIONS

- **Associated radial head:** These make up 5–10% of cases.
- **Associated medial or lateral epicondyle (12% to 34%):** They may result in mechanical block following closed reduction owing to entrapment of fragment.
- **Associated coronoid process (5% to 10%):** These are secondary to avulsion by brachialis muscle and are most common with posterior dislocation.
  - ☐ **Types I, II, and III (Regan and Morrey), based on size of fragment (Fig. 18.4):**
    - Type I, avulsion of the tip of the coronoid process
    - Type II, a single or comminuted fragment involving 50% of the coronoid process or less

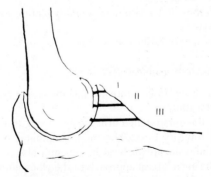

FIGURE 18.4 Regan and Morrey classification of coronoid fractures. (From Regan W, Morrey BF. Fractures of coronoid process of the ulna. *J Bone Joint Surg.* 1989;71:1348–1354, with permission.)

- Type III, a single or comminuted fragment involving >50% of the process

■ Elbow dislocations that are associated with one or more intra-articular fractures are at greater risk for recurrent or chronic instability.

■ Fracture-dislocations of the elbow usually occur in one of several distinct, recognizable injury patterns, including
  □ Posterior dislocation with a fracture of the radial head
  □ Posterior dislocation with fractures of the radial head and coronoid process—the so-called terrible triad injury
  □ Varus posteromedial rotational instability pattern injuries, associated with anteromedial facet of the coronoid fractures
  □ Anterior olecranon fracture-dislocations
  □ Posterior olecranon fracture-dislocations

■ The following observations may be useful in guiding treatment:
  □ Terrible triad injuries nearly always have a type I or II coronoid fracture including the anterior capsular attachment. Much less commonly, the coronoid fracture is type III.
  □ In the setting of an olecranon fracture-dislocation, the coronoid fracture can be one simple large fragment, it can be fragmented into two or three large pieces (anteromedial facet, central, and lesser sigmoid notch) with or without a tip fragment, or it can be more comminuted.

Types of Elbow Instability

■ Posterolateral rotatory instability (elbow dislocations with or without associated fractures)

■ Varus posteromedial rotational instability (anteromedial coronoid facet fractures)

■ Olecranon fracture-dislocations

Posterolateral Rotatory Instability (Fig. 18.5)

■ May range from radiocapitellar instability to complete ulno-umeral dislocation.

■ A fall onto the outstretched arm creates a valgus, axial, and posterolateral rotatory force. The radius supinates away from the humerus and dislocate posteriorly. This may also be caused iatrogenically during a lateral approach to the elbow joint, if the ulnar band of the LCL is taken down and left unrepaired.

■ This may result in injury to the radial head or coronoid.

■ The soft tissue injury proceeds from lateral to medial, with the anterior band of the MCL being the last structure injured.

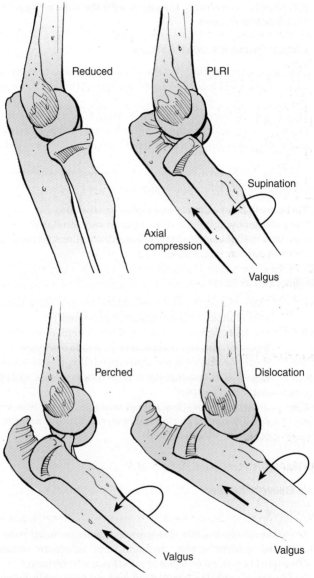

FIGURE 18.5 Posterolateral rotatory instability (PLRI) occurs in several stages. Elbow dislocation is the final stage. (From Bucholz RW, Heckman JD, Court-Brown C, et al., eds. *Rockwood and Green's Fractures in Adults*. 6th ed. Philadelphia: Lippincott Williams & Wilkins; 2006.)

- It is possible to dislocate the elbow with the anterior band of the MCL remaining intact.

Varus Posteromedial Rotational Instability

- This occurs with a fall onto the outstretched arm that creates a varus stress, axial load, and posteromedial rotational force to the elbow.
- This results in fracture of the anteromedial facet of the coronoid process and (1) injury to the lateral collateral ligament, (2) fracture of the olecranon, or (3) an additional fracture of the coronoid at its base.

Anterior Olecranon Fracture-Dislocations

- These result from a direct blow to the flexed elbow.
- Some authors suggest that these injuries may result from the same mechanism that usually creates elbow dislocations, particularly in older osteopenic individuals.

Instability Scale (Morrey)

Type I: Posterolateral rotatory instability; positive pivot shift test; lateral ulnar collateral ligament disrupted

Type II: Perched condyles; varus instability; lateral ulnar collateral ligament, anterior and posterior capsule disrupted

Type IIIa: Posterior dislocation; valgus instability; lateral ulnar collateral ligament, anterior and posterior capsule, and posterior MCL disrupted

Type IIIb: Posterior dislocation; grossly unstable; lateral ulnar collateral ligament, anterior and posterior capsule, anterior and posterior MCL disrupted

TREATMENT

Simple Elbow Dislocation

Nonoperative

- Acute simple elbow dislocations should undergo closed reduction with the patient under sedation and adequate analgesia. Alternatively, general or regional anesthesia may be used.
- Correction of medial or lateral displacement followed by longitudinal traction and flexion is usually successful for posterior dislocations (Fig. 18.6).
- For posterior dislocations, reduction should be performed with the elbow flexed while providing distal traction.

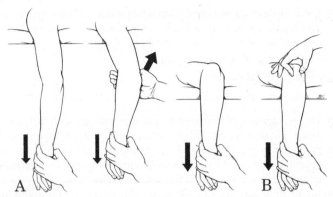

FIGURE 18.6 (A) Parvin's method of closed reduction of an elbow dislocation. The patient lies prone on a stretcher, and the physician applies gentle downward traction of the wrist for a few minutes. As the olecranon begins to slip distally, the physician lifts up gently on the arm. No assistant is required, and if the maneuver is done gently, no anesthesia is required. **(B)** In Meyn and Quigley's method of reduction, only the forearm hangs from the side of the stretcher. As gentle downward traction is applied on the wrist, the physician guides reduction of the olecranon with the opposite hand. **(A,** redrawn from Parvin RW. Closed reduction of common shoulder and elbow dislocations without anesthesia. *Arch Surg.* 1957;75:972–975. **B,** redrawn from Meyn MA, Quigley TB. Reduction of posterior dislocation of the elbow by traction on the dangling arm. *Clin Orthop.* 1974;103:106–108.)

- Neurovascular status should be reassessed, followed by evaluation of stable range of elbow motion.
- Postreduction radiographs are essential.
- Postreduction management should consist of a posterior splint at 90 degrees and elevation.
- Early, gentle, active, or active-assisted range of elbow motion is associated with better long-term results. Prolonged immobilization is associated with unsatisfactory results and greater flexion contracture.
- A hinged elbow brace through a stable arc of motion may be indicated in cases of instability without associated fracture.
- Recovery of motion and strength may require 3 to 6 months.

Operative

- When the elbow cannot be held in a concentrically reduced position, redislocates before postreduction radiography, or dislocates later in spite of splint immobilization, the dislocation is deemed unstable, and operative treatment is required.

■ **There are three general approaches to this problem:** (1) open reduction and repair of soft tissues back to the distal humerus, (2) hinged external fixation, or (3) cross-pinning of the joint.

Elbow Fracture-Dislocations

Nonoperative

■ This is a reasonable treatment option in patients with dislocation and a non or minimally displaced fracture of the radial head only.

■ Patients who elect nonoperative treatment need to be aware of the potential for instability and the substantial potential for restriction of motion or arthrosis from the radial head fracture.

■ Under close supervision, it is reasonable to remove the splint and begin active motion at the patient's first visit to the office, typically about a week after injury.

Operative

■ This includes repair or replacement of the radial head and lateral collateral ligament repair.

■ Most authors do not support acute MCL reconstruction.

■ Some authors, however, stress the importance of the lateral collateral ligament to elbow stability and advocate reattachment of this ligament to the lateral epicondyle.

■ When the lateral collateral ligament is repaired, immediate active motion is usually possible (particularly if radiocapitellar contact has also been restored), but up to 10 days of immobilization is reasonable.

"Terrible Triad" Fracture-Dislocations

■ The addition of a coronoid fracture, no matter how small, to a dislocation of the elbow and fracture of the radial head dramatically increases the instability and the potential for problems.

■ Not all terrible triad injuries will be unstable, but it may be difficult to predict which injuries will be unstable.

■ Good results have been reported with repair of the coronoid or anterior capsule, repair or replacement of the radial head, and lateral collateral ligament repair.

■ This algorithm has been shown to restore stability in most cases, but in some patients, either MCL repair or a lateral hinged external fixator may also be necessary if instability persists after reconstruction of the lateral side (Fig. 18.7).

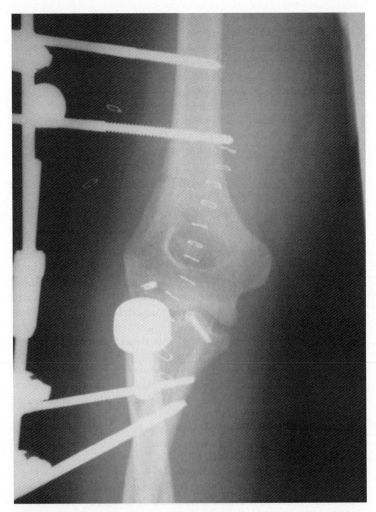

FIGURE 18.7 Example of a fracture-dislocation of the elbow treated with a stepwise approach of coronoid repair, radial head replacement, lateral ligamentous repair, and hinged external fixation.

COMPLICATIONS

- **Loss of motion (stiffness):** Stiffness following complicated or uncomplicated elbow dislocation is usually the rule. Immobilization of the elbow should generally not go beyond 2 weeks.

- **Neurologic compromise:** Sustained neurologic deficits at the time of injury should be observed.
  - □ Spontaneous recovery usually occurs; a decline in nerve function (especially after manipulation) and severe pain in nerve distribution are indications for exploration and decompression.
  - □ Exploration is recommended if no recovery is seen after 3 months following electromyography.
  - □ Late ulnar neuropathy may be seen and is associated with loss of elbow extension and scarring in the cubital tunnel.
- **Vascular injury:** The brachial artery is most commonly disrupted during injury.
  - □ Prompt recognition of vascular injury is essential, with closed reduction to re-establish perfusion.
  - □ If, after reduction, perfusion is not re-established, angiography is indicated to identify the lesion, with arterial reconstruction when indicated.
- **Compartment syndrome (Volkmann contracture):** This may result from massive swelling due to soft tissue injury. Postreduction care must include elevation and avoidance of hyperflexion of the elbow. Serial neurovascular examinations and compartment pressure monitoring may be necessary, with forearm fasciotomy when indicated.
- **Persistent instability/redislocation:** This is rare after isolated, traumatic posterior elbow dislocation; the incidence is increased in the presence of an associated coronoid process and radial head fracture (terrible triad of the elbow). It may necessitate capsuloligamentous reconstruction, internal fixation, prosthetic replacement of the radial head, or hinged external fixation.
- **Arthrosis:** May result from persistent elbow instability over a period of time. Associated more with fracture-dislocation of the elbow than with simple dislocation.
- **Heterotopic bone/myositis ossificans:**
  - □ Anteriorly it forms between the brachialis muscle and the capsule; posteriorly it may form medially or laterally between the triceps and the capsule.
  - □ The risk is increased with multiple reduction attempts, a greater degree of soft tissue trauma, or the presence of associated fractures.
  - □ It may result in significant loss of function.
  - □ Forcible manipulation or passive stretching increases soft tissue trauma and should be avoided.
  - □ Indomethacin or local radiation therapy is recommended for prophylaxis after surgery and in the presence of significant soft tissue injury and/or associated fractures.

Olecranon

EPIDEMIOLOGY

- Bimodal distribution is seen, with younger individuals as a result of high-energy trauma and with older individuals as a result of a simple fall.
- The incidence of olecranon fractures in the adult population is 11.5 per 100,000 population per year.
- Accounts for 8% to 10% of all elbow fractures.

ANATOMY

- The coronoid process delineates the distal border of the greater sigmoid (semilunar) notch of the ulna, which articulates with the trochlea. This articulation allows motion only about the flexion-extension axis, thus providing intrinsic stability to the elbow joint.
- The articular cartilage surface is interrupted by a transverse ridge known as the "bare area."
- Posteriorly, the triceps tendon envelops the articular capsule before it inserts onto the olecranon. A fracture of the olecranon with displacement represents a functional disruption of the triceps mechanism, resulting in loss of active extension of the elbow.
- The ossification center for the olecranon appears at 10 years and is fused by about age 16. There can be persistent epiphyseal plates in adults; these are usually bilateral and demonstrate familial inheritance.
- The subcutaneous position of the olecranon makes it vulnerable to direct trauma.

MECHANISM OF INJURY

Two common mechanisms are seen, each resulting in a predictable fracture pattern:

- **Direct:** A fall on the point of the elbow or direct trauma to the olecranon typically results in a comminuted olecranon fracture (less common).
- **Indirect:** A strong, sudden eccentric contraction of the triceps upon a flexed elbow typically results in a transverse or oblique fracture (more common).

■ A combination of these may produce displaced, comminuted fractures, or, in cases of extreme violence, fracture-dislocation with anterior displacement of the distal ulnar fragment and radial head.

CLINICAL EVALUATION

■ Patients typically present with the upper extremity supported by the contralateral hand with the elbow in relative flexion. Abrasions over the olecranon or hand may be indicative of the mechanism of injury.

■ Physical examination may demonstrate a palpable defect at the fracture site. An inability to extend the elbow actively against gravity indicates discontinuity of the triceps mechanism.

■ A careful neurosensory evaluation should be performed, because associated ulnar nerve injury is possible, especially with comminuted fractures resulting from high-energy injuries.

RADIOGRAPHIC EVALUATION

■ Standard anteroposterior and lateral radiographs of the elbow should be obtained. A true lateral radiograph is imperative, because this will demonstrate the extent of the fracture, the degree of comminution, the degree of articular surface involvement, and displacement of the radial head, if present.

■ The anteroposterior view should be evaluated to exclude associated fractures or dislocations. The distal humerus may obscure osseous details of the olecranon fracture.

CLASSIFICATION

Mayo Classification (Fig. 19.1)

This distinguishes three factors that have a direct influence on treatment: (1) fracture displacement, (2) comminution, and (3) ulnohumeral stability.

■ Type I fractures are nondisplaced or minimally displaced and are subclassified as either noncomminuted (type 1A) or comminuted (type 1B). Treatment is nonoperative.

■ Type II fractures have displacement of the proximal fragment without elbow instability; these fractures require operative treatment.

  □ Type IIA fractures, which are noncomminuted, can be treated by tension band wire fixation.

  □ Type IIB fractures are comminuted and may require plate fixation.

Type I Undisplaced

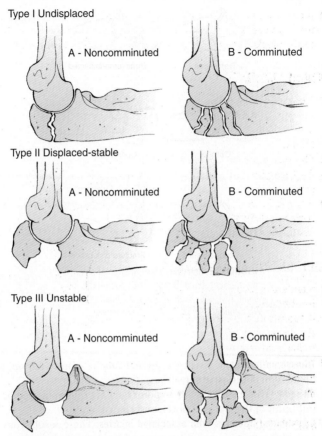

A - Noncomminuted

B - Comminuted

Type II Displaced-stable

A - Noncomminuted

B - Comminuted

Type III Unstable

A - Noncomminuted

B - Comminuted

FIGURE 19.1 The Mayo classification of olecranon fractures divides fractures according to displacement, comminution, and subluxation/dislocation. (From Bucholz RW, Heckman JD, Court-Brown C, et al., eds. *Rockwood and Green's Fractures in Adults.* 6th ed. Philadelphia: Lippincott Williams & Wilkins; 2006.)

- Type III fractures feature instability of the ulnohumeral joint and require surgical treatment.

Schatzker (Based on Fracture Pattern) (Fig. 19.2)

- **Transverse:** This occurs at the apex of the sigmoid notch and represents an avulsion fracture from a sudden, violent pull of both triceps and brachialis, and uncommonly from direct trauma.

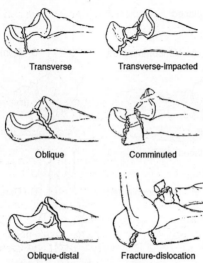

FIGURE 19.2 Schatzker classification of olecranon fractures. (From Browner BD, Jupiter JB, Levine AM, eds. *Skeletal Trauma*. Philadelphia: WB Saunders; 1992:1137, with permission.)

- **Transverse-impacted:** A direct force leads to comminution and depression of the articular surface.
- **Oblique:** This results from hyperextension injury; it begins at midpoint of the sigmoid notch and runs distally.
- **Comminuted fractures with associated injuries:** These result from direct high-energy trauma; fractures of the coronoid process may lead to instability.
- **Oblique-distal:** Fractures extend distal to the coronoid and compromise elbow stability.
- **Fracture-dislocation:** It is usually associated with severe trauma.

OTA Classification of Proximal Radius/Ulna Fractures

See Fracture and Dislocation Classification Compendium at http://www.ota.org/ compendium/compendium.html.

TREATMENT OBJECTIVES

- Restoration of the articular surface
- Restoration and preservation of the elbow extensor mechanism

- Restoration of elbow motion and prevention of stiffness
- Prevention of complications

TREATMENT

Nonoperative

- Is reserved for nondisplaced fractures and some displaced fractures in low-functioning older individuals.
- Immobilization in a long arm cast or splint with the elbow in 45 to 90 degrees of flexion is favored by many authors, although in reliable patients a posterior splint or orthosis with gradual initiation of range of motion after 5 to 7 days may be used.
- Follow-up radiographs should be obtained within 5 to 7 days after treatment to rule out fracture displacement. Osseous union is usually not complete until 6 to 8 weeks.
- In general, there is adequate fracture stability at 3 weeks to remove the cast and allow protected range-of-motion exercises, avoiding active extension and flexion past 90 degrees.

Operative

- Indications for surgery
  - □ Disruption of extensor mechanism (any displaced fracture)
  - □ Articular incongruity
- **Types of operative treatment:**
  - □ **Tension band wiring in combination with two parallel Kirschner wires remains the treatment of choice:** This counteracts the tensile forces and converts them to compressive forces and is indicated for avulsion-type olecranon fractures (Fig. 19.3).

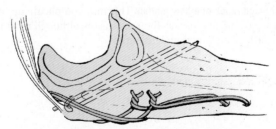

FIGURE 19.3 The Kirschner wires are bent 180 degrees and are impacted into the olecranon beneath the triceps insertion. (From Bucholz RW, Heckman JD, Court-Brown C, et al., eds. *Rockwood and Green's Fractures in Adults.* 6th ed. Philadelphia: Lippincott Williams & Wilkins; 2006.)

☐ **Intramedullary fixation:** 6.5-mm cancellous lag screw fixation. The screw must be of sufficient length to engage the distal intramedullary canal for adequate fixation. This may be used in conjunction with tension band wiring (described later).
- With screw techniques, beware of bowing of the ulna intramedullary canal that may shift the fracture with screw advancement.

☐ **Plate and screws:** They are used for comminuted olecranon fractures, Monteggia fractures, and olecranon fracture-dislocations. A plate should also be used for fractures that extend distal to the coronoid.
- Fewer problems with plate prominence are noted when it is placed laterally.

☐ **Excision (with repair of the triceps tendon):** This is indicated for nonunited fractures, extensively comminuted fractures, fractures in elderly individuals with severe osteopenia and low functional requirements, and extra-articular fractures.

■ **Postoperative management:** The patient should be placed in a posterior elbow splint. With a stable repair, one should initiate early range-of-motion exercises.

COMPLICATIONS

■ Symptomatic hardware may occur in up to 80% of patients.
   ☐ From 34% to 66% may require hardware removal.
■ Hardware failure occurs in 1% to 5%.
■ Infection occurs in 0% to 6%.
■ Pin migration occurs in 15%.
■ Ulnar neuritis occurs in 2% to 12%.
■ Heterotopic ossification occurs in 2% to 13%.
■ Nonunion occurs in 5%.
■ **Decreased range of elbow motion:** This may complicate up to 50% of cases, particularly loss of elbow extension, although most patients note little if any functional limitation.

20 Radial Head

EPIDEMIOLOGY

- Radial head fractures account for 1.7% to 5.4% of all fractures, and one-third of all elbow fractures.
- One-third of patients have associated injuries such as fracture or ligamentous damage of the shoulder, humerus, forearm, wrist, or hand.

ANATOMY

- The capitellum and the radial head are reciprocally curved.
- Force transmission across the radiocapitellar articulation takes place at all angles of elbow flexion and is greatest in full extension.
- Full rotation of the head of the radius requires accurate anatomic positioning in the lesser sigmoid notch.
- The radial head plays a role in valgus stability of the elbow, but the degree of conferred stability remains disputed.
- The radial head is a secondary restraint to valgus forces and seems to function by shifting the center of varus-valgus rotation laterally, so the moment arm and forces on the medial ligaments are smaller.
- Clinically, the radial head is most important when there is injury to both the ligamentous and muscle-tendon units about the elbow.
- The radial head acts in concert with the interosseous ligament of the forearm to provide longitudinal stability.
- Proximal migration of the radius can occur after radial head excision if the interosseous ligament is disrupted.

MECHANISM OF INJURY

- Most of these injuries are the result of a fall onto the outstretched hand, the higher-energy injuries representing falls from a height or during sports.
- The radial head fractures when it impacts the capitellum. This may occur with a pure axial load, with a posterolateral rotatory force, or as the radial head dislocates posteriorly as part of a posterior Monteggia fracture or posterior olecranon fracture-dislocation.
- It is frequently associated with injury to the ligamentous structures of the elbow.
- It is less commonly associated with fracture of the capitellum.

CLINICAL EVALUATION

- Patients typically present with limited elbow and forearm motion and pain on passive rotation of the forearm.
- Well-localized tenderness overlying the radial head may be present, as well as an elbow effusion.
- The ipsilateral distal forearm and wrist should be examined. Tenderness to palpation or stress at the distal radioulnar joint (DRUJ) may indicate the presence of an Essex-Lopresti lesion (radial head fracture-dislocation with associated interosseous ligament and DRUJ disruption).
- Medial collateral ligament competence should be tested, especially with type IV radial head fractures in which valgus instability may result. This may be difficult in the acute setting.
- Aspiration of the hemarthrosis through a direct lateral approach with injection of lidocaine will decrease acute pain and allow evaluation of passive range of motion. This can help identify a mechanical block to motion.

RADIOGRAPHIC EVALUATION

- Standard anteroposterior (AP) and lateral radiographs of the elbow should be obtained, with oblique views (Greenspan view) for further fracture definition or in cases in which fracture is suspected but not apparent on AP and lateral views.
- A Greenspan view is taken with the forearm in neutral rotation and the radiographic beam angled 45 degrees cephalad; this view provides visualization of the radiocapitellar articulation (Fig. 20.1).
- Nondisplaced fractures may not be readily appreciable, but they may be suggested by a positive fat pad sign (posterior more sensitive than anterior) on the lateral radiograph, especially if clinically suspected.
- Complaints of forearm or wrist pain should be assessed with appropriate radiographic evaluation.
- Computed tomography of the elbow may be utilized for further fracture definition for preoperative planning, especially in cases of comminution or fragment displacement.

CLASSIFICATION

Mason (Fig. 20.2)

Type I: Nondisplaced fractures
Type II: Marginal fractures with displacement (impaction, depression, angulation)

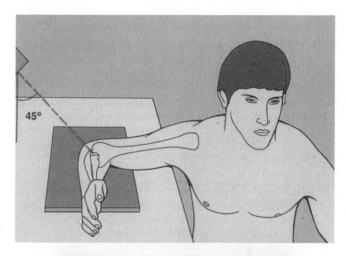

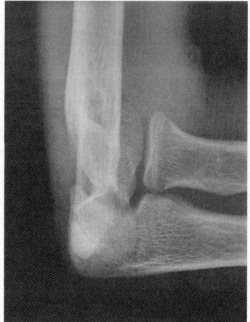

FIGURE 20.1 Schematic and radiograph demonstrating the radial head-capitellum view. (Reproduced with permission from Greenspan A. *Orthopedic Imaging*. Philadelphia: Lippincott Williams & Wilkins; 2004.)

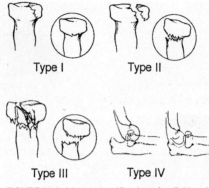

FIGURE 20.2 Mason classification of radial head and neck fractures. (From Broberg MA, Morrey BF. Results of treatment of fracture-dislocations to the elbow. *Clin Orthop.* 1987;216:109.)

Type III: Comminuted fractures involving the entire head
Type IV: Associated with dislocation of the elbow (Johnston)

OTA Classification of Proximal Radius/Ulna Fractures

See Fracture and Dislocation Classification Compendium at http://www.ota.org/ compendium/compendium.html.

TREATMENT GOALS

- Correction of any block to forearm rotation
- Early range of elbow and forearm motion
- Stability of the forearm and elbow
- Limitation of the potential for ulnohumeral and radiocapitellar arthrosis, although the latter seems uncommon

TREATMENT

Nonoperative

- Most isolated fractures of the radial head can be treated nonoperatively.
- Symptomatic management consists of a sling and early range of motion 24 to 48 hours after injury as pain subsides.
- Aspiration of the radiocapitellar joint with or without injection of local anesthesia has been advocated by some authors for pain relief.

■ Persistent pain, contracture, and inflammation may represent capitellar fracture (possibly osteochondral) that was not appreciated on radiographs and can be assessed by magnetic resonance imaging.

Operative

Isolated Partial Radial Head Fractures

■ The one accepted indication for operative treatment of a displaced partial radial head fracture (Mason II) is a block to motion. This can be assessed by lidocaine injection into the elbow joint.

■ A relative indication is displacement of a large fragment >2 mm without a block to motion.

■ A Kocher exposure can be used to approach the radial head; one should take care to protect the uninjured lateral collateral ligament complex. Hardware should be placed only within the 90-degree arc between the radial styloid and Lister tubercle (safe zone) (Fig. 20.3).

■ The anterolateral aspect of the radial head is usually involved and is readily exposed through these intervals.

■ After the fragment has been reduced, it is stabilized using one or two small screws.

Partial Radial Head Fracture as Part of a Complex Injury

■ Partial head fragments that are part of a complex injury are often displaced and unstable with little or no soft tissue attachments.

■ Open reduction and internal fixation may be performed when stable, reliable fixation can be achieved. This is reserved for simple patterns only.

■ In an unstable elbow or forearm injury, it may be preferable to resect the remaining intact radial head and replace it with a metal prosthesis.

Fractures Involving the Entire Head of the Radius

■ When treating a fracture-dislocation of the forearm or elbow with an associated fracture involving the entire head of the radius and/or radial neck, open reduction and internal fixation should only be considered a viable option if stable, reliable fixation can be achieved. Otherwise, prosthetic replacement is indicated.

■ The optimal fracture for open reduction and internal fixation has three or fewer articular fragments without impaction or deformity, each should be of sufficient size and bone quality to accept screw fixation, and there should be little or no metaphyseal bone loss.

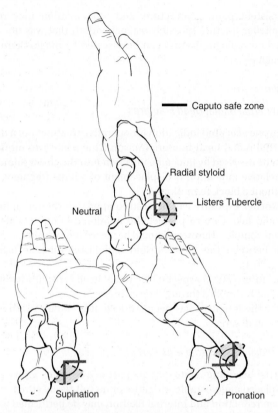

FIGURE 20.3 The nonarticular area of the radial head—or the so-called safe zone for the application of internal fixation devices—has been defined in various ways. Smith and Hotchkiss defined it based on lines bisecting the radial head made in full supination, full pronation, and neutral. Implants can be placed as far as halfway between the middle and posterior lines and a few millimeters beyond halfway between the middle and anterior lines. Caputo and colleagues recommended using the radial styloid and Lister tubercle as intraoperative guides to this safe zone, but this describes a slightly different zone. (From Bucholz RW, Heckman JD, Court-Brown C, et al., eds. *Rockwood and Green's Fractures in Adults*. 6th ed. Philadelphia: Lippincott Williams & Wilkins; 2006.)

■ Once reconstructed with screws, the radial head is secured to the radial neck with a plate.
■ The plate should be placed posteriorly with the forearm supinated; otherwise, it may impinge on the ulna and restrict forearm rotation (Fig. 20.3).

Prosthetic Replacement

- The rationale for use is as a spacer to prevent proximal migration of the radius.
- Long-term studies of fracture-dislocations and Essex-Lopresti lesions demonstrated poor function with silicone implants. Metallic (titanium, vitallium) radial head implants have been used with increasing frequency and are the prosthetic implants of choice in the unstable elbow.
- A problem with a radial head prosthesis is oversizing the radial head implant and thus potentially "overstuffing" the joint.

Radial Head Excision

- Is rarely indicated anymore for isolated injuries in the acute phase and never in a potentially unstable situation (fracture-dislocation, Essex-Lopresti, or Monteggia).
- A direct lateral approach is preferred; the posterior interosseous nerve is at risk with this approach. The level of the excision should be kept proximal to the annular ligament.
- Patients generally have few complaints, mild occasional pain, and nearly normal range of motion; the DRUJ is rarely symptomatic, with proximal migration averaging 2 mm (except with associated Essex-Lopresti lesion). Symptomatic migration of the radius may necessitate radioulnar synostosis.
- Late excision for Mason type II and III fractures produces good-to-excellent results in 80% of cases.

Essex-Lopresti Lesion

- This is defined as longitudinal disruption of forearm interosseous ligament, usually combined with radial head fracture and/or dislocation *plus* DRUJ injury.
- It is difficult to diagnose; wrist pain is the most sensitive sign of DRUJ injury.
- One should assess the DRUJ on the lateral x-ray view.
- Treatment requires restoring stability of both elbow and DRUJ components of injury.
- Radial head excision in this injury will result in proximal migration of the radius.
- Treatment is repair or replacement of the radial head with evaluation of the DRUJ.

Postoperative Care

■ With stable fixation, it is essential to begin early active or active-assisted flexion-extension and supination-pronation exercises.

COMPLICATIONS

■ Contracture may occur secondary to prolonged immobilization or in cases with unremitting pain, swelling, and inflammation, even after seemingly minimal trauma. These may represent unrecognized capitellar osteochondral injuries. After a brief period of immobilization, the patient should be encouraged to do flexion-extension and supination-pronation exercises. The outcome may be maximized by a formal, supervised therapy regimen.

■ Chronic wrist pain may represent an unrecognized interosseous ligament, DRUJ, or triangular fibrocartilage complex injury. Recognition of such injuries is important, especially in Mason type III or IV fractures in which radial head excision is considered. Proximal migration of the radius may require radioulnar synostosis to prevent progressive migration.

■ **Posttraumatic Radio-Capitellar osteoarthritis:** This may occur especially in the presence of articular incongruity or with free osteochondral fragments.

■ **Complex regional pain syndrome:** This may occur following nonoperative or operative management of radial head fractures and may be related to the injury itself.

■ **Missed fracture-dislocation:** Unrecognized (occult) fracture-dislocation of the elbow may result in a late dislocation owing to a failure to address associated ligamentous injuries of the elbow.

21 Radius and Ulna Shaft

EPIDEMIOLOGY

- Forearm fractures are more common in men than in women, secondary to the higher incidence in men of motor vehicle accidents, contact athletic participation, altercations, and falls from a height.
- The ratio of open fractures to closed fractures is higher for the forearm than for any other anatomic area except the tibia.

ANATOMY

- The forearm acts as a ring; a fracture that shortens either the radius or the ulna results either in a fracture or in a dislocation of the other forearm bone at the proximal or distal radioulnar joint. Direct injuries ("nightstick") are an exception.
- The ulna, which is relatively straight, acts as an axis around which the laterally bowed radius rotates in supination and pronation. A loss of supination and pronation may result from radial shaft fractures in which the lateral curvature ("radial bow") has not been restored.
- The interosseous membrane occupies the space between the radius and the ulna. The central band is approximately 3.5 cm wide running obliquely from its proximal origin on the radius to its distal insertion on the ulna. Sectioning of the central band alone reduces stability by 71% (Fig. 21.1).
- **Fracture location dictates deforming forces:**
  - □ Radial fractures distal to the supinator muscle insertion but proximal to the pronator teres insertion tend to result in supination of the proximal fragment owing to unopposed pull of the supinator and biceps brachii muscles.
  - □ Radial fractures distal to the supinator and pronator teres muscles tend to result in neutral rotational alignment of the proximal fragment.

FRACTURES OF BOTH THE RADIUS AND ULNA SHAFTS

Mechanism of Injury

- These fractures are most commonly associated with high-energy (MVC, MCA) accidents, although they are also commonly caused

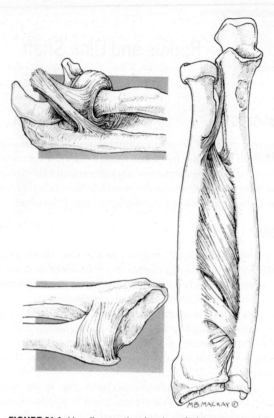

FIGURE 21.1 Line diagram showing the soft tissue connections of the radius and the ulna to each other. The proximal radioulnar joint is stabilized by the annular ligament. The distal radioulnar joint is stabilized by the dorsal and volar radioulnar ligaments and the triangular fibrocartilage complex. (From Richards RR. Chronic disorders of the forearm. *J Bone Joint Surg.* 1996;78A:916–930, with permission.)

by direct trauma (while protecting one's head), gunshot wounds, and falls either from a height or during an athletic competition.
■ Pathologic fractures in this area are uncommon.

Clinical Evaluation

■ Patients typically present with gross deformity of the involved forearm, pain, swelling, and loss of hand and forearm function.

- A careful neurovascular examination is essential, with assessment of radial and ulnar pulses, as well as median, radial, and ulnar nerve function.
- One must carefully assess open wounds because the ulna border is subcutaneous, and even superficial wounds can expose the bone.
- Excruciating, unremitting pain, tense forearm compartments, or pain on passive stretch of the fingers should raise suspicions of impending or present compartment syndrome. Compartment pressure monitoring should be performed, with urgent fasciotomy indicated for diagnosed compartment syndrome.

Radiographic Evaluation

- Anteroposterior (AP) and lateral views of the forearm should be obtained, with oblique views obtained as necessary for further fracture definition.
- Radiographic evaluation should include the ipsilateral wrist and elbow to rule out the presence of associated fracture or dislocation.
- The radial head must be aligned with the capitellum on all views.

Classification

Descriptive

- Closed versus open
- Location
- Comminuted, segmental, multifragmented
- Displacement
- Angulation
- Rotational alignment

OTA Classification of Fractures of the Radial and Ulna Shaft

See Fracture and Dislocation Classification Compendium at http://www.ota.org/compendium/compendium.html.

Treatment

Nonoperative

- The rare, nondisplaced fracture of both the radius and the ulna may be treated with a well-molded, long arm cast in neutral rotation with the elbow flexed to 90 degrees.
- The patient should have frequent follow-up to evaluate for possible loss of fracture reduction.

Operative

■ Because the forearm can be considered a "joint," responsible for motion, open reduction and internal fixation is the procedure of choice for displaced forearm fractures involving the radius and ulna in adults.

■ Internal fixation involves the use of compression plating (3.5-mm dynamic compression plate) with or without bone grafting.

■ **Principles of plate fixation:**
  □ Restore ulnar and radial length (prevents subluxation of either the proximal or distal radioulnar joint).
  □ Restore rotational alignment.
  □ Restore radial bow (essential for rotational function of the forearm).

■ A volar Henry approach may be used for fixation of the entire length of the radius with plate placement on the flat volar surface. Midshaft fractures may be approached and stabilized via a dorsal safely. Dorsal plating elsewhere is associated with plate prominence (distal) and is the potential for PIN injury (proximal).

■ The ulna may be plated on either the volar or the dorsal aspect, depending on the location of the fragments and contour of the ulna surrounding the fracture site. Using two separate incisions decreases the incidence of radioulnar synostosis.

■ One should consider acute grafting if substantial comminution or bone loss exists.

■ Open fractures may receive primary open reduction and internal fixation after debridement, except in severe open injuries. This approach restores stability, limits dead space, and improves wound care. The timing of bone grafting of open fractures is controversial; it can be performed at the time of delayed primary closure or at 6 weeks after injury.

■ External fixation may be used in cases with severe bone or soft tissue loss, gross contamination, infected nonunion, or in cases of open elbow fracture-dislocations with soft tissue loss.

■ Good results have been reported with locked intramedullary nail fixation. However, the indications for intramedullary nailing over plate and screws have not been clearly defined and are technically more demanding. Some of the reported indications are segmental fractures, open fractures with bone or soft tissue loss, pathologic fractures, and failed plate fixation.

Complications

■ **Nonunion and malunion:** These are uncommon, most often related to infection and errors of surgical technique. Patients may require removal of hardware, bone grafting, and revision internal fixation.

- **Infection:** The incidence is only 3% with open reduction and internal fixation. It necessitates surgical drainage, debridement, copious irrigation, wound cultures, and antibiotics. If internal fixation is found to be stable, it does not necessarily need to be removed because most fractures will unite despite infection. Infections, not responsive with severe soft tissue and osseous compromise, may necessitate external fixation with wounds left open and serial debridements.

- **Neurovascular injury:** This is uncommon, associated with gunshot injury or iatrogenic causes. Nerve palsies can generally be observed for 3 months, with surgical exploration indicated for failure of return of nerve function. Injuries to the radial or ulnar arteries may be addressed with simple ligation if the other vessel is patent.

- **Volkmann ischemia:** This devastating complication follows a missed compartment syndrome. Clinical suspicion should be followed by compartment pressure monitoring with emergency fasciotomy if a compartment syndrome is diagnosed.

- **Posttraumatic radioulnar synostosis:** This is uncommon (3% to 9% incidence); the risk increases with massive crush injuries or closed head injury. It may necessitate surgical excision if functional limitations of supination and pronation result, although a nonarticular synostosis excision is rarely successful in the proximal forearm. Separate incisions for bony fixation are best for avoiding this complication.
  - ☐ Risk factors include
    - Fracture of both bones at the same level (11% incidence)
    - Closed head injury
    - Surgical delay >2 weeks
    - Single incision for fixation of both bone forearm fractures
    - Penetration of the interosseous membrane by bone graft or screws, bone fragments, or surgical instruments
    - Crush injury
    - Infection

FRACTURES OF THE ULNA SHAFT

- These include nightstick and Monteggia fractures, as well as stress fractures in athletes.
- A *Monteggia* lesion denotes a fracture of the proximal ulna accompanied by radial head dislocation.

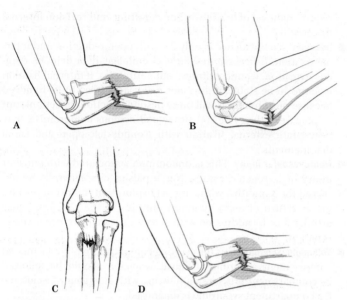

FIGURE 21.2 The Bado classification of Monteggia fractures. **(A)** Type I. An anterior dislocation of the radial head with associated anteriorly angulated fracture of the ulna shaft. **(B)** Type II. Posterior dislocation of the radial head with a posteriorly angulated fracture of the ulna. **(C)** Type III. A lateral or antero-lateral dislocation of the radial head with a fracture of the ulnar metaphysic. **(D)** Type IV. Anterior dislocation of the radial head with a fracture of the radius and ulna. (From Bado JL. The Monteggia lesion. *Clin Orthop Related Res.* 1967; 50:70–86, with permission.)

Mechanism of Injury

■ Ulna *nightstick* fractures result from direct trauma to the ulna along its subcutaneous border, classically as a victim attempts to protect the head from assault.

■ Monteggia fractures are produced by various mechanisms (by Bado classification) (Fig. 21.2):

Type I: Forced pronation of the forearm
Type II: Axial loading of the forearm with a flexed elbow
Type III: Forced abduction of the elbow
Type IV: Type I mechanism in which the radial shaft additionally fails

Clinical Evaluation

■ Patients with a nightstick fracture typically present with focal swelling, pain, tenderness, and variable abrasions at the site of trauma.

- Patients with Monteggia fractures present with elbow swelling, deformity, crepitus, and painful range of elbow motion, especially supination and pronation.
- A careful neurovascular examination is essential, because nerve injury, especially to the radial or posterior interosseous nerve, is common. Most nerve injuries have been described with type II Bado fractures.

Radiographic Evaluation

- AP and lateral views of the forearm (additional views should include the wrist and elbow) are required.
- Oblique views may aid in fracture definition.
- **Normal radiographic findings:**
  - □ A line drawn through the radial head and shaft should always line up with the capitellum.
  - □ **Supinated lateral:** Lines drawn tangential to the radial head anteriorly and posteriorly should enclose the capitellum.

Classification of Ulna Fractures

Descriptive

- Closed versus open
- Location
- Comminuted, segmental, multifragmented
- Displacement
- Angulation
- Rotational alignment

Bado Classification of Monteggia Fractures (Fig. 21.2)

Type I:	Anterior dislocation of the radial head with fracture of ulnar diaphysis at any level with anterior angulation
Type II:	Posterior/posterolateral dislocation of the radial head with fracture of ulnar diaphysis with posterior angulation
Type III:	Lateral/anterolateral dislocation of the radial head with fracture of ulnar metaphysis
Type IV:	Anterior dislocation of the radial head with fractures of both radius and ulna within proximal third at the same level

Classification

OTA Classification of Fractures of the Ulna Shaft

See Fracture and Dislocation Classification Compendium at http://www.ota.org/compendium/compendium.html.

Treatment

Nightstick Fractures

- Nondisplaced or minimally displaced ulna fractures may be treated with plaster immobilization in a sugar-tong splint for 7 to 10 days. Depending on the patient's symptoms, this may be followed by functional bracing for 8 weeks with active range-of-motion exercises for the elbow, wrist, and hand, or simple immobilization in a sling with a compression wrap.
- Displaced fractures (>10-degree angulation in any plane or >50% displacement of the shaft) may be treated with open reduction and internal fixation using a 3.5-mm dynamic compression plate.

Monteggia Fractures

- Closed reduction and casting of Monteggia fractures should be reserved only for the pediatric population.
- Monteggia fractures require operative treatment, open reduction, and internal fixation of the ulna shaft with a 3.5-mm dynamic compression plate or pre-contoured plate of sufficient strength. Closed reduction of the radial head with restoration of ulnar length is the rule. Plate application on the tension side (dorsal) is recommended especially in Bado type II fracture.
- After fixation of the ulna, the radial head is usually stable (>90%).
- Failure of the radial head to reduce with ulna reduction and stabilization is usually the result of inaccurate reduction of the ulna. Secondarily, an interposed annular ligament or rarely the radial nerve.
- Associated radial head fractures may require fixation or replacement.
- Postoperatively, the patient is placed in a posterior elbow splint for 5 to 7 days. With stable fixation, physical therapy can be started with active flexion-extension and supination-pronation exercises. If fixation or radial head stability is questionable, the patient may be placed in longer-term immobilization with serial radiographic evaluation to determine healing, followed by a supervised physical therapy regimen.

Complications

- **Nonunion:** is seen most often with Bado type II fractures.
- **Nerve injury:** most commonly associated with Bado type II and III injuries involving the radial and/or median nerves, as well as their respective terminal branches, the posterior and anterior interosseous nerves. These may also complicate open reduction

owing to overzealous traction or reduction maneuvers. Surgical exploration is indicated for failure of nerve palsy recovery after a 3-month period of observation.

■ **Radial head instability:** uncommon following anatomic reduction of the ulna. If redislocation occurs <6 weeks postoperatively with a nonanatomic reduction of the ulnar, repeat reduction and fixation of the ulna with an open reduction of the radial head may be considered. Dislocation of the radial head >6 weeks postoperatively is best managed by radial head excision.

FRACTURES OF THE RADIAL SHAFT

■ Fractures of the proximal two-thirds of the radius without associated injuries may be considered to be truly isolated. However, radial fractures involving the distal third involve the distal radioulnar joint until proven otherwise.

■ A *Galeazzi* refers to a fracture of the radial diaphysis at the junction of the middle and distal thirds with associated disruption of the distal radioulnar joint. It has also been referred to as the "fracture of necessity," because it requires open reduction and internal fixation to achieve a good result. This lesion is approximately three times as common as Monteggia fractures.
  □ **Variants:** Fracture can occur anywhere along the radius or associated with fractures of both radius and ulna with distal radioulnar joint disruption.

■ Four major deforming forces contribute to a loss of reduction if the fracture is treated by nonoperative means:
  1. **Weight of the hand:** This results in dorsal angulation of the fracture and subluxation of the distal radioulnar joint.
  2. **Pronator quadratus insertion:** This tends to pronate the distal fragment with proximal and volar displacement.
  3. **Brachioradialis:** This tends to cause proximal displacement and shortening.
  4. **Thumb extensors and abductors:** They result in shortening and relaxation of the radial collateral ligament, allowing displacement of the fracture despite immobilization of the wrist in ulnar deviation.

■ A *reverse Galeazzi fracture* denotes a fracture of the distal ulna with associated disruption of the distal radioulnar joint.

Mechanism of Injury

■ Radial diaphyseal fractures may be caused by direct trauma or indirect trauma, such as a fall onto an outstretched hand.

- The radial shaft in the proximal two-thirds is well padded by the extensor musculature; therefore, most injuries severe enough to result in proximal radial shaft fractures typically result in ulna fracture as well. In addition, the anatomic position of the radius in most functional activities renders it less vulnerable to direct trauma than the ulna.
- Galeazzi fractures may result from direct trauma to the wrist, typically on the dorsolateral aspect, or a fall onto an outstretched hand with forearm pronation.
- Reverse Galeazzi fractures may result from a fall onto an outstretched hand with forearm supination.

Clinical Evaluation

- Patient presentation is variable and is related to the severity of the injury and the degree of fracture displacement. Pain, swelling, and point tenderness over the fracture site are typically present.
- Elbow range of motion, including supination and pronation, should be assessed; rarely, limited forearm rotation may suggest a radial head dislocation in addition to the diaphyseal fracture.
- Galeazzi fractures typically present with wrist pain or midline forearm pain that is exacerbated by stressing of the distal radioulnar joint in addition to the radial shaft fracture.
- Neurovascular injury is rare.

Radiographic Evaluation

- AP and lateral radiographs of the forearm, elbow, and wrist should be obtained.
- Radiographic signs of distal radioulnar joint injury are
  - ☐ Fracture at base of the ulnar styloid
  - ☐ Widened distal radioulnar joint on AP x-ray
  - ☐ Subluxed ulna on lateral x-ray
  - ☐ >5 mm radial shortening

Classification

OTA Classification of Fractures of the Radial Shaft

See Fracture and Dislocation Classification Compendium at http://www.ota.org/compendium/compendium.html.

Treatment

Proximal Radius Fracture

- Nondisplaced fractures may be managed in a long arm cast. Any evidence of loss of radial bow is an indication for open reduction and internal fixation. The cast is continued until radiographic evidence of healing occurs.

■ Displaced fractures are best managed by open reduction and plate fixation using a 3.5-mm dynamic compression plate.

Galeazzi Fractures

■ Open reduction and internal fixation comprise the treatment of choice, because closed treatment is associated with a high failure rate.

■ Plate and screw fixation (3.5-mm dynamic compression plate) is the treatment of choice.

■ An anterior Henry approach (interval between the flexor carpi radialis and the brachioradialis) typically provides adequate exposure of the radius fracture, with plate fixation on the flat, volar surface of the radius.

■ The distal radioulnar joint injury typically results in dorsal instability; therefore, a dorsal capsulotomy may be utilized to gain access to the distal radioulnar joint if it remains dislocated after fixation of the radius. Kirschner wire fixation may be necessary to maintain reduction of the distal radioulnar joint if unstable. If the distal radioulnar joint is believed to be stable, however, postoperative plaster immobilization may suffice.

■ **Postoperative management:**
  □ If the distal radioulnar joint is stable, early motion is recommended.
  □ If the distal radioulnar joint is unstable, immobilize the forearm in supination for 4 to 6 weeks in a long arm splint or cast.
  □ Distal radioulnar joint pins, if needed, are removed at 6 to 8 weeks.

Complications

■ **Malunion:** Nonanatomic reduction of the radius fracture with a failure to restore rotational alignment or lateral bow may result in a loss of supination and pronation, as well as painful range of motion. This may require osteotomy or distal ulnar shortening for cases in which symptomatic shortening of the radius results in ulnocarpal impaction.

■ **Nonunion:** This is uncommon with stable fixation, but it may require bone grafting.

■ **Compartment syndrome:** Clinical suspicion should be followed by compartment pressure monitoring with emergency fasciotomy if a compartment syndrome is diagnosed.
  □ One should assess all three forearm compartments and the carpal tunnel.

- **Neurovascular injury:**
  - □ This is usually iatrogenic.
  - □ Superficial radial nerve injury (beneath the brachioradialis) is at risk with anterior radius approaches.
  - □ Posterior interosseous nerve injury (in the supinator) is at risk with proximal radius approaches.
  - □ If no recovery occurs, explore the nerve at 3 months.
- **Radioulnar synostosis:** This is uncommon (3% to 9% incidence).
  - □ See previous discussion.
  - □ The worst prognosis is with distal synostosis, and the best is with diaphyseal synostosis.
- **Recurrent dislocation:** This may arise as a result of radial malreduction. It emphasizes the need for anatomic restoration of the radial fracture to ensure adequate healing and biomechanical function of the distal radioulnar joint.

22   Distal Radius

 # extra-articular deformities

EPIDEMIOLOGY

- Distal radius fractures are among the most common fractures of the upper extremity.
- More than 650,000 occur annually in the United States.
- Fractures of the distal radius represent approximately one-sixth of all fractures treated in emergency departments. *1/6*
- The incidence of distal radius fractures in the elderly correlates with osteopenia and rises in incidence with increasing age, nearly in parallel with the increased incidence of hip fractures.
- In males aged 35 years and older, the incidence is approximately 90 per 100,000 population per year and remains relatively constant until the age of 70 where a slight increase is seen.
- Risk factors for fractures of the distal radius in the elderly include decreased bone mineral density, female sex, white race, family history, and early menopause.

ANATOMY

*→ remember:
scaphoid fx
at route/PIN*

- The metaphysis of the distal radius is composed primarily of cancellous bone. The articular surface has a biconcave surface for articulation with the proximal carpal row (scaphoid and lunate fossae), as well as a notch for articulation with the distal ulna.
- Eighty percent of axial load is supported by the distal radius and 20% by the ulna and the triangular fibrocartilage complex (TFCC).
- Reversal of the normal palmar tilt results in load transfer onto the ulna and TFCC; the remaining load is then borne eccentrically by the distal radius and is concentrated on the dorsal aspect of the scaphoid fossa.
- Numerous ligamentous attachments exist to the distal radius; these often remain intact during distal radius fracture, facilitating reduction through "ligamentotaxis."
- The volar ligaments are stronger and confer more stability to the radiocarpal articulation than the dorsal ligaments. *volar lig > dorsal lig.*

MECHANISM OF INJURY

- Common mechanisms in younger individuals include falls from a height, motor vehicle accident, or injuries sustained during athletic articipation. In elderly individuals, distal radial fractures may arise from low-energy mechanisms, such as a simple fall from a standing height.

- The most common mechanism of injury is a fall onto an outstretched hand with the wrist in dorsiflexion.
- Fractures of the distal radius are produced when the dorsiflexion of the wrist varies between 40 and 90 degrees, with lesser degrees of force required at smaller angles.
- The radius initially fails in tension on the volar aspect, with the fracture propagating dorsally, whereas bending moment forces induce compression stresses resulting in dorsal comminution. Cancellous impaction of the metaphysis further compromises dorsal stability. Additionally, shearing forces influence the injury pattern, often resulting in articular surface involvement.
- High-energy injuries (e.g., vehicular trauma) may result in significantly displaced or highly comminuted unstable fractures to the distal radius.

CLINICAL EVALUATION

- Patients typically present with variable wrist deformity and displacement of the hand in relation to the wrist (dorsal in Colles or dorsal Barton fractures and volar in Smith-type fractures). The wrist is typically swollen with ecchymosis, tenderness, and painful range of motion.
- The ipsilateral elbow and shoulder should be examined for associated injuries.
- A careful neurovascular assessment should be performed, with particular attention to median nerve function. Carpal tunnel compression symptoms are common (13% to 23%) owing to traction during forced hyperextension of the wrist, direct trauma from fracture fragments, hematoma formation, or increased compartment pressure.

RADIOGRAPHIC EVALUATION

- Posteroanterior and lateral views of the wrist should be obtained, with oblique views for further fracture definition, if necessary. Shoulder or elbow symptoms should be evaluated radiographically.
- Contralateral wrist views may help to assess the patient's normal ulnar variance and scapholunate angle.
- Computed tomography scan may help to demonstrate the extent of intra-articular involvement.
- **Normal radiographic relationships (Fig. 22.1):**
  □ **Radial inclination:** averages 23 degrees (range, 13 to 30 degrees)
  □ **Radial length:** averages 11 mm (range, 8 to 18 mm)
  □ **Palmar (volar) tilt:** averages 11 to 12 degrees (range, 0 to 28 degrees)

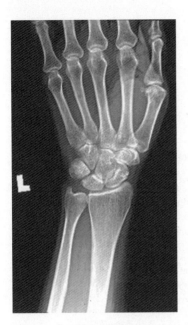
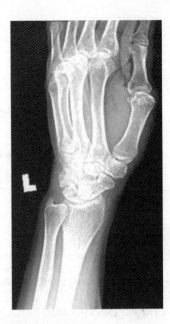
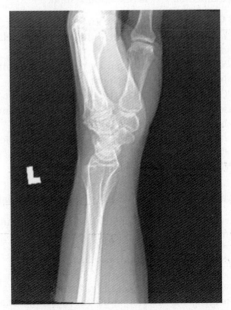

FIGURE 22.1 The normal radiographic measurements of the distal radius. (Reproduced with permission from the Orthopaedic Trauma Association.)

CLASSIFICATION

Descriptive

Open versus closed
Displacement
Angulation
Comminution
Loss of radial length

Frykman Classification of Colles Fractures

This is based on the pattern of intra-articular involvement (Fig. 22.2).

Fracture	Distal Ulna Fracture	
	Absent	Present
Extra-articular	I	II
Intra-articular involving radiocarpal joint	III	IV
Intra-articular involving distal radioulnar joint (DRUJ)	V	VI
Intra-articular involving radiocarpal and DRUJ	VII	VIII

Fernandez Classification

This is a mechanism-based classification system.

Type I: Metaphyseal bending fracture with the inherent problems of loss of palmar tilt and radial shortening relative to the ulna (DRUJ injury)

Type II: Shearing fracture requiring reduction and often buttressing of the articular segment

Type III: Compression of the articular surface *without the characteristic fragmentation*; also the potential for significant interosseous ligament injury

Type IV: Avulsion fracture or radiocarpal fracture-dislocation

Type V: Combined injury with significant soft tissue involvement owing to high-energy injury

OTA Classification of Fractures of the Distal Radius and Ulna

See Fracture and Dislocation Classification Compendium at http://www.ota.org/compendium/compendium.html.

Eponyms (Fig. 22.3)

■ Colles fracture
   □ The original description was for extra-articular fractures. Present usage of eponym includes both extra-articular and

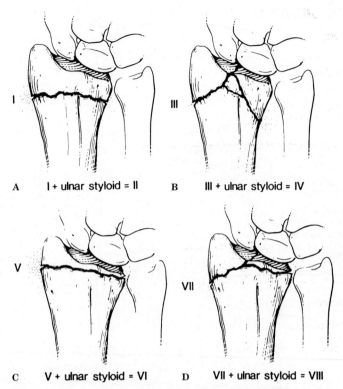

FIGURE 22.2 Frykman classification of distal radius fractures. **(A)** Frykman Type I/II, extra-articular. **(B)** Frykman Type III/IV, intra-articular radiocarpal joint. **(C)** Frykman Type V/VI, intra-articular distal radioulnar joint. **(D)** Frykman Type VII/VIII, intra-articular radiocarpal and distal radioulnar joints. (From Rockwood CA Jr, Green DP, Bucholz RW, Heckman JD, eds. *Rockwood and Green's Fractures in Adults.* Vol 1. 4th ed. Philadelphia: Lippincott–Raven; 1996:771.)

　　intra-articular distal radius fractures demonstrating various combinations of dorsal angulation (apex volar), dorsal displacement, radial shift, and radial shortening.

☐ Clinically, it has been described as a "dinner fork" deformity.

☐ More than 90% of distal radius fractures are of this pattern.

☐ The mechanism of injury is a fall onto a hyperextended, radially deviated wrist with the forearm in pronation.

☐ Intra-articular fractures are generally seen in the younger age group secondary to higher-energy forces; concomitant injuries (i.e., to nerve, carpus, and distal ulna) are more frequent, as is involvement of both the radiocarpal joint and the DRUJ.

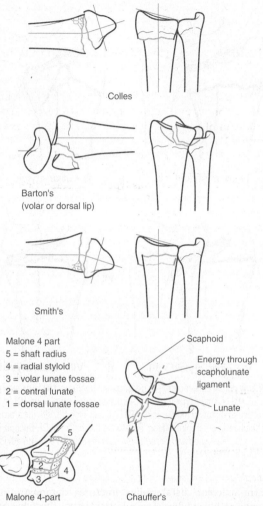

FIGURE 22.3 Eponymic classification of five basic types of distal radius fractures: four classic (Colles, Barton, Smith, and Chauffer's) fracture descriptions, and the Malone four-part fracture, which was described more recently and represents an increasing understanding of the importance of the distal radioulnar joint and the ulnar column of the radius.

- ■ Smith fracture (reverse Colles fracture)
  - □ This describes a fracture with volar angulation (apex dorsal) of the distal radius with a "garden spade" deformity or volar displacement of the hand and distal radius.

- ☐ The mechanism of injury is a fall onto a flexed wrist with the forearm fixed in supination.
- ☐ This is an unstable fracture pattern; it often requires open reduction and internal fixation because of difficulty in maintaining adequate closed reduction.
- ■ Barton fracture
  - ☐ This is a shearing mechanism of injury that results in a fracture-dislocation or subluxation of the wrist in which the dorsal or volar rim of the distal radius is displaced with the hand and carpus. Volar involvement is more common.
  - ☐ The mechanism of injury is a fall onto a dorsiflexed wrist with the forearm fixed in pronation.
  - ☐ Almost all fractures of this type are unstable and require open reduction and internal fixation with a buttress plate to achieve stable, anatomic reduction.
- ■ Radial styloid fracture (chauffeur's fracture, backfire fracture, Hutchinson fracture)
  - ☐ This is an avulsion fracture with extrinsic ligaments remaining attached to the styloid fragment. It may also be secondary to a direct blow.
  - ☐ The mechanism of injury is compression of the scaphoid against the styloid with the wrist in dorsiflexion and ulnar deviation.
  - ☐ It may involve the entire styloid or only the dorsal or volar portion.
  - ☐ It is often associated with intercarpal ligamentous injuries (i.e., scapholunate dissociation, perilunate dislocation).
  - ☐ Open reduction and internal fixation are often necessary.

TREATMENT

- ■ Factors affecting treatment include
  - ☐ Fracture pattern
  - ☐ **Local factors:** bone quality, soft tissue injury, fracture comminution, fracture displacement, and energy of injury
  - ☐ **Patient factors:** physiologic patient age, lifestyle, occupation, hand dominance, associated medical conditions, associated injuries, and compliance
- ■ Radiographic alignment parameters for acceptable reduction in an active, healthy patient include
  - ☐ **Radial length:** within 2 to 3 mm of the contralateral wrist
  - ☐ **Palmar tilt:** neutral tilt (0 degrees), but up to 10 degrees dorsal angulation
  - ☐ **Intra-articular step-off:** <2 mm
  - ☐ **Radial inclination:** <5-degree loss

- Carpal alignment after distal radius fracture may have the most influence on outcome following distal radius fracture.
  - □ **Carpal alignment is measured by the intersection of two lines on the lateral radiograph:** one parallel and through the middle of the radial shaft and the other through and parallel to the capitate. If the two lines intersect within the carpus, then the carpus is aligned. If the two lines intersect out with the carpus, then the carpus is malaligned.
- **Several factors have been associated with redisplacement following closed manipulation of a distal radius fracture:**
  - □ **The initial displacement of the fracture:** The greater the degree of displacement (particularly radial shortening), the more energy is imparted to the fracture resulting in a higher likelihood that closed treatment will be unsuccessful.
  - □ **The age of the patient:** Elderly patients with osteopenic bones tend to displace, particularly late.
  - □ The extent of metaphyseal comminution (the metaphyseal defect), as evidenced by either plain radiograph or computerized tomography.
  - □ Displacement following closed treatment is a predictor of instability, and repeat manipulation is unlikely to result in a successful radiographic outcome.

Nonoperative

- All displaced fractures should undergo closed reduction, even if it is expected that surgical management will be needed.
  - □ Fracture reduction helps to limit post injury swelling, provides pain relief, and relieves compression on the median nerve.
- Cast immobilization is indicated for
  - □ Nondisplaced or minimally displaced fractures
  - □ Displaced fractures with a stable fracture pattern, which can be expected to unite within acceptable radiographic parameters
  - □ Low-demand elderly patients in whom future functional impairment is less of a priority than immediate health concerns and/or operative risks
- Hematoma block with supplemental intravenous sedation, Bier block, or conscious sedation can be used to provide analgesia for closed reduction.
- **Technique of closed reduction (dorsally tilted fracture):**
  - □ The distal fragment is hyperextended.
  - □ Traction is applied to reduce the distal to the proximal fragment with pressure applied to the distal radius.
  - □ A well-molded long arm ("sugar-tong") splint is applied, with the wrist in neutral to slight flexion.

- ☐ One must avoid extreme positions of the wrist and hand.
- ☐ The cast should leave the metacarpophalangeal joints free.
- Once swelling has subsided, a well-molded cast is applied.
- The ideal forearm position, duration of immobilization, and need for a long arm cast remain controversial; no prospective study has demonstrated the superiority of one method over another.
- Extreme wrist flexion should be avoided, because it increases carpal canal pressure (and thus median nerve compression) as well as digital stiffness. Fractures that require extreme wrist flexion to maintain reduction may require operative fixation.
- The cast should be worn for approximately 6 weeks or until radiographic evidence of union has occurred.
- Frequent radiographic examination is necessary to detect loss of reduction.

Operative

- Indications
  - ☐ High-energy injury
  - ☐ Secondary loss of reduction
  - ☐ Articular comminution, step-off, or gap
  - ☐ Metaphyseal comminution or bone loss
  - ☐ Loss of volar buttress with displacement
  - ☐ DRUJ incongruity
  - ☐ Open fractures

Operative Techniques

- **Percutaneous pinning:** This is primarily used for extra-articular fractures or two-part intra-articular fractures.
  - ☐ It may be accomplished using two or three Kirschner wires placed across the fracture site, generally from the radial styloid, directed proximally and from the dorsoulnar side of the distal radial fragment directed proximally. Transulnar pinning with multiple pins has also been described.
  - ☐ Percutaneous pinning is generally used to supplement short arm casting or external fixation. The pins may be removed 6 to 8 weeks postoperatively, with the cast maintained for an additional 2 to 3 weeks.
- Kapandji "intrafocal" pinning
  - ☐ This is a technique of trapping the distal fragment by buttressing to prevent displacement.
  - ☐ The wires are inserted both radially and dorsally directly into the fracture site. The wires are then levered up and then directed into the proximal intact opposite cortex.

- ☐ The fragments are thus buttressed from displacing dorsally or proximally.
- ☐ In addition to being relatively simple and inexpensive, this technique has been shown to be very effective, particularly in elderly patients.
- ■ **External fixation:** Its use has diminished in popularity since the advent of volar locked plating despite low complication rates.
  - ☐ Spanning external fixation
    - Ligamentotaxis is used to restore radial length and radial inclination, but it rarely restores palmar tilt.
    - External fixation alone is not sufficiently stable to prevent some degree of collapse and loss of palmar tilt during the course of healing. Supplemental K-wire fixation is needed.
    - Overdistraction should be avoided because it may result in finger stiffness and may be recognized by increased intercarpal distance on intraoperative fluoroscopy.
    - Pins are retained for 6 to 8 weeks of external fixation.
  - ☐ Nonspanning external fixation
    - A nonspanning fixator is one that stabilizes the distal radius fracture by securing pins in the radius alone, proximal to and distal to the fracture site.
    - It requires a sufficiently large intact segment of intact distal radius.
    - May be better to preserve volar tilt, prevent carpal malalignment, and result in improved grip strength and hand function than spanning external fixation.
- ■ Open reduction and internal fixation
  - ☐ **Dorsal plating:** This has several theoretic advantages.
    - It is technically familiar to most surgeons, and the approach avoids the neurovascular structures on the palmar side.
    - The fixation is on the compression side of the fracture and provides a buttress against collapse.
    - Initial reports of the technique demonstrated successful outcomes with the theoretic advantages of earlier return of function and better restoration of radial anatomy than seen with external fixation.
    - Dorsal plating has been associated with extensor tendon complications.
  - ☐ Volar nonlocked plating
    - The primary indication is a buttress plate for the shear fracture of the volar Barton.
    - This construct may be unable to maintain fracture reduction in the presence of dorsal comminution.
  - ☐ Volar locked plating

- Locked volar plating has increased in popularity because this implant has been shown to stabilize distal radius fractures with dorsal comminution.
- Has surpassed external fixation as the most popular mode of fracture fixation of the distal radius.
- The dorsal side of the radius may be accessed through an extension of the volar approach.
  □ Fragment specific plating
  - Has been advocated for more complex fracture patterns involving several aspects of the radial and ulnar columns.
- Adjunctive fixation
  □ Supplemental graft may be autograft, allograft, or synthetic graft.
  □ Adjunctive Kirschner wire fixation may be helpful with smaller fragments.
- Arthroscopically assisted intra-articular fracture reduction
  □ Although arthroscopy has been invaluable at enhancing existing knowledge of associated soft tissue lesions in distal radius fractures, it is controversial whether this technique provides outcomes superior to those of conventional techniques.
  □ Fractures that may benefit most from adjunctive arthroscopy are (1) articular fractures without metaphyseal comminution, particularly those with central impaction fragments; and (2) fractures with evidence of substantial interosseous ligament or TFCC injury without large ulnar styloid base fracture.
- **Ulna styloid fractures:** Indications for fixation of ulna styloid are controversial. Some authors have advocated fixation for displaced fractures at the base of the ulna styloid.

COMPLICATIONS

- **Median nerve dysfunction:** Management is controversial, although there is general agreement about the following:
  □ A complete median nerve lesion with no improvement following fracture reduction requires surgical exploration (rare).
  □ Median nerve dysfunction developing after reduction mandates release of the splint and positioning of the wrist in neutral position; if there is no improvement, exploration and release of the carpal tunnel should be considered.
  □ An incomplete lesion in a fracture requiring operative intervention is a relative indication for carpal tunnel release.
- **Malunion or nonunion:** This typically results from inadequate fracture reduction or stabilization; it may require internal fixation with or without osteotomy with bone graft. Malunion in the elderly without functional disturbance is generally the rule.

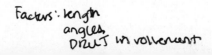
Factors: length
angles
DRUJ involvement

- Complications of external fixation include reflex sympathetic dystrophy, pin tract infection, wrist and finger stiffness, fracture through a pin site, and radial sensory neuritis. Open pin placement is advisable to allow visualization of the superficial radial nerve.

- **Posttraumatic osteoarthritis:** This is a consequence of radiocarpal and radioulnar articular injury, thus emphasizing the need for anatomic restoration of the articular surface.

- **Finger, wrist, and elbow stiffness:** This occurs especially with prolonged immobilization in a cast or with external fixation; it emphasizes the need for aggressive occupational therapy to mobilize the digits and elbow while wrist immobilization is in place, as well as a possible supervised therapy regimen once immobilization has been discontinued.

- Tendon rupture, most commonly extensor pollicis longus, may occur as an early or late complication of distal radius fractures, even in cases of minimally displaced injuries. Degeneration of the tendon, owing to vascular disruption of the tendon sheath as well as mechanical impingement on the callus, results in attrition of tendon integrity. Dorsal plating has been most often associated with extensor tendon complications.

- Midcarpal instability (i.e., dorsal or volar intercalated segmental instability) may result from radiocarpal ligamentous injury or a dorsal or volar rim distal radius disruption.

Wrist

EPIDEMIOLOGY

- **Approximate incidences of carpal fractures are as follows:**
  - Scaphoid (68.2%)
  - Triquetrum (18.3%)
  - Trapezium (4.3%)
  - Lunate (3.9%)
  - Capitate (1.9%)
  - Hamate (1.7%)
  - Pisiform (1.3%)
  - Trapezoid (0.4%)
- The annual incidence of carpal fractures in the United States was reported at more than 678,000 in 1995, of which approximately 70% are scaphoid fractures—fractures to bones of the proximal row.

ANATOMY

- The distal radius has articular facets for the scaphoid and lunate separated by a ridge. The sigmoid notch articulates with the distal ulna.
- The distal ulna articulates with the sigmoid notch of the distal radius. The fovea (base) of the ulna styloid process serves as the attachment for the triangular fibrocartilage complex (TFCC).
- Carpal bones (Fig. 23.1)
  - **Proximal row:** This consists of the scaphoid (an oblique strut that spans both rows), lunate, triquetrum, and pisiform.
  - **Distal row:** The trapezium, trapezoid, capitate, and hamate are connected to one another and to the base of the metacarpals by strong ligaments, making the distal row relatively immobile.
  - The lunate is the key to carpal stability.
    - It is connected to both scaphoid and triquetrum by strong interosseous ligaments.
    - Injury to the scapholunate or lunotriquetral ligaments leads to asynchronous motion of the lunate and dissociative carpal instability patterns. SL = DISI (dorsal intercalated segmental instability) and LT tear = VISI (volar intercalated segmental instability)

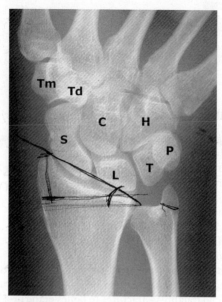

FIGURE 23.1 The wrist is composed of two rows of bones that provide motion and transfer forces: scaphoid (*S*), lunate (*L*), triquetrum (*T*), pisiform (*P*), trapezium (*Tm*), trapezoid (*Td*), capitate (*C*), hamate (*H*). (From Bucholz RW, Heckman JD, Court-Brown C, et al., eds. *Rockwood and Green's Fractures in Adults.* 6th ed. Philadelphia: Lippincott Williams & Wilkins; 2006.)

- The main articulations are the distal radioulnar, radiocarpal, and midcarpal.
- Normal anatomic relationships (see Fig. 23.1)
  - **Radial inclination:** averages 23 degrees (range, 13 to 30 degrees)
  - **Radial length:** averages 11 mm (range, 8 to 18 mm)
  - **Palmar (volar) tilt:** averages 11 to 12 degrees (range, 0 to 28 degrees)
  - **The 0-degree capitolunate angle:** a straight line drawn down the third metacarpal shaft, capitate, lunate, and shaft of radius with wrist in neutral position
  - The 47-degree scapholunate angle (normal range, 30 to 70 degrees); <3 mm scapholunate space
- Wrist ligaments (Figs. 23.2 and 23.3)
  - Extrinsic ligaments connect the radius to the carpus and the carpus to the metacarpals.

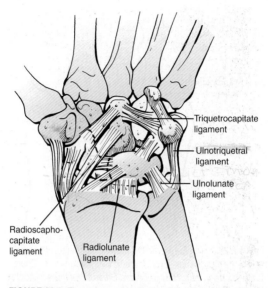

Triquetrocapitate
ligament

Ulnotriquetral
ligament

Ulnolunate
ligament

Radioscapho-
capitate
ligament

Radiolunate
ligament

FIGURE 23.2 The palmar capsule consists of two major ligamentous inclusions: The radiolunate ligament is the deeper of
the two, which proceeds to the triquetrum and composes in
effect the radiolunotriquetral ligament. The more distal and
superficial component is often referred to as the arcuate ligament or distal V. The radial component of this ligament is the
radioscaphocapitate ligament. The ulnar component of the arcuate ligament is the triquetrocapitate ligament. (From Bucholz
RW, Heckman JD, Court-Brown C, et al., eds. *Rockwood and
Green's Fractures in Adults*. 6th ed. Philadelphia: Lippincott
Williams & Wilkins; 2006.)

☐ Intrinsic ligaments connect carpal bone to carpal bone (e.g.,
scapholunate and lunotriquetral ligaments).
☐ In general, the volar ligaments are stronger than the dorsal
ligaments.
☐ Important volar ligaments include
  • The radioscaphocapitate (guides scaphoid kinematics)
  • The radioscapholunate also called the ligament of Testut (not
    a strong ligament, a neurovascular tuft of synovium)
  • The short radiolunate
  • The radiolunotriquetral (supports the proximal row, stabilizes
    the radiolunate and lunotriquetral joints)
    – The important dorsal ligaments are
    – The dorsal intercarpal (from trapezium to triquetrum)
    – The radiocarpal (from the triquetrum to the radius)

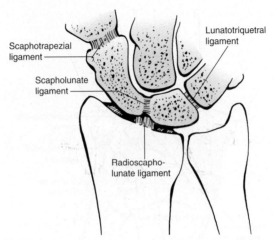

FIGURE 23.3 The intra-articular intrinsic ligaments connect adjacent carpal bones. (From Bucholz RW, Heckman JD, Court-Brown C, et al., eds. *Rockwood and Green's Fractures in Adults.* 6th ed. Philadelphia: Lippincott Williams & Wilkins; 2006.)

- □ The proximal and distal carpal rows are attached by capsular ligaments on each side of the lunocapitate joint.
  - ● Injury to these ligaments leads to abnormal motion between the two rows and to nondissociative wrist instability patterns.
- □ **Space of Poirier:** This ligament-free area in the palmar aspect of the capitolunate space is an area of potential weakness.
- □ The TFCC is a major stabilizer of the ulnar carpus and distal radioulnar joint.
  - ● The TFCC absorbs about 20% of the axial load across the wrist joint.
  - ● It consists of several components, including the ulnotriquetral ligament, themeniscal homologue, articular disc, ulnolunate ligament, and ulnar collateral ligament.
- ■ Vascular supply (Fig. 23.4)
  - □ The radial, ulnar, and anterior interosseous arteries combine to form a network of transverse arterial arches both dorsal and volar to the carpus.
  - □ The blood supply to the scaphoid is derived primarily from the radial artery, both dorsally and volarly. The volar scaphoid branches supply the distal 20% to 30% of the scaphoid, whereas branches entering the dorsal ridge supply the proximal 70% to 80%.

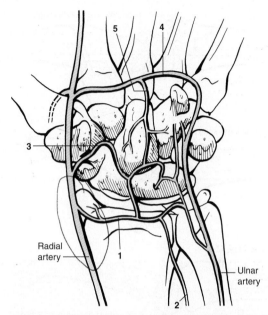

FIGURE 23.4 Schematic drawing of the arterial supply of the palmar aspect of the carpus. Circulation of the wrist is obtained through the radial, ulnar, and anterior interosseous arteries and the deep palmar arch: *1,* palmar radiocarpal arch; *2,* palmar branch of anterior interosseous artery; *3,* palmar intercarpal arch; *4,* deep palmar arch; and *5,* recurrent artery. (From Bucholz RW, Heckman JD, Court-Brown C, et al., eds. *Rockwood and Green's Fractures in Adults.* 6th ed. Philadelphia: Lippincott Williams & Wilkins; 2006.)

- ☐ The lunate receives blood supply from both its volar and dorsal surfaces in most cases (80%). About 20% of lunates have only a volar blood supply.
- ■ Kinematics
  - ☐ The global motion of the wrist is composed of flexion and extension, radioulnar deviation at the radiocarpal joint, and axial rotation around the distal radioulnar joint.
  - ☐ The radiocarpal articulation acts as a universal joint allowing a small degree of intercarpal motion related to rotation of individual carpal bones.
  - ☐ The forearm accounts for about 140 degrees of rotation.
  - ☐ Radiocarpal joint motion is primarily flexion and extension of nearly equal proportions (70 degrees), and radial and ulnar deviation of 20 and 40 degrees, respectively.

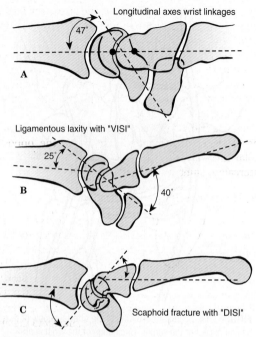

FIGURE 23.5 Schematic drawing of carpal instability. **(A)** Normal longitudinal alignment of the carpal bones with the scaphoid axis at a 47-degree angle to the axes of the capitate, lunate, and radius. **(B)** A volar intercalated segmental instability (VISI) deformity is usually associated with disruption of the lunatotriquetral ligament. **(C)** A dorsal intercalated segmental instability (DISI) deformity is associated with scapholunate ligament disruption or a displaced scaphoid fracture. (From Bucholz RW, Heckman JD, Court-Brown C, et al., eds. *Rockwood and Green's Fractures in Adults.* 6th ed. Baltimore: Lippincott Williams & Wilkins; 2005.)

- ☐ The scaphoid rests on the radioscaphocapitate ligament at its waist. Using the ligament as an axis, it rotates from a volar flexed perpendicular position to a dorsiflexed longitudinal position. With the wrist in radial deviation, the scaphoid flexes; with ulnar deviation, the scaphoid extends.
- ■ Pathomechanics (Fig. 23.5)
  - ☐ Classically, the radius, lunate, and capitate have been described as a central "link" that is colinear in the sagittal plane.

- ☐ The scaphoid serves as a connecting strut. Any flexion moment transmitted across the scaphoid is balanced by an extension moment at the triquetrum.
- ☐ When the scaphoid is destabilized by fracture or scapholunate ligament disruption, the lunate and triquetrum assume a position of excessive dorsiflexion (dorsal intercalated segmental instability [DISI]) and the scapholunate angle becomes abnormally high (>70 degrees).
- ☐ When the triquetrum is destabilized (usually by disruption of the lunotriquetral ligament complex), the opposite pattern (volar intercalated segmental instability [VISI]) is seen as the intercalated lunate segment volar flexes.

MECHANISM OF INJURY

- ■ The most common mechanism of carpal injury is a fall onto the outstretched hand, resulting in an axial compressive force with the wrist in hyperextension. The volar ligaments are placed under tension with compression and shear forces applied dorsally, especially when the wrist is extended beyond its physiologic limits.
- ■ Excessive ulnar deviation and intercarpal supination result in a predictable pattern of perilunate injury, progressing from the radial side of the carpus to the mid carpus and finally to the ulnar carpus.

CLINICAL EVALUATION

- ■ The clinical presentation of individual carpal injuries is variable, but in general, the most consistent sign of carpal injury is well-localized tenderness.
- ■ Gross deformity may be present, ranging from displacement of the carpus to prominence of individual carpal bones.
- ■ Provocative tests may reproduce or exacerbate pain, crepitus, or displacement indicative of individual carpal injuries (see specific carpal injuries).

RADIOGRAPHIC EVALUATION

- ■ Posteroanterior (PA) and lateral x-rays are each taken in the neutral position.
  - ☐ *Gilula lines* (three smooth radiographic arcs) should be examined on the PA view. Disruption of these arcs indicates ligamentous instability.
- ■ **For further diagnosis of carpal and mainly scaphoid fractures:**
  - ☐ A scaphoid view (anteroposterior [AP] x-ray with wrist supinated 30 degrees and in ulnar deviation) is obtained.
  - ☐ A pronated oblique view is indicated.

- If there is the suspicion of carpal instability, additional views in maximal radial and ulnar deviation are recommended as well as a clenched-fist PA.
- Further views can be done in maximal flexion and extension.
- Arthrography, magnetic resonance (MR), wrist arthrography, videoradiography, and arthroscopy can assist in the diagnosis of carpal ligament injuries.
- Computed tomography (CT) scans are helpful in evaluating carpal fractures, malunion, nonunion, and bone loss.
- MRI scans are sensitive to detect occult fractures and osteonecrosis of the carpal bones as well as detecting soft tissue injury, including ruptures of the scapholunate ligament and TFCC.

CLASSIFICATION

OTA Classification of Carpal Fractures and Fracture-Dislocations

See Fracture and Dislocation Classification Compendium at http://www.ota.org/compendium/compendium.html.

SPECIFIC FRACTURES

Scaphoid

- Fractures of the scaphoid are common and account for about 50% to 80% of carpal injuries.
- Anatomically, the scaphoid is divided into proximal and distal poles, a tubercle, and a waist; 80% of the scaphoid is covered with articular cartilage (Fig. 23.6).
- Ligamentous attachments to the scaphoid include the radioscaphocapitate ligament, which variably attaches to the ulnar aspect of the scaphoid waist, and the dorsal intercarpal ligament, which provides the primary vascular supply to the scaphoid.
- The major vascular supply is derived from scaphoid branches of the radial artery, entering the dorsal ridge and supplying 70% to 80% of the scaphoid, including the proximal pole. The remaining distal aspect is supplied through branches entering the tubercle. Fractures at the scaphoid waist or proximal third depend on fracture union for revascularization (Fig. 23.7).
- The most common mechanism is a fall onto the outstretched hand that imposes a force of dorsiflexion, ulnar deviation, and intercarpal supination.
- Clinical evaluation.

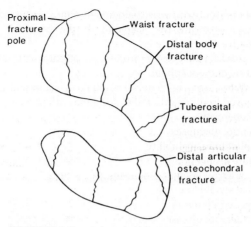

FIGURE 23.6 Types of scaphoid fractures. The scaphoid is susceptible to fractures at any level. (From Bucholz RW, Heckman JD, Court-Brown C, et al., eds. *Rockwood and Green's Fractures in Adults.* Vol 1. 4th ed. Philadelphia: Lippincott–Raven; 1996:826.)

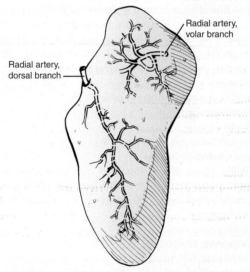

FIGURE 23.7 The vascular supply of the scaphoid is provided by two vascular pedicles. (From Bucholz RW, Heckman JD, Court-Brown C, et al., eds. *Rockwood and Green's Fractures in Adults.* 6th ed. Philadelphia: Lippincott Williams & Wilkins; 2006.)

- Patients present with wrist pain and swelling, with tenderness to palpation overlying the scaphoid in the anatomic snuffbox. Provocative tests include
  - □ **The scaphoid shift test:** reproduction of pain with dorsal-volar shifting of the scaphoid.
  - □ **The Watson test:** painful dorsal scaphoid displacement as the wrist is moved from ulnar to radial deviation with palmar pressure on the tuberosity.
- Differential diagnoses
  - □ Scapholunate instability
  - □ Lunate dislocation
  - □ Flexor carpi radialis tendon rupture
  - □ Radial styloid fracture
  - □ Trapezium fracture
  - □ De Quervain disease
  - □ Carpometacarpal (basal) joint arthrosis
- Radiographic evaluation
  - □ This includes a PA view of the wrist in ulnar deviation to extend the scaphoid, a lateral, a supinated AP and pronated oblique-view, and a clenched supinated view in ulnar deviation.
  - □ Initial films are nondiagnostic in up to 25% of cases.
  - □ If the clinical examination suggests fracture but radiographs are not diagnostic, a trial of immobilization with follow-up radiographs 1 to 2 weeks after injury may demonstrate the fracture.
  - □ Technetium bone scan, MRI, CT, and ultrasound evaluation may be used to diagnose occult scaphoid fractures.
- Classification
  - □ Based on fracture pattern (Russe)
    - Horizontal oblique
    - Transverse
    - Vertical oblique
  - □ Based on displacement
    - **Stable:** nondisplaced fractures with no step-off in any plane
    - **Unstable:** displacement with 1 mm or more step-off scapholunate angulation >60 degrees or radiolunate angulation >15 degrees
  - □ Based on location
    - **Tuberosity:** 17% to 20%
    - **Distal pole:** 10% to 12%
    - **Waist:** 66% to 70%
      Horizontal oblique: 13% to 14%
      Vertical oblique: 8% to 9%
      Transverse: 45% to 48%
    - **Proximal pole:** 5% to 7%

Treatment

- ■ Indications for nonoperative treatment
  - □ Nondisplaced distal third fracture
  - □ Tuberosity fractures
- ■ Nonoperative treatment
  - □ Long arm thumb spica cast for 6 weeks; limit forearm rotation
  - □ Immobilization in slight flexion and slight radial deviation
  - □ Replacement with short arm thumb spica cast at 6 weeks until united
  - □ **Expected time to union:**
    - • **Distal third:** 6 to 8 weeks
    - • **Middle third:** 8 to 12 weeks
    - • **Proximal third:** 12 to 24 weeks
- ■ Management of suspected scaphoid fractures
  - □ In patients with an injury and positive examination findings but normal x-rays, immobilization for 1 to 2 weeks (thumb spica) is indicated.
  - □ Repeat x-rays if the patient is still symptomatic.
  - □ If pain is still present but x-rays continue to be normal, consider MRI.
  - □ If an acute diagnosis is necessary, consider MRI or CT immediately.
- ■ **Healing rates with nonoperative treatment depends on fracture location:**

Tuberosity and distal third	100%
Waist	80% to 90%
Proximal Pole	60% to 70%

Proximal fractures are prone to nonunion and osteonecrosis

- ■ Operative treatment
  - □ Indications for surgery
    - • Fracture displacement >1 mm
    - • Radiolunate angle >15 degrees
    - • Scapholunate angle >60 degrees
    - • "Humpback" deformity
    - • Nonunion
  - □ Surgical techniques
    - • Most involve the insertion of screws.
    - • Controversy exists about open versus percutaneous techniques.
    - • Open techniques are needed for nonunions and fractures with unacceptable displacement.
    - • Closed techniques are appropriate for acute fractures with minimal displacement.

- □ The volar approach between the flexor carpi radialis and the radial artery provides good exposure for open reduction and internal fixation and repair of the radioscapholunate ligament. The volar approach is the least damaging to the vascular supply of the vulnerable proximal pole.
- □ Postoperative immobilization consists of a short arm thumb spica cast for 6 weeks.
- ■ Complications
  - □ **Delayed union, nonunion, and malunion:** These are reported to occur with greater frequency when there is a delay in treatment, as well as with proximal scaphoid fractures. They may necessitate operative fixation with bone grafting to achieve union.
  - □ **Osteonecrosis:** This occurs especially with fractures of the proximal pole, owing to the tenuous vascular supply.

Lunate

- ■ The lunate is the fourth most fractured carpal bone after the scaphoid, triquetrum, and trapezium.
- ■ The lunate has been referred to as the "carpal keystone," because it rests in the well-protected concavity of the lunate fossa of the distal radius, anchored by interosseous ligaments to the scaphoid and triquetrum, and distally is congruent with the convex head of the capitate.
- ■ Its vascular supply is derived from the proximal carpal arcade dorsally and volarly, with three variable intralunate anastomoses.
- ■ The mechanism of injury is typically a fall onto an outstretched hand with the wrist in hyperextension, or a strenuous push with the wrist in extension.
- ■ Clinical evaluation reveals tenderness to palpation on the dorsal wrist overlying the distal radius and lunate, as well as painful range of motion.
- ■ **Radiographic evaluation:** PA and lateral views of the wrist are often inadequate to establish the diagnosis of lunate fracture because osseous details are frequently obscured by overlapping densities.
  - □ Oblique views may be helpful, but CT scanning best demonstrates fractures.
  - □ MRI has been used with increasing frequency to appreciate the vascular changes associated with injury and healing and is the imaging test of choice for evaluation of Kienbock disease.
- ■ **Classification:** Acute fractures of the lunate can be classified into five groups:
  - □ Frontal fractures of the palmar pole with involvement of the palmar nutrient arteries

- ☐ Osteochondral fractures of the proximal articular surface without substantial damage to the nutrient vessels
- ☐ Frontal fractures of the dorsal pole
- ☐ Transverse fractures of the body
- ☐ Transarticular frontal fractures of the body of the lunate
- ■ Treatment
  - ☐ Nondisplaced fractures should be treated in a short or long arm cast or splint with follow-up at close intervals to evaluate progression of healing.
  - ☐ Displaced or angulated fractures should be treated surgically to allow adequate apposition for formation of vascular anastomoses.
- ■ Complications
  - ☐ **Osteonecrosis:** Depending on the degree of involvement, osteonecrosis may represent the most devastating complication of lunate fractures, with advanced collapse and radiocarpal degeneration. This may require further operative intervention for pain relief, including radial shortening, radial wedge osteotomy, ulnar lengthening, or salvage procedures such as proximal row carpectomy, wrist denervation, or arthrodesis. (Note: Most cases of Kienbock disease are idiopathic.)

Triquetrum

- ■ The triquetrum is the carpal bone that is most commonly fractured after the scaphoid.
- ■ Most fractures of the triquetrum are avulsion or impaction injuries that may be associated with ligament damage.
- ■ Most commonly, injury occurs with the wrist in extension and ulnar deviation, resulting in an impingement shear fracture by the ulnar styloid against the dorsal triquetrum.
- ■ Clinical evaluation reveals tenderness to palpation on the dorsoulnar aspect of the wrist, directly dorsal to the pisiform, as well as painful range of wrist motion.
- ■ Radiographic evaluation
  - ☐ Transverse fractures of the body can generally be identified on the PA view.
  - ☐ Dorsal triquetral fractures are not easily appreciated on AP and lateral views of the wrist owing to superimposition of the lunate. An oblique, pronated lateral view may help to visualize the dorsal triquetrum.
- ■ Treatment
  - ☐ Nondisplaced fractures of the body or dorsal chip fractures may be treated in a short arm cast or splint for 6 weeks.

□ Displaced fractures may be amenable to open reduction and internal fixation.

Pisiform

■ Fractures of the pisiform are rare.

■ The mechanism of injury is either a direct blow to the volar aspect of the wrist or a fall onto an outstretched, dorsiflexed hand.

■ Clinical evaluation demonstrates tenderness on the volar aspect of the ulnar wrist with painful passive extension of the wrist as the flexor carpus ulnaris is placed under tension.

■ **Radiographic evaluation:** Pisiform fractures are not well visualized on standard views of the wrist; special views include a lateral view of the wrist with forearm supination of 20 to 45 degrees (beware of getting called to the ED for a carpal bone dislocation that is just the pisiform being seen on the supinated lateral film!) or a carpal tunnel view (20-degree supination oblique view demonstrating an oblique projection of the wrist in radial deviation and semisupination).

■ Treatment of nondisplaced or minimally displaced fractures consists of a short arm splint or short arm cast for 6 weeks. Displaced fractures may require fragment excision, either early, in the case of a severely displaced fragment, or late, in the case of a pisiform fracture that has resulted in painful nonunion.

Trapezium

■ Fractures of the trapezium comprise approximately 3% to 5% of all carpal bone fractures.

■ About 60% of the reported cases have an unsatisfactory outcome secondary to degenerative changes.

■ Most are ridge avulsion fractures or vertical fractures of the body.

■ The mechanism of injury is axial loading of the adducted thumb, driving the base of the first metacarpal onto the articular surface of the trapezium.

□ Avulsion fractures may occur with forceful deviation, traction, or rotation of the thumb.

□ Direct trauma to the palmar arch may result in avulsion of the trapezial ridge by the transverse carpal ligament.

■ Clinical evaluation reveals tenderness to palpation of the radial wrist, accompanied by painful range of motion at the first carpometacarpal joint.

■ **Radiographic evaluation:** Fractures are usually identifiable on standard PA and lateral views.

□ Superimposition of the first metacarpal base may be eliminated by obtaining a Robert view, or a true PA view of the first carpometacarpal joint and trapezium, taken with the hand in maximum pronation.

☐ A carpal tunnel view may be necessary for adequate visualization of dorsal ridge fractures.

■ Treatment

☐ Nondisplaced fractures are generally amenable to thumb spica splinting or casting to immobilize the first carpometacarpal joint for 6 weeks.

☐ Indications for open reduction and internal fixation include articular involvement of the carpometacarpal articulation, comminuted fractures, and displaced fractures.

☐ Comminuted fractures may require supplemental bone grafting.

■ Complications

☐ Posttraumatic osteoarthritis may result in decreased or painful range of motion at the first carpometacarpal joint. Irreparable joint damage may necessitate fusion or excisional arthroplasty.

Trapezoid

■ Because of the shape and position of the trapezoid, fractures are rare. An axial load transmitted through the second metacarpal may lead to dislocation, more often dorsal, with associated capsular ligament disruption.

■ Direct trauma from blast or crush injuries may cause trapezoid fracture, although this is often in conjunction with other injuries.

■ Clinical evaluation demonstrates tenderness proximal to the base of the second metacarpal with a variable dorsal prominence representing a dislocated trapezoid. Range of motion of the second carpometacarpal joint is painful and limited.

■ **Radiographic evaluation:** Fractures can be identified on the PA radiograph based on a loss of the normal relationship between the second metacarpal base and the trapezoid. Comparison with the contralateral, uninjured wrist may aid in the diagnosis. The trapezoid, or fracture fragments, may be superimposed over the trapezium or capitate, and the second metacarpal may be proximally displaced.

☐ Oblique views or CT may aid in the diagnosis if osseous details are obscured by overlap.

■ Treatment

☐ Nondisplaced fractures may be treated with a splint or short arm cast for 6 weeks.

☐ Indications for open reduction and internal fixation include displaced fractures, especially those involving the carpometacarpal articulation. These may be addressed with open reduction and internal fixation with Kirschner wires with attention to restoration of articular congruity.

- ■ Complications
  - □ Posttraumatic osteoarthritis may result at the second carpometacarpal articulation if joint congruity is not restored.

Capitate

- ■ Isolated injury to the capitate is uncommon, owing to its relatively protected position.
- ■ A fracture of the capitate is more commonly associated with greater arc injury pattern (transscaphoid transcapitate perilunate fracture-dislocation). A variation of this is the "naviculocapitate syndrome," in which the capitate and scaphoid are fractured without associated dislocation.
- ■ The mechanism of injury is typically direct trauma or a crushing force that results in associated carpal or metacarpal fractures.
- ■ Clinical evaluation reveals point tenderness as well as variable painful dorsiflexion of the wrist as the capitate impinges on the dorsal rim of the radius.
- ■ Fractures of the capitate can usually be identified on standard scaphoid views.
- ■ Diagnosis may require a CT scan.
- ■ **Treatment:** Capitate fractures require reduction to diminish the risk of osteonecrosis. If closed reduction is unattainable, open reduction and internal fixation are indicated, usually with Kirschner wires or lag screws, to restore normal anatomy.
- ■ Complications
  - □ **Midcarpal arthritis:** This is caused by capitate collapse as a result of displacement of the proximal pole.
  - □ **Osteonecrosis:** This is rare but results in functional impairment; it emphasizes the need for accurate diagnosis and stable reduction.

Hamate

- ■ The hamate may be fractured through its distal articular surface, through other articular surfaces, or through its hamulus, or hook.
- ■ A distal articular fracture accompanied by fifth metacarpal subluxation may occur when axial force is transmitted down the shaft of the metacarpal, such as with a fist strike or a fall.
- ■ Fractures of the body of the hamate generally occur with direct trauma or crush injuries to the hand.
- ■ Fracture of the hook of the hamate is a frequent athletic injury sustained when the palm of the hand is struck by an object (e.g., baseball bat, golf club, hockey stick). Generally, it occurs at the base of the hook, although avulsion fractures of the tip may occur.

- **Clinical evaluation:** Patients typically present with pain and tenderness over the hamate. Ulnar and median neuropathy can also be seen, as well as rare injuries to the ulnar artery, which is located in proximity to the hook of the hamate, in Guyon's canal, along with the ulnar nerve.

- **Radiographic evaluation:** The diagnosis of hamate fracture can usually be made on the basis of the PA view of the wrist. A fracture of the hook of the hamate can be visualized on the carpal tunnel or a 20-degree supination oblique view (oblique projection of the wrist in radial deviation and semisupination). The CT scan is the best radiographic test to visualize the fracture. A hamate fracture should not be confused with an os hamulus proprium, which represents an ossification center that has failed to fuse.

- The classification of hamate fractures is descriptive.

- Treatment
  - □ Nondisplaced hamate fractures may be treated with immobilization in a short arm splint or cast for 6 weeks.
  - □ Displaced fractures of the body may be amenable to Kirschner wire or screw fixation. Fractures of the hook of the hamate may be treated with excision of the fragment for displaced fragments or in cases of symptomatic nonunion.

- Complications
  - □ **Symptomatic nonunion:** This may be treated with excision of the nonunited fragment.
  - □ **Ulnar or median neuropathy:** This is related to the proximity of the hamate to these nerves and may require surgical exploration and release.
  - □ **Ruptures of the flexor tendons to the small finger:** They result from attritional wear at the fracture site.

PERILUNATE DISLOCATIONS AND FRACTURE-DISLOCATIONS

- The lunate, which is normally securely attached to the distal radius by ligamentous attachments, is commonly referred to as the "carpal keystone."

- **Greater arc injury:** This passes through the scaphoid, capitate, triquetrum, or distal radial styloid and often results in transscaphoid, transscaphoid transcapitate, or transradial styloid perilunate fracture-dislocations (Fig. 23.8).

- **Lesser arc injury:** This follows a curved path around the lunate, involving only the soft tissues through the midcarpal joint, scapholunate, and lunatotriquetral ligaments and results in perilunate and lunate dislocations.

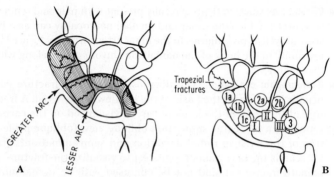

FIGURE 23.8 Vulnerable zones of the carpus. **(A)** A lesser arch injury follows a curved path through the radial styloid, midcarpal joint, and the lunatotriquetral space. A greater arc injury passes through the scaphoid, capitate, and triquetrum. **(B)** Lesser and greater arc injuries can be considered as three stages of the perilunate fracture or ligament instabilities. (From Johnson RP. The acutely injured wrist and its residuals. *Clin Orthop.* 1980;149:33–44.)

- The most common injury is transscaphoid perilunate fracture-dislocation (de Quervain injury).
- Mechanism of injury
  - **Perilunate injuries:** Load is applied to the thenar eminence, forcing the wrist into extension.
  - **Injury progresses through several stages (Mayfield progression):**
    - It usually begins radially through the body of scaphoid (fracture) or through scapholunate interval (dissociation), although both are possible in the same injury (rare).
    - Force is then transmitted ulnarly through the space of Poirier (between the lunate and the capitate).
    - Subsequently, force transmission disrupts the lunotriquetral articulation (Fig. 23.9).
    - Finally, the lunate can dislocate volarly out of the lunate fossa of the distal radius, in which case it is called the lunate dislocation.
- **Clinical evaluation:** Scapholunate or perilunate injuries typically cause tenderness just distal to Lister tubercle. Swelling is generalized about the wrist with variable dorsal prominence of the entire carpus in cases of dorsal perilunate dislocations.
- **Radiographic evaluation:** PA and lateral views should be obtained to confirm the diagnosis and rule out associated injuries. A CT scan may be useful in further defining the injury pattern.
  - **PA view:** The dislocated lunate appears to be wedge-shaped and more triangular, with an elongated volar lip.

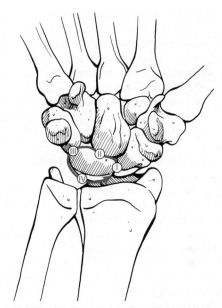

FIGURE 23.9 Mayfield stages of progressive peri-ilunate instability. Stage I results in scapholunate instability. Stages II to IV result in progressively worse perilunate instability. (From Bucholz RW, Heckman JD, Court-Brown C, et al., eds. *Rockwood and Green's Fractures in Adults.* 6th ed. Philadelphia: Lippincott Williams & Wilkins; 2006.)

□ Loss of normal carpal colinear "Gilula lines" and abnormal widening of the scapholunate interval >3 mm are noted.

□ Look for associated fractures, such as "transscaphoid" injuries.

□ **Lateral view (most important view):** Carefully look at the outline of the capitate and the lunate. The "spilled tea cup sign" occurs with volar dislocation of the lunate.

□ A clenched-fist PA view obtained after closed reduction of the midcarpal joint is useful for checking residual scapholunate or lunotriquetral dissociation as well as fractures.

■ **Classification (Mayfield):** A sequence of progressive perilunate instability is seen as the injury spreads:

□ From the scapholunate joint (radioscapholunate ligament) → midcarpal joint (radioscaphocarpal ligament) → lunotriquetral joint (distal limb of radiolunotriquetral ligament) → dorsal radiolunotriquetral ligament → volar dislocation of the lunate.

Stage I: **Disruption of the scapholunate joint:** The radioscapholunate and interosseous scapholunate ligaments are disrupted.

Stage II: **Disruption of the midcarpal (capitolunate) joint:** The radioscaphocapitate ligament is disrupted.

Stage III: **Disruption of the lunotriquetral joint:** The distal limb of the radiolunotriquetral ligament is disrupted.

Stage IV: **Disruption of the radiolunate joint:** The dorsal radiolunotriquetral ligament is disrupted, ultimately causing volar dislocation of the lunate.

- Treatment
  - □ Closed reduction should be performed with adequate sedation.
  - □ Technique of closed reduction
    - Longitudinal traction is applied for 5 to 10 minutes.
    - For dorsal perilunate injuries, the wrist is hyperextended, and volar pressure is applied to the lunate.
    - Wrist palmar flexion and traction then reduces the capitate into the concavity of the lunate.
  - □ Early surgical reconstruction is performed if swelling allows. Immediate surgery is needed if there are progressive signs of median nerve compromise.
  - □ Closed reduction and pinning—for patients who can't tolerate ORIF
    - The lunate is reduced and pinned to the radius in neutral alignment.
    - The triquetrum or scaphoid can then be pinned to the lunate.
  - □ Transscaphoid perilunate dislocation
    - This requires reduction and stabilization of the fractured scaphoid.
    - Most of these injuries are best treated by open volar and dorsal reduction and repair of the injured structures.
    - Open repair may be supplemented by pin fixation.
  - □ Delayed reconstruction is indicated if early intervention is not feasible.
- Complications
  - □ **Median neuropathy:** This may result from carpal tunnel compression, necessitating surgical release.
  - □ **Posttraumatic arthritis:** This may result from the initial injury or secondarily from small, retained osseous fragments and cartilage damage.
  - □ **Chronic perilunate injury:** This may result from untreated or inadequately treated dislocation or fracture-dislocation resulting in chronic pain, instability, and wrist deformity, often associated with tendon rupture or increasing nerve symptoms. Repair may be possible, but a salvage procedure, such as proximal row

carpectomy or radiocarpal fusion, may be necessary after a
delay in treatment for 1 to 2 months.

CARPAL DISLOCATIONS

- Carpal dislocations represent a continuum of perilunate dislocations, with frank lunate dislocation representing the final stage. All
  such injuries reflect significant ligamentous injury.
- Associated fractures are common and may represent avulsion
  injuries (e.g., VISI or DISI with associated radial rim fracture).
- **Mechanism of injury:** A fall onto an outstretched hand represents the
  most common cause, although direct force can cause traumatic
  carpal dislocations as well.
- **Clinical evaluation:** Patients typically present with painful, limited
  wrist range of motion. Median neuropathy may be present. Specific
  tests for carpal instability include the following:
  - □ **Midcarpal stress test:** Dorsal-palmar stressing of the midcarpal
    joint results in a pathologic clunk representing subluxation of
    the lunate.
  - □ **Dynamic test for midcarpal instability:** Wrist extension with
    radioulnar deviation produces a "catchup" clunk as the proximal
    row snaps from flexion to extension.
- **Radiographic evaluation:** Most dislocations may be diagnosed on PA
  and lateral views of the wrist.
  - □ CT and MRI may aid in further injury definition.
- Treatment of carpal dislocations consists of closed reduction of the
  midcarpal joint, which is often accomplished with traction, com-
  bined with direct manual pressure over the capitate and the lunate.
  - □ Irreducible dislocations or unstable injuries should be treated
    with open reduction and internal fixation utilizing a combined
    dorsal and volar approach. Dorsally, the osseous anatomy is re-
    stored and stabilized with possible ligamentous repair and dorsal
    capsulodesis. The repair is protected using Kirschner wire fixa-
    tion for 8 to 12 weeks. Volarly, the dislocation is reduced, median
    nerve is decompressed, if necessary, and soft tissues are repaired.
- Complications
  - □ **Posttraumatic arthritis:** This may result from unrecognized associ-
    ated fractures or malreduction, with subsequent functional
    limitation and pain.
  - □ **Recurrent instability:** This may result from inadequate repair of
    ligamentous structures on the volar aspect or insufficient
    fixation dorsally.

SCAPHOLUNATE DISSOCIATION

- This is the ligamentous analog of a scaphoid fracture; it represents the most common and significant ligamentous disruption of the wrist.
- The underlying pathologic process is a disruption of the radioscapholunate and the scapholunate interosseous ligaments.
- The mechanism of injury is loading of the extended carpus in ulnar deviation.
- Clinical findings include ecchymosis and tenderness of the wrist. The proximal pole of the scaphoid may be prominent dorsally. Signs of scapholunate dissociation include pain with a vigorous grasp, decreasing repetitive grip strength, a positive Watson test (see earlier, under scaphoid fractures), and painful flexion-extension or ulnar-radial deviation of the wrist.
- **Radiographic evaluation:** PA, lateral, clenched-fist supinated PA, and radial and ulnar deviation views are obtained. Classic signs of scapholunate dissociation on the PA view include
  - **The "Terry Thomas sign":** widening of the scapholunate space >3 mm (normal <2 mm)
  - The "cortical ring sign" caused by the abnormally flexed scaphoid
  - A scapholunate angle of >70 degrees visualized on the lateral view
- Treatment
  - Arthroscopically assisted reduction with percutaneous pin fixation has been described with variable results.
  - An inability to obtain or maintain reduction is an indication for open reduction and internal fixation. This may be accomplished by a combined dorsal and volar approach with reduction and stabilization of the scapholunate interval dorsally, by repair of SL interosseous ligament, if possible, and dorsal capsulodesis. The construct is held together using Kirschner wires. Wrist ligaments can be repaired via the volar approach, if necessary.
- Complications
  - **Recurrent instability:** Failure of closed or open reduction and internal fixation with ligament repair may necessitate ligament augmentation, intercarpal fusion, proximal row carpectomy, or wrist fusion. It may progress to a DISI pattern or a scaphoid-lunate advanced collapse of the wrist.

LUNOTRIQUETRAL DISSOCIATION

- These injuries involve disruption of the distal limb of the volar radiolunotriquetral ligament either as a stage III lesser arc injury of perilunate instability or as a result of a force causing excessive radial deviation and intercarpal pronation. The lunotriquetral interosseous and dorsal radiolunotriquetral ligaments are also injured.

- Clinical findings include swelling over the peritriquetral area and tenderness dorsally, typically one fingerbreadth distal to the ulnar head.
  - □ **Ballottement test (shear or shuck test):** Dorsal-volar displacement of the triquetrum on the lunate results in increased excursion as compared with the normal, contralateral side, as well as painful crepitus.
- **Radiographic evaluation:** PA radiographs of the hand rarely reveal frank gapping of the lunotriquetral space, but a break in the normal smooth contour of the proximal carpal row can be appreciated.
  - □ **Radial deviation view:** This may demonstrate the triquetrum to be dorsiflexed with the intact scapholunate complex palmarflexed. A lateral projection may reveal a volar intercalated segmental instability pattern.
- Treatment
  - □ Acute lunotriquetral dissociation with minimal deformity may be treated with a short arm cast or splint for 6 to 8 weeks.
  - □ Closed reduction with pinning of the lunate to the triquetrum may be necessary to maintain reduction.
  - □ Angular deformity or unacceptable reduction from nonoperative treatment may necessitate open reduction and internal fixation utilizing a combined dorsal and volar approach, with pinning of the triquetrum to the lunate and ligamentous repair.
- Complications
  - □ Recurrent instability may necessitate ligament reconstruction with capsular augmentation. If recurrent instability persists, lunotriquetral fusion may be necessary, with possible concomitant ulnar shortening to tension the volar ulnocarpal ligaments.

ULNOCARPAL DISSOCIATION

- Avulsion or rupture of the TFCC from the ulnar styloid results in a loss of "sling" support for the ulnar wrist.
- The lunate and triquetrum "fall away" relative to the distal ulna and assume a semisupinated and palmar-flexed attitude, with the distal ulna subluxed dorsally.
- Clinical evaluation reveals dorsal prominence of the distal ulna and volar displacement of the ulnar carpus.
- **Radiographic evaluation:** The PA view may reveal avulsion of the ulnar styloid. Dorsal displacement of the distal ulna on true lateral

views suggests disruption of the TFCC in the absence of an ulnar styloid avulsion fracture.

☐ MRI may demonstrate a tear of the TFCC and may additionally provide evidence of chondral lesions and effusion.

■ **Treatment:** Operative repair of the TFCC may be achieved via a dorsal approach between the fifth and sixth extensor compartments.

☐ Open reduction and internal fixation of large displaced ulnar styloid fragments may be necessary if they involve the base or fovea.

■ Complications

☐ **Recurrent instability:** This may occur with or without previous operative intervention and may result in pain and functional debilitation that may be progressive.

☐ **Ulnar neuropathy:** Transient sensory symptoms may result from irritation of the ulnar nerve in Guyon canal or its dorsal sensory branch. Permanent damage is rare, but persistence of symptoms beyond 12 weeks may necessitate exploration.

24 Hand

EPIDEMIOLOGY

- Metacarpal and phalangeal fractures are common, comprising 10% of all fractures; >50% of these are work related.
- The 1998 United States National Hospital Ambulatory Medical Care Survey found phalangeal (23%) and metacarpal (18%) fractures to be the second and third most common hand and forearm fractures following radius fractures. They constitute anywhere from 1.5% to 28% of all emergency department visits, depending on survey methods.
- **Location:** Border digits are most commonly involved with approximate incidence as follows:
  - Distal phalanx (45%)
  - Metacarpal (30%)
  - Proximal phalanx (15%)
  - Middle phalanx (10%)
- Male-to-female ratios run from 1.8:1 to 5.4:1, with higher ratios seen in the age groups associated with the greatest incidence (sports injuries in the early third decade and workplace injuries in the fifth decade).

ANATOMY

Metacarpals

- They are bowed, concave on palmar surface.
- They form the longitudinal and transverse arches of the hand.
- The index and long finger carpometacarpal articulation is rigid.
- The ring and small finger carpometacarpal articulation is flexible.
- Three palmar and four dorsal interosseous muscles arise from metacarpal shafts and flex the metacarpophalangeal (MCP) joints.
- These muscles create deforming forces in the case of metacarpal fractures, typically flexing the fracture (apex dorsal angulation).

Phalanges

- Proximal phalanx fractures usually angulate into extension (apex volar).
  - The proximal fragment is flexed by the interossei.

    ❑ The distal fragment is extended by the central slip.
- Middle phalanx fractures are unpredictable.
- Distal phalanx fractures usually result from crush injuries and are comminuted tuft fractures.

MECHANISM OF INJURY

- A high degree of variation in mechanism of injury accounts for the broad spectrum of patterns seen in skeletal trauma sustained by the hand.
- Axial load or "jamming" injuries are frequently sustained during ball sports or sudden reaches made during everyday activities such as to catch a falling object. Patterns frequently resulting from this mechanism are shearing articular fractures or metaphyseal compression fractures.
- Axial loading along the upper extremity must also make one suspicious of associated injuries to the carpus, forearm, elbow, and shoulder girdle.
- Diaphyseal fractures and joint dislocations usually require a bending component in the mechanism of injury, which can occur during ball-handling sports or when the hand is trapped by an object and is unable to move with the rest of the arm.
- Individual digits can easily be caught in clothing, furniture, or workplace equipment to sustain torsional mechanisms of injury, resulting in spiral fractures or more complex dislocation patterns.
- Industrial settings or other environments with heavy objects and high forces lead to crushing mechanisms that combine bending, shearing, and torsion to produce unique patterns of skeletal injury and associated soft tissue damage.

CLINICAL EVALUATION

- **History:** A careful history is essential as it may influence treatment. This should include the patient's
  - ❑ Age
  - ❑ Hand dominance
  - ❑ Occupation
  - ❑ Systemic illnesses
  - ❑ **Mechanism of injury:** crush, direct trauma, twist, tear, laceration, etc.
  - ❑ Time of injury (for open fractures)
  - ❑ **Exposure to contamination:** barnyard, brackish water, animal/human bite
  - ❑ **Treatment provided:** cleansing, antiseptic, bandage, tourniquet
  - ❑ **Financial issues:** workers' compensation

- Physical examination includes
  - □ Digital viability (capillary refill should be <2 seconds).
  - □ Neurologic status (documented by two-point discrimination [normal is 6 mm] and individual muscle testing).
  - □ Rotational and angulatory deformity.
  - □ Range of motion (documented by goniometer).
  - □ Malrotation at one bone segment is best represented by the alignment of the next more distal segment. This alignment is best demonstrated when the intervening joint is flexed to 90 degrees. Comparing nail plate alignment is an inadequate method of evaluating rotation.

RADIOGRAPHIC EVALUATION

- Posteroanterior, lateral, and oblique radiographs of the affected digit or hand should be obtained. Injured digits should be viewed individually to minimize overlap of other digits over the area of interest.

CLASSIFICATION

Descriptive

- Open versus closed injury (see later)
- Bone involved
- Location within bone
- **Fracture pattern:** comminuted, transverse, spiral, vertical split
- Presence or absence of displacement
- Presence or absence of deformity (rotation and/or angulation)
- Extra-articular versus intra-articular fracture
- Stable versus unstable

Open Fractures

Swanson, Szabo, and Anderson

Type I: Clean wound without significant contamination or delay in treatment and no systemic illness

Type II: One or more of the following:
- Contamination with gross dirt/debris, human or animal bite, warm lake/river injury, barnyard injury
  - □ Delay in treatment >24 hours
- Significant systemic illness, such as diabetes, hypertension, rheumatoid arthritis, hepatitis, or asthma

Rate of infection: Type I injuries (1.4%)
                          Type II injuries (14%)

- Neither primary internal fixation nor immediate wound closure is associated with increased risk of infection in type I injuries. Primary internal fixation is not associated with increased risk of infection in type II injuries.
- Primary wound closure is appropriate for type I injuries, with delayed closure appropriate for type II injuries.

OTA Classification of Metacarpal Fractures

See Fracture and Dislocation Classification Compendium at http://www.ota.org/compendium/compendium.html.

OTA Classification of Phalangeal Fractures

See Fracture and Dislocation Classification Compendium at http://www.ota.org/compendium/compendium.html.

TREATMENT: GENERAL PRINCIPLES

- **"Fight-bite" injuries:** Any short, curved laceration overlying a joint in the hand, particularly the metacarpophalangeal joint, must be suspected of having been caused by a tooth. These injuries must be assumed to be contaminated with oral flora and should be addressed with broad-spectrum antibiotics (need anaerobic coverage) and irrigation and debridement.
- **Animal bites:** Antibiotic coverage is needed for *Pasterella* and *Eikenella*.
- There are essentially five major treatment alternatives:
  - □ Immediate motion
  - □ Temporary splinting
  - □ Closed reduction and internal fixation (CRIF)
  - □ Open reduction and internal fixation (ORIF)
  - □ Immediate reconstruction
- The general advantages of entirely nonoperative treatment are lower cost and avoidance of the risks and complications associated with surgery and anesthesia. The disadvantage is that stability is less assured than with some form of operative fixation.
- CRIF is expected to prevent overt deformity but not to achieve an anatomically perfect reduction. Pin tract infection is the prime complication that should be mentioned to patients in association with CRIF, unless K-wires are buried.
- Open treatments are considered to add the morbidity of surgical tissue trauma, titrated against the presumed advantages of the most anatomic and stable reduction.
- Critical elements in selecting between nonoperative and operative treatment are the assessments of rotational malalignment and stability.

- ☐ If carefully sought, rotational discrepancy is relatively easy to determine.
- ☐ Defining stability is somewhat more difficult. Some authors have used what seems to be the very reasonable criterion of maintenance of fracture reduction when the adjacent joints are taken through at least 30% of their normal motion.
- ■ Contraction of soft tissues begins approximately 72 hours following injury. Motion should be instituted by this time for all joints stable enough to tolerate rehabilitation.
- ■ General indications for surgery include
  - ☐ Open fractures
  - ☐ Unstable fractures
  - ☐ Irreducible fractures
  - ☐ Multiple fractures
  - ☐ Fractures with bone loss
  - ☐ Fractures with tendon lacerations
- ■ **Treatment of stable fractures:**
  - ☐ Buddy taping or splinting is performed, with repeat radiographs in 1 week.
  - ☐ **Initially unstable fractures that are reduced and then converted into a stable position:** External immobilization (cast, cast with outrigger splint, gutter splint, or anterior–posterior splints) or percutaneous pinning prevents displacement and permits earlier mobilization.
- ■ **Treatment of unstable fractures:**
  - ☐ Unstable fractures that are irreducible by closed means or exhibit continued instability despite closed treatment require CRIF or ORIF, including Kirschner wire fixation, interosseous wiring, tension band technique, interfragmentary screws alone, or plates and screws.
- ■ Fractures with segmental bone loss
  - ☐ These continue to be problematic. The primary treatment should be directed to the soft tissues, maintaining length with Kirschner wires or external fixation. These injuries usually require secondary procedures, including bone grafting.

MANAGEMENT OF SPECIFIC FRACTURE PATTERNS

Metacarpals

Metacarpal Head

- ■ Fractures include
  - ☐ Epiphyseal fractures
  - ☐ Collateral ligament avulsion fractures
  - ☐ Oblique, vertical, and horizontal head fractures

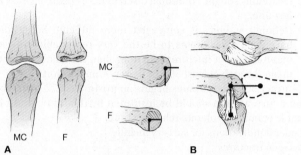

A   **B**

FIGURE 24.1 Left: The collateral ligaments of the metacarpophalangeal joints are relaxed in extension, permitting lateral motion, but they become taut when the joint is fully flexed. This occurs because of the unique shape of the metacarpal head, which acts as a cam. Right: The distance from the pivot point of the metacarpal to the phalanx in extension is less than the distance in flexion, so the collateral ligament is tight when the joint is flexed. (From Rockwood CA Jr, Green DP, Bucholz RW, Heckman JD, eds. *Rockwood and Green's Fractures in Adults.* Vol 1. 4th ed. Philadelphia: Lippincott–Raven; 1996:659.)

  ☐ Comminuted fractures
  ☐ Boxer's fractures with joint extension
  ☐ Fractures associated with bone loss
 ■ Most require anatomic reduction (if possible) to re-establish joint congruity and to minimize posttraumatic arthrosis.
  ☐ Stable reductions of fractures may be splinted in the "protected position," consisting of metacarpal-phalangeal flexion >70 degrees to minimize joint stiffness (Fig. 24.1).
  ☐ Displaced metacarpal head fractures usually require open reduction internal fixation with K-wires or headless compression screws.
 ■ Early range of motion is essential.

Metacarpal Neck

 ■ Fractures result from direct trauma with volar comminution and dorsal apex angulation. Most of these fractures can often be reduced closed, but maintenance of reduction may be difficult (Fig. 24.2).
 ■ **The degree of acceptable deformity varies according to the metacarpal injured:**
  ☐ Less than 10-degree angulation for the second and third metacarpals.

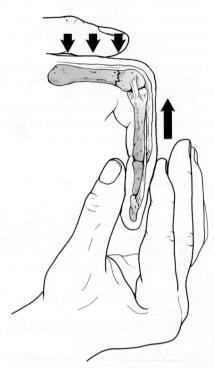

FIGURE 24.2 Reduction of metacarpal fractures can be accomplished by using the digit to control the distal fragment, but the proximal interphalangeal joint should be extended rather than flexed. (From Bucholz RW, Heckman JD, Court-Brown C, et al., eds. *Rockwood and Green's Fractures in Adults*. 6th ed. Philadelphia: Lippincott Williams & Wilkins; 2006.)

- □ Less than 30- to 40-degree angulation for the fourth and fifth metacarpals.
- ■ Unstable fractures require operative intervention with either percutaneous pins (may be intramedullary or transverse into the adjacent metacarpal) or plate fixation.

Metacarpal Shaft

- ■ Nondisplaced or minimally displaced fractures can be reduced and splinted in the protected position. Central metacarpal fractures (third and fourth) are usually more stable due to the intermetacarpal ligaments.

- Operative indications include rotational deformity, dorsal angulation >10 degrees for second and third metacarpals, and >20 degrees for fourth and fifth metacarpals.
- Generally, malrotation is not acceptable. Ten degrees of malrotation (which risks as much as 2 cm of overlap at the digital tip) should represent the upper tolerable limit.
- Operative fixation may be achieved with either closed reduction and percutaneous intermetacarpal pinning, or open reduction internal fixation with interfragmentary screws, intramedullary nails, or plate and screws.

Metacarpal Base

Fingers
- Fractures of the bases of the second through fifth metacarpals may be associated with carpometacarpal fracture-dislocations. In addition to a PA radiograph, it is important to get a true lateral and a 30-degree pronated from lateral view. Displaced fractures require CRIF versus ORIF.
- The reverse Bennett fracture is a fracture-dislocation of the base of the fifth metacarpal/hamate.
  - □ The proximal metacarpal fragment is displaced proximally by the pull of the extensor carpi ulnaris.
  - □ This fracture often requires surgical intervention with CRIF versus ORIF.

Thumb
- **Extra-articular fractures:** These are usually transverse or oblique. Most can be held by closed reduction and casting, but some unstable fractures require closed reduction and percutaneous pinning. The basal joint of the thumb is quite forgiving, and an anatomic reduction of an angulated shaft fracture is not essential.
- **Intra-articular fractures (Figs. 24.3 and 24.4):**

Type I: **Bennett fracture:** Fracture line separates major part of metacarpal from volar lip fragment, producing a disruption of the first carpometacarpal (CMC) joint; first metacarpal is pulled proximally by the abductor pollicis longus.

Type II: **Rolando fracture:** It requires greater force than a Bennett fracture; presently used to describe a comminuted Bennett fracture, a "Y" or "T" fracture, or a fracture with dorsal and palmar fragments.

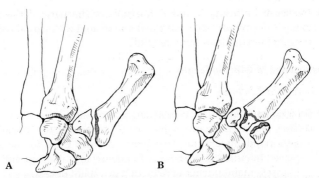

A   **B**

FIGURE 24.3 The most recognized patterns of thumb metacarpal base intra-articular fractures are **(A)** the partial articular Bennett fracture and **(B)** the complete articular Rolando fracture. (From Bucholz RW, Heckman JD, Court-Brown C, et al., eds. *Rockwood and Green's Fractures in Adults.* 6th ed. Philadelphia: Lippincott Williams & Wilkins; 2006.)

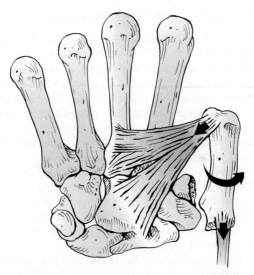

FIGURE 24.4 Displacement of Bennett fractures is driven primarily by the abductor pollicis longus and the adductor pollicis resulting in flexion, supination, and proximal migration. (From Bucholz RW, Heckman JD, Court-Brown C, et al., eds. *Rockwood and Green's Fractures in Adults.* 6th ed. Philadelphia: Lippincott Williams & Wilkins; 2006.)

■ **Treatment:** Both type I and II fractures of the base of the first metacarpal are unstable and should be treated with closed reduction and percutaneous pins, or ORIF.

Proximal and Middle Phalanges

Intra-articular Fractures

■ **Condylar fractures:** single, bicondylar, osteochondral
  □ They require anatomic reduction; CRIF versus ORIF should be performed for any displacement. Consider CRIF for nondisplaced fractures since they are frequently unstable and difficult to assess maintainence of reduction in a splint or cast.
  □ Comminuted intra-articular phalangeal fractures should be treated with reconstruction of the articular surface, if possible. Severely comminuted fractures that are deemed nonreconstructible may be treated closed with early protected mobilization. The surgeon should discuss with the patient the possibility of secondary procedures.

Proximal Interphalangeal (PIP) Fracture-Dislocations

■ Volar lip fracture of middle phalangeal base (dorsal fracture-dislocation)
  □ **Treatment is controversial and depends on percentage of articular surface fractured:**
    • **Hyperextension injuries without a history of dislocation with <30% to 35% articular (nondisplaced) involvement:** 20-degree dorsal block splint and buddy tape to the adjacent digit × 3 weeks, then buddy tape active and active assisted range of motion.
    • **Forty percent or more articular involvement:** usually unstable. Dynamic external fixator (Suzuki/Slade with 0.045 in K-wires and rubber bands). Add ORIF if fragments need further reduction. If too comminuted or chronic and 40% to 50% articular involvement: volar plate arthroplasty versus hemi-hamate arthroplasty. >50% articular involvement: hemi-hamate arthroplasty.
■ Dorsal lip fracture of middle phalangeal base (volar fracture-dislocation)
  □ Usually this is the result of a central slip avulsion.
  □ **Fractures with <1 mm of displacement:** may be treated closed with splinting, as in a boutonniere injury.
  □ **Fractures with >1 mm of displacement or volar subluxation of the PIP joint:** operative stabilization of the fracture is indicated. CRIF versus ORIF.
  □ Pilon fractures (Suzuki/Slade with 0.045 in K-wires and rubber bands). Add ORIF if fragments need further reduction.

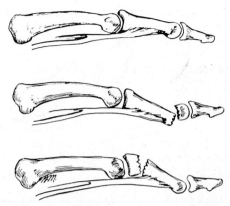

FIGURE 24.5 Top: A lateral view, showing the prolonged insertion of the superficialis tendon into the middle phalanx. Center: A fracture through the neck of the middle phalanx is likely to have a volar angulation because the proximal fragment is flexed by the strong pull of the superficialis. Bottom: A fracture through the base of the middle phalanx is more likely to have a dorsal angulation because of the extension force of the central slip on the proximal fragment and a flexion force on the distal fragment by the superficialis. (From Rockwood CA Jr, Green DP, Bucholz RW, Heckman JD, eds. *Rockwood and Green's Fractures in Adults.* Vol 1. 4th ed. Philadelphia: Lippincott–Raven; 1996:627.)

Extra-articular Fractures

Add: Shaft fractures. If displaced or unstable, CRIF versus ORIF. Epibasilar proximal phalanx fractures are usually apex volar. Consider CRIF with trans-MCP joint pin while flexing MCP joint.

- Fractures at the base of the middle phalanx tend to angulate apex dorsal, whereas fractures at the neck angulate the apex volarly owing to the pull of the sublimis tendon (Fig. 24.5). Closed reduction should be attempted initially with finger-trap traction followed by splinting.
- Fractures in which a stable closed reduction cannot be achieved or maintained should be addressed with closed reduction and percutaneous pinning or ORIF with minifragment implants.

Distal Phalanx (Fig. 24.6)

Intra-articular Fractures

- Dorsal lip
  - □ A mallet finger may result from a fracture of the dorsal lip with disruption of the extensor tendon. Alternatively, a mallet finger

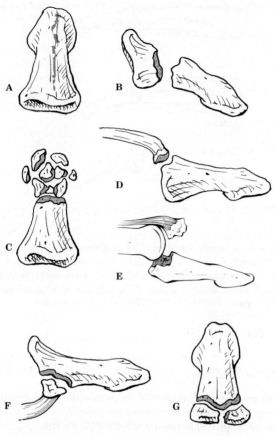

FIGURE 24.6 Fracture patterns seen in the distal phalanx include **(A)** longitudinal shaft, **(B)** transverse shaft, **(C)** tuft, **(D)** dorsal base avulsion, **(E)** dorsal base shear, **(F)** volar base, and **(G)** complete articular. (From Bucholz RW, Heckman JD, Court-Brown C, et al., eds. *Rockwood and Green's Fractures in Adults.* 6th ed. Philadelphia: Lippincott Williams & Wilkins; 2006.)

may result from a purely tendinous disruption and may therefore not be radiographically apparent.

☐ Treatment remains somewhat controversial.

- Some recommend nonoperative treatment for all mallet fingers with full-time extension splinting for 6 to 8 weeks, including those with a significant articular fracture and joint subluxation.

- Others recommend CRIF for displaced dorsal base fractures with subluxation. Various closed pinning techniques are possible, but the mainstay is extension block pinning.
- Volar lip
  - This is associated with flexor digitorum profundus rupture ("jersey finger": seen in football and rugby players, most commonly involving the ring finger).
  - Treatment is primary repair, especially with large, displaced bony fragments.

Extra-articular Fractures

- These are transverse, longitudinal, and comminuted (nail matrix injury is very common).
- Treatment consists of closed reduction and splinting.
- The splint should leave the PIP joint free but usually needs to cross the distal interphalangeal (DIP) joint to provide adequate stability. Aluminum and foam splints or plaster of Paris are common materials chosen.
- CRIF is indicated for shaft fractures with wide displacement because of the risk for nailbed incongruity and later nail plate non-adherence.

Nailbed Injuries (Fig. 24.7)

- These are frequently overlooked or neglected in the presence of an obvious fracture, but failure to address such injuries may result in growth disturbances of the nail.
- Acute subungual hematomas may be evacuated with cautery or a hot paper clip.
- If the nailplate has been avulsed at its base, it should be removed, cleansed with povidone-iodine, and retained to replace under the eponychium.
- Nailbed disruptions should be carefully sutured with 6-0 chromic catgut under magnification.
- The aluminum suture package material may be used if the original nailplate is not usable as a biologic dressing.

CMC Joint Dislocations and Fracture-Dislocations

- Dislocations at the finger CMC joints are usually high-energy injuries with involvement of associated structures, including neurovascular injury.
- Overlap on the lateral x-ray obscures accurate depiction of the injury pattern. A 30-degree pronated view from lateral will help elucidate.

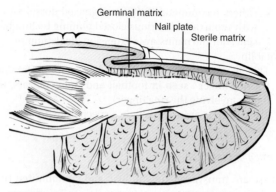

FIGURE 24.7 An intimate relationship exists between the three layers of the dorsal cortex of the distal phalanx, the nail matrix (both germinal and sterile), and the nail plate. (From Bucholz RW, Heckman JD, Court-Brown C, et al., eds. *Rockwood and Green's Fractures in Adults*. 6th ed. Philadelphia: Lippincott Williams & Wilkins; 2006.)

- When fracture-dislocations include the dorsal cortex of the hamate, computed tomography may be necessary to better evaluate the pathoanatomy.
- Most thumb CMC joint injuries are fracture-dislocations rather than pure dislocations. Terms associated with these fracture-dislocations are Bennett (partial articular) and Rolando (complete articular) fractures.
- Dorsal finger CMC fracture-dislocations cannot usually be held effectively with external splints/casts alone. CRIF versus ORIF is the treatment of choice.

Metacarpophalangeal (MCP) Joint Dislocations (Fig. 24.8)

- Dorsal dislocations are the most common.
- Simple dislocations are reducible and present with a hyperextension posture.
- They are really subluxations, because some contact usually remains between the base of proximal phalanx and the metacarpal head.
- Reduction can be achieved with simple flexion of the joint; excessive longitudinal traction on the finger should be avoided, since this could interpose the volar plate. Wrist flexion to relax the flexor tendons may assist reduction.

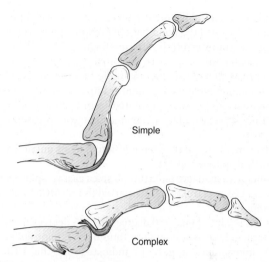

Simple

Complex

FIGURE 24.8 Simple metacarpophalangeal joint dislocations are spontaneously reducible and usually present in an extended posture with the articular surface of P1 sitting on the dorsum of the metacarpal head. Complex dislocations have bayonet apposition with volar plate interposition that prevents reduction. (From Bucholz RW, Heckman JD, Court-Brown C, et al., eds. *Rockwood and Green's Fractures in Adults.* 6th ed. Philadelphia: Lippincott Williams & Wilkins; 2006.)

■ The other variety of MCP joint dislocation is a complex dislocation, which is by definition irreducible, most often the result of volar plate interposition.
  □ Complex dislocations occur most frequently in the index finger.
  □ A pathognomonic x-ray sign of complex dislocation is the appearance of a sesamoid in the joint space.
■ Most dorsal dislocations are stable following reduction and do not need surgical repair of the ligaments or volar plate.
■ Volar dislocations are rare but are particularly unstable.
■ Volar dislocations are at risk for late instability and should have repair of the ligaments.
■ Open dislocations may be either reducible or irreducible.

Thumb Metacarpophalangeal (MCP) Joint Dislocations

■ The thumb MCP joint, in addition to its primary plane of flexion and extension, allows abduction-adduction and a slight amount of rotation (pronation with flexion).
■ With a one-sided collateral ligament injury, the phalanx tends to subluxate volarly in a rotatory fashion, pivoting around the opposite intact collateral ligament.

- The ulnar collateral ligament may have a two-level injury consisting of a fracture of the ulnar base of proximal phalanx with the ligament also ruptured off the fracture fragment.
- Of particular importance is the proximal edge of the adductor aponeurosis that forms the anatomic basis of the Stener lesion. The torn ulnar collateral ligament stump comes to lie dorsal to the aponeurosis and is thus prevented from healing to its anatomic insertion on the volar, ulnar base of the proximal phalanx (Fig. 24.9).
- The true incidence of the Stener lesion remains unknown, because of widely disparate reports.
- Nonoperative management (thumb spica cast vs. splint × 6 weeks) is the mainstay of treatment for partial thumb MCP joint collateral ligament injuries.
- If the MCP joint opens >30 degrees or >15 degrees from the contralateral side, it is a complete thumb MCP joint collateral ligament injury and surgery is indicated for the UCL and is

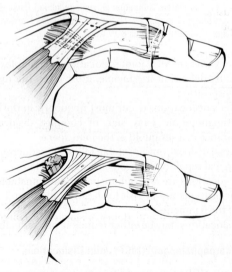

FIGURE 24.9 The Stener lesion: The adductor aponeurosis proximal edge functions as a shelf that blocks the distal phalangeal insertion of the ruptured ulnar collateral ligament of the thumb metacarpophalangeal joint from returning to its natural location for healing after it comes to lie on top of the aponeurosis. (From Bucholz RW, Heckman JD, Court-Brown C, et al., eds. *Rockwood and Green's Fractures in Adults.* 6th ed. Philadelphia: Lippincott Williams & Wilkins; 2006.)

controversial for the RCL. The ligament can be repaired with a bone suture anchor. If the injury is chronic and there is not adequate ligament to repair, a free tendon graft through bone tunnels may be employed.

Proximal Interphalangeal (PIP) Joint Dislocations

- Dislocations of the PIP joint have a high rate of missed diagnoses that are passed off as "sprains."
- Although large numbers of incomplete injuries occur (especially in ball-handling sports), complete disruptions of the collateral ligaments and the volar plate are also frequent (50% occur in the long finger followed in frequency by the ring finger).
- Congruence on the lateral radiograph is the key to detecting residual subluxation.
- Residual instability is quite rare in pure dislocations, as opposed to fracture-dislocations, in which it is the primary concern.
- Recognized patterns of dislocation other than complete collateral ligament injury are dorsal dislocation, pure volar dislocation, and rotatory volar dislocation.
- Dorsal dislocations involve volar plate injury (usually distally, with or without a small flake of bone).
- For pure volar dislocations, the pathologic findings are consistently damage to the volar plate, one collateral ligament, and the central slip.
- Volar or lateral dislocations may be irreducible if the head of proximal phalanx passes between the central slip and the lateral bands, which can form a noose effect and prevent reduction.
- In pure dislocations, stiffness is the primary concern. Stiffness can occur following any injury pattern.
- Chronic missed dislocations require open reduction with a predictable amount of subsequent stiffness.
- Treatment
  - □ Once reduced, rotatory volar dislocations, isolated collateral ligament ruptures, and dorsal dislocations congruent in full extension on the lateral radiograph can all begin immediate active range of motion with adjacent digit strapping.
  - □ Dorsal dislocations that are subluxated on the extension lateral radiograph require a few weeks of extension block splinting.
  - □ Volar dislocations with central slip disruptions require 4 to 6 weeks of PIP extension splinting, followed by nighttime static extension splinting for 2 additional weeks. The DIP joint should be unsplinted and actively flexed throughout the entire recovery period.

- ☐ Open dorsal dislocations usually have a transverse rent in the skin at the flexion crease. Debridement of this wound should precede reduction of the dislocation.

Distal Interphalangeal (DIP) and Thumb Interphalangeal (IP) Joint Dislocations

- ■ Dislocations at the DIP/IP joint are often not diagnosed initially and present late.
- ■ Injuries are considered chronic after 3 weeks.
- ■ Pure dislocations without tendon rupture are rare, usually result from ball-catching sports, are primarily dorsal in direction, and may occur in association with PIP joint dislocations.
- ■ Transverse open wounds in the volar skin crease are frequent.
- ■ Injury to a single collateral ligament or to the volar plate alone at the DIP joint is rare.

Nonoperative Treatment

- ■ Reduced dislocations that are stable may begin immediate active range of motion.
- ■ The rare unstable dorsal dislocation should be immobilized in 20 degrees of flexion for up to 3 weeks before instituting active range of motion.
  - ☐ The duration of the immobilization should be in direct proportion to the surgeon's assessment of joint stability following reduction.
  - ☐ Complete collateral ligament injuries should be protected from lateral stress for at least 4 weeks.
- ■ Should pin stabilization prove necessary because of recurrent instability, a single longitudinal Kirschner wire is usually sufficient.

Operative Treatment

- ■ Delayed presentation (>3 weeks) of a subluxated joint may require open reduction to resect scar tissue and to allow tension-free reduction.
- ■ Open dislocations require thorough debridement to prevent infection.
- ■ The need for fixation with a Kirschner wire should be based on the assessment of stability, and it is not necessarily required for all open dislocations.
- ■ The duration of pinning should not be >4 weeks, and the wire may be left through the skin for easy removal.

COMPLICATIONS

- **Malunion:** Angulation can disturb intrinsic balance and also can result in prominence of metacarpal heads in the palm with pain on gripping. Rotational or angulatory deformities, especially of the second and third metacarpals, may result in functional and cosmetic disturbances, emphasizing the need to maintain as near anatomic relationships as possible.
- **Nonunion:** This is uncommon, but it may occur with extensive soft tissue injury and bone loss, as well as with open fractures with gross contamination and infection. It may necessitate debridement, bone grafting, or flap coverage.
- **Infection:** Grossly contaminated wounds require meticulous debridement and appropriate antibiotics depending on the injury setting (e.g., barnyard contamination, contaminated water, bite wounds), local wound care with debridement as necessary, and possible delayed closure.
- **Metacarpophalangeal joint extension contracture:** This may result if splinting is not in the protected position (i.e., MCP joints at >70 degree) leading to soft tissue contracture.
- **Loss of motion:** This is secondary to tendon adherence, especially at the level of the PIP joint.
- **Posttraumatic osteoarthritis:** This may result from a failure to restore articular congruity.

PART IV

Lower Extremity
Fractures and Dislocations

25 Pelvis

EPIDEMIOLOGY

- The incidence of pelvic fractures in the United States has been estimated to be 37 cases per 100,000 population per year.
- In persons younger than 35 years, males sustain more pelvic fractures than females; in persons older than 35 years, women sustain more pelvic fractures than men.
- Most pelvic fractures that occur in younger patients result from high-energy mechanisms, whereas pelvic fractures sustained in the elderly population occur from minimal trauma, such as a low fall.

ANATOMY

- The *pelvic ring* is composed of the sacrum and two innominate bones joined anteriorly at the symphysis and posteriorly at the paired sacroiliac joints (Figs. 25.1A and 25.1B).
- The *innominate* bone is formed at maturity by the fusion of three ossification centers: the ilium, the ischium, and the pubis through the triradiate cartilage at the dome of the acetabulum.
- The *pelvic brim* is formed by the arcuate lines that join the sacral promontory posteriorly and the superior pubis anteriorly. Below this is the *true* or *lesser* pelvis in which are contained the pelvic viscera. Above this is the *false* or *greater* pelvis that represents the inferior aspect of the abdominal cavity.
- Inherent stability of the pelvis is conferred by ligamentous structures. These may be divided into two groups according to the ligamentous attachments:
  1. **Sacrum to ilium:** The strongest and most important ligamentous structures occur in the posterior aspect of the pelvis connecting the sacrum to the innominate bones.
     - The *sacroiliac ligamentous complex* is divided into posterior (short and long) and anterior ligaments. Posterior ligaments provide most of the stability.
     - The *sacrotuberous ligament* runs from the posterolateral aspect of the sacrum and the dorsal aspect of the posterior iliac spine to the ischial tuberosity. This ligament, in association with the posterior sacroiliac ligaments, is especially important in helping maintain vertical stability of the pelvis.

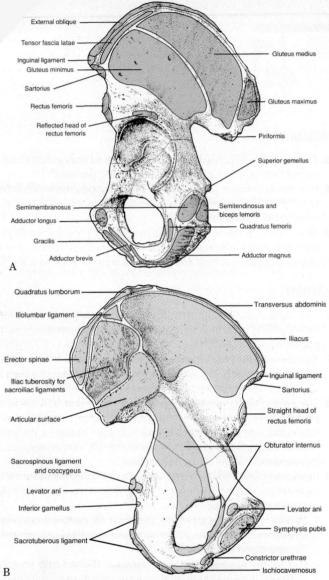

FIGURE 25.1 (A) Lateral projection of the left innominate bone. Note the muscular attachments to the ilium, ischium, and pubis. **(B)** Medial projection of the left innominate bone with muscle attachments and outline of the sacroiliac joint surface. (From Bucholz RW, Heckman JD, Court-Brown C, et al., eds. *Rockwood and Green's Fractures in Adults.* 6th ed. Philadelphia: Lippincott Williams & Wilkins; 2006.)

- The *sacrospinous ligament* is triangular, running from the lateral margins of the sacrum and coccyx and inserting on the ischial spine. It is more important in maintaining rotational control of the pelvis if the posterior sacroiliac ligaments are intact.

2. **Pubis to pubis:** Symphyseal ligaments.

■ Additional stability is conferred by ligamentous attachments between the lumbar spine and the pelvic ring:

1. The *iliolumbar ligaments* originate from the L4 and L5 transverse processes and insert on the posterior iliac crest.

2. The *lumbosacral ligaments* originate from the transverse process of L5 to the ala of the sacrum.

■ The transversely placed ligaments resist rotational forces and include the short posterior sacroiliac, anterior sacroiliac, iliolumbar, and sacrospinous ligaments.

■ The vertically placed ligaments resist shear forces (vertical shear, VS) and include the long posterior sacroiliac, sacrotuberous, and lateral lumbosacral ligaments.

PELVIC STABILITY

■ A stable injury is defined as one that can withstand normal physiologic forces without abnormal deformation.

■ Penetrating trauma infrequently results in pelvic ring destabilization.

■ An unstable injury may be characterized by the type of displacement as:

□ Rotationally unstable (open and externally rotated, or compressed and internally rotated).

□ Vertically unstable.

■ Sectioned ligaments of the pelvis determine relative contributions to pelvic stability (these included bony equivalents to ligamentous disruptions):

□ **Symphysis alone:** pubic diastasis <2.5 cm

□ **Symphysis and sacrospinous ligaments:** >2.5 cm of pubic diastasis (note that these are rotational movements and not vertical or posterior displacements)

□ **Symphysis, sacrospinous, sacrotuberous, and posterior sacroiliac:** unstable vertically, posteriorly, and rotationally

MECHANISM OF INJURY

■ These may be divided into low-energy injuries, which typically result in fractures of individual bones, or high-energy fractures, which may result in pelvic ring disruption.

□ Low-energy injuries may result from sudden muscular contractions in young athletes that cause an avulsion injury, a low-energy fall, or a straddle-type injury.

□ High-energy injuries typically result from a motor vehicle accident, pedestrian-struck mechanism, motorcycle accident, fall from heights, or crush mechanism.

■ Impact injuries result when a moving victim strikes a stationary object or vice versa. Direction, magnitude, and nature of the force all contribute to the type of fracture.

■ Crush injuries occur when a victim is trapped between the injurious force, such as motor vehicle, and an unyielding environment, such as the ground or pavement. In addition to those factors mentioned previously, the position of the victim, the duration of the crush, and whether the force was direct or a "rollover" (resulting in a changing force vector) are important to understanding the fracture pattern.

■ **Specific injury patterns vary by the direction of force application:**

1. Anteroposterior (AP) force (motorcycle crash)

   □ This results in external rotation of the hemipelvis.

   □ The pelvis springs open, hinging on the intact posterior ligaments.

2. **Lateral compression (LC) force (fall onto side, "T-bone" in motor vehicle crash):** This is most common and results in impaction of cancellous bone through the sacroiliac joint and sacrum. The injury pattern depends on location of force application:

   • **Posterior half of the ilium:** This is classic LC with minimal soft tissue disruption. This is often a stable configuration.

   • **Anterior half of the iliac wing:** This rotates the hemipelvis inward. It may disrupt the posterior sacroiliac ligamentous complex. If this force continues to push the hemipelvis across to the contralateral side, it will push the contralateral hemipelvis out into external rotation, producing LC on the ipsilateral side and an external rotation injury on the contralateral side.

   • **Greater trochanteric region:** This may be associated with a transverse acetabular fracture.

   • **External rotation abduction force:** This is common in motorcycle accidents.

     – Force application occurs through the femoral shafts and head when the leg is externally rotated and abducted.

     – This tends to tear the hemipelvis from the sacrum.

   • Shear force

     – This leads to a completely unstable fracture with triplanar instability secondary to disruption of the sacrospinous, sacrotuberous, and sacroiliac ligaments.

     – In the elderly individual, bone strength will be less than ligamentous strength and will fail first.

– In a young individual, bone strength is greater, and thus ligamentous disruptions usually occur.

CLINICAL EVALUATION

Perform patient primary assessment (ABCDE): airway, breathing, circulation, disability, and exposure. This should include a full trauma evaluation.

- **Initiate resuscitation:** Address life-threatening injuries.
- Evaluate injuries to head, chest, abdomen, and spine.
- Identify all injuries to extremities and pelvis, with careful assessment of distal neurovascular status.
- Pelvic instability may result in a leg-length discrepancy involving shortening on the involved side or a markedly internally or externally rotated lower extremity.
- The AP–LC test for pelvic instability should be performed once only, and involves rotating the pelvis internally and externally.
  - □ "The first clot is the best clot." Once disrupted, subsequent thrombus formation of a retroperitoneal hemorrhage is difficult because of hemodilution by administered intravenous fluid and exhaustion of the body's coagulation factors by the original thrombus.
- Massive flank or buttock contusions and swelling with hemorrhage are indicative of significant bleeding.
- Palpation of the posterior aspect of the pelvis may reveal a large hematoma, a defect representing the fracture, or a dislocation of the sacroiliac joint. Palpation of the symphysis may also reveal a defect.
- The perineum must be carefully inspected for the presence of a lesion representing an open fracture.
- Digital rectal in all and a vaginal exam in women should be performed in all trauma patients who present with a pelvic ring disruption. A missed rectal or vaginal perforation in association with a pelvic ring injury has a poor prognosis.

HEMODYNAMIC STATUS

Retroperitoneal hemorrhage may be associated with massive intravascular volume loss. The usual cause of retroperitoneal hemorrhage secondary to pelvic fracture is a disruption of the venous plexus in the posterior pelvis. It may also be caused by a large-vessel injury, such as external or internal iliac disruption. Large-vessel injury causes rapid, massive hemorrhage with frequent loss of the distal pulse and marked hemodynamic instability. This often necessitates immediate surgical exploration to gain proximal control of the vessel before repair. The superior gluteal artery is occasionally injured and can be managed with rapid fluid resuscitation, appropriate stabilization of the pelvic ring, and embolization.

■ Options for immediate hemorrhage control include
1. Application of military antishock trousers (MAST). This is typically performed in the field.
2. Application of an anterior external fixator.
3. Wrapping of a pelvic binder circumferentially around the pelvis (or sheet if a binder is not available) (Fig. 25.2). Should be applied at the level of the trochanters to provide access to the abdomen.
4. Application of a bean bag.
5. Application of a pelvic C-clamp (posterior).
6. **Open reduction and internal fixation (ORIF):** This may be undertaken if the patient is undergoing emergency laparotomy for other indications; it is frequently contraindicated by itself because loss of the tamponade effect may encourage further hemorrhage.
7. Open packing of the retroperitoneum is an option in the unstable patient who is brought to the operating room for laparotomy and exploration.

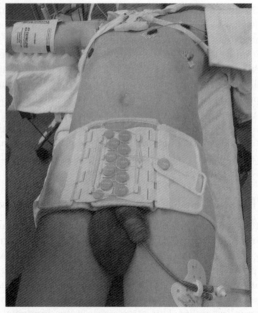

FIGURE 25.2 Pelvic Binder. (From Bucholz RW, Heckman JD, Court-Brown C, et al., eds. *Rockwood and Green's Fractures in Adults.* 6th ed. Philadelphia: Lippincott Williams & Wilkins; 2006.)

   8. Consider angiography or embolization if hemorrhage continues
       despite closing of the pelvic volume.

NEUROLOGIC INJURY

■ Lumbosacral plexus and nerve root injuries may be present, but
   they may not be apparent in an unconscious patient.
■ Higher incidence with more medial sacral fractures (Denis
   classification)

GENITOURINARY AND GASTROINTESTINAL INJURY

■ **Bladder injury:** 20% incidence occurs with pelvic trauma.
   □ **Extraperitoneal:** treated with a foley or suprapubic tube if unable
      to pass
   □ **Intraperitoneal:** requires repair
■ **Urethral injury:** 10% incidence occurs with pelvic fractures, in male
   patients much more frequently than in female patients.
   □ Examine for blood at the urethral meatus or blood on catheteri-
      zation.
   □ Examine for a high-riding or "floating" prostate on rectal exami-
      nation.
   □ Clinical suspicion should be followed by a retrograde urethrogram.

Bowel Injury

Perforations in the rectum or anus owing to osseous fragments are
technically open injuries and should be treated as such. Infrequently,
entrapment of bowel in the fracture site with gastrointestinal obstruction may occur. If either is present, the patient should undergo diverting
colostomy.

RADIOGRAPHIC EVALUATION

Standard trauma radiographs include an AP view of the chest, a lateral
view of the cervical spine, and an AP view of the pelvis.

■ **AP of the pelvis (Fig. 25.3):**
   □ **Anterior lesions:** pubic rami fractures and symphysis displace-
      ment
   □ Sacroiliac joint and sacral fractures
   □ Iliac fractures
   □ L5 transverse process fractures
■ Special views of the pelvis include
   □ **Obturator and iliac oblique views:** They may be utilized in sus-
      pected acetabular fractures (see Chapter 26).

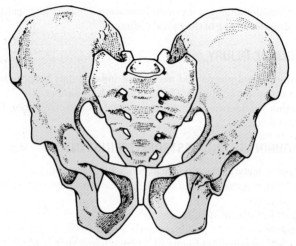

FIGURE 25.3 Anteroposterior view of the pelvis. (From Bucholz RW, Heckman JD, Court-Brown C, et al., eds. *Rockwood and Green's Fractures in Adults.* 6th ed. Philadelphia: Lippincott Williams & Wilkins; 2006.)

Inlet radiograph (Fig. 25.4): This is taken with the patient supine with the tube directed 60 degrees caudally, perpendicular to the pelvic brim.

- This is useful for determining anterior or posterior displacement of the sacroiliac joint, sacrum, or iliac wing.
- It may determine internal rotation deformities of the ilium and sacral impaction injuries.

☐ **Outlet radiograph (Fig. 25.5):** This is taken with the patient supine with the tube directed 45 degrees cephalad.

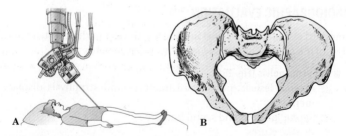

FIGURE 25.4 Inlet view of the pelvis: technique **(A)** and artist's sketch **(B)**. (Modified from Tile M. *Fractures of the Pelvis and Acetabulum.* 2nd ed. Baltimore: Williams & Wilkins; 1995.)

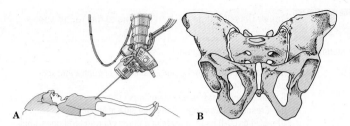

FIGURE 25.5 Outlet view of the pelvis: technique **(A)** and artist's sketch **(B)**. (Modified from Tile M. *Fractures of the Pelvis and Acetabulum.* 2nd ed. Baltimore: Williams & Wilkins; 1995.)

- This is useful for determination of vertical displacement of the hemipelvis.
- It may allow for visualization of subtle signs of pelvic disruption, such as a slightly widened sacroiliac joint, discontinuity of the sacral borders, nondisplaced sacral fractures, or disruption of the sacral foramina.
- **Computed tomography:** This is excellent for assessing the posterior pelvis, including the sacrum and sacroiliac joints.
- **Magnetic resonance imaging:** It has limited clinical utility owing to restricted access to a critically injured patient, prolonged duration of imaging, and equipment constraints. However, it may provide superior imaging of genitourinary and pelvic vascular structures.
- **Stress views:** Push–pull radiographs are performed while the patient is under general anesthesia to assess vertical stability.
  - Tile-defined instability as ≥0.5 cm of motion.
  - Bucholz, Kellam, and Browner consider ≥1 cm of vertical displacement unstable.
- Radiographic signs of instability include
  - Sacroiliac displacement of 5 mm in any plane.
  - Posterior fracture gap (rather than impaction).
  - Avulsion of the fifth lumbar transverse process, the lateral border of the sacrum (sacrotuberous ligament), or the ischial spine (sacrospinous ligament).

CLASSIFICATION

Young and Burgess

The Young and Burgess system (Table 25.1 and Fig. 25.6) is based on the mechanism of injury.

TABLE 25.1	Injury Classification Keys According to the Young and Burgess System
Category	Distinguishing Characteristics
LC	Transverse fracture of pubic rami, ipsilateral or contralateral to posterior injury I—Sacral compression on side of impact II—Crescent (iliac wing) fracture on side of impact III—LC-I or LC-II injury on side of impact; contralateral open-book (APC) injury
APC	Symphyseal diastasis or longitudinal rami fractures I—Slight widening of pubic symphysis or anterior sacroiliac joint; stretched but intact anterior sacroiliac, sacrotuberous, and sacrospinous ligaments; intact posterior sacroiliac ligaments II—Widened anterior sacroiliac joint; disrupted anterior sacroiliac, sacrotuberous, and sacrospinous ligaments; intact posterior sacroiliac ligaments III—Complete sacroiliac joint disruption with lateral displacement, disrupted anterior sacroiliac, sacrotuberous, and sacrospinous ligaments; disrupted posterior sacroiliac ligaments
VS	Symphyseal diastasis or vertical displacement anteriorly and posteriorly, usually through the sacroiliac joint, occasionally through the iliac wing or sacrum
CM	Combination of other injury patterns, LC/VS being the most common

Modified from Bucholz RW, Heckman JD, eds. *Rockwood and Green's Fractures in Adults*. 5th ed. Baltimore: Lippincott Williams & Wilkins; 2002:1487.

1. **LC:** This is an implosion of the pelvis secondary to laterally applied force that shortens the anterior sacroiliac, sacrospinous, and sacrotuberous ligaments. One may see oblique fractures of the pubic rami, ipsilateral or contralateral to the posterior injury.

Type I: Sacral impaction on the side of impact. Transverse fractures of the pubic rami are stable.

Type II: Posterior iliac wing fracture (crescent) on the side of impact with variable disruption of the posterior ligamentous structures resulting in variable mobility of the anterior fragment to internal rotation stress. It maintains vertical stability and may be associated with an anterior sacral crush injury.

Type III: LC-I or LC-II injury on the side of impact; force continued to contralateral hemipelvis to produce an external rotation injury (windswept pelvis) owing to sacroiliac, sacrotuberous, and sacrospinous ligamentous disruption. Instability may result with hemorrhage and neurologic injury secondary to traction injury on the side of sacroiliac injury.

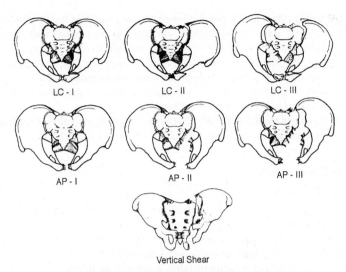

LC - I   LC - II   LC - III

AP - I   AP - II   AP - III

Vertical Shear

FIGURE 25.6 Young and Burgess classification of pelvic ring fractures. (From Young JWR, Burgess AR. *Radiologic Management of Pelvic Ring Fractures.* Baltimore: Urban & Schwarzenberg; 1987, with permission.)

2. **AP compression (APC):** This is anteriorly applied force from direct impact or indirectly transferred via the lower extremities or ischial tuberosities resulting in external rotation injuries, symphyseal diastasis, or longitudinal rami fractures.

    Type I: Less than 2.5 cm of symphyseal diastasis. Vertical fractures of one or both pubic rami occur, with intact posterior ligaments.

    Type II: More than 2.5 cm of symphyseal diastasis; widening of sacroiliac joints; caused by anterior sacroiliac ligament disruption. Disruption of the sacrotuberous, sacrospinous, and symphyseal ligaments with intact posterior sacroiliac ligaments results in an "open book" injury with internal and external rotational instability; vertical stability is maintained.

    Type III: Complete disruption of the symphysis, sacrotuberous, sacrospinous, and sacroiliac ligaments resulting in extreme rotational instability and lateral displacement; no cephaloposterior displacement. It is completely unstable with the highest rate of associated vascular injuries and blood loss.

3. **VS:** Vertically or longitudinally applied forces caused by falls onto an extended lower extremity, impacts from above, or motor vehicle

accidents with an extended lower extremity against the floorboard or dashboard. These injuries are typically associated with complete disruption of the symphysis, sacrotuberous, sacrospinous, and sacroiliac ligaments and result in extreme instability, most commonly in a cephaloposterior direction because of the inclination of the pelvis. They have a highly associated incidence of neurovascular injury and hemorrhage.

4. **Combined mechanical (CM):** Combination of injuries often resulting from crush mechanisms. The most common are VS and LC.

Tile Classification

Type A:	Stable
A1:	Fractures of the pelvis not involving the ring; avulsion injuries
A2:	Stable, minimal displacement of the ring
Type B:	Rotationally unstable, vertically stable
B1:	External rotation instability; open-book injury
B2:	LC injury; internal rotation instability; ipsilateral only
B3:	LC injury; bilateral rotational instability (bucket handle)
Type C:	Rotationally and vertically unstable
C1:	Unilateral injury
C2:	Bilateral injury, one side rotationally unstable, with the contralateral side vertically unstable
C3:	Bilateral injury, both sides rotationally and vertically unstable with an associated acetabular fracture

OTA Classification of Pelvic Fractures

See Fracture and Dislocation Classification Compendium at http://www.ota.org/compendium/compendium.html.

FACTORS INCREASING MORTALITY

- Type of pelvic ring injury
  - Posterior disruption is associated with higher mortality (APC-III, VS, LC-III).
- High Injury Severity Score (Tile, 1980; McMurty, 1980)
- Associated injuries
  - Head and abdominal, 50% mortality
- Hemorrhagic shock on admission (Gilliland, 1982)
- Requirement for large quantities of blood (McMurty, 1980)
- Perineal lacerations, open fractures (Hanson, 1991)
- Increased age (Looser, 1976)

Associated Morel–Lavallé Lesion (Skin Degloving Injury)

■ Colonized in up to one-third of cases
■ Requires thorough debridement before definitive surgery

TREATMENT

■ The recommended management of pelvic fractures varies from institution to institution, a finding highlighting that these are difficult injuries to treat and require an algorithmic approach (Fig. 25.7).

Nonoperative

Fractures amenable to nonoperative treatment include

■ Most LC-1 and APC-1 fractures.
■ Gapping of pubic symphysis <2.5 cm.
■ Rehabilitation
  □ Protect weight bearing typically with a walker or crutches initially.
  □ Serial radiographs are required after mobilization has begun to monitor for subsequent displacement.
  □ If secondary displacement of the posterior ring >1 cm is noted, weight bearing should be stopped. Operative treatment should be considered for gross displacement.

Absolute Indications for Operative Treatment

■ Open pelvic fractures or those in which there is an associated visceral perforation requiring operative intervention.
■ Open-book fractures or vertically unstable fractures with associated patient hemodynamic instability.

Relative Indications for Operative Treatment

■ Symphyseal diastasis >2.5 cm (loss of mechanical stability)
■ Leg-length discrepancy >1.5 cm
■ Rotational deformity
■ Sacral displacement >1 cm.
■ Intractable pain

Operative Techniques

■ **External fixation:** This can be applied as a construct mounted on two to three 5-mm pins spaced 1 cm apart along the anterior iliac crest, or with the use of single pins placed in the supra-acetabular area in an AP direction (Hanover frame).

External fixation is a resuscitative fixation and can only be used for definitive fixation of anterior pelvis injuries; it cannot be used as definitive fixation of posteriorly unstable injuries.

- **Internal fixation:** This significantly increases the forces resisted by the pelvic ring compared with external fixation.
  - □ **Iliac wing fractures:** Open reduction and stable internal fixation are performed using lag screws and neutralization plates.
  - □ **Diastasis of the pubic symphysis:** Plate fixation is most commonly used. Presence of an open injury, rectal or bladder injury, requires coordination between orthopaedics, trauma, and genitourinary surgery services to identify the best care plan.
  - □ **Sacral fractures:** Transiliac bar fixation may be inadequate or may cause compressive neurologic injury; in these cases, plate fixation or noncompressive iliosacral screw fixation may be indicated.
  - □ **Unilateral sacroiliac dislocation:** Direct fixation with iliosacral screws or anterior sacroiliac plate fixation is used.
  - □ **Bilateral posterior unstable disruptions:** Fixation of the displaced portion of the pelvis to the sacral body may be accomplished by posterior screw fixation. In addition, lumbopelvic fixation may be utilized in these cases.

Special Considerations

- **Open fractures:** In addition to fracture stabilization, hemorrhage control, and resuscitation, priority must be given to evaluation of the anus, rectum, vagina, and genitourinary system.
  - □ Anterior and lateral wounds generally are protected by muscle and are not contaminated by internal sources.
  - □ Posterior and perineal wounds may be contaminated by rectal and vaginal tears and genitourinary injuries.
  - □ Colostomy may be necessary for large bowel perforations or injuries to the anorectal region. Colostomy is indicated for any open injury where the fecal stream will contact the open area.
- Urologic injury
  - □ The incidence is up to 20%.
  - □ Blood at the meatus or a high-riding prostate may be noted.
  - □ Retrograde urethrogram is indicated in patients with suspicion of urologic injury, but one should ensure hemodynamic stability as embolization may be difficult because of dye extravasation.
  - □ Intraperitoneal bladder ruptures are repaired. Extraperitoneal ruptures may be observed.
  - □ Urethral injuries are repaired on a delayed basis.
- Neurologic injury
  - □ L2 to S4 are possible.

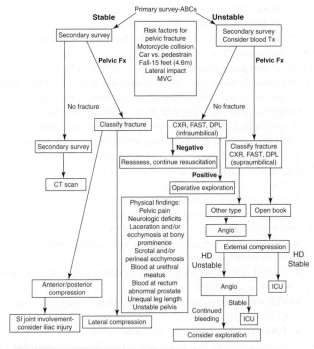

FIGURE 25.7 NYU Hospital for Joint Diseases algorithm for evaluation of a patient who presents to the ED with a suspected pelvic fracture.

☐ L5 and S1 are most common.
☐ Neurologic injury depends on the location of the fracture and the amount of displacement.
☐ **Sacral fractures:** neurologic injury
  • **Lateral to foramen (Denis I):** 6% injury
  • **Through foramen (Denis II):** 28% injury
  • **Medial to foramen (Denis III):** 57% injury
☐ Decompression of sacral foramen may be indicated if progressive loss of neural function occurs.
☐ It may take up to 3 years for recovery.
■ **Hypovolemic shock:** origin
☐ Intrathoracic bleeding
☐ Intraperitoneal bleeding
  • Diagnostic tables
  • Ultrasound
  • Peritoneal tap
  • Computed tomography
☐ Retroperitoneal bleeding

- ☐ Blood loss from open wounds
- ☐ Bleeding from multiple extremity fractures
- ■ AP injuries are associated with the largest amount of blood loss and greatest mortality.
- ■ **Postoperative management:** In general, early mobilization is desired.
  - ☐ Aggressive pulmonary toilet should be pursued with incentive spirometry, early mobilization, encouraged deep inspirations and coughing, and suctioning or chest physical therapy, if necessary.
  - ☐ Prophylaxis against thromboembolic phenomena should be undertaken, with a combination of elastic stockings, sequential compression devices, and chemoprophylaxis if hemodynamic and injury status allows.
  - ☐ High-risk patients unable to be chemically anticoagulated should undergo vena caval filter placement.
    - • Newer designs are retrievable up to 6 months after placement.
  - ☐ Weight-bearing status may be advanced as follows:
    - • Full weight bearing on the uninvolved lower extremity/sacral side occurs within several days.
    - • Partial weight bearing on the involved side is recommended for at least 6 weeks.
    - • Full weight bearing on the affected side without crutches is indicated by 12 weeks.
    - • Patients with bilateral unstable pelvic fractures should be mobilized from bed to chair with aggressive pulmonary toilet until radiographic evidence of fracture healing is noted. Partial weight bearing on the "less" injured side is generally tolerated by 12 weeks.

COMPLICATIONS

- ■ **Infection:** The incidence is variable, ranging from 0% to 25%, although the presence of wound infection does not preclude a successful result. The presence of contusion or shear injuries to soft tissues (Morel lesion) is a risk factor for infection if a posterior approach is used. This risk is minimized by a percutaneous posterior ring fixation.
- ■ **Thromboembolism:** Disruption of the pelvic venous vasculature and immobilization constitute major risk factors for the development of deep venous thromboses.
- ■ **Malunion:** Significant disability may result, with complications including chronic pain, limb length inequalities, gait disturbances, sitting difficulties, low back pain, and pelvic outlet obstruction.
- ■ **Nonunion:** This is rare, although it tends to occur more in younger patients (average age 35 years) with possible sequelae of pain, gait

abnormalities, and nerve root compression or irritation. Stable fixation and bone grafting are usually necessary for union.

■ Mortality
  □ Hemodynamically stable patients 3%
  □ Hemodynamically unstable patients 38%
  □ **LC:** head injury major cause of death
  □ **APC:** pelvic and visceral injury major cause of death
  □ **AP3 (comprehensive posterior instability):** 37%: death
  □ **VS:** 25% death

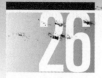

Acetabulum

EPIDEMIOLOGY

- The incidence of acetabular fractures is 3 per 100,000 population per year.
- Neurologic injuries occur in up to 30% of cases are usually partial injuries to the sciatic nerve, with the peroneal division more commonly injured than the tibial division.

ANATOMY

- From the lateral aspect of the pelvis, the innominate osseous structural support of the acetabulum may be conceptualized as a two-columned construct (Judet and Letournel) forming an inverted Y (Fig. 26.1).
- **Anterior column (iliopubic component):** This extends from the iliac crest to the symphysis pubis and includes the anterior wall of the acetabulum.
- **Posterior column (ilioischial component):** This extends from the superior gluteal notch to the ischial tuberosity and includes the posterior wall of the acetabulum.
- **Acetabular dome:** This is the superior weight-bearing portion of the acetabulum at the junction of the anterior and posterior columns, including contributions from each.
- Corona mortis
  - A vascular communication between the external iliac or deep inferior epigastric and the obturator may be visualized within the second window of the ilioinguinal approach.
  - Present in up to 10–15% of patients
  - May extend over the superior pubic ramus; average distance from the symphysis to corona 6 cm
- Ascending branch of medial circumflex
  - Main blood supply to femoral head
  - Deep to quadratus femoris
- Superior gluteal neurovascular bundle
  - Emerges from the greater sciatic notch

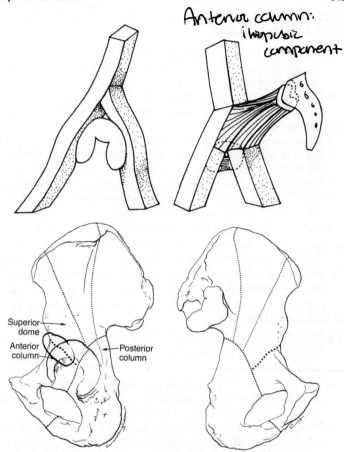

Handwritten annotation: *Anterior column: iliopubic component*

FIGURE 26.1 **(A)** A diagram of the two columns as an inverted Y supporting the acetabulum. **(B)** The two columns are linked to the sacral bone by the "sciatic buttress." **(C)** Lateral aspect of the hemipelvis and acetabulum. The posterior column is characterized by the dense bone at the greater sciatic notch and follows the *dotted line* distally through the center of the acetabulum, the obturator foramen, and the inferior pubic ramus. The anterior column extends from the iliac crest to the symphysis pubis and includes the entire anterior wall of the acetabulum. Fractures involving the anterior column commonly exit below the anterior-inferior iliac spine as shown by the *heavy dotted line*. **(D)** The hemipelvis from its medial aspect, showing the columns from the quadrilateral plate. The area between the posterior column and the *heavy dotted line*, representing a fracture through the anterior column, is often considered the superior dome fragment. (From Letournel E, Judet R. *Fractures of the Acetabulum.* New York: Springer-Verlag; 1964.)

MECHANISM OF INJURY

- Like pelvis fractures, these injuries are mainly caused by high-energy trauma secondary to a motor vehicle, motorcycle accident, or fall from a height.
- The fracture pattern depends on the position of the femoral head at the time of injury, the magnitude of force, and the age of the patient.
- Direct impact to the greater trochanter with the hip in neutral position can cause a transverse type of acetabular fracture (an abducted hip causes a low transverse fracture, whereas an adducted hip causes a high transverse fracture). An externally rotated and abducted hip anterior column injury. An internally rotated hip causes posterior column injury.
- With indirect trauma (e.g., a "dashboard"-type injury to the flexed knee), as the degree of hip flexion increases, the posterior wall is fractured in an increasingly inferior position. Similarly, as the degree of hip flexion decreases, the superior portion of the posterior wall is more likely to be involved.

CLINICAL EVALUATION

- Trauma evaluation is usually necessary, with attention to airway, breathing, circulation, disability, and exposure, depending on the mechanism of injury.
- Patient factors, such as patient age, degree of trauma, presence of associated injuries, and general medical condition are important because they affect treatment decisions as well as prognosis.
- Careful assessment of neurovascular status is necessary because sciatic nerve injury may be present in up to 40% of posterior column disruptions. In rare cases, maybe entrapped within the posterior column fracture. Femoral nerve involvement with anterior column injury is rare, although compromise of the femoral artery by a fractured anterior column has been described.
- The presence of associated ipsilateral injuries must be ruled out, with particular attention to the ipsilateral knee in which posterior instability and patellar fractures are common.
- Soft tissue injuries (e.g., abrasions, contusions, presence of subcutaneous hemorrhage, Morel lesion) may provide insight into the mechanism of injury.

RADIOGRAPHIC EVALUATION

- An anteroposterior (AP) and two Judet views (iliac and obturator oblique views) should be obtained.

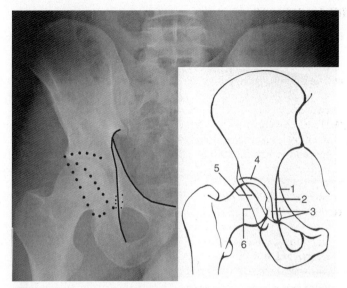

FIGURE 26.2 Diagram outlining the major landmarks: the iliopectineal line (anterior column), the ilioischial line (posterior column), the anterior lip of the acetabulum, and the posterior lip of the acetabulum. (From Bucholz RW, Heckman JD, eds. *Rockwood and Green's Fractures in Adults.* 5th ed. Baltimore: Lippincott Williams & Wilkins; 2002.)

- **AP view:** Anatomic landmarks include the iliopectineal line (limit of anterior column), the ilioischial line (limit of posterior column), the anterior lip, the posterior lip, and the line depicting the superior weight-bearing surface of the acetabulum terminating as the medial teardrop (Fig. 26.2).
- **Iliac oblique radiograph (45-degree external rotation view):** This best demonstrates the posterior column (ilioischial line), the iliac wing, and the anterior wall of the acetabulum (Fig. 26.3).
- **Obturator oblique view (45-degree internal rotation view):** This is best for evaluating the anterior column and posterior wall of the acetabulum (Fig. 26.4).
- **Computed tomography (CT):** This provides additional information regarding size and position of column fractures, impacted fractures of the acetabular wall, retained bone fragments in the joint, degree of comminution, and sacroiliac joint disruption. Three-dimensional reconstruction allows for digital subtraction of the femoral head, resulting in full delineation of the acetabular surface.

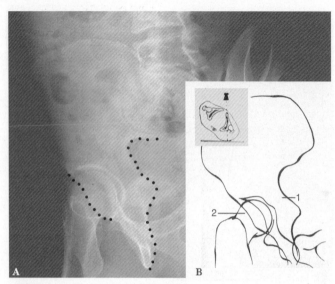

FIGURE 26.3 Iliac oblique view **(A)**. This view is taken by rotating the patient into 45 degrees of external rotation by elevating the uninjured side on a wedge. **(B)** Diagram of the anatomic landmarks of the left hemipelvis on the iliac oblique view. This view best demonstrates the posterior column of the acetabulum, outlined by the ilioischial line, the iliac crest, and the anterior lip of the acetabulum. (From Tile M. *Fractures of the Pelvis and Acetabulum.* 2nd ed. Baltimore: Williams & Wilkins; 1995.)

CLASSIFICATION

Judet–Letournel

Based on degree of columnar damage, there are 10 fracture patterns, 5 "elementary" and 5 "associated" (Fig. 26.5).

Elementary Fractures	Associated Fractures
Posterior wall	T-shaped
Posterior column	Posterior column and posterior wall
Anterior wall	Transverse and posterior wall
Anterior column	Anterior column/posterior hemitransverse
Transverse	Both-column

Elementary Fractures

- Posterior wall fracture
  - □ This involves a separation of posterior articular surface.
  - □ Most of the posterior column is undisturbed.

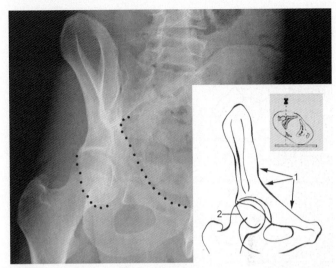

FIGURE 26.4 Obterator oblique view **(A)**. This view is taken by elevating the affected hip 45 degrees to the horizontal by means of a wedge and directing the beam through the hip joint with a 15-degree upward tilt. **(B)** Diagram of the anatomy of the pelvis on the obturator oblique view. (From Bucholz RW, Heckman JD, eds. *Rockwood and Green's Fractures in Adults*. 5th ed. Baltimore: Lippincott Williams & Wilkins; 2002.)

- □ It is often associated with posterior femoral head dislocation.
- □ The posterior wall fragment is best visualized on the obturator oblique view.
- □ "Marginal impaction" is often present in posterior fracture–dislocations (articular cartilage impacted into underlying cancellous bone).
  - • Marginal impaction is identified in 25% of posterior fracture–dislocations requiring open reduction. This is best appreciated on CT scan.
- ■ Posterior column fracture
  - □ The ischium is disrupted.
  - □ The fracture line originates at the greater sciatic notch, travels across the retroacetabular surface, and exits at the obturator foramen.
  - □ The ischiopubic ramus is fractured.
  - □ Medial displacement of the femoral head can occur.
- ■ Anterior wall fracture
  - □ Disruption of a small portion of the anterior roof and acetabulum occurs.

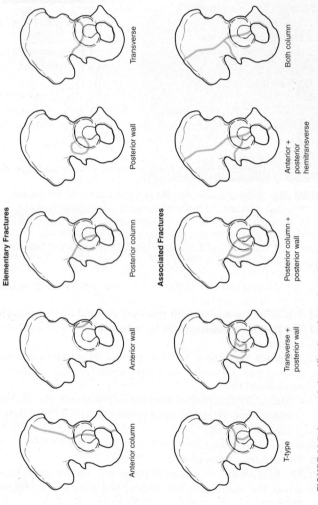

Elementary Fractures

Anterior column

Anterior wall

Posterior column

Posterior wall

Transverse

Associated Fractures

T-type

Transverse + posterior wall

Posterior column + posterior wall

Anterior + posterior hemitransverse

Both column

FIGURE 26.5 Letournel classification of acetabular fractures.

- ☐ Much of anterior column is undisturbed.
- ☐ The ischiopubic ramus is not fractured.
- ☐ The teardrop is often displaced medially with respect to the ilioischial line.
- ■ Anterior column fracture
  - ☐ This is associated with disruption of the iliopectineal line.
  - ☐ It is often associated with anteromedial displacement of the femoral head.
  - ☐ It is classified according to the level at which the superior margin of the fracture line divides the innominate bone: low, intermediate, or high pattern.
  - ☐ The more superiorly the fracture line ascends, the greater the involvement of the weight-bearing aspect of the acetabulum.
  - ☐ CT may be helpful in delineating the degree of articular surface involvement.
- ■ Transverse fracture
  - ☐ The innominate bone is separated into two fragments, dividing the acetabular articular surface in one of three ways:
    1. Transtectal: through the acetabular dome
    2. Juxtatectal: through the junction of the acetabular dome and fossa acetabuli
    3. Infratectal: through the fossa acetabuli
  - ☐ The more superior the fracture line, the greater the displacement of the acetabular dome will be.
  - ☐ The femoral head follows the inferior ischiopubic fragment and may dislocate centrally.
  - ☐ The ilioischial line and teardrop maintain a normal relationship.
  - ☐ CT typically demonstrates an AP fracture line.

Associated Fractures

- ■ Associated posterior column and posterior wall fracture
  - ☐ Two elementary fracture patterns are present. The posterior wall is usually markedly displaced/rotated in relation to the posterior column. This injury represents one pattern of posterior hip dislocation that is frequently accompanied by injury to the sciatic nerve.
- ■ T-shaped fracture
  - ☐ This combines a transverse fracture of any type (transtectal, juxtatectal, or infratectal) with an additional vertical fracture line that divides the ischiopubic fragment into two parts. The vertical component, or stem, may exit anteriorly, inferiorly, or posteriorly depending on the vector of the injurious force. The vertical component is best seen on the obturator oblique view.

- Associated transverse and posterior wall fracture
  - □ The obturator oblique view best demonstrates the position of the transverse component as well as the posterior wall element. By CT, in two-thirds of cases, the femoral head dislocates posteriorly; in one-third of cases, the head dislocates centrally.
  - □ Marginal impaction may exist; this is best evaluated by CT.
- Associated anterior column and posterior hemitransverse fracture
  - □ This combines an anterior wall or anterior column fracture (of any type) with a fracture line that divides the posterior column exactly as it would a transverse fracture. It is termed a hemitransverse because the "transverse" component involves only one column.
  - □ Importantly, in this fracture a piece of acetabular articular surface remains nondisplaced and is the key for operative reduction of other fragments.
- Both-column fracture
  - □ This is the most complex type of acetabular fracture, formerly called a "central acetabular fracture."
  - □ Both columns are separated from each other and from the axial skeleton, resulting in a "floating" acetabulum.
  - □ The "spur" sign above the acetabulum on an obturator oblique radiograph is diagnostic.

OTA Classification of Acetabular Fractures

See Fracture and Dislocation Classification Compendium at http://www.ota.org/compendium/compendium.html.

TREATMENT

The goal of treatment is anatomic restoration of the articular surface to prevent posttraumatic arthritis (Fig. 26.6).

Initial Management

The patient is usually placed in skeletal traction to minimize further soft tissue damage, allow associated injuries to be addressed, maintain the length of the limb, and maintain femoral head reduction within the acetabulum.

Nonoperative

- A system for roughly quantifying the acetabular dome following fracture can be employed using three measurements: (1) the medial, (2) anterior, and (3) posterior roof arcs, measured on the AP, obturator oblique, and the iliac oblique views, respectively.

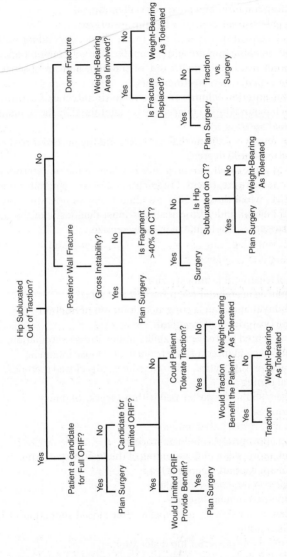

FIGURE 26.6 Treatment algorithm for acetabular fractures. (From Bucholz RW, Heckman JD, eds. *Rockwood and Green's Fractures in Adults*. 5th ed. Baltimore: Lippincott Williams & Wilkins; 2002.)

- □ The roof arc is formed by the angle between two lines, one drawn vertically through the geometric center of the acetabulum, the other from the fracture line to the geometric center.
- □ Roof arc angles are of limited utility for evaluation of both-column fractures and posterior wall fractures.
- Nonoperative treatment may be appropriate in
  - □ Displacement of <2 to 5 mm in the dome, depending on the location of the fracture and patient factors, with maintenance of femoral head congruency out of traction, and an absence of intra-articular osseous fragments.
  - □ Distal anterior column or transverse (infratectal) fractures in which femoral head congruency is maintained by the remaining medial buttress.
  - □ Maintenance of the medial, anterior, and the posterior roof arcs greater than 45 degrees.
  - □ For posterior wall fractures, size has been a major determinant for operative treatment. Fragments <20% are generally nonoperative, while those >50% are almost always operative. Stress examination under fluoroscopy is most diagnostic of the need for surgery in fragments of in-between size.

Operative

- Surgical treatment is indicated for
  - □ Displaced acetabular fractures (>2 to 3 mm).
  - □ Inability to maintain a congruent joint out of traction.
  - □ Large posterior wall fragment.
  - □ Documented posterior instability under stress examination.
  - □ Removal of an interposed intra-articular loose fragment.
  - □ A fracture–dislocation that is irreducible by closed methods.
- Surgical timing
  - □ Surgery should be performed within 2 weeks of injury.
  - □ It requires
    - A well-resuscitated patient
    - An appropriate radiologic workup
    - An appropriate understanding of the fracture pattern
    - An appropriate operative team
  - □ Surgical emergencies include
    - Open acetabular fracture.
    - New-onset sciatic nerve palsy after closed reduction of hip dislocation.
    - Irreducible posterior hip dislocation.
    - Medial dislocation of femoral head against cancellous bone surface of intact ilium.

- Morel–Lavallé lesion (skin degloving injury)
  - ☐ This is infected in one-third of cases with this lesion.
  - ☐ This requires thorough debridement before definitive fracture surgery.
- Not been shown to be predictive of clinical outcome
  - ☐ Fracture pattern
  - ☐ Posterior dislocation
  - ☐ Initial displacement
  - ☐ Presence of intra-articular fragments
  - ☐ Presence of acetabular impaction
- Has been shown to be predictive of clinical outcome
  - ☐ Injury to cartilage or bone of femoral head
    - **Damage:** 60% good/excellent result
    - **No damage:** 80% good/excellent result
  - ☐ Anatomic reduction
  - ☐ Posterior wall comminution
  - ☐ **Age of patient:** predictive of the ability to achieve an anatomic reduction

Stability

- Instability is most common in posterior fracture types but may be present when large fractures of the quadrilateral plate allow central subluxation of the femoral head or anterior with major anterior wall fractures.
- Central instability results when a quadrilateral plate fracture is of sufficient size to allow for central subluxation of the femoral head. A medial buttress with a spring plate or cerclage wire is necessary to restore stability.
- Anterior instability results from a large anterior wall fracture or as part of an anterior type fracture with posterior hemitransverse fracture.

Congruity

- Incongruity of the hip may result in early degenerative changes and posttraumatic osteoarthritis. Evaluation is best made by CT. Acceptance of incongruity is based on the location within the acetabulum.
- Displaced dome fractures rarely reduce with traction; surgery is usually necessary for adequate restoration of the weight-bearing surface.
- High transverse or T-type fractures are shearing injuries that are grossly unstable when they involve the superior, weight-bearing

dome. Nonoperative reduction is virtually impossible, whereas operative reduction can be extremely difficult.

■ **Displaced both-column fractures (floating acetabulum):** Surgery is indicated for restoration of congruence if the roof fragment is displaced and secondary congruence cannot be obtained or if the posterior column is grossly displaced.

■ Retained osseous fragments may result in incongruity or an inability to maintain concentric reduction of the femoral head. Avulsions of the ligamentum teres need not be removed unless they are of substantial size.

■ Femoral head fractures generally require open reduction and internal fixation to maintain sphericity and congruity.

■ Soft tissue interposition may necessitate operative removal of the interposed tissues.

■ Assessment of reduction includes
  □ Restoration of pelvic lines.
  □ Comparison to contralateral hip on the AP pelvis X-ray
  □ Concentric reduction on all three views
  □ The goal of anatomic reduction

Surgical Approaches

Approaches to the acetabulum include the Kocher–Langenbach ilioinguinal and extended iliofemoral. No single approach provides ideal exposure of all fracture types. Proper preoperative classification of the fracture configuration is essential to selecting the best surgical approach.

■ Kocher–Langenbach
  □ Indications
    • Posterior wall fractures
    • Posterior column fractures
    • Posterior column/posterior wall fractures
    • Juxtatectal/infratectal transverse or transverse with posterior wall fractures
    • Some T-type fractures
  □ Access
    • Entire posterior column
    • Greater and lesser sciatic notches
    • Ischial spine
    • Retroacetabular surface
    • Ischial tuberosity
    • Ischiopubic ramus
  □ Limitations
    • Superior acetabular region

- Anterior column
  - Fractures high in greater sciatic notch
  □ Complications
  - **Sciatic nerve palsy:** 10%
  - **Infection:** 3%
  - **Heterotopic ossification:** 8% to 25%
- Ilioinguinal
  □ Indications
  - Anterior wall
  - Anterior column
  - Transverse with significant anterior displacement
  - Anterior column/posterior hemitransverse
  - Both-column
  □ Access
  - Sacroiliac joint
  - Internal iliac fossa
  - Pelvic brim
  - Quadrilateral surface
  - Superior pubic ramus
  - Limited access to external iliac wing
  □ Complications
  - **Direct hernia:** 1%
  - **Significant lateral femoral circumflex artery nerve numbness:** 23%
  - **External iliac artery thrombosis:** 1%
  - **Hematoma:** 5%
  - **Infection:** 2%
- Modified Stoppa
  □ Indications
  - Anterior wall
  - Anterior column
  - Transverse with significant anterior displacement
  - Anterior column/posterior hemitransverse
  - Both-column
  □ Access
  - Sacroiliac joint
  - Internal iliac fossa
  - Pelvic brim
  - Quadrilateral surface
  - Superior pubic ramus
  - Limited access to external iliac wing
  □ Complications
  - Rectus hernia
  - Hematoma
  - Infection

■ Extended iliofemoral
  □ Indications
    • Transtectal transverse plus posterior wall or T-shaped fractures
    • Transverse fractures with extended posterior wall
    • T-shaped fractures with wide separations of the vertical stem of the "T" or those with associated pubic symphysis dislocations
    • Certain associated both-column fractures
    • Associated fracture patterns or transverse fractures operated on more than 21 days following injury
  □ Access
    • External aspect of the ilium
    • Anterior column as far medial as the iliopectineal eminence
    • Posterior column to the upper ischial tuberosity
■ Complications
    • **Infection:** 2% to 5%
    • **Sciatic nerve palsy:** 3% to 5%
    • **Heterotopic ossification:** 20% to 50% without prophylaxis

Postoperative Care

■ Indomethacin or irradiation is indicated for heterotopic ossification prophylaxis.
■ Chemical prophylaxis, sequential compression devices, and compressive stockings for thromboembolic prophylaxis are recommended. Inferior vena cava (IVC) filter for those not amenable to chemical prophylaxis.
■ Mobilization out of bed is indicated as associated injuries allow, with pulmonary toilet and incentive spirometry.
■ Full weight bearing on the affected extremity should be withheld until radiographic signs of union are present, generally by 8 to 12 weeks postoperatively.

COMPLICATIONS

■ **Surgical wound infection:** The risk is increased secondary to the presence of associated abdominal and pelvic visceral injuries. Local soft tissue injury from the original impact force may cause closed degloving or local abrasions. Postoperative hematoma formation occurs frequently, further contributing to potential wound infection.
■ Nerve injury
  □ **Sciatic nerve:** The Kocher–Langenbach approach with prolonged or forceful traction can cause sciatic nerve palsy (most often the peroneal branch; incidence, 16% to 33%).

- ☐ **Femoral nerve:** The ilioinguinal approach may result in traction injury to the femoral nerve. Rarely, the femoral nerve may be lacerated by an anterior column fracture.
- ☐ **Superior gluteal nerve:** This is most vulnerable in the greater sciatic notch. Injury to this nerve during trauma or surgery may result in paralysis of the hip abductors, often causing severe disability.
- ■ **Heterotopic ossification:** The incidence ranges from 3% to 69%, highest with the extended iliofemoral approach and second highest with the Kocher–Langenbach. The highest risk is a young male patient undergoing a posterolateral extensile approach in which muscle is removed. The lowest risk is with use of the ilioinguinal approach. Both indomethacin and low-dose radiation have been helpful in reducing the incidence of this complication.
- ■ **Avascular necrosis:** This devastating complication occurs in 6.6% of cases, mostly with posterior types associated with dislocations.
- ■ **Chondrolysis:** This may occur with nonoperative or operative treatment, resulting in posttraumatic osteoarthritis. Concentric reduction with restoration of articular congruity may minimize this complication.

Hip Dislocations

EPIDEMIOLOGY

- Up to 50% of patients sustain concomitant fractures elsewhere at the time of hip dislocation.
- Unrestrained motor vehicle accident occupants are at a significantly higher risk for sustaining a hip dislocation than passengers wearing a restraining device.
- Anterior dislocations constitute 10% to 15% of traumatic dislocations of the hip, with posterior dislocations accounting for the remainder.
- The incidence of femoral head osteonecrosis is between 2% and 17% of patients, while 16% of patients develop posttraumatic arthritis.
- Sciatic nerve injury is present in 10% to 20% of posterior dislocations (Fig. 27.1).

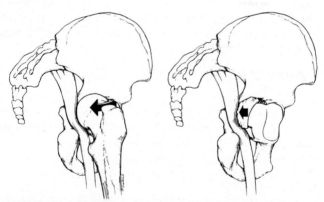

FIGURE 27.1 Left: Sciatic nerve impingement by the posteriorly dislocated femoral head. Right: Sciatic nerve impingement by a posterior acetabular fracture fragment in a posterior fracture–dislocation of the hip. (From Rockwood CA Jr, Green DP, Bucholz RW, Heckman JD, eds. *Rockwood and Green's Fractures in Adults*. Vol 1. 4th ed. Philadelphia: Lippincott-Raven; 1996:1756.)

ANATOMY

- The hip articulation has a ball-and-socket configuration with stability conferred by bony and ligamentous restraints, as well as the congruity of the femoral head with the acetabulum.
- The acetabulum is formed from the confluence of the ischium, ilium, and pubis at the triradiate cartilage.
- Forty percent of the femoral head is covered by the bony acetabulum at any position of hip motion. The effect of the labrum is to deepen the acetabulum and increase the stability of the joint.
- The hip joint capsule is formed by thick longitudinal fibers supplemented by much stronger ligamentous condensations (iliofemoral, pubofemoral, and ischiofemoral ligaments) that run in a spiral fashion, preventing excessive hip extension (Fig. 27.2).
- The main vascular supply to the femoral head originates from the medial and lateral femoral circumflex arteries, branches of the profunda femoral artery. An extracapsular vascular ring is formed at the base of the femoral neck with ascending cervical branches that pierce the hip joint at the level of the capsular insertion. These branches ascend along the femoral neck and enter the bone just inferior to the cartilage of the femoral head. The artery of the ligamentum teres, a branch of the obturator artery, may contribute blood supply to the epiphyseal region of the femoral head (Fig. 27.3).
- The sciatic nerve exits the pelvis at the greater sciatic notch. A certain degree of variability exists in the relationship of the nerve with the piriformis muscle and short external rotators of the hip. Most frequently, the sciatic nerve exits the pelvis deep to the muscle belly of the piriformis.

MECHANISM OF INJURY

- Hip dislocations almost always result from high-energy trauma, such as motor vehicle accident, fall from a height, or industrial accident. Force transmission to the hip joint occurs with application to one of three common sources:
  - ☐ The anterior surface of the flexed knee striking an object
  - ☐ The sole of the foot, with the ipsilateral knee extended
  - ☐ The greater trochanter
- Less frequently, the dislocating force may be applied to the posterior pelvis with the ipsilateral foot or knee acting as the counterforce.
- Direction of dislocation—anterior versus posterior—is determined by the direction of the pathologic force and the position of the lower extremity at the time of injury.

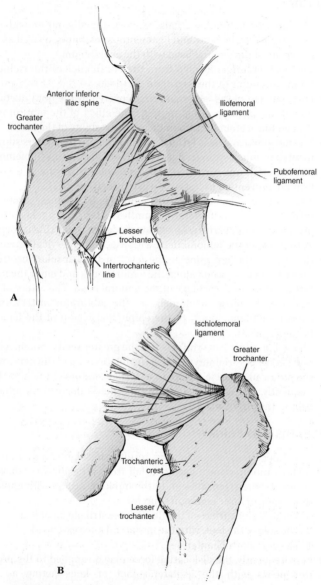

FIGURE 27.2 The hip capsule and its thickenings (ligaments) as visualized anteriorly **(A)** and posteriorly **(B)**. (From Bucholz RW, Heckman JD, Court-Brown C, et al., eds. *Rockwood and Green's Fractures in Adults*. 6th ed. Philadelphia: Lippincott Williams & Wilkins; 2006.)

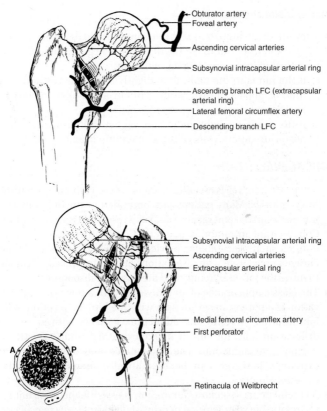

FIGURE 27.3 Vascular anatomy of the femoral head and neck. Top: Anterior aspect. Bottom: Posterior aspect. *LFC*, lateral femoral circumflex artery. (From Rockwood CA Jr, Green DP, Bucholz RW, Heckman JD, eds. *Rockwood and Green's Fractures in Adults.* Vol 2. 4th ed. Philadelphia: Lippincott-Raven; 1996:1662.)

Anterior Dislocations

- These comprise 10% to 15% of traumatic hip dislocations.
- They result from external rotation and abduction of the hip.
- The degree of hip flexion determines whether a superior or inferior type of anterior hip dislocation results.
  - Inferior (obturator) dislocation is the result of simultaneous abduction, external rotation, and hip flexion.
  - Superior (iliac or pubic) dislocation is the result of simultaneous abduction, external rotation, and hip extension.

Posterior Dislocations

- They are much more frequent than anterior hip dislocations.
- They result from trauma to the flexed knee (e.g., dashboard injury), with the hip in varying degrees of flexion.
  - □ If the hip is in the neutral or slightly adducted position at the time of impact, a dislocation without acetabular fracture will likely occur.
  - □ If the hip is in slight abduction, an associated fracture of the posterior-superior rim of the acetabulum usually occurs.

CLINICAL EVALUATION

- Full trauma survey is essential because of the high-energy nature of these injuries. Many patients are obtunded or unconscious when they arrive in the emergency room as a result of associated injuries. Concomitant intra-abdominal, chest, and other musculoskeletal injuries, such as acetabular, pelvic, or spine fractures, are common.
- Patients presenting with dislocations of the hip typically are unable to move the lower extremity and are in severe discomfort.
- The classic appearance of an individual with a posterior hip dislocation is a patient in severe pain with the hip in a position of flexion, internal rotation, and adduction. Patients with an anterior dislocation hold the hip in marked external rotation with mild flexion and abduction. The appearance and alignment of the extremity, however, can be dramatically altered by ipsilateral extremity injuries.
- A careful neurovascular examination is essential because injury to the sciatic nerve or femoral neurovascular structures may occur at time of dislocation. Sciatic nerve injury may occur with stretching of the nerve over the posteriorly dislocated femoral head. Posterior wall fragments from the acetabulum have the potential to injure the nerve. Usually, the peroneal portion of the nerve is affected, with little if any dysfunction of the tibial nerve. Rarely, injury to the femoral artery, vein, or nerve may occur as a result of an anterior dislocation. Ipsilateral knee, patella, and femur fractures are common. Pelvic fractures and spine injuries may also be seen.

RADIOGRAPHIC EVALUATION

- An anteroposterior (AP) radiograph of the pelvis is essential, as well as a cross-table lateral view of the affected hip.
- On the AP view of the pelvis
  - □ The femoral heads should appear similar in size, and the joint spaces should be symmetric throughout. In posterior dislocations,

the affected femoral head will appear smaller than the normal femoral head. In anterior dislocation, the femoral head will appear slightly larger than the normal hip because of magnification of the femoral head to the x-ray cassette.

☐ The Shenton line should be smooth and continuous.

☐ The relative appearance of the greater and lesser trochanters may indicate pathologic internal or external rotation of the hip. The adducted or abducted position of the femoral shaft should also be noted.

☐ One must evaluate the femoral neck to rule out the presence of a femoral neck fracture before any manipulative reduction.

■ A cross-table lateral view of the affected hip may help distinguish a posterior from an anterior dislocation.

■ Use of 45-degree oblique (Judet) views of the hip may be helpful to ascertain the presence of osteochondral fragments, the integrity of the acetabulum, and the congruence of the joint spaces. Femoral head depressions and fractures may also be seen.

■ Computed tomography (CT) scans may be obtained following closed reduction of a dislocated hip. If closed reduction is not possible and an open reduction is planned, a CT scan should be obtained to detect the presence of intra-articular fragments and to rule out associated femoral head and acetabular fractures.

■ The role of magnetic resonance imaging in the evaluation of hip dislocations has not been established; it may prove useful in the evaluation of the integrity of the labrum and the vascularity of the femoral head.

CLASSIFICATION

Hip dislocations are classified based on (1) the relationship of the femoral head to the acetabulum and (2) whether or not associated fractures are present.

Thompson and Epstein Classification of Posterior Hip Dislocations (Fig. 27.4)

Type I:	Simple dislocation with or without an insignificant posterior wall fragment
Type II:	Dislocation associated with a single large posterior wall fragment
Type III:	Dislocation with a comminuted posterior wall fragment
Type IV:	Dislocation with fracture of the acetabular floor
Type V:	Dislocation with fracture of the femoral head (Pipkin classification)

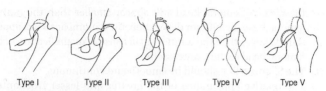

| Type I | Type II | Type III | Type IV | Type V |

FIGURE 27.4 Thompson and Epstein classification of posterior hip dislocations.

Epstein Classification of Anterior Hip Dislocations (Fig. 27.5)

Type I: Superior dislocations, including pubic and subspinous
IA: No associated fractures
IB: Associated fracture or impaction of the femoral head
IC: Associated fracture of the acetabulum
Type II: Inferior dislocations, including obturator, and perineal
IIA: No associated fractures
IIB: Associated fracture or impaction of the femoral head
IIC: Associated fracture of the acetabulum

OTA Classification of Hip Dislocations

See Fracture and Dislocation Classification Compendium at http://www.ota.org/compendium/compendium.html.

TREATMENT

- One should reduce the hip on an urgent basis to minimize the risk of osteonecrosis of the femoral head; it remains controversial whether this should be accomplished by closed or open methods. Most authors recommend an immediate attempt at a closed reduction, although some believe that all fracture–dislocations should have immediate open surgery to remove fragments from the joint and to reconstruct fractures.

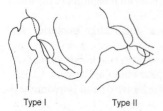

Type I   Type II

FIGURE 27.5 Epstein classification of anterior hip dislocations. (From Rockwood CA Jr, Green DP, eds. *Rockwood and Green's Fractures in Adults.* 3rd ed. Philadelphia: Lippincott-Raven; 1996:1576–1579.)

■ The long-term prognosis worsens if reduction (closed or open) is delayed more than 12 hours. Associated acetabular or femoral head fractures can be treated in the subacute phase.

Closed Reduction

Regardless of the direction of the dislocation, the reduction can be attempted with in-line traction with the patient lying supine. The preferred method is to perform a closed reduction using general anesthesia, but if this is not feasible, reduction under conscious sedation is possible. There are three popular methods of achieving closed reduction of the hip:

1. **ALLIS METHOD.** This consists of traction applied in line with the deformity. The patient is placed supine with the surgeon standing above the patient on the stretcher or table. Initially, the surgeon applies in-line traction while the assistant applies countertraction by stabilizing the patient's pelvis. While increasing the traction force, the surgeon should slowly increase the degree of flexion to approximately 70 degrees. Gentle rotational motions of the hip as well as slight adduction will often help the femoral head to clear the lip of the acetabulum. A lateral force to the proximal thigh may assist in reduction. An audible "clunk" is a sign of a successful closed reduction (Fig. 27.6).

2. **STIMSON GRAVITY TECHNIQUE.** The patient is placed prone on the stretcher with the affected leg hanging off the side of the stretcher. This brings the extremity into a position of hip flexion and knee flexion of 90 degrees each. In this position, the assistant immobilizes the pelvis, and the surgeon applies an anteriorly directed force on the proximal calf. Gentle rotation of the limb may assist in reduction (Fig. 27.7). This technique is difficult to perform in the emergency department.

3. **BIGELOW AND REVERSE BIGELOW MANEUVERS.** These have been associated with iatrogenic femoral neck fractures and are not as frequently used as reduction techniques. In the Bigelow maneuver, the patient is supine, and the surgeon applies longitudinal traction on the limb. The adducted and internally rotated thigh is then flexed at least 90 degrees. The femoral head is then levered into the acetabulum by abduction, external rotation, and extension of the hip. In the reverse Bigelow maneuver, used for anterior dislocations, traction is again applied in the line of the deformity. The hip is then adducted, sharply internally rotated, and extended.

   □ Following closed reduction, AP pelvis radiographs should be obtained to confirm the adequacy of reduction. The hip should be examined for stability while the patient is still sedated or

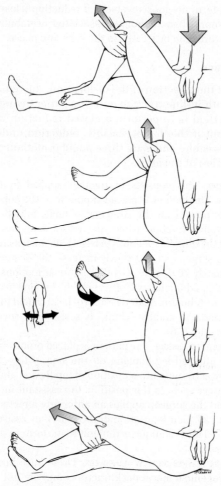

FIGURE 27.6 The Allis reduction technique for posterior hip dislocations. (From Bucholz RW, Heckman JD, Court-Brown C, et al., eds. *Rockwood and Green's Fractures in Adults*. 6th ed. Philadelphia: Lippincott Williams & Wilkins; 2006.)

under anesthesia. If there is an obvious large displaced acetabular fracture, the stability examination need not be performed.

- Stability is checked by flexing the hip to 90 degrees in neutral position. A posteriorly directed force is then applied. If any sensation of subluxation is detected, the patient will require

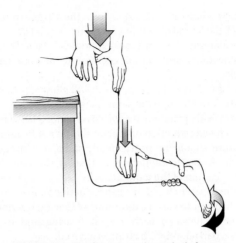

FIGURE 27.7 The Stimson gravity method of re-
duction (From Bucholz RW, Heckman JD, Court-
Brown C, et al., eds. *Rockwood and Green's
Fractures in Adults.* 6th ed. Philadelphia: Lippincott
Williams & Wilkins; 2006.)

additional diagnostic studies and possibly surgical exploration or traction.
- Following successful closed reduction and completion of the
  stability examination, the patient should undergo CT
  evaluation.

Open Reduction

- Indications for open reduction of a dislocated hip include
  □ Dislocation irreducible by closed means.
  □ Nonconcentric reduction.
  □ Fracture of the acetabulum or femoral head requiring excision
    or open reduction and internal fixation.
  □ Ipsilateral femoral neck fracture.
- A standard posterior approach (Kocher–Langenbeck) will allow
  exploration of the sciatic nerve, removal of posteriorly incarcerated fragments, treatment of major posterior labral disruptions or
  instability, and repair of posterior acetabular fractures.
- An anterior (Smith-Peterson) approach is recommended for isolated
  femoral head fractures. A concern when using an anterior approach
  for a posterior dislocation is the possibility of complete vascular
  disruption. By avoiding removal of the capsule from the femoral

neck and trochanters (i.e., taking down the capsule from the acetabular side), the lateral circumflex artery be preserved.

- An anterolateral (Watson-Jones) approach is useful for most anterior dislocations and combined fracture of both femoral head and neck.
- A direct lateral (Hardinge) approach will allow exposure anteriorly and posteriorly through the same incision.
- In the case of an ipsilateral displaced or nondisplaced femoral neck fracture, closed reduction of the hip should not be attempted. The hip fracture should be provisionally stabilized through a lateral approach. A gentle reduction is then performed, followed by definitive fixation of the femoral neck.
- Management after closed or open reduction ranges from short periods of bed rest to various durations of skeletal traction. No correlation exists between early weight bearing and osteonecrosis. Therefore, partial weight bearing is advised.
  - □ **If reduction is concentric and stable:** A short period of bed rest is followed by protected weight bearing for 4 to 6 weeks.
  - □ **If reduction is concentric but unstable:** Skeletal traction for 4 to 6 weeks is followed by protective weight bearing.

PROGNOSIS

- The outcome following hip dislocation ranges from an essentially normal hip to a severely painful and degenerated joint.
- Most authors report a 70% to 80% good or excellent outcome in simple posterior dislocations. When posterior dislocations are associated with a femoral head or acetabular fracture, however, the associated fractures generally dictate the outcome.
- Anterior dislocations of the hip are noted to have a higher incidence of associated femoral head injuries (transchondral or indentation types). The only patients with excellent results in most authors' series are those without an associated femoral head injury.

COMPLICATIONS

- **Osteonecrosis:** This is observed in 5% to 40% of injuries, with increased risk associated with increased time until reduction (>6 to 24 hours); however, some authors suggest that osteonecrosis may result from the initial injury and not from prolonged dislocation. Osteonecrosis may become clinically apparent several years after injury. Repeated reduction attempts may also increase its incidence.

- **Posttraumatic osteoarthritis:** This is the most frequent long-term complication of hip dislocations; the incidence is dramatically higher when dislocations are associated with acetabular fractures or transchondral fractures of the femoral head.
- **Recurrent dislocation:** This is rare (<2%), although patients with decreased femoral anteversion may sustain a recurrent posterior dislocation, whereas those with increased femoral anteversion may be prone to recurrent anterior dislocations.
- **Neurovascular injury:** Sciatic nerve injury occurs in 10% to 20% of hip dislocations. It is usually caused by a stretching of the nerve from a posteriorly dislocated head or from a displaced fracture fragment. Prognosis is unpredictable, but most authors report 40% to 50% full recovery. Electromyographic studies are indicated at 3 to 4 weeks for baseline information and prognostic guidance. If no clinical or electrical improvement is seen by 1 year, surgical intervention may be considered. If a sciatic nerve injury occurs after closed reduction is performed, then entrapment of the nerve is likely and surgical exploration is indicated. Injury to the femoral nerve and femoral vascular structures has been reported with anterior dislocations.
- **Femoral head fractures:** These occur in 10% of posterior dislocations (shear fractures) and in 25% to 75% of anterior dislocations (indentation fractures).
- **Heterotopic ossification:** This occurs in 2% of patients and is related to the initial muscular damage and hematoma formation. Surgery increases its incidence. Prophylaxis choices include indomethacin for 6 weeks or use of radiation.
- **Thromboembolism:** This may occur after hip dislocation owing to traction-induced intimal injury to the vasculature. Patients should be given adequate prophylaxis consisting of compression stockings, sequential compression devices, and chemoprophylaxis, particularly if they are placed in traction.

AVN:
- 0:
- I: XR: WNL, MRI: edema + groin pain
- II: Sclerosis/cysts XR
- III: crescent sign + concave collapse
- IV:

28 Femoral Head

EPIDEMIOLOGY

- Almost all are associated with hip dislocations.
- These fractures complicate 10% of posterior hip dislocations.
- Most are shear or cleavage type, although recently, more indentation-type or crush-type fractures have been recognized with the increased use of computed tomography (CT).
- Impaction fractures are more commonly associated with anterior hip dislocations (25% to 75%).

ANATOMY

- The femoral head receives its blood supply from three sources (Fig. 28.1):
  - □ The medial femoral circumflex artery supplies the majority of the superior weight-bearing portion.
  - □ The lateral femoral circumflex artery and the artery of the ligamentum teres supply the remainder.
- Seventy percent of the femoral head articular surface is involved in load transfer, and thus damage to this surface may lead to the development of posttraumatic arthritis.

MECHANISM OF INJURY

- Most femoral head fractures are secondary to motor vehiclecrashes, with axial load transmission proximally through the femur.
- If the thigh is neutral or adducted, a posterior hip dislocation with or without a femoral head fracture may result. These fractures may be the result of avulsion by the ligamentum teres or cleavage by the posterior acetabular edge.
- In anterior dislocations, impacted femoral head fractures may occur because of a direct blow from the acetabular margin.

CLINICAL EVALUATION

- Formal trauma evaluation is necessary because most femoral head fractures are a result of high-energy trauma.
- Ninety-five percent of patients have injuries that require inpatient management independent of femoral head fracture.

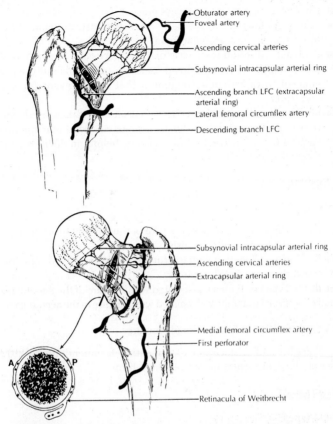

FIGURE 28.1 Vascular anatomy of the femoral head and neck. Top: Anterior aspect. Bottom: Posterior aspect. *LFC*, lateral femoral circumflex artery. (From Rockwood CA Jr, Green DP, Bucholz RW, Heckman JD, eds. *Rockwood and Green's Fractures in Adults.* Vol 2. 4th ed. Philadelphia: Lippincott-Raven; 1996:1662.)

- In addition to hip dislocation, femoral head fractures are also associated with acetabular fractures, knee ligament injuries, patella fractures, and femoral shaft fractures.
- A careful neurovascular examination is essential because posterior hip dislocations may result in neurovascular compromise.

RADIOGRAPHIC EVALUATION

- Anteroposterior (AP) and Judet (45-degree oblique) views of the pelvis should be obtained.

- Hip dislocation is almost always present.
- The AP radiograph of the pelvis may demonstrate femoral head fragments in the acetabular fossa.
- If closed reduction is successful, CT is necessary to evaluate the reduction of the femoral head fracture and to rule out the presence of intra-articular fragments that may prevent hip joint congruity.
- Some authors recommend CT evaluation even if the closed reduction is unsuccessful to evaluate associated acetabular fractures.
- Sagittal CT reconstruction may also be helpful in delineating the femoral head fracture.

CLASSIFICATION

Pipkin (Fig. 28.2)

Type I: Hip dislocation with fracture of the femoral head inferior to the fovea capitis femoris

Type II: Hip dislocation with fracture of the femoral head superior to the fovea capitis femoris

Type III: Type I or II injury associated with fracture of the femoral neck

Type IV: Type I or II injury associated with fracture of the acetabular rim

OTA Classification of Femoral Head Fractures

See Fracture and Dislocation Classification Compendium at http://www.ota.org/compendium/compendium.html.

TREATMENT

Pipkin Type I

The femoral head fracture is inferior to the fovea. These fractures occur in the non–weight-bearing surface.

- If reduction is adequate (<1 mm step-off) and the hip is stable, closed treatment is recommended.
- If the reduction is not adequate, open reduction and internal fixation with small subarticular screws using an anterior approach are recommended.
- Small fragments may be excised if they do not sacrifice stability.

Pipkin Type II

The femoral head fracture is superior to the fovea. These fractures involve the weight-bearing surface.

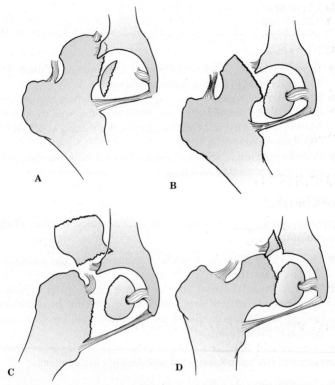

FIGURE 28.2 The Pipkin classification of dislocations with femoral head fractures. **(A)** Type I. **(B)** Type II. **(C)** Type III. **(D)** Type IV. (From Bucholz RW, Heckman JD, Court-Brown C, et al., eds. *Rockwood and Green's Fractures in Adults.* 6th ed. Philadelphia: Lippincott Williams & Wilkins; 2006.)

- The same recommendations apply for the nonoperative treatment of Type II fractures as for Type I fractures, except that only an anatomic reduction as seen on CT and repeat radiographs can be accepted for nonoperative care.
- Open reduction and internal fixation generally comprise the treatment of choice through an anterior approach (Smith-Peterson).
- Mini-fragment implants must be countersunk and/or headless screws utilized. Care must be taken to bury the implants below the articular cartilage.

Pipkin Type III

A femoral head fracture occurs with an associated fracture of the femoral neck.

- The prognosis for this fracture is poor and depends on the degree of displacement of the femoral neck fracture.
- In younger individuals, emergency open reduction and internal fixation of the femoral neck are performed, followed by internal fixation of the femoral head. This can be done using an anterolateral (Watson-Jones) approach.
- In older individuals with a displaced femoral neck fracture, prosthetic replacement is indicated.

Pipkin Type IV

A femoral head fracture occurs with an associated fracture of the acetabulum.

- This fracture must be treated in tandem with the associated acetabular fracture.
- The acetabular fracture should dictate the surgical approach (although this may not be possible), and the femoral head fracture, even if nondisplaced, should be internally fixed to allow early motion of the hip joint.

Femoral Head Fractures Associated with Anterior Dislocations

- These fractures are difficult to manage.
- Impaction fractures, typically located on the superior aspect of the femoral head, require no specific treatment, but the fracture size and location have prognostic implications.
- Displaced transchondral fractures that result in a nonconcentric reduction require open reduction and either excision or internal fixation, depending on fragment size and location.

COMPLICATIONS

- Osteonecrosis
  - □ Patients with posterior hip dislocations with an associated femoral head fracture are at high risk for developing osteonecrosis and posttraumatic degenerative arthritis. The prognosis for these injuries varies. Pipkin Types I and II are reported to have the same prognosis as a simple dislocation (1% to 10% if dislocated <6 hours). Pipkin Type IV injuries seem to have roughly the same prognosis as acetabular fractures without a femoral head

fracture. Pipkin Type III injuries have a poor prognosis, with a 50% rate of posttraumatic osteonecrosis.

☐ Ten percent of patients with anterior dislocations develop osteonecrosis. Risk factors include a time delay in reduction and repeated reduction attempts.

■ **Posttraumatic osteoarthritis:** Risk factors include transchondral fracure, indentation fracture greater than 4 mm in depth, and osteonecrosis.

29 Femoral Neck Fractures

EPIDEMIOLOGY

- More than 250,000 hip fractures occur in the United States each year (50% involve the femoral neck), and this number is projected to double by the year 2040.
- Eighty percent occur in women, and the incidence doubles every 5 to 6 years in women age >30 years.
- There is a bimodal incidence. The incidence in younger patients is very low and is associated mainly with high-energy trauma. The majority occurs in the elderly with the average age being 72, as a result of low-energy falls.
- The incidence of femoral neck fractures in the United States is 63.3 and 27.7 per 100,000 population per year for women and men, respectively.
- Risk factors include female sex, white race, increasing age, poor health, tobacco and alcohol use, previous fracture, fall history, and low estrogen level.

ANATOMY

- The upper femoral epiphysis closes by age 16 years.
- **Neck-shaft angle:** 130 ± 7 degrees
- **Femoral anteversion:** 10 ± 7 degrees
- There is minimal periosteum about the femoral neck; thus, any callus that forms must do so by endosteal proliferation.
- **Calcar femorale:** This is a vertically oriented plate from the postero-medial portion of the femoral shaft radiating superiorly toward the greater trochanter.
- The capsule is attached anteriorly to the intertrochanteric line and posteriorly 1 to 1.5 cm proximal to the intertrochanteric line.
- **Three ligaments attach in this region:**
  1. **Iliofemoral:** Y-ligament of Bigelow (anterior)
  2. **Pubofemoral:** anterior
  3. **Ischiofemoral:** posterior
- Vascular supply (Fig. 28.1)
- Forces acting across the hip joint
  - **Straight leg raise:** 1.5 × body weight
  - **One-legged stance:** 2.5 × body weight

□ **Two-legged stance:** $0.5 \times$ body weight
□ **Running:** $5.0 \times$ body weight
■ **Internal anatomy:** The direction of the trabeculae parallels the direction of compressive forces. The bony trabeculae are laid down along the lines of internal stress. A set of vertically oriented trabeculae results from the weight-bearing forces across the femoral head, and a set of horizontally oriented trabeculae results from the force of the abductor muscles. These two trabeculae systems cross each other at right angles.

MECHANISM OF INJURY

■ Low-energy trauma; most common in older patients
  □ **Direct:** A fall onto the greater trochanter (valgus impaction) or forced external rotation of the lower extremity impinges an osteoporotic neck onto the posterior lip of the acetabulum (resulting in posterior comminution).
  □ **Indirect:** Muscle forces overwhelm the strength of the femoral neck.
■ **High-energy trauma:** This accounts for femoral neck fractures in both younger and older patients, such as motor vehicle accident or fall from a significant height.
■ **Cyclical loading-stress fractures:** These are seen in athletes, military recruits, ballet dancers; patients with osteoporosis and osteopenia are at particular risk.

CLINICAL EVALUATION

■ Patients with displaced femoral neck fractures typically are non-ambulatory on presentation, with shortening and external rotation of the lower extremity. Patients with impacted or stress fractures may however demonstrate subtle findings, such as anterior capsular tenderness, pain with axial compression, and lack of deformity, and they may be able to bear weight.
■ Those involved in high-energy trauma should be subject to standard ATLS protocols.
■ Pain is evident on attempted range of hip motion, with pain on axial compression and tenderness to palpation of the groin.
■ An accurate history is important in the low-energy fracture that usually occurs in older individuals. Obtaining a history of loss of consciousness, prior syncopal episodes, medical history, chest pain, prior hip pain (pathologic fracture), and preinjury ambulatory status is essential and critical in determining optimal treatment and disposition.

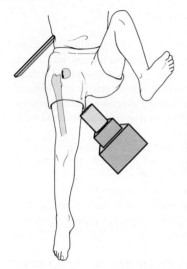

FIGURE 29.1 A cross-table lateral view of the affected hip is obtained by flexing the uninjured hip and knee 90 degrees and aiming the beam into the groin, parallel to the floor and perpendicular to the femoral neck (not the shaft). This allows orthogonal assessment of the femoral neck without the painful and possible injurious manipulation of the affected hip required for a "frog-leg" lateral view. (From Bucholz RW, Heckman JD, eds. *Rockwood and Green's Fractures in Adults.* 5th ed. Baltimore: Lippincott Williams & Wilkins; 2002.)

- All patients should undergo a thorough secondary survey to evaluate for associated injuries.

RADIOGRAPHIC EVALUATION

- An anteroposterior (AP) view of the pelvis and an AP and a cross-table lateral view of the involved proximal femur are indicated (Fig. 29.1).
- A physician assisted internal rotation view of the injured hip may be helpful to further clarify the fracture pattern and determine treatment plans.
- Computed tomography (CT) scan is of value in the trauma patient. Abdominal–pelvic CT cuts can be scanned for nondisplaced femoral neck fractures.
- Magnetic resonance imaging is currently the imaging study of choice in delineating nondisplaced or occult fractures that are not apparent on plain radiographs (Fig 29.2). Bone scans or CT scanning is reserved for those who have contraindications to MRI.

CLASSIFICATION

Anatomic Location

- Subcapital (most common)
- Transcervical
- Basicervical

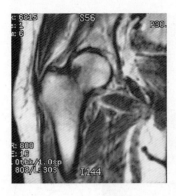

FIGURE 29.2 An MRI scan depicting a nondisplaced femoral neck fracture.

Pauwel

This is based on the angle of fracture from the horizontal (Fig. 29.3).

Type I: >30 degrees
Type II: 30 to 70 degrees
Type III: >70 degrees

Increasing shear forces with increasing angle lead to more fracture instability.

Garden

This is based on the degree of valgus displacement (Fig. 29.4).

Type I: Incomplete/valgus impacted
Type II: Complete and nondisplaced on AP and lateral views

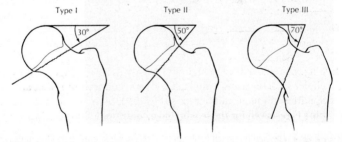

FIGURE 29.3 The Pauwel classification of femoral neck fractures is based on the angle the fracture forms with the horizontal plane. As a fracture progresses from Type I to Type III, the obliquity of the fracture line increases, and, theoretically, the shear forces at the fracture site also increase. (From Rockwood CA Jr, Green DP, Bucholz RW, Heckman JD, eds. *Rockwood and Green's Fractures in Adults*. Vol 2. 4th ed. Philadelphia: Lippincott-Raven; 1996:1670.)

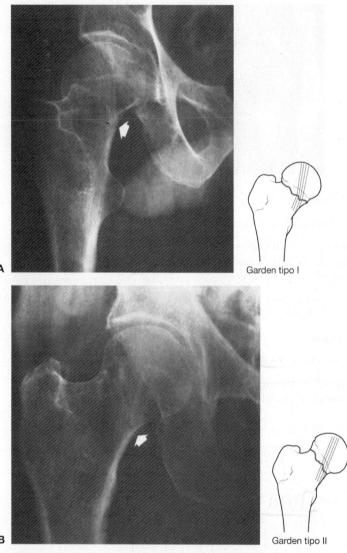

Garden tipo I

Garden tipo II

FIGURE 29.4 The Garden classification of femoral neck fractures. Type I fractures can be incomplete, but much more typically they are impacted into valgus and retroversion **(A)**. Type II fractures are complete, but nondisplaced. These rare fractures have a break in the trabeculations, but no shift in alignment **(B)**. Type III fractures have marked angulation, but usually minimal to no proximal translation of the shaft **(C)**. In the Garden Type IV fracture, there is complete displacement between fragments, and the shaft translates proximally **(D)**. *(Continued)*

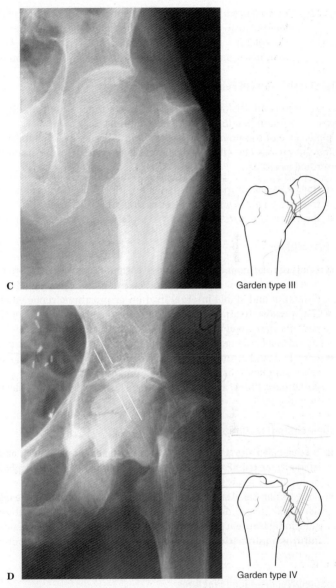

C   Garden type III

D   Garden type IV

FIGURE 29.4 (Continued) The head is free to realign itself within the acetabulum, and the primary compressive trabeculae of the head and acetabulum realign (*white lines*). (From Bucholz RW, Heckman JD, Court-Brown C, et al., eds. *Rockwood and Green's Fractures in Adults.* 6th ed. Baltimore: Lippincott Williams & Wilkins; 2005.)

Type III: Complete with partial displacement; trabecular pattern of the femoral head does not line up with that of the acetabulum

Type IV: Completely displaced; trabecular pattern of the head assumes a parallel orientation with that of the acetabulum

OTA Classification of Femoral Neck Fractures

See Fracture and Dislocation Classification Compendium at http://www.ota.org/compendium/compendium.html.

Because of too poor intraobserver and interobserver reliability in using the various classifications, femoral neck fractures are commonly described as either:

- **Nondisplaced:** Impacted valgus femoral neck fractures/stress fractures: This is a much better prognostic situation.
- **Displaced:** Characterized by any detectable fracture displacement.

TREATMENT

- Goals of treatment are to minimize patient discomfort, restore hip function, and allow rapid mobilization by obtaining early anatomic reduction and stable internal fixation or prosthetic replacement.
- Nonoperative treatment for traumatic fractures is indicated only for patients who are at extreme medical risk for surgery; it may also be considered for demented nonambulators who have minimal hip pain.
- Early bed to chair mobilization is essential to avoid increased risks and complications of prolonged recumbency, including poor pulmonary toilet, atelectasis, venous stasis, and pressure ulceration (Fig. 29.5).

Fatigue/Stress Fractures

- **Tension-sided stress fractures (seen at the superior lateral neck on an internally rotated AP view):** These are at significant risk for displacement; in situ screw fixation is recommended.
- **Compression-sided stress fractures (seen as a haze of callus at the inferior neck):** These are at minimal risk for displacement without additional trauma; protective crutch ambulation is recommended until asymptomatic. Surgery is reserved for painful, refractory fractures.

Impacted/Nondisplaced Fractures

- Up to 40% of "impacted" or nondisplaced fractures will displace without internal stabilization, decreasing to <5% with internal fixation.
- Less than 5% develop osteonecrosis.

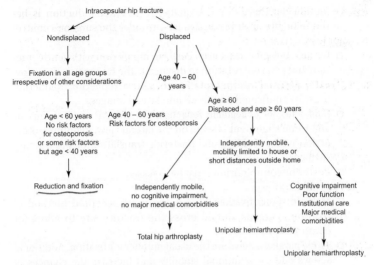

FIGURE 29.5 Algorithm for treatment of intracapsular femoral neck fractures.

H type I / III = 3 cancellous screws

- In situ fixation with three cancellous screws is indicated; exceptions are pathologic fractures, severe osteoarthritis/rheumatoid arthritis, Paget disease, and other metabolic conditions; may require prosthetic replacement.

Displaced Fractures

- **Young patient with high-energy injury and normal bone:** Urgent closed or open reduction with internal fixation and capsulotomy is performed. Fixed-angle implant may be indicated in these fractures.
- **Elderly patients:** Treatment is controversial.
  - □ **High functional demands and good bone density:** Almost all should receive a total hip replacement. Open or closed reduction and fixation may be considered, with a 40% reoperation rate in these patients.
  - □ **Low demand and poor bone quality:** Perform hemiarthroplasty using a cemented unipolar prosthesis.
  - □ **Severely ill, demented, bedridden patients:** Consider nonoperative treatment or prosthetic replacement for intolerable pain.

Operative Treatment Principles

- Fracture reduction should be achieved in a timely fashion. Risk of osteonecrosis may increase with increasing time to fracture reduction. Furthermore, the quality of fracture reduction is believed to be the most predictive factor under the surgeon's control for loss of fixation.

- ☐ **Fracture reduction maneuver:** Perform hip flexion with gentle traction and external rotation to disengage the fragments, then slow extension and internal rotation to achieve reduction. Reduction must be confirmed on the AP and lateral images.
- ☐ **Guidelines for acceptable reduction:** On the AP view, valgus or anatomic alignment is seen; on the lateral view, maintain anteversion while avoiding any posterior translation of the fracture surfaces.
- ☐ Posterior comminution must be assessed.

■ Internal fixation
- ☐ **Multiple screw fixation:** This is the most accepted method of fixation. Threads should cross the fracture site to allow for compression.
- ☐ Three parallel screws are the usual number for fixation. Additional screws add no additional stability and increase the chances of penetrating the joint. The screws should be in an inverted triangular configuration with one screw adjacent to the inferior femoral neck and one adjacent to the posterior femoral neck.
- ☐ Avoid screw insertion distal to the lesser trochanter secondary to a stress riser effect and risk of subsequent subtrochanteric fracture.

■ **Sliding-screw sideplate devices:** If they are used, a second pin or screw should be inserted superiorly to control rotation during screw insertion. Improve resistance to shear forces in high Pauwel's angle fractures.

■ Prosthetic replacement
- ☐ Advantages over open reduction and internal fixation
  - It may allow faster full weight bearing.
  - It eliminates nonunion, osteonecrosis, failure of fixation risks (>20% to 40% of cases with open reduction and internal fixation require secondary surgery).
- ☐ Disadvantages
  - It is a more extensive procedure with greater blood loss.
- ☐ Bipolar versus unipolar implants
  - No proven benefit of bipolar implants over unipolar implants
  - Over time, the bipolar implant may lose motion at its inner bearing and functionally become unipolar.
  - Unipolar implant is a less expensive implant.
- ☐ Cement versus noncemented
  - Lower incidence of intraoperative fracture

- • Risk of intraoperative hypotension and death with pressurization of cement
- ☐ Primary total hip replacement
  - • Recent enthusiasm has been reported with the use of total hip replacement for acute treatment of displaced femoral neck fractures. Becoming the standard in active patients.
  - • Studies have reported better functional results compared with hemiarthroplasty and internal fixation.
  - • It eliminates the potential for acetabular erosion seen with hemiarthroplasty.

COMPLICATIONS

- ■ **Nonunion (ORIF):** This is usually apparent by 12 months as groin or buttock pain, pain on hip extension, or pain with weight bearing. It may complicate up to 5% of nondisplaced fractures and up to 25% of displaced fractures. Elderly individuals presenting with nonunion may be adequately treated with arthroplasty, whereas younger patients may benefit from proximal femoral osteotomy. Cancellous bone grafting or muscle pedicle graft has fallen out of favor.
- ■ **Osteonecrosis (ORIF):** This may present as groin, buttock, or proximal thigh pain; it complicates up to 10% of nondisplaced fractures and up to 30% of displaced fractures. Not all cases develop evidence of radiographic collapse. Treatment is guided by symptoms.
  - ☐ **Early without x-ray changes:** Protected weight bearing or possible core decompression.
  - ☐ **Late with x-ray changes:** Elderly individuals may be treated with arthroplasty, whereas younger patients may be treated with osteotomy, arthrodesis, or arthroplasty.
- ■ **Fixation failure (ORIF):** This is usually related to osteoporotic bone or technical problems (malreduction, poor implant insertion). It may be treated with attempted repeat open reduction and internal fixation or prosthetic replacement.
- ■ Prominent hardware may occur secondary to fracture collapse and screw backout.
- ■ **Dislocation:** Seen with prosthetic replacement, total hip arthroplasty has a greater incidence than hemiarthroplasty. Overall 1% to 2%.

30 Intertrochanteric Fractures

EPIDEMIOLOGY

- Intertrochanteric fractures account for nearly 50% of all fractures of the proximal femur.
- Average patient age of incidence is 66 to 76 years. Younger than femoral neck fracture patients.
- There are approximately 150,000 intertrochanteric fractures annually in the United States with an annual incidence of 63 and 34 per 100,000 population per year for elderly females and males, respectively.
- The ratio of women to men ranges from 2:1 to 8:1, likely because of postmenopausal metabolic changes in bone.
- In the United States, the annual rate of intertrochanteric fractures in elderly women is about 63 per 100,000; in men, it is 34 per 100,000.
- Some of the factors associated with intertrochanteric rather than femoral neck fractures include advancing age, increased number of comorbidities, increased dependency in activities of daily living, and a history of other osteoporosis-related (fragility) fractures.

ANATOMY

- Intertrochanteric fractures occur in the region between the greater and lesser trochanters of the proximal femur, occasionally extending into the subtrochanteric region.
- These extracapsular fractures occur in cancellous bone with an abundant blood supply. As a result, nonunion and osteonecrosis are not major problems, as in femoral neck fractures.
- Deforming muscle forces will usually produce shortening, external rotation, and varus position at the fracture.
  - □ Abductors tend to displace the greater trochanter laterally and proximally.
  - □ The iliopsoas displaces the lesser trochanter medially and proximally.
  - □ The hip flexors, extensors, and adductors pull the distal fragment proximally.
- Fracture stability is determined by the presence of posteromedial bony contact, which acts as a buttress against fracture collapse.

MECHANISM OF INJURY

- Intertrochanteric fractures in younger individuals are usually the result of a high-energy injury such as a motor vehicle accident or fall from a height.
- Ninety percent of intertrochanteric fractures in the elderly result from a simple fall.
- Most fractures result from a direct impact to the greater trochanteric area.

CLINICAL EVALUATION

- Same as femoral neck fractures see Chapter 29.
- Patients may have experienced a delay before hospital presentation, time usually spent on the floor and without oral intake. The examiner must therefore be cognizant of potential dehydration, nutritional depletion, venous thromboembolic disease (VTE), and pressure ulceration issues as well as hemodynamic instability because intertrochanteric fractures may be associated with as much as a full unit of hemorrhage into the thigh.

RADIOGRAPHIC EVALUATION

- An anteroposterior (AP) view of the pelvis and an AP and a cross-table lateral view of the involved proximal femur are obtained.
- A physician assisted internal rotation view of the injured hip may be helpful to clarify the fracture pattern further.
- Magnetic resonance imaging (MRI) is currently the imaging study of choice in delineating nondisplaced or occult fractures that are not apparent on plain radiographs. Bone scans or CT scanning is reserved for those who have contraindications to MRI.

CLASSIFICATION

Evans (Fig. 30.1)

- This is based on prereduction and postreduction stability, that is, the convertibility of an unstable fracture configuration to a stable reduction.
- In stable fracture patterns, the posteromedial cortex remains intact or has minimal comminution, making it possible to obtain and maintain a stable reduction.
- Unstable fracture patterns are characterized by greater comminution of the posteromedial cortex. Although they are inherently

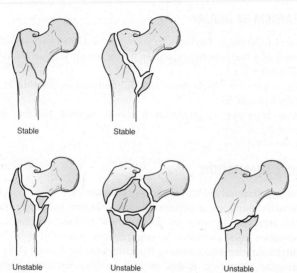

Stable   Stable

Unstable   Unstable   Unstable

FIGURE 30.1 The Evans classification of intertrochanteric fractures. In stable fracture patterns, the posteromedial cortex remains intact or has minimal comminution, making it possible to obtain and maintain a reduction. Unstable fracture patterns, conversely, are characterized by greater comminution of the posteromedial cortex. The reverse obliquity pattern is inherently unstable because of the tendency for medial displacement of the femoral shaft. (From Bucholz RW, Heckman JD, Court-Brown C, et al., eds. *Rockwood and Green's Fractures in Adults.* 6th ed. Philadelphia: Lippincott Williams & Wilkins; 2006.)

unstable, these fractures can be converted to a stable reduction if medial cortical opposition is obtained.
- The reverse obliquity pattern is inherently unstable because of the tendency for medial displacement of the femoral shaft.
- The adoption of this system was important not only because it emphasized the important distinction between stable and unstable fracture patterns, but also because it helped define the characteristics of a stable reduction.

OTA Classification of Intertrochanteric Fractures

See Fracture and Dislocation Classification Compendium at http://www.ota.org/compendium/compendium.html.

- Several studies have documented poor reproducibility of results based on the various intertrochanteric fracture classification systems.

■ Many investigators simply classify intertrochanteric fractures as either stable or unstable, depending on the status of the postero-medial cortex. Unstable fracture patterns comprise those with comminution of the posteromedial cortex, subtrochanteric exten-sion, or a reverse obliquity pattern.

UNUSUAL FRACTURE PATTERNS

Basicervical Fractures — *Treat as intertrochanteric fx AND likely to sustain rotation of fem head*

■ Basicervical neck fractures are located just proximal to or along the intertrochanteric line (Fig. 30.2).
■ Although anatomically, femoral neck fractures, basicervical frac-tures are usually extracapsular and thus behave and are treated as intertrochanteric fractures. *# treat basicervical line IT fx*
■ They are at greater risk for osteonecrosis than the more distal intertrochanteric fractures. *↓ 2/2*
■ They lack the cancellous interdigitation seen with fractures through the intertrochanteric region and are more likely to sustain rotation of the femoral head during implant insertion.

Reverse Obliquity Fractures → *↑ chance for medial displacement* *↗ subtroch.*

■ Reverse obliquity intertrochanteric fractures are unstable fractures characterized by an oblique fracture line extending from the me-dial cortex proximally to the lateral cortex distally (Fig. 30.3).
■ The location and direction of the fracture line result in a ten-dency to medial displacement from the pull of the adductor muscles. → *medial displacement of distal segment*
■ These fractures should be treated as subtrochanteric hip fractures.

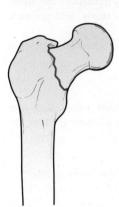

FIGURE 30.2 Basicervical neck fractures are located just proximal to or along the intertrochanteric line. (From Bucholz RW, Heckman JD, Court-Brown C, et al., eds. *Rockwood and Green's Fractures in Adults.* 6th ed. Philadelphia: Lippincott Williams & Wilkins; 2006.)

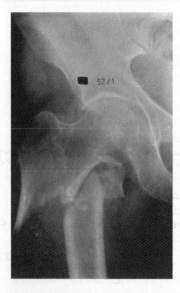

FIGURE 30.3 Anteroposterior x-ray demonstrating a reverse obliquity right intertrochanteric fracture. (From Bucholz RW, Heckman JD, Court-Brown C, et al., eds. *Rockwood and Green's Fractures in Adults.* 6th ed. Philadelphia: Lippincott Williams & Wilkins; 2006.)

TREATMENT

Nonoperative

- This is indicated only for patients who are at extreme medical risk for surgery; it may also be considered for demented nonambulatory patients with mild hip pain.
- Nondisplaced fractures can be considered for nonoperative treatment because unlike with femoral neck fractures, displacement changes neither the operation type nor outcome.
- Early bed to chair mobilization is important to avoid increased risks and complications of prolonged recumbency, including poor pulmonary toilet, atelectasis, venous stasis, and pressure ulceration.
- Resultant hip deformity is both expected and accepted in cases of displacement.

Operative

- The goal is stable internal fixation to allow early mobilization and full weight-bearing ambulation. Stability of fracture fixation depends on:
  - ☐ Bone quality
  - ☐ Fracture pattern
  - ☐ Fracture reduction
  - ☐ Implant design
  - ☐ Implant placement

Timing of Surgery

- Abundant evidence exists that surgery should be performed in a timely fashion, once the patient has been medically stabilized.

Fixation Implants

Sling Hip Screw

- This has historically been the most commonly used device for both stable and unstable fracture patterns. It is available in plate angles from 130 to 150 degrees (Fig. 30.4).
- The most important technical aspects of screw insertion are (1) placement within 1 cm of subchondral bone to provide secure fixation and (2) central position in the femoral head (Tip-apex distance).
- The tip-apex distance can be used to determine lag screw position within the femoral head. This measurement, expressed in millimeters, is the sum of the distances from the tip of the lag screw to the apex of the femoral head on both the AP and lateral radiographic views (after controlling for radiographic

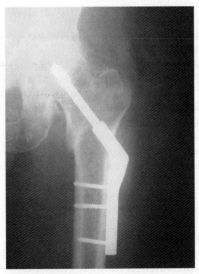

FIGURE 30.4 X-ray of a sliding hip screw. (From Bucholz RW, Heckman JD, Court-Brown C, et al., eds. *Rockwood and Green's Fractures in Adults.* 6th ed. Philadelphia: Lippincott Williams & Wilkins; 2006.)

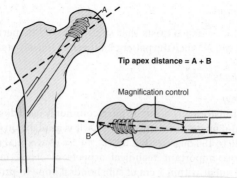

FIGURE 30.5 The tip-apex distance (TAD), expressed in millimeters, is the sum of the distances from the tip of the lag screw to the apex of the femoral head on both the anteroposterior and lateral radiographic views. (From Baumgaertner MR, Chrostowski JH, Levy RN. Intertrochanteric hip fractures. In: Browner BD, Levine AM, Jupiter JB, Trafton PG, eds. *Skeletal Trauma*. Vol 2. Philadelphia: WB Saunders; 1992:1833–1881.)

magnification) (Fig. 30.5). The sum should be <25 mm to minimize the risk of lag screw cutout.

- Biomechanical and clinical studies have shown no advantage of four screws over two to stabilize the sideplate.
- At surgery, the surgeon must be prepared to address any residual varus angulation, posterior sag, or malrotation.
- There is a 4% to 12% incidence of loss of fixation is reported, most commonly with unstable fracture patterns.
- Most failures of fixation are attributable to technical problems of screw placement and/or inadequate impaction of the fracture fragments at the time of screw insertion.
- Clinically, more shortening and deformity is seen with the use of sliding hip screw (SHS) in unstable patterns.

Intramedullary Hip Screw Nail

- This implant combines the features of an SHS and an intramedullary nail (IMN) (Fig. 30.6).
- **Advantages are both technical and mechanical:** Theoretically, these implants can be inserted in a closed manner with limited fracture exposure, decreased blood loss, and less tissue damage than an SHS. In addition, these devices are subjected to a lower

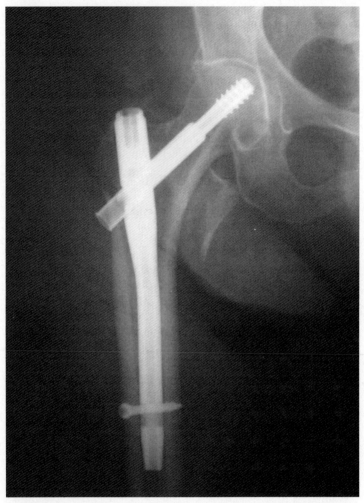

FIGURE 30.6 Unstable intertrochanteric fracture stabilized with a cephalomedullary nail.

bending moment than the SHS owing to their intramedullary location.

■ Use of the intramedullary hip screw limits the amount of fracture collapse, compared with an SHS.

■ Most studies have demonstrated no clinical advantage of the intramedullary hip screw compared with the SHS in stable fracture patterns.

- Use of intramedullary hip screws has been most effective in intertrochanteric fractures with subtrochanteric extension and in reverse obliquity fractures.
- Use of older design intramedullary hip screws has been associated with an increased risk of femur fracture at the nail tip or distal locking screw insertion point.

Prosthetic Replacement

- This has been used successfully for patients in whom ORIF have failed and who are unsuitable candidates for repeat internal fixation.
- A calcar replacement hemiarthroplasty may be needed because of the level of the fracture.
- Primary prosthetic replacement for comminuted, unstable intertrochanteric fractures has yielded up to 94% good functional results in limited series.
- Disadvantages include morbidity associated with a more extensive operative procedure, the internal fixation problems with greater trochanteric reattachment, and the risk of postoperative prosthetic dislocation.

External Fixation

- This is not commonly considered for the treatment of intertrochanteric femur fractures.
- Early experiences with external fixation for intertrochanteric fractures were associated with postoperative complications such as pin loosening, infection, and varus collapse.
- Recent studies have reported good results using hydroxyapatite-coated pins.

Special Considerations

- With use of an SHS, greater trochanteric displacement should be fixed utilizing tension band techniques or a trochanteric stabilizing plate and screw construct.
- Basicervical fractures treated with an SHS or IMN may require a supplemental antirotation screw or pin during implant insertion.
- Reverse obliquity fractures are best treated as subtrochanteric fractures with either a 95-degree fixed angle implant or an intramedullary device.
- Ipsilateral fractures of the femoral shaft, although more common in association with femoral neck fractures, should be ruled out when the injury is caused by high-energy trauma.

Rehabilitation

- Early patient mobilization with weight bearing as tolerated ambulation is indicated.

COMPLICATIONS

- **Loss of fixation:** This most commonly results from varus collapse of the proximal fragment with cutout of the lag screw from the femoral head; the incidence of fixation failure is reported to be as high as 20% in unstable fracture patterns. Lag screw cutout from the femoral head generally occurs within 3 months of surgery and is usually caused by one the following:
  - Eccentric placement of the lag screw within the femoral head (most common).
  - Improper reaming that creates a second channel.
  - Inability to obtain a stable reduction.
  - Excessive fracture collapse such that the sliding capacity of the device is exceeded.
  - Inadequate screw-barrel engagement, which prevents sliding.
  - Severe osteopenia, which precludes secure fixation.
    - Management choices include (1) acceptance of the deformity, (2) revision ORIF, which may require methylmethacrylate, and (3) conversion to prosthetic replacement.
- **Nonunion:** Rare, occurring in <2% of patients, especially in patients with unstable fracture patterns. The diagnosis should be suspected in a patient with persistent hip pain and radiographs revealing a persistent radiolucency at the fracture site 4 to 7 months after fracture fixation. With adequate bone stock, repeat internal fixation combined with a valgus osteotomy and bone grafting may be considered. In most elderly individuals, conversion to a calcar replacement prosthesis is preferred.
- **Malrotation deformity:** This results from internal rotation of the distal fragment at the time of internal fixation. When it is severe and interferes with ambulation, revision surgery with plate removal and rotational osteotomy of the femoral shaft should be considered.
- With full-length intramedullary nails, impingement or perforation of the distal aspect of the nail on the anterior femoral cortex can occur, secondary to a mismatch of the nail curvature and femoral bow.
- Z-Effect Seen most commonly with dual screw cephalomedullary trochanteric nails, :failure can result with the most proximal screw penetrating the hip joint and the distal screw backing out of the femoral head.

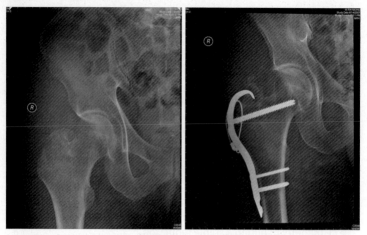

FIGURE 30.7A, B 55-year-old male who fell and sustained a displaced greater trochanteric fracture **(A)** was treated with a trochanteric hook plate and tension band wire **(B)**.

- **Osteonecrosis of the femoral head:** This is rare following intertrochanteric fracture.
- Lag screw-sideplate dissociation.
- Traumatic laceration of the superficial femoral artery by a displaced lesser trochanter fragment.

Greater Trochanteric Fractures

- Isolated greater trochanteric fractures, although rare, typically occur in older patients as a result of an eccentric muscle contraction or less commonly a direct blow.
- Treatment of greater trochanteric fractures is usually nonoperative.
- Operative management can be considered in younger, active patients who have a widely displaced greater trochanter.
- ORIF with a tension band wiring of the displaced fragment and the attached abductor muscles or plate and screw fixation with a "hook plate" are the preferred techniques. (Fig. 30.7A, B)

Lesser Trochanteric Fractures

- These are most common in adolescence, typically secondary to forceful iliopsoas contracture.
- In the elderly, isolated lesser trochanter fractures have been recognized as pathognomonic for pathologic lesions of the proximal femur.

31

Subtrochanteric Fractures

EPIDEMIOLOGY

■ Subtrochanteric fractures account for approximately 10% to 30% of all hip fractures, and they affect persons of all ages.

ANATOMY

■ A subtrochanteric femur fracture is a fracture between the lesser trochanter and a point 5 cm distal to the lesser trochanter.
■ The subtrochanteric segment of the femur is subject to high biomechanical stresses. The medial and posteromedial cortices are the sites of high compressive forces, whereas the lateral cortex experiences high tensile forces (Fig. 31.1).
■ The subtrochanteric area of the femur is composed mainly of cortical bone. Therefore, there is less vascularity in this region, and the potential for healing is diminished as compared with intertrochanteric fractures.
■ The deforming muscle forces on the proximal fragment include abduction by the gluteus, external rotation by the short rotators, and flexion by the psoas. The distal fragment is pulled proximally and into varus by the adductors (Fig. 31.2).

Mechanism of Injury

■ **Low-energy mechanisms:** Elderly individuals sustain a minor fall in which the fracture occurs through weakened bone (pathologic).
■ **High-energy mechanisms:** Younger adults with normal bone sustain injuries related to motor vehicle accidents, gunshot wounds, or falls from a height.
■ **Pathologic fracture:** The subtrochanteric region is also a frequent site for pathologic fractures, accounting for 17% to 35% of all subtrochanteric fractures.
■ Ten percent of higher-energy subtrochanteric fractures result from gunshot injuries.

CLINICAL EVALUATION

■ Patients involved in high-energy trauma should receive full trauma evaluation.

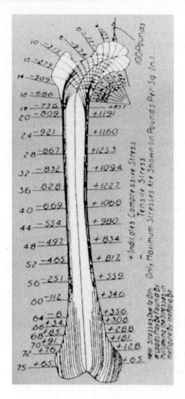

FIGURE 31.1 Koch's diagram showing the compression stress on the medial side and the tension stress on the lateral side of the proximal femur. (From Bucholz RW, Heckman JD, Court-Brown C, et al., eds. *Rockwood and Green's Fractures in Adults.* 6th ed. Philadelphia: Lippincott Williams & Wilkins; 2006.)

- Patients typically are unable to walk and have varying degrees of gross deformity of the lower extremity.
- Hip motion is painful, with tenderness to palpation and swelling of the proximal thigh.
- Because substantial forces are required to produce this fracture pattern in younger patients, associated injuries should be expected and carefully evaluated.
- Field dressings or splints should be completely removed, with the injury site examined for evidence of soft tissue compromise or open injury.
- The thigh represents a compartment into which volume loss from hemorrhage may be significant; monitoring for hypovolemic shock should thus be undertaken, with invasive monitoring as necessary.
- Provisional splinting (i.e., traction pin) until definitive fixation should be performed to limit further soft tissue damage and hemorrhage.
- A careful neurovascular examination is important to rule out associated injuries, although neurovascular compromise related to the subtrochanteric fracture is uncommon.

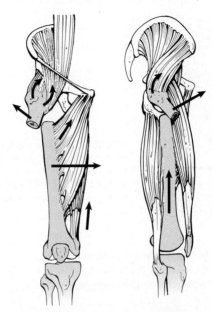

FIGURE 31.2 The deforming force by the unopposed pull of the iliopsoas causes the proximal femur in flexion and external rotation. (From Bucholz RW, Heckman JD, Court-Brown C, et al., eds. *Rockwood and Green's Fractures in Adults*. 6th ed. Philadelphia: Lippincott Williams & Wilkins; 2006.)

RADIOGRAPHIC EVALUATION

- An anteroposterior (AP) view of the pelvis and AP and lateral views of the hip and femur should be obtained.
- One should assess the entire femur including the knee.
- Associated injuries should be evaluated, and if suspected, appropriate radiographic studies ordered.
- A contralateral scanogram is helpful to determine femoral length in highly comminuted fractures.

CLASSIFICATION

Fielding

This is based on the location of the primary fracture line in relation to the lesser trochanter (Fig. 31.3).

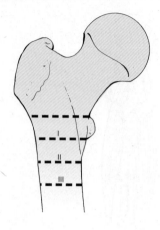

FIGURE 31.3 Fielding classification of subtrochanteric fractures. (From Bucholz RW, Heckman JD, Court-Brown C, et al., eds. *Rockwood and Green's Fractures in Adults.* 6th ed. Philadelphia: Lippincott Williams & Wilkins; 2006.)

Type I:	At the level of the lesser trochanter
Type II:	<2.5 cm below the lesser trochanter
Type III:	2.5 to 5 cm below the lesser trochanter

Seinsheimer

This is based on the number of major bone fragments and the location and shape of the fracture lines (Fig. 31.4).

Type I:	Nondisplaced fracture or any fracture with <2 mm of displacement of the fracture fragments, regardless of pattern
Type II:	Two-part fractures
IIA:	Two-part transverse femoral fracture
IIB:	Two-part spiral fracture with the lesser trochanter attached to the proximal fragment
IIC:	Two-part spiral fracture with the lesser trochanter attached to the distal fragment (reverse obliquity pattern)
Type III:	Three-part fractures
IIIA:	Three-part spiral fracture in which the lesser trochanter is part of the third fragment, which has an inferior spike of cortex of varying length
IIIB:	Three-part spiral fracture of the proximal third of the femur, with the third part a butterfly fragment
Type IV:	Comminuted fracture with four or more fragments
Type V:	Subtrochanteric–intertrochanteric fracture, including any subtrochanteric fracture with extension through the greater trochanter

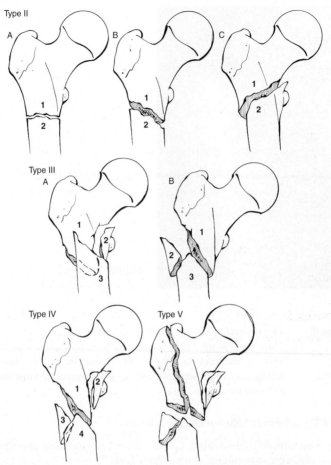

FIGURE 31.4 Seinsheimer classification of subtrochanteric fractures. (From Bucholz RW, Heckman JD, Court-Brown C, et al., eds. *Rockwood and Green's Fractures in Adults*. 6th ed. Philadelphia: Lippincott Williams & Wilkins; 2006.)

Russell-Taylor

This was created in response to the development of first-generation and second-generation (cephalomedullary) interlocked nails as a guide to implant choice (may be obsolete now).

Type I: Fractures with an intact piriformis fossa:
A: The lesser trochanter is attached to the proximal fragment (Fig 31.5).
B: The lesser trochanter is detached from the proximal fragment.

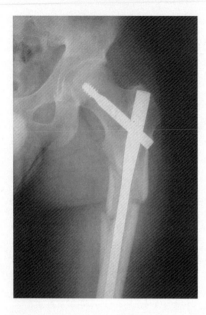

FIGURE 31.5 A subtrochanteric fracture fixed with an IM nail.

Type II: Fractures that extend into the piriformis fossa.
A: Have a stable medial construct (posteromedial cortex).
B: Have comminution of the piriformis fossa and lesser trochanter, associated with varying degrees of femoral shaft comminution.

OTA Classification of Subtrochanteric Fractures

See Fracture and Dislocation Classification Compendium at http://www.ota.org/compendium/compendium.html.

TREATMENT

Nonoperative (Historical)

- This involves skeletal traction in the 90/90-degree position followed by spica casting or cast bracing.
- This is reserved only for those elderly individuals who are not operative candidates, and for children.
- Nonoperative treatment generally results in increased morbidity and mortality in adults, as well as in nonunion, delayed union, and malunion with varus angulation, rotational deformity, and shortening.

Operative

- Operative treatment is indicated in most subtrochanteric fractures.

Implants

Interlocking Nail

- First-generation (centromedullary) nails are indicated for sub-trochanteric fractures with both trochanters intact.
- Second-generation cephalomedullary (i.e., reconstruction) nails are indicated for all fractures, especially those with loss of the posteromedial cortex. May be trochanteric or piriformis starting types.
- Second-generation nails can also be used for fractures extending into the piriformis fossae; trochanteric types are recommended.
- With use of an intramedullary nail, one must monitor for the nail exiting posteriorly out of the proximal fragment. One must also monitor for the common malalignment of varus and flexion of the proximal fragment. Distally, anterior perforation can occur due to nail femur radius of curvature mismatch.

Ninety-Five-Degree Fixed Angle Device

- The 95-degree fixed angle plates are best suited for fractures involving both trochanters; an accessory screw can be inserted beneath the fixed angle blade or screw into the calcar to increase proximal fixation (Fig. 31.6).
- These devices function as a tension band when the posteromedial cortex is restored.
- A dynamic condylar screw is technically easier to insert than a blade plate.
- Proximal femur precontoured locking plates are a newer alternative to traditional fixed angle plates and screws.
- One must take care not to devitalize the fracture fragments during fracture reduction and fixation.

Sliding Hip Screw

- This implant is a poor choice for subtrochanteric fractures.

Bone Grafting

- Closed reduction techniques have decreased the need for bone grafting because fracture fragments are not devascularized to the same extent as in open reduction.
- If needed, it should be inserted through the fracture site, usually before plate application.

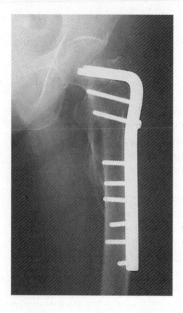

FIGURE 31.6 A subtrochanteric fracture fixed with a fixed-angle blade plate and bone graft on the posteromedial cortex. (From Bucholz RW, Heckman JD, Court-Brown C, et al., eds. *Rockwood and Green's Fractures in Adults*. 6th ed. Philadelphia: Lippincott Williams & Wilkins; 2006.)

Open Subtrochanteric Fractures

- These are rare, almost always associated with either penetrating injury or high-energy trauma from a motor vehicle accident or a fall from a height.
- Treatment consists of immediate surgical debridement and osseous stabilization.

COMPLICATIONS

Loss of Fixation

- With plate and screw devices, implant failure usually occurs secondary to screw cutout from the femoral head and neck in patients with osteopenic bone or plate breakage.
- With interlocked nails, loss of fixation is commonly related to failure to lock the device statically, comminution of the entry portal, or use of smaller-diameter nails. Cephalomedullary nails tend to fail when healing does not occur. The nail tends to fail by fatiguing through the lag screw hole in the nail (Fig 31.7).
- Fixation failure involves removal of hardware, revision internal fixation with either plate and screws or an interlocked nail, and bone grafting.

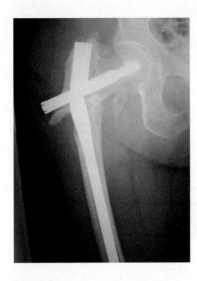

FIGURE 31.7 71-year-old female who is one year out from a right sub-trochanteric femur fracture with a nonunion and failure of hardware through the lag screw hole in the nail.

Nonunion

- This may be evident by a patient's inability to resume full weight bearing within 4 to 6 months.
- Symptoms are pain about the proximal thigh and pain on attempted weight bearing.
- Nonunion usually is accompanied by deformity of the fracture.
- Nonunions that develop following intramedullary nailing can be treated by implant removal followed by repeat reaming and placement of a larger-diameter intramedullary nail.
- Correction of varus or flexion deformity is critical to success of nonunion surgery for subtrochanteric fracture nonunions.

Malunion

- The patient may complain of a limp, leg length discrepancy, or rotational deformity.
- Coxa varus is mainly the result of the uncorrected abduction deformity of the proximal segment caused by the hip abductors.
- A valgus osteotomy and revision internal fixation with bone grafting are the usual treatment for a varus malreduction.
- Leg length discrepancy is a complex problem that is more likely to occur following a fracture with extensive femoral shaft comminution stabilized with a dynamically locked rather than a statically locked nail.
- Malrotation may occur with use of plate and screws or an intramedullary nail if the surgeon is not alert to this potential complication.

32 Femoral Shaft

EPIDEMIOLOGY

- The highest age- and gender-specific incidences of femoral shaft fracture are seen in males from 15 to 24 years of age and in females 75 years of age or older.
- Femoral shaft fractures occur most frequently in young men after high-energy trauma and elderly women after a low-energy fall.
- The bimodal distribution peaks at 25 and 65 years of age with an overall incidence of approximately 10 per 100,000 population per year.

ANATOMY

- The femur is the largest tubular bone in the body and is surrounded by the largest mass of muscle. An important feature of the femoral shaft is its anterior bow.
- The medial cortex is under compression, whereas the lateral cortex is under tension.
- The isthmus of the femur is the region with the smallest intramedullary (IM) diameter; the diameter of the isthmus affects the size of the IM nail that can be inserted into the femoral shaft.
- The femoral shaft is subjected to major muscular deforming forces (Fig. 32.1).
  - □ **Abductors (gluteus medius and minimus):** They insert on the greater trochanter and abduct the proximal femur following subtrochanteric and proximal shaft fractures.
  - □ **Iliopsoas:** It flexes and externally rotates the proximal fragment by its attachment to the lesser trochanter.
  - □ **Adductors:** They span most shaft fractures and exert a strong axial and varus load to the bone by traction on the distal fragment.
  - □ **Gastrocnemius:** It acts on distal shaft fractures and supracondylar fractures by flexing the distal fragment.
  - □ **Fascia lata:** It acts as a tension band by resisting the medial angulating forces of the adductors.
- **The thigh musculature is divided into three distinct fascial compartments (Fig. 32.2):**

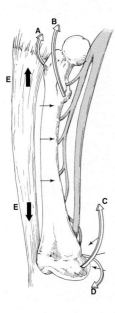

FIGURE 32.1 Deforming muscle forces on the femur; abductors *(A)*, iliopsoas *(B)*, adductors *(C)*, and gastrocnemius origin *(D)*. The medial angulating forces are resisted by the fascia lata *(E)*. Potential sites of vascular injury after fracture are at the adductor hiatus and the perforating vessels of the profunda femoris. (From Bucholz RW, Heckman JD, eds. *Rockwood and Green's Fractures in Adults.* 5th ed. Baltimore: Lippincott Williams & Wilkins; 2002.)

1. **Anterior compartment:** This is composed of the quadriceps femoris, iliopsoas, sartorius, and pectineus, as well as the femoral artery, vein, and nerve, and the lateral femoral cutaneous nerve.
2. **Medial compartment:** This contains the gracilis, adductor longus, brevis, magnus, and obturator externus muscles along with the obturator artery, vein, and nerve, and the profunda femoris artery.
3. **Posterior compartment:** This includes the biceps femoris, semitendinosus, and semimembranosus, a portion of the adductor magnus muscle, branches of the profunda femoris artery, the sciatic nerve, and the posterior femoral cutaneous nerve

- Because of the large volume of the three fascial compartments of the thigh, compartment syndromes are much less common than in the lower leg.
  - The vascular supply to the femoral shaft is derived mainly from the profunda femoral artery. The one to two nutrient vessels usually enter the bone proximally and posteriorly along the linea aspera. This artery then arborizes proximally and distally to provide the endosteal circulation to the shaft. The periosteal vessels also enter the bone along the linea aspera and supply blood to the outer one-third of the cortex.

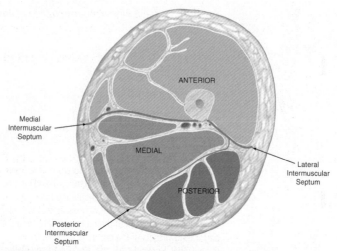

FIGURE 32.2 Cross-sectional diagram of the thigh demonstrates the three major compartments. (From Bucholz RW, Heckman JD, Court-Brown C, et al., eds. *Rockwood and Green's Fractures in Adults.* 6th ed. Philadelphia: Lippincott Williams & Wilkins; 2006.)

The endosteal vessels supply the inner two-thirds of the cortex.

☐ Following most femoral shaft fractures, the endosteal blood supply is disrupted, and the periosteal vessels proliferate to act as the primary source of blood for healing. The medullary supply is eventually restored late in the healing process.

☐ Reaming may further obliterate the endosteal circulation, but it returns fairly rapidly, in 3 to 4 weeks.

■ Femoral shaft fractures heal readily if the blood supply is not excessively compromised. Therefore, it is important to avoid excessive periosteal stripping, especially posteriorly, where the arteries enter the bone at the linea aspera.

MECHANISM OF INJURY

■ Femoral shaft fractures in adults are almost always the result of high-energy trauma. These fractures result from motor vehicle accident, gunshot injury, or fall from a height.

■ Pathologic fractures, especially in the elderly, commonly occur at the relatively weak metaphyseal–diaphyseal junction. Any fracture that is inconsistent with the degree of trauma should arouse suspicion for pathologic fracture.

■ Stress fractures occur mainly in military recruits or runners. Most patients report a recent increase in training intensity just before the onset of thigh pain.

■ Recently, insufficiency fractures of the femur have been reported with extended use of bisphosphonates.

CLINICAL EVALUATION

■ Because these fractures tend to be the result of high-energy trauma, a full trauma survey is indicated.

■ The diagnosis of femoral shaft fracture is usually obvious, with the patient presenting nonambulatory with pain, variable gross deformity, swelling, and shortening of the affected extremity.

■ A careful neurovascular examination is essential, although neurovascular injury is uncommonly associated with femoral shaft fractures.

■ Thorough examination of the ipsilateral hip and knee should be performed, including systematic inspection and palpation. Range-of-motion or ligamentous testing is often not feasible in the setting of a femoral shaft fracture and may result in displacement. Knee ligament injuries are common, however, and need to be assessed after fracture fixation.

■ Major blood loss into the thigh may occur. The average blood loss in one series was greater than 1200 mL, and 40% of patients ultimately required transfusions. Therefore, a careful preoperative assessment of hemodynamic stability is essential, regardless of the presence or absence of associated injuries.

■ No or low energy mechanisms should alert the examiner to pathologic causes.

ASSOCIATED INJURIES

■ Associated injuries are common and may be present in up to 5% to 15% of cases, with patients presenting with multisystem trauma, spine, pelvis, and ipsilateral lower extremity injuries.

■ Ligamentous and meniscal injuries of the ipsilateral knee are present in 50% of patients with closed femoral shaft fractures.

RADIOGRAPHIC EVALUATION

■ Anteroposterior (AP) and lateral views of the femur, hip, and knee as well as an AP view of the pelvis should be obtained.

■ The radiographs should be critically evaluated to determine the fracture pattern, the bone quality, the presence of bone loss, associated comminution, the presence of air in the soft tissues, and the amount of fracture shortening.

■ One must evaluate the region of the proximal femur for evidence of an associated femoral neck or intertrochanteric fracture.

■ If a computed tomography scan of the abdomen and/or pelvis is obtained for other reasons, this should be reviewed because it may provide evidence of injury to the ipsilateral acetabulum or femoral neck.

CLASSIFICATION

Descriptive

■ Open versus closed injury
■ **Location:** proximal, middle, or distal one-third
■ **Location:** isthmal, infraisthmal, or supracondylar
■ **Pattern:** spiral, oblique, or transverse
■ Comminuted, segmental, or butterfly fragment
■ Angulation or rotational deformity
■ **Displacement:** shortening or translation

Winquist and Hansen (Fig. 32.3)

■ This is based on fracture comminution.
■ It was used before routine placement of statically locked IM nails.
Type I: Minimal or no comminution
Type II: Cortices of both fragments at least 50% intact

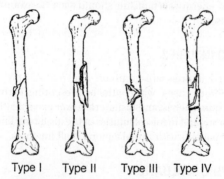

Type I   Type II   Type III   Type IV

FIGURE 32.3 Winquist and Hansen classification of femoral shaft fractures. (From Browner BD, Jupiter JB, Levine AM, et al. *Skeletal Trauma.* Philadelphia: WB Saunders; 1992:1537.)

Type III: 50% to 100% cortical comminution
Type IV: Circumferential comminution with no cortical contact

OTA Classification of Femoral Shaft Fractures

See Fracture and Dislocation Classification Compendium at http://www.ota.org/compendium/compendium.html.

TREATMENT

Nonoperative

Skeletal Traction

- Currently, closed management as definitive treatment for femoral shaft fractures is largely limited to adult patients with such significant medical comorbidities that operative management is contraindicated.
- The goal of skeletal traction is to restore femoral length, limit rotational and angular deformities, reduce painful spasms, and minimize blood loss into the thigh.
- Skeletal traction is usually used as a temporizing measure before surgery to stabilize the fracture and prevent fracture shortening.
- A general rule of thumb is use of 1/9 or 15% body weight (usually 20 to 40 lb) of traction is usually applied to the extremity. A lateral radiograph checked to assess fracture length.
- Distal femoral pins should be placed in an extracapsular location to avoid the possibility of septic arthritis. Proximal tibia pins are typically positioned at the level of the tibial tubercle and are placed in a bicortical location.
- Safe pin placement is usually from medial to lateral at the distal femur (directed away from the femoral artery) and from lateral to medial at the proximal tibia (directed away from the peroneal nerve).
- Problems with use of skeletal traction for definitive fracture treatment include knee stiffness, limb shortening, heterotopic ossification of the quadriceps, prolonged hospitalization, respiratory and skin ailments, and malunion.

Operative

- Operative stabilization is the standard of care for most femoral shaft fractures.
- Surgical stabilization should occur within 24 hours, if possible.

- Early stabilization of long bone injuries appears to be particularly important in the multiply injured patient.
- Stabilization should follow resuscitation efforts.

Intramedullary Nailing

- This is the standard of care for femoral shaft fractures.
- Its IM location results in lower tensile and shear stresses on the implant than plate fixation. Benefits of IM nailing over plate fixation include less extensive exposure and dissection, lower infection rate, and less quadriceps scarring.
- Closed IM nailing in closed fractures has the advantage of maintaining both the fracture hematoma and the attached periosteum. If reaming is performed, these elements provide a combination of osteoinductive and osteoconductive materials to the site of the fracture.
- Other advantages include early functional use of the extremity, restoration of length and alignment with comminuted fractures, rapid and high union (>95%), and low refracture rates.

Antegrade Inserted Intramedullary Nailing

- Surgery can be performed on a fracture table or on a radiolucent table with or without skeletal traction.
- The patient can be positioned supine or lateral. Supine positioning allows unencumbered access to the entire patient. Lateral positioning facilitates identification of the piriformis starting point but may be contraindicated in the presence of pulmonary compromise.
- One can use either a piriformis fossa or greater trochanteric starting point. The advantage of a piriformis starting point is that it is in line with the medullary canal of the femur. However, it is easier to locate the greater trochanteric starting point. Use of a greater trochanteric starting point requires use of a nail with a valgus proximal bow to negotiate the off starting point axis.
- With the currently available nails, the placement of large-diameter nails with an intimate fit along a long length of the medullary canal is no longer necessary. At this point in time most studies support reaming prior to nail placement.
- The role of unreamed IM nailing for the treatment of femoral shaft fractures remains unclear. The potentially negative effects of reaming for insertion of IM nails include elevated IM pressures, elevated pulmonary artery pressures, increased fat embolism, and increased pulmonary dysfunction. The potential advantages of reaming

rate include the ability to place a larger implant, increased union, and decreased hardware failure. At this point in time most studies support reaming prior to nail placement.

- All IM nails should be statically locked to maintain femoral length and control rotation. The number of distal interlocking screws necessary to maintain the proper length, alignment, and rotation of the implant bone construct depends on numerous factors including fracture comminution, fracture location, implant size, patient size, bone quality, and patient activity.

Retrograde Inserted Intramedullary Nailing

- The major advantage with a retrograde entry portal is the ease in properly identifying the starting point.
- Relative indications include
  □ Ipsilateral injuries such as femoral neck, pertrochanteric, acetabular, patellar, or tibial shaft fractures.
  □ Bilateral femoral shaft fractures.
  □ Morbidly obese patient.
  □ Pregnant woman.
  □ Periprosthetic fracture above a total knee arthroplasty.
  □ Ipsilateral through knee amputation in a patient with an associated femoral shaft fracture.
- Contraindications include
  □ Restricted knee motion <60 degrees.
  □ Patella baja.

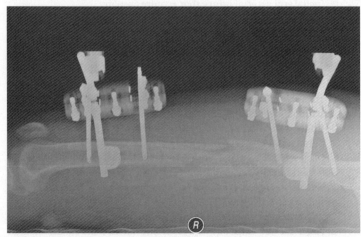

FIGURE 32.4 Comminuted femur fracture stabilized with a bridging external fixator.

External Fixation

- Use as definitive treatment for femoral shaft fractures has limited indications.
- Its use is most often provisional (damage control) (Fig. 32.4).
- **Advantages include the following:**
  - ☐ The procedure is rapid; a temporary external fixator can be applied in less than 30 minutes.
  - ☐ The vascular supply to the femur is minimally damaged during application.
  - ☐ No additional foreign material is introduced in the region of the fracture.
  - ☐ It allows access to the medullary canal and the surrounding tissues in open fractures with significant contamination.
  - ☐ Allows for transfer of patients to and from ICU for testing while maintaining skeletal stabilization.
  - ☐ Up to 2 weeks to convert to IM fixation.
- **Disadvantages:** Most are related to use of this technique as a definitive treatment and include
  - ☐ Pin tract infection.
  - ☐ Loss of knee motion.
  - ☐ Angular malunion and femoral shortening.
  - ☐ Limited ability to adequately stabilize the femoral shaft.
  - ☐ Potential infection risk associated with conversion to an IM nail.
- Indications for use of external fixation include
  - ☐ Use as a temporary bridge to IM nailing in the severely injured patient.
  - ☐ Ipsilateral arterial injury that requires repair.
  - ☐ Patients with severe soft tissue contamination in whom a second debridement would be limited by other devices.

Plate Fixation

Plate fixation for femoral shaft stabilization has decreased with the use of IM nails.

- Advantages to plating include
  - ☐ Ability to obtain an anatomic reduction in appropriate fracture patterns.
  - ☐ Lack of additional trauma to remote locations such as the femoral neck, the acetabulum, and the distal femur.
  - ☐ Newer implants allow for minimally invasive insertion techniques.
- Disadvantages compared with IM nailing include
  - ☐ Need for an extensive surgical approach with its associated blood loss, risk of infection, and soft tissue insult. This can result

in quadriceps scarring and its effects on knee motion and quadriceps strength.

☐ Decreased vascularization beneath the plate and the stress shielding of the bone spanned by the plate.

☐ The plate is a load-bearing implant; therefore, a higher rate of implant failure potentially exists.

■ Indications include

☐ Extremely narrow medullary canal where IM nailing is impossible or difficult.

☐ Fractures that occur adjacent to or through a previous malunion.

☐ Obliteration of the medullary canal due to infection or previously closed management.

☐ Fractures that have associated proximal or distal extension into the pertrochanteric or condylar regions.

☐ In patients with an associated vascular injury, the exposure for the vascular repair frequently involves a wide exposure of the medial femur. If rapid femoral stabilization is desired, a plate can be applied quickly through the medial open exposure.

■ An open or a submuscular technique may be applicable.

■ As the fracture comminution increases, so should the plate length such that at least four to five screw holes of plate length are present on each side of the fracture.

■ The routine use of cancellous bone grafting in plated femoral shaft fractures is questionable if indirect reduction techniques are used.

Femur Fracture in Multiply Injured Patient

■ The impact of femoral nailing and reaming is controversial in the polytrauma patient.

■ In a specific subpopulation of patients with multiple injuries, early IM nailing is associated with elevation of certain proinflammatory markers.

■ It has been recommended that early external fixation of long bone fractures followed by delayed IM nailing may minimize the additional surgical impact in patients at high risk for developing complications (i.e., patients in extremis or underresuscitated) (Fig. 32.5).

Ipsilateral Fractures of the Proximal or Distal Femur

■ Concomitant femoral neck fractures occur in 3% to 5% of patients with femoral shaft fractures. Options for operative fixation include antegrade IM nailing with multiple screw fixation of the femoral neck, retrograde femoral nailing with multiple screw fixation of the femoral neck, and compression plating with screw

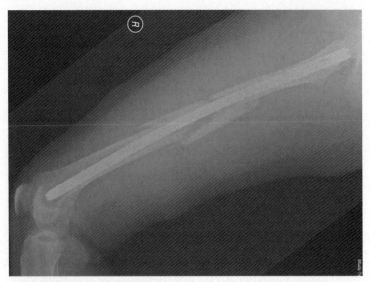

FIGURE 32.5 This fracture was eventually definitively stabilized with an IM nail.

fixation of the femoral neck. The sequence of surgical stabilization is controversial.

■ Ipsilateral fractures of the distal femur may exist as a distal extension of the shaft fracture or as a distinct fracture. Options for fixation include fixation of both fractures with a single plate, fixation of the shaft and distal femoral fractures with separate plates, IM nailing of the shaft fracture with plate fixation of the distal femoral fracture, or interlocked IM nailing spanning both fractures (high supracondylar fractures).

Open Femoral Shaft Fractures

■ These are typically the result of high-energy trauma. Automatically a type 3 injury due to soft tissue stripping.
■ Patients frequently have multiple other orthopaedic injuries and involvement of several organ systems.
■ Treatment is urgent debridement with skeletal stabilization as patient condition allows.
■ Stabilization can usually involve placement of a reamed IM nail.

REHABILITATION

■ Early patient mobilization out of bed is recommended.
■ Early range of knee motion is indicated.

- Weight bearing on the extremity is guided by a number of factors including the patient's associated injuries, soft tissue status, type of implant, and the location of the fracture.

COMPLICATIONS

- **Nerve injury:** This is uncommon because the femoral and sciatic nerves are encased in muscle throughout the length of the thigh. Most injuries occur as a result of traction or compression during surgery.
- **Vascular injury:** This may result from tethering of the femoral artery at the adductor hiatus.
- **Compartment syndrome:** This occurs only with significant bleeding. It presents as pain out of proportion, tense thigh swelling, numbness or paresthesias to medial thigh (saphenous nerve distribution), or painful passive quadriceps stretch.
- **Infection (<1% incidence in closed fractures):** The risk is greater with open versus closed IM nailing. Types I, II, and IIIA open fractures carry a low risk of infection with IM nailing, whereas fractures with gross contamination, exposed bone, and extensive soft tissue injury (types IIIB and IIIC) have a higher risk of infection regardless of treatment method.
- **Refracture:** Patients are vulnerable during early callus formation and after hardware removal. It is usually associated with plate or external fixation.
- **Nonunion and delayed union:** This is unusual. Delayed union is defined as healing taking longer than 6 months, usually related to insufficient blood supply (i.e., excessive periosteal stripping), uncontrolled repetitive stresses, infection, and heavy smoking. Nonunion is diagnosed once the fracture has no further potential to unite.
- **Malunion:** This is usually varus, internal rotation, and/or shortening owing to muscular deforming forces or surgical technique leading to malalignment.
- **Fixation device failure:** This results from nonunion or "cycling" of device, especially with plate fixation.
- Heterotopic ossification may occur proximally at site of nail insertion or within the quadriceps.

33

Distal Femur

EPIDEMIOLOGY

- Distal femoral fractures account for about 7% of all femur fractures.
- If hip fractures are excluded, one-third of femur fractures involve the distal portion.
- A bimodal age distribution exists, with a high incidence in young adults from high-energy trauma, such as motor vehicle or motorcycle accidents or falls from a height, and a second peak in the elderly from minor falls.
- Open fractures occur in 5% to 10% of all distal femur fractures.

ANATOMY

- The distal femur includes both the supracondylar and condylar regions (Fig. 33.1).
- The supracondylar area of the femur is the zone between the femoral condyles and the junction of the metaphysis with the femoral shaft. This area comprises the distal 10 to 15 cm of the femur.

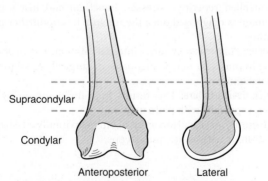

Supracondylar

Condylar

Anteroposterior   Lateral

FIGURE 33.1 Schematic drawing of the distal femur. (Adapted from Wiss D. *Master Techniques in Orthopaedic Surgery.* Philadelphia: Lippincott-Raven; 1998.)

- The distal femur broadens from the cylindric shaft to form two curved condyles separated by an intercondylar groove.
- The medial condyle extends more distally and is more convex than the lateral femoral condyle. This accounts for the physiologic valgus of the femur.
- When viewing the lateral femur, the femoral shaft is aligned with the anterior half of the lateral condyle (Fig. 33.2).
- When viewing the distal surface of the femur end on, the condyles are wider posteriorly, thus forming a trapezoid.
- Normally, the knee joint is parallel to the ground. On average, the anatomic axis (the angle between the shaft of the femur and

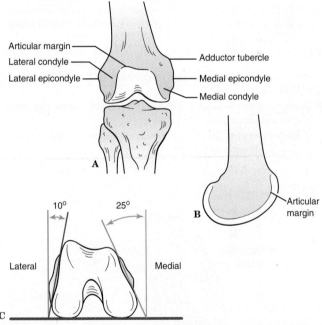

FIGURE 33.2 Anatomy of the distal femur. **(A)** Anterior view. **(B)** Lateral view. The shaft of the femur is aligned with the anterior half of the lateral condyle. **(C)** Axial view. The distal femur is trapezoidal. The anterior surface slopes downward from lateral to medial, the lateral wall inclines 10 degrees, and the medial wall inclines 25 degrees. (Adapted from Wiss D, Watson JT, Johnson EE. Fractures of the knee. In: Rockwood CA, Green DP, Bucholz RW, et al., eds. *Rockwood and Green's Fractures in Adults.* 4th ed. Philadelphia: Lippincott-Raven; 1996.)

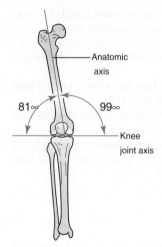

FIGURE 33.3 Alignment of the lower extremity. The knee joint is parallel to the ground. The knee joint is in 9 degree valgus to the knee joint. (Adapted from Browner BD, Levine AM, Jupiter JB. *Skeletal Trauma: Fractures, Dislocations, Ligamentous Injuries.* 2nd ed. Philadelphia: WB Saunders; 1997.)

the knee joint) has a valgus angulation of 9 degrees (range, 7 to 11 degrees) (Fig. 33.3).

■ Deforming forces from muscular attachments cause characteristic displacement patterns (Fig. 33.4).

□ **Gastrocnemius:** This flexes the distal fragment, causing posterior displacement and angulation.

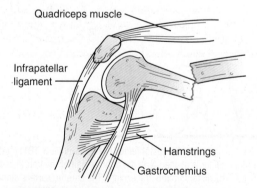

FIGURE 33.4 Lateral view showing muscle attachments and resulting deforming forces. These result in posterior displacement and angulation at the fracture site. (Adapted from Browner BD, Levine AM, Jupiter JB. *Skeletal Trauma: Fractures, Dislocations, Ligamentous Injuries.* 2nd ed. Philadelphia: WB Saunders; 1997.)

☐ **Quadriceps and hamstrings:** They exert proximal traction, resulting in shortening of the lower extremity.

MECHANISM OF INJURY

- Most distal femur fractures are the result of a severe axial load with a varus, valgus, or rotational force.
- In young adults, this force is typically the result of high-energy trauma such as motor vehicle collision or fall from a height.
- In the elderly, the force may result from a minor slip or fall onto a flexed knee.

CLINICAL EVALUATION

- Patients typically are unable to ambulate with pain, swelling, and variable deformity in the lower thigh and knee.
- Assessment of neurovascular status is mandatory. The proximity of the neurovascular structures to the fracture area is an important consideration. Unusual and tense swelling in the popliteal area and the usual signs of pallor and lack of pulse suggest rupture of a major vessel.
- Compartment syndrome of the thigh is uncommon and is associated with major bleeding into the thigh.
- Examination of the ipsilateral hip, knee, leg, and ankle is essential, especially in the obtunded or polytraumatized patient.
- When a distal femoral fracture is associated with an overlying laceration or puncture wound, greater than 120 cc's mL or more of saline should be injected into the knee from a remote location to determine continuity with the wound. CT scanning of the knee will demonstrate free air if the wound communicates with the joint.

RADIOGRAPHIC EVALUATION

- Anteroposterior, lateral, and two 45-degree oblique radiographs of the distal femur should be obtained.
- Radiographic evaluation should include the entire femur.
- Traction views may be helpful to better determine the fracture pattern and intra-articular extension.
- Contralateral views may be helpful for comparison and serve as a template for preoperative planning.
- Complex intra-articular fractures and osteochondral lesions may require additional imaging with computed tomography to assist in completing the diagnostic assessment and preoperative planning.

- Magnetic resonance imaging may be of value in evaluating associated injuries to ligamentous or meniscal structures.
- Arteriography may be indicated with dislocation of the knee, as 40% of dislocations are associated with vascular disruption. This is due to the fact that the popliteal vascular bundle is tethered proximally at the adductor hiatus and distally at the soleus arch. By contrast, the incidence of vascular disruption with isolated supracondylar fractures is between 2% and 3%.

CLASSIFICATION

Descriptive

- Open versus closed
- **Location:** supracondylar, intercondylar, condylar
- **Pattern:** spiral, oblique, or transverse
- Articular involvement
- Comminuted, segmental, or butterfly fragment
- Angulation or rotational deformity
- **Displacement:** shortening or translation

Neer

- Based on direction of displacement of distal fragments.
- Does not take into account intra-articular displacement.

OTA Classification of Distal Femoral Fractures

See Fracture and Dislocation Classification Compendium at http://www.ota.org/compendium/compendium.html.

TREATMENT

Nonoperative

- Indications include nondisplaced or incomplete fractures, impacted stable fractures in elderly patients, severe osteopenia, advanced underlying medical conditions, or select gunshot injuries.
- In stable, nondisplaced fractures, treatment is mobilization of the extremity in a hinged knee brace, with partial weight bearing.

■ In displaced fractures, nonoperative treatment entails a 6- to 12-week period of casting with acceptance of resultant deformity followed by bracing. The objective is not absolute anatomic reduction, but restoration of the knee joint axis to a normal relationship with the hip and ankle. Potential drawbacks include varus and internal rotation deformity, knee stiffness, and the necessity for prolonged hospitalization and bed rest.

Operative

■ Most displaced distal femur fractures are best treated with operative stabilization.

■ Most of these fractures can be temporized in a bulky cotton dressing and a knee immobilizer; in significantly shortened fractures, atibial pin traction may be considered.

■ Articular fractures require anatomic reconstruction of the joint surface and fixation with interfragmentary lag screws.

■ The articular segment is then fixed to the proximal segment, in an effort to restore the normal anatomic relationships. These should encompass all angular, translational, and rotational relationships.

■ In elderly patients with severe osteopenia or those with contralateral amputation, length may be sacrificed for fracture stability and bony contact.

■ With the advent of more biologic techniques of fracture stabilization, the necessity for bone grafting has diminished.

■ Polymethylmethacrylate cement or calcium phosphate cement may be utilized in extremely osteoporotic bone to increase the fixation capability of screws and/or fill bony voids.

Implants

■ **Screws:** In most cases, they are used in addition to other fixation devices. In noncomminuted, unicondylar fractures in young adults with good bone stock, interfragmentary screws alone can provide adequate fixation.

■ **Plates:** To control alignment (particularly varus and valgus) of the relatively short distal articular segment, a fixed angle implant is most stable.

  □ **A 95-degree condylar blade plate:** This provides excellent fracture control but is technically demanding.

  □ **Dynamic condylar screw (DCS):** This is technically easier to insert than a condylar blade plate, and interfragmentary compression is also possible through its lag screw design. Disadvantages of the DCS are the bulkiness of the device and the poorer rotational control than with the blade plate.

□ **Locking plates (with fixed angle screws):** The development of locking plates made the nonlocking periarticular plate relatively obsolete. Locking plates are an alternative to the DCS and blade plate. Like the DCS and the blade plate, locking plates are fixed-angle devices. The screws lock to the plate and therefore provide angular stability to the construct.

□ **Nonlocking periarticular plates (condylar buttress plates):** Are virtually obsolete.

■ Intramedullary (IM) nails

□ **Antegrade inserted IM nail:** It has limited use owing to the distal nature of the fracture. It is best used in supracondylar type fractures with a large distal segment.

□ **Retrograde inserted IM nail:** It has the advantage of improved distal fixation. The disadvantages are the further insult to the knee joint and the potential of knee sepsis if the nailing is complicated by infection. Retrograde nails should bypass the isthmus proximally.

■ External fixation

□ In patients whose medical condition requires rapid fracture stabilization or in patients with major soft tissue lesions, spanning external fixation allows for rapid fracture stabilization while still allowing access to the limb and patient mobilization.

□ Definitive external fixation, although rarely used, can be in the form of a unilateral half-pin fixator or a hybrid frame.

□ Problems include pin tract infection, quadriceps scarring, delayed or nonunion, and loss of reduction after device removal.

Associated Vascular Injury

■ The incidence is estimated to be about 2%.

■ If arterial reconstruction is necessary, it should be done following temporary stabilization and before definitive skeletal stabilization.

■ Definitive fracture management can proceed after the vascular procedure if the patient's condition allows.

■ Fasciotomy of the lower leg should be performed in all cases.

Supracondylar Fractures After Total Knee Replacement

■ Classified according to fracture extent and implant stability.

■ These are increasing in incidence and are related to osteopenia, rheumatoid arthritis, prolonged corticosteroid usage, anterior notching of the femur, and revision arthroplasty.

- Treatment is based on the status of the arthroplasty implants (well-fixed or loose) and the patient's preinjury function.
- Surgical options include
  - **Retrograde IM nailing:** Open box designs, dependent upon amount of bone distally.
  - **Plate fixation:** Allow for treatment of most fractures, especially if no access through femoral component.
  - **Revision arthroplasty:** For implants that are aseptically loosened with associated fractures.

Postoperative Management

- The injured extremity is typically placed on a continuous passive motion device in the immediate postoperative period if the skin and soft tissues will tolerate.
- Physical therapy consists of active range-of-motion exercises and non–weight bearing or touch down weight bearing with crutches 2 to 3 days after stable fixation may be allowed.
- A cast brace may be used if fixation is tenuous.
- Weight bearing may be advanced with radiographic evidence of healing (6 to 12 weeks).
- Healing in the elderly may be delayed beyond 12 weeks.

COMPLICATIONS

- **Fixation failure:** This is usually a result of one of the following: poor bone stock, patient noncompliance with postoperative care, or inadequate surgical planning and execution.
- **Malunion:** This usually results from malalignment at the time of surgery. More common with use of IM nails. Varus is the most common deformity. Malunion with the articular surface in extension may result in relative hyperextension of the knee, whereas malunion in flexion may result in a functional loss of full extension. Malunion resulting in functional disability may be addressed with osteotomy.
- **Nonunion:** This is infrequent because of the rich vascular supply to this region and the predominance of cancellous bone. Greater incidence in the elderly.
- **Posttraumatic osteoarthritis:** This may result as a failure to restore articular congruity, especially in younger patients. It also may reflect chondral injury at the time of trauma.
- **Infection:** Open fractures require meticulous debridement and copious irrigation (serial, if necessary) with intravenous antibiotics.

Open injuries contiguous with the knee necessitate formal irrigation and debridement to prevent knee sepsis.

■ **Loss of knee motion:** This is the most common complication as a result of scarring, quadriceps damage, or articular disruption during injury. If significant, it may require lysis of adhesions or quadricepsplasty for restoration of joint motion. It is best prevented by anatomic reduction, early range of motion and adequate pain control.

34

Knee Dislocation (Femorotibial)

EPIDEMIOLOGY

- Traumatic knee dislocation is an uncommon injury that may be limb-threatening; it should therefore be treated as an orthopaedic emergency.
- True incidence is probably underreported.
  - □ From 20% to 50% spontaneously reduced.
- Most knee dislocations are the result of high-energy injuries, such as motor vehicle or industrial accidents. They also can occur with low-energy injuries, such as those that occur in sports.

ANATOMY

- **The ginglymoid (hinge joint) consists of three articulations:** (1) patellofemoral, (2) tibiofemoral, and (3) tibiofibular. Under normal cyclic loading, the knee may experience up to five times body weight per step. The normal range of motion is from 0 degrees of extension to 140 degrees of flexion with 8 to 12 degrees of rotation through the flexion-extension arc. The dynamic and static stability of the knee is conferred mainly by soft tissues (ligaments, muscles, tendons, menisci) in addition to the bony articulations.
- Significant soft tissue injury is necessary for knee dislocation, including ruptures of at least three of four major ligamentous structures of the knee. The anterior and posterior cruciate ligaments (ACL and PCL) are disrupted in most cases, with a varying degree of injury to the collateral ligaments, capsular elements, and menisci.
- The popliteal vascular bundle courses through a fibrous tunnel at the level of the adductor hiatus. Within the popliteal fossa, the five geniculate branches are given off, after which the vascular structures run deep to the soleus and through another fibrous canal. It is this tethering effect that leaves the popliteal vessels vulnerable to tenting and injury, especially at the moment of dislocation.
- Associated fractures of the tibial eminence, tibial tubercle, fibular head or neck, and capsular avulsions are common and should be suspected.

MECHANISM OF INJURY

■ **High-energy:** A motor vehicle accident with a "dashboard" injury involves axial loading to a flexed knee.

■ **Low-energy:** This includes athletic injuries and falls. The latter will usually occur in an obese patient.

■ Hyperextension with or without varus/valgus leads to anterior dislocation.

■ Flexion plus posterior force leads to posterior dislocation (dashboard injury).

  □ Associated injuries include fractures of the femur, acetabulum, and tibial plateau.

CLINICAL EVALUATION

■ Patients present with gross knee distortion unless the knee underwent spontaneous reduction. Immediate reduction should be undertaken without waiting for radiographs. Of paramount importance is the arterial supply, with secondary consideration given to neurologic status.

■ Patients who sustain a knee dislocation that spontaneously reduces may have a relatively normal-appearing knee. Subtle signs of injury such as mild abrasions, or a minimal effusion, or complaints of knee pain may be the only abnormalities.

■ The extent of ligamentous injury is related to the degree of displacement, with injury occurring with displacement greater than 10% to 25% of the resting length of the ligament. Gross instability may be realized after reduction.

■ Isolated ligament examination

  □ ACL

    • Lachman at 30 degrees

  □ PCL

    • Posterior drawer at 90 degrees

  □ Lateral collateral ligament (LCL)/posterolateral corner (PLC)

    • Varus stress at 30 degrees and full extension

    • Increased tibial external rotation at 30 degrees

    • Increased posterior tibial (PT) translation at 30 degrees

  □ Medial collateral ligament (MCL)

    • Valgus stress at 30 degrees

■ Combined ligament examination

  □ LCL/PLC and cruciate

    • Increased varus in full extension and at 30 degrees

  □ MCL and cruciate

    • Increased valgus in full extension and at 30 degrees

poor results. Bracing and/or tendon transfer may be necessary for treatment of muscular deficiencies.

RADIOGRAPHIC EVALUATION

- A knee dislocation is a potentially limb-threatening condition. Because of the high incidence of neurovascular compromise, immediate reduction is recommended before radiographic evaluation. Following reduction, anteroposterior (AP) and lateral views of the knee should be obtained to assess the reduction and evaluate associated injuries. Widened knee joint spaces may indicate soft tissue interposition and the need for open reduction.
- Plain radiographs
  - □ AP and lateral
  - □ 45-degree oblique and/or plateau views if an associated fracture is suspected.
  - □ Findings
    - Obvious dislocation
    - Irregular/asymmetric joint space
    - Lateral capsular sign (Segund)
    - Avulsions
    - Osteochondral defects
- The use of angiography in every case of knee dislocation is controversial. Vascular compromise is an indication for operative intervention. Identifying intimal tears in a neurovascularly intact limb may be unnecessary because most do not result in thrombosis and vascular occlusion. Some authors advocate selective arteriography only if the ankle brachial index is (ABI) <0.9. Regardless, the patient should be closely observed for evidence of vascular insufficiency.
- MRI
  - □ Valuable diagnostic tool
    - Preoperative planning
    - Identification of ligament avulsions
    - **MCL:** injury location (femur, tibia, midsubstance)
    - **Lateral structures:** popliteus, LCL, biceps
    - Meniscal pathology
      Displaced in notch an indication for early surgery
      Limited arthroscopy secondary to extravasation
    - Articular cartilage lesions

CLASSIFICATION

Descriptive

This is based on displacement of the proximal tibia in relation to the distal femur. It also should include open versus closed, reducible versus irreducible. It may be classified as occult, indicating a knee dislocation with spontaneous reduction.

Anterior: Forceful knee hyperextension beyond –30 degrees; most common (30% to 50%); associated with posterior (and possibly anterior) cruciate ligament tear, with increasing incidence of popliteal artery disruption with increasing degree of hyperextension (Fig. 34.1)

Posterior: Posteriorly directed force against proximal tibia of flexed knee (25%); "dashboard" injury; accompanied by anterior and posterior ligament disruption as well as popliteal artery compromise with increasing proximal tibial displacement

Lateral: Valgus force (13%); medial supporting structures disrupted, often with tears of both cruciate ligaments

Medial: Varus force (3%); lateral and posterolateral structures disrupted

Rotational: Varus/valgus with rotatory component (4%); usually results in buttonholing of the femoral condyle through the articular capsule

Anatomic Classification (Schenck, 1992)

I	Single cruciate + collateral	ACL + collateral
		PCL + collateral
II	ACL/PCL	Collaterals intact
IIIM	ACL/PCL/MCL	LCL + PLC intact
IIIL	ACL/PCL/LCL + PLC	MCL intact
IV	ACL/PCL/MCL/LCL + PLC	
V	Fracture–dislocation	
C	Arterial injury	
N	Nerve injury	

Utility of Anatomic Classification

- It requires the surgeon to focus on what is torn.
- It directs treatment to what is injured.
- It leads to accurate discussion of injuries among clinicians.
- Comparison of similar injuries can be made within the wide spectrum of knee dislocations.

TREATMENT

- Immediate closed reduction is essential, even in the field and especially in the compromised limb. Direct pressure on the popliteal space should be avoided during or after reduction. Reduction maneuvers for specific dislocations.

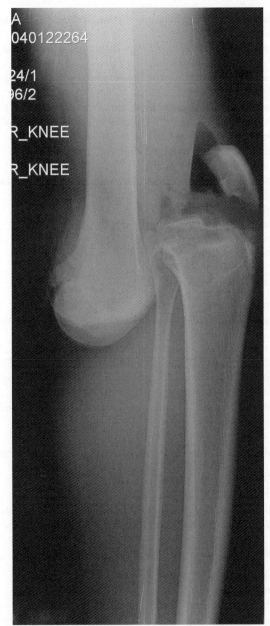

FIGURE 34.1 A lateral radiograph which demonstrates an anterior knee dislocation.

- □ **Anterior:** Axial limb traction is combined with lifting of the distal femur.
- □ **Posterior:** Axial limb traction is combined with extension and lifting of the proximal tibia.
- □ **Medial/lateral:** Axial limb traction is combined with lateral/medial translation of the tibia.
- □ **Rotatory:** Axial limb traction is combined with derotation of the tibia.
- ■ The posterolateral dislocation is believed to be "irreducible" owing to buttonholing of the medial femoral condyle through the medial capsule, resulting in a dimple sign over the medial aspect of the limb; it requires open reduction.
- ■ The knee should be splinted at 20 to 30 degrees of flexion. The knee must be perfectly reduced in the splint.
- ■ External fixation.
  - □ This approach is better for the grossly unstable knee.
  - □ Protects vascular repair.
  - □ Permits skin care for open injuries.

General Treatment Considerations

- ■ Most authors recommend repair of the torn structures.
- ■ Nonoperative treatment has been associated with poor results.
- ■ Period of immobilization
  - □ A shorter period leads to improved motion and residual laxity.
  - □ A longer period leads to improved stability and limited motion.
- ■ Recent clinical series have reported better results with operative treatment. High rates of heterotopic ossification.
- ■ No prospective, controlled, randomized trials of comparable injuries have been reported.
- ■ Once stiffness occurs, it is very difficult to treat.
- ■ Complete PLC disruption is best treated with early open repair.
  - □ Late reconstruction is difficult.
- ■ Reconstitution of the PCL is important.
  - □ It allows tibiofemoral positioning.
  - □ Collateral and ACL surgery evolves around PCL reconstitution.
  - □ ACL reconstruction before PCL treatment is never indicated.

Nonoperative

- ■ Immobilization in extension for 6 weeks
- ■ External fixation
  - □ "Unstable" or subluxation in brace
  - □ Obese patient
  - □ Multitrauma patient
  - □ Head injury
  - □ Vascular repair

- ☐ Fasciotomy or open wounds
- ☐ Removal of fixator under anesthesia
- ■ Arthroscopy
  - ☐ Manipulation for flexion
  - ☐ Assessment of residual laxity

Operative

- ■ Indications for operative treatment of knee dislocation include
  - ☐ Unsuccessful closed reduction.
  - ☐ Residual soft issue interposition.
  - ☐ Open injuries.
  - ☐ Vascular injuries.
- ■ Vascular injuries require external fixation and vascular repair with a reverse saphenous vein graft from the contralateral leg; amputation rates as high as 86% have been reported when there is a delay beyond 8 hours with documented vascular compromise to limb. A fasciotomy should be performed at time of vascular repair for limb ischemia times longer than 6 hours.
- ■ **Ligamentous repair is controversial:** The current literature favors acute repair of lateral ligaments followed by early motion and functional bracing. Timing of surgical repair depends on the condition of both the patient and the limb. Meniscal injuries should also be addressed at the time of surgery.

Treatment Recommendations of Specific Patterns

- ■ ACL + MCL (class I knee dislocation)
  - ☐ **MCL:** Predictable healing
  - ☐ Cylinder cast immobilization in extension for 2 weeks
  - ☐ Hinged brace permitting to range of motion
  - ☐ Delayed ACL reconstruction
    - • Motion restored
    - • Residual laxity and desired activity level
- ■ ACL + LCL/PLC (class I knee dislocation)
  - ☐ Delayed surgery at 14 days
    - • Capsular healing
    - • Identification of lateral structures
  - ☐ **Arthroscopic ACL:** femoral fixation
    - • Instruments and experience with open techniques
    - • Femoral fixation
  - ☐ Tibial fixation/ACL tensioned after LCL/PLC
  - ☐ Open posterolateral repair/reconstruction
- ■ ACL + PLC (class II knee dislocation)
  - ☐ Collateral ligaments intact

- □ Hinged brace and early range of motion
  - Extension stop at 0 degrees
- □ Arthroscopic reconstruction after 6 weeks
  - PCL only in most cases
  - ACL/PCL limited to high-demand patient
- □ **Sedentary individuals:** No surgery
- ACL + PLC + MCL (class IIIM knee dislocation)
  - □ Immobilization in extension
  - □ Early surgery (2 weeks)
    - Examination under anesthesia and limited diagnostic arthroscopy (MRI)
    - Single straight medial parapatellar incision
    - Open PCL reconstruction or repair
    - MCL repair
- ACL + PLC + LCL/PLC (class IIIL knee dislocation)
  - □ Immobilization in extension
  - □ Delayed surgery at 14 days
    - Diagnostic arthroscopy
    - Arthroscopic or open PCL
    - Open LCL/PLC
  - □ **Incisions critical:** Avoidance of the midline
    - **PCL:** medial (open or arthroscopic)
    - Straight posterolateral

COMPLICATIONS

- **Limited range of motion:** This is most common, related to scar formation and capsular tightness. This reflects the balance between sufficient immobilization to achieve stability versus mobilization to restore motion. If it is severely limiting, lysis of adhesions may be undertaken to restore range of motion.
- **Ligamentous laxity and instability:** Redislocation is uncommon, especially after ligamentous reconstruction and adequate immobilization.
- **Vascular compromise:** This may result in atrophic skin changes, hyperalgesia, claudication, and muscle contracture. Recognition of popliteal artery injury is of paramount importance, particularly 24 to 72 hours after the initial injury, when late thrombosis related to intimal injury may be overlooked.
- **Nerve traction injury:** Injury resulting in sensory and motor disturbances portends a poor prognosis because exploration in the acute (<24 hours), subacute (1 to 2 weeks), and long-term settings (3 months) has yielded poor results. Bracing or muscle tendon transfers may be necessary to improve function.

35 Patella and Extensor Mechanism Injuries

PATELLAR FRACTURES

Epidemiology

- Represent 1% of all skeletal injuries
- Male-to-female ratio 2:1
- Most common age group 20 to 50 years old
- Bilateral injuries uncommon

Anatomy

- The patella is the largest sesamoid bone in the body.
- The quadriceps tendon inserts on the superior pole and the patellar ligament originates from the inferior pole of the patella.
- There are seven articular facets; the lateral facet is the largest (50% of the articular surface).
- The articular cartilage may be up to 1 cm thick.
- The medial and lateral extensor retinacula are strong longitudinal expansions of the quadriceps and insert directly onto the tibia. If these remain intact in the presence of a patella fracture, then active extension will be preserved (Fig. 35.1).

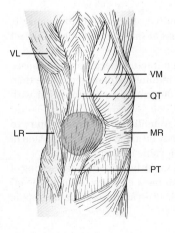

FIGURE 35.1 Soft tissue anatomy of the patella. *VL*, vastus lateralis; *LR*, lateral retinaculum; *VM*, vastus medialis; *QT*, quadriceps tendon; *MR*, medial retinaculum; *PT*, patellar tendon. (From Bucholz RW, Heckman JD, Court-Brown C, et al., eds. *Rockwood and Green's Fractures in Adults.* 6th ed. Philadelphia: Lippincott Williams & Wilkins; 2006.)

■ The function of the patella is to increase the mechanical advantage and leverage of the quadriceps tendon, aid in nourishment of the femoral articular surface, and protect the femoral condyles from direct trauma.

■ The blood supply arises from the geniculate arteries, which form an anastomosis circumferentially around the patella.

Mechanism of Injury

■ **Direct:** Trauma to the patella may produce incomplete, simple, stellate, or comminuted fracture patterns. Displacement is typically minimal owing to preservation of the medial and lateral retinacular expansions. Abrasions over the area or open injuries are common. Active knee extension may be preserved.

■ **Indirect (most common):** This is secondary to forcible eccentric quadriceps contraction while the knee is in a semiflexed position (e.g., in a "stumble" or "fall"). The intrinsic strength of the patella is exceeded by the pull of the musculotendinous and ligamentous structures. A transverse fracture pattern is most commonly seen with this mechanism, with variable inferior pole comminution. The degree of displacement of the fragments suggests the degree of retinacular disruption. Active knee extension is usually lost.

■ **Combined direct/indirect mechanisms:** These may be caused by trauma in which the patient experiences direct and indirect trauma to the knee, such as in a fall from a height.

Clinical Evaluation

■ Patients typically present with limited or no ambulatory capacity with pain, swelling, and tenderness of the involved knee. A defect at the patella may be palpable.

■ It is important to rule out an open fracture because these constitute a surgical urgency; this may require instillation of more than 100 mL saline into the knee to determine communication with overlying lacerations.

■ Active knee extension should be evaluated to determine injury to the retinacular expansions. This may be aided by decompression of hemarthrosis or intra-articular lidocaine injection.

■ Associated lower extremity injuries may be present in the setting of high-energy trauma. The physician must carefully evaluate the ipsilateral hip, femur, tibia, and ankle, with appropriate radiographic evaluation, if indicated.

Radiographic Evaluation

- Anteroposterior (AP) and lateral views of the knee should be obtained.
  - □ **AP view:** A bipartite patella (8% of the population) may be mistaken for a fracture; it usually occurs in the superolateral position and has smooth margins; it is bilateral in 50% of individuals.
  - □ **Lateral view:** Displaced fractures usually are obvious.
  - □ **Axial view (sunrise):** This may help identify osteochondral or vertical marginal fractures. This view may be difficult to obtain in the acute setting, however.
- Computed tomography scanning may be used to better delineate fracture patterns, marginal fractures, or free osteochondral fragments.

CLASSIFICATION

Descriptive

Open versus closed
Nondisplaced versus displaced
Pattern: stellate, comminuted, transverse, vertical (marginal), polar
Osteochondral (Fig. 35.2)

Undisplaced   Transverse   Lower or   Multifragmented
                             upper pole   undisplaced (stellate)

Multifragmented   Vertical   Osteochondral
displaced

FIGURE 35.2 Classification of patella fractures. (From Bucholz RW, Heckman JD, Court-Brown C, et al., eds. *Rockwood and Green's Fractures in Adults*. 6th ed. Philadelphia: Lippincott Williams & Wilkins; 2006.)

OTA Classification of Patellar Fractures

See Fracture and Dislocation Classification Compendium at http://www.ota.org/compendium/compendium.html.

Treatment

Nonoperative

- Indications include nondisplaced or minimally displaced (2 to 3 mm) fractures with minimal articular disruption (1 to 2 mm). This requires an intact extensor mechanism.
- A cylinder cast or knee immobilizer is used for 4 to 6 weeks. Early weight bearing in extension is encouraged, advancing to full weight bearing with crutches as tolerated by the patient. Early straight leg raising and isometric quadriceps strengthening exercises should be started within a few days. After radiographic evidence of healing, progressive active flexion and extension strengthening exercises are begun with a hinged knee brace initially locked in extension for ambulation.

Operative

Open Reduction and Internal Fixation

- Indications for open reduction and internal fixation include loss of active extension, an extensor lag, >2-mm articular incongruity, >3-mm fragment displacement, or open fracture.
- There are multiple methods of operative fixation, including tension banding (using parallel longitudinal Kirschner wires or cannulated screws) (Figs. 35.3A and 35.3B) as well as circumferential cerclage wiring. Retinacular disruption should be repaired at the time of surgery. Comminuted fractures may require multiple small fragment or mini-fragment screws or wires.
- Postoperatively, the patient should be placed in a splint for 3 to 6 days until skin healing, with early institution of knee motion. The patient should perform active assisted range-of-motion exercises, progressing to partial and full weight bearing by 6 weeks.
- Severely comminuted or marginally repaired fractures, particularly in older individuals, may necessitate immobilization for 3 to 6 weeks.
- Weightbearing as tolerated in extension is allowed. Knee immobilizer is removed for range of knee motion. Hinged bracing is not indicated.

Patellectomy

- Partial patellectomy
  - □ Indications for partial patellectomy are limited, but include the presence of a large, salvageable fragment in the presence of smaller, comminuted polar fragments in which it is believed

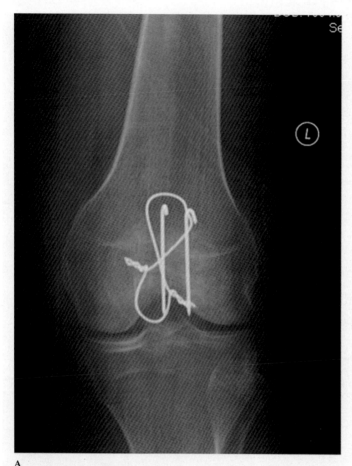

A

FIGURE 35.3 Example of a transverse patella fracture fixed with a K-wire tension band construct.

impossible to restore the articular surface or to achieve stable fixation. Excision of distal fragments will lead to patella baja.
- □ The patellar tendon may be reattached nonabsorbable sutures placed longitudinally along the long axis.
- ■ Total patellectomy
  - □ Total patellectomy is reserved for extensive and severely comminuted fractures and is rarely indicated.
  - □ Peak torque of the quadriceps is reduced by 50%.
  - □ Repair of medial and lateral retinacular injuries at the time of patellectomy is essential.

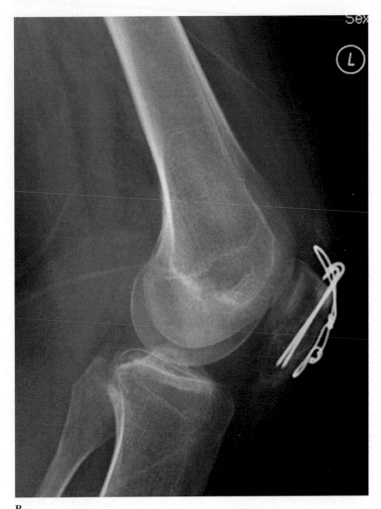

B

FIGURE 35.3 (Continued)

- Following partial or total patellectomy, the knee should be immobilized in a long leg cast at 10 degrees of flexion for 3 to 6 weeks.

Complications

- **Postoperative infection:** Uncommon and is related to open injuries that may necessitate serial debridements. Relentless infection may require excision of nonviable fragments and repair of the extensor mechanism.

- **Fixation failure:** Incidence is increased in osteoporotic bone or after failure to achieve compression at fracture site.
- **Refracture (1% to 5%):** Secondary to decreased inherent strength at the fracture site.
- **Nonunion (2%):** Most patients retain good function, although one may consider partial patellectomy for painful nonunion. Consider revision osteosynthesis in active, younger individuals.
- **Osteonecrosis (proximal fragment):** Associated with greater degrees of initial fracture displacement. Treatment consists of observation only, with spontaneous revascularization occurring by 2 years.
- **Posttraumatic osteoarthritis:** Present in more than 50% of patients in long-term studies. Intractable patellofemoral pain may require Maquet tibial tubercle advancement.
- **Loss of knee motion:** Secondary to prolonged immobilization or postoperative scarring.
- **Painful retained hardware:** Due to the subcutaneous nature of the fixation. May necessitate removal for adequate pain relief.
- **Loss of extensor strength and extensor lag:** Most patients will experience a loss of knee extension of approximately 5 degrees, although this is rarely clinically significant.
- Patellar instability.

PATELLA DISLOCATION

Epidemiology

- Patellar dislocation is more common in women, owing to physiologic laxity, as well as in patients with hypermobility and connective tissue disorders (e.g., Ehlers–Danlos or Marfan syndrome).

Anatomy

- The "Q angle" is defined as the angle subtended by a line drawn from the anterior superior iliac spine through the center of the patella, with a second line from the center of the patella to the tibial tubercle (Fig. 35.3). The Q angle ensures that the resultant vector of pull with quadriceps action is laterally directed; this lateral moment is normally counterbalanced by patellofemoral, patellotibial, and retinacular structures as well as patellar engagement within the trochlear groove. An increased Q angle predisposes to patella dislocation.
- Dislocations are associated with patella alta, congenital abnormalities of the patella and trochlea, hypoplasia of the vastus medialis, and hypertrophic lateral retinaculum.

Mechanism of Injury

- **Lateral dislocation:** Forced internal rotation of the femur on an externally rotated and planted tibia with knee in flexion is the usual cause. It is associated with a 5% risk of osteochondral fractures.
- Medial instability is rare and usually iatrogenic, congenital, traumatic, or associated with atrophy of the quadriceps musculature.
- **Intra-articular dislocation:** This is uncommon but may occur following knee trauma in adolescent male patients. The patella is avulsed from quadriceps tendon and is rotated around horizontal axis, with the proximal pole lodged in the intercondylar notch.
- **Superior dislocation:** This occurs in elderly individuals from forced hyperextension injuries to the knee with the patella locked on an anterior femoral osteophyte.

Clinical Evaluation

- Patients with an unreduced patella dislocation will present with hemarthrosis, an inability to flex the knee, and a displaced patella on palpation.
- Lateral dislocations may also cause medial retinacular pain.
- Patients with reduced or chronic patella dislocation may demonstrate a positive "apprehension test" in which a laterally directed force applied to the patella with the knee in extension reproduces the sensation of impending dislocation, causing pain and quadriceps contraction to limit patella mobility.

Radiographic Evaluation

- AP and lateral views of the knee should be obtained. In addition, an axial (sunrise) view of both patellae should be obtained. Various axial views have been described by several authors (Fig. 35.4):
  - □ **Hughston 55 degrees of knee flexion:** Sulcus angle, patellar index
  - □ **Merchant 45 degrees of knee flexion:** Sulcus angle, congruence angle
  - □ **Laurin 20 degrees of knee flexion:** Patellofemoral index, lateral patellofemoral angle
- Assessment of patella alta or baja is based on the lateral radiograph of the knee:
  - □ **Blumensaat line:** The lower pole of the patella should lie on a line projected anteriorly from the intercondylar notch on lateral radiograph with the knee flexed to 30 degrees.
  - □ **Insall–Salvati ratio:** The ratio of the length of the patellar ligament (LL; from the inferior pole of the patella to the tibial tubercle) to the patellar length (LP; the greatest diagonal length

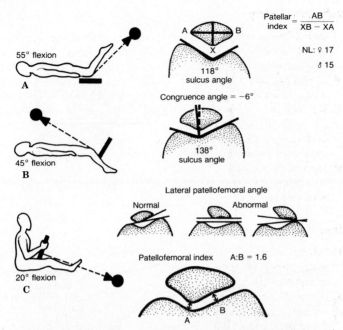

FIGURE 35.4 Representation of the **(A)** Hughston (knee flexed to 55 degrees) **(B)** Merchant (knee flexed to 45 degrees), and **(C)** Laurin (knee flexed to 20 degrees) patellofemoral views. (From Bucholz RW, Heckman JD, eds. *Rockwood and Green's Fractures in Adults.* 5th ed. Baltimore: Lippincott Williams & Wilkins; 2002.)

of the patella) should be 1.0. A ratio of 1.2 indicates patella alta, whereas 0.8 indicates patella baja (Fig. 35.5).

Classification

Reduced versus unreduced
Congenital versus acquired
Acute (traumatic) versus chronic (recurrent)
Lateral, medial, intra-articular, superior

Treatment

Nonoperative

■ Reduction and casting or bracing in knee extension may be undertaken with or without arthrocentesis for comfort.

■ The patient may ambulate in locked extension for 3 weeks, at which time progressive flexion can be instituted with physical

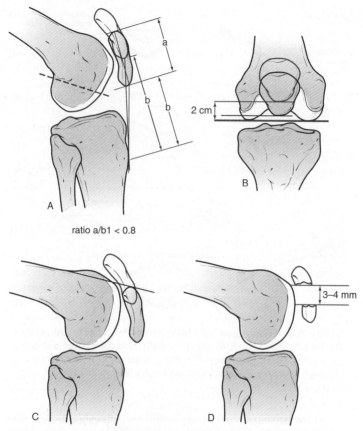

FIGURE 35.5 Insall–Salvati technique for measuring patellar height. (Modified from Insall NJ. *Surgery.* New York: Churchill Livingstone; 1984.)

therapy for quadriceps strengthening. After a total of 6 to 8 weeks, the patient may be weaned from the brace as tolerated.

- Surgical intervention for acute dislocations may be indicated depending upon activity level and involves repair of the medial patellofemoral ligament. Surgery is also indicated in conjunction with a displaced osteochondral fracture.
- Intra-articular dislocations may require reduction with the patient under anesthesia.
- Functional taping has been described in the physical therapy literature with moderate success.

Operative

- This is primarily used with recurrent dislocations.
- No single procedure corrects all patellar malalignment problems; the patient's age, diagnosis, level of activity, and condition of the patellofemoral articulation must be taken into consideration.
- Patellofemoral instability should be addressed by correction of all malalignment factors.
- Degenerative articular changes influence the selection of the realignment procedure.
- Surgical interventions include

   Lateral release: Indicated for patellofemoral pain with lateral tilt, lateral retinacular pain with lateral patellar position, and lateral patellar compression syndrome. It may be performed arthroscopically or as an open procedure.

   Medial plication: This may be performed at the time of lateral release to centralize patella.

   Proximal patella realignment: Medialization of the proximal pull of the patella is indicated when a lateral release/medial plication fails to centralize the patella. The release of tight proximal lateral structures and reinforcement of the pull of medial supporting structures, especially the vastus medialis obliquus, are performed in an effort to decrease lateral patellar tracking and improve congruence of the patellofemoral articulation. Indications include recurrent patellar dislocations that have not responded to nonoperative therapy and acute dislocations in young, athletic patients, especially with medial patellar avulsion fractures or radiographic lateral subluxation/tilt after closed reduction.

   Distal patella realignment: Reorientation of the patellar ligament and tibial tubercle is indicated when an adult patient experiences recurrent dislocations and patellofemoral pain with malalignment of the extensor mechanism. This is contraindicated in patients with open physes and normal Q angles. It is designed to advance and medialize tibial tubercle, thus correcting patella alta and normalizing the Q angle.

Complications

- **Redislocation:** The risk is higher in patients younger than 20 years at the time of the first episode. Recurrent dislocation is an indication for surgical intervention.
- **Loss of knee motion:** This may result from prolonged immobilization. Surgical intervention may lead to scarring with resultant arthrofibrosis. This emphasizes the need for aggressive physical therapy to

increase quadriceps tone to maintain patella alignment and to maintain knee motion.

■ **Patellofemoral pain:** This may result from retinacular disruption at the time of dislocation or from chondral injury.

QUADRICEPS TENDON RUPTURE

■ Typically occurs in patients >40 years old. Due to an eccentric quadriceps contraction.
■ It usually ruptures within 2 cm proximal to superior pole of patella.
■ Rupture level is often associated with the patient's age.
  □ Rupture occurs at the bone–tendon junction in most patients >40 years old.
  □ Rupture occurs at the midsubstance in most patients <40 years old.
■ Risk factors for quadriceps rupture
■ Tendinitis
  □ Anabolic steroid use
  □ Local steroid injection
  □ Diabetes mellitus
  □ Inflammatory arthropathy
  □ Chronic renal failure
■ History
  □ Sensation of a sudden pop while stressing the extensor mechanism
  □ Pain at the site of injury
  □ Inability/difficulty weight bearing
■ Physical examination
  □ Knee joint effusion
  □ Tenderness at the upper pole of patella
  □ Loss of active knee extension
    • With partial tears, intact active extension
  □ Palpable defect proximal to the superior pole of the patella
    • If defect present but patient able to extend the knee, then intact extensor retinaculum
    • If no active extension, then both tendon and retinaculum completely torn
■ Radiographic examination
  □ AP, lateral, and tangential (sunrise, Merchant)
  □ Distal displacement of the patella
  □ Patellofemoral relationship
    • This is based on a lateral x-ray with the knee in 30 degrees of flexion.

- The lower pole of the patella should be at the level of the line projected anteriorly from the intercondylar notch (Blumensaat line).
- Patella alta possible with patellar tendon rupture and patella baja with quadriceps tendon rupture.
  □ MRI or ultrasound
  - Useful for unclear diagnosis
- Treatment
  □ Nonoperative
  - Reserved for incomplete tears in which active, full knee extension is preserved.
  - The leg is immobilized in extension for approximately 4 to 6 weeks.
  - Progressive physical therapy may be required to regain strength and motion.
- Operative
  □ Indicated for complete ruptures.
  □ Reapproximation of tendon to bone using nonabsorbable sutures passed through bone tunnels.
  □ Repair the tendon close to the articular surface to avoid patellar tilting.
  □ Midsubstance tears may undergo end-to-end repair after edges are freshened and slightly overlapped (Fig. 35.6).
  □ The patient may benefit from reinforcement from a distally based partial-thickness quadriceps tendon turned down across the repair site (Scuderi technique).
  □ Chronic tears may require a V-Y advancement of a retracted quadriceps tendon (Codivilla V-Y-plasty technique).
- Postoperative management
  □ A knee immobilizer or cylinder cast is used for 5 to 6 weeks.
  □ Immediate weight bearing in extension as tolerated is allowed.
  □ Hinged knee bracing has almost no use in extensor mechanism injuries of the knee.
- Complications
  □ Rerupture
  □ Persistent quadriceps atrophy/weakness
  □ Loss of knee motion
  □ Infection

PATELLA TENDON RUPTURE

- Less common than quadriceps tendon rupture
- Most common in patients <40 years old
- Associated with degenerative changes of the tendon (calcification may be seen radiographically)

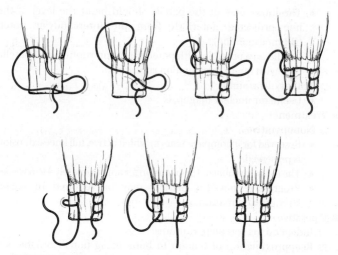

FIGURE 35.6 Sequential steps of placing Krackow locking loop ligament sutures for tendon or ligament repair. (Modified from Krackow KA, Thomas SC, Jones LC. A new stitch for ligament tendon fixation: brief note. *J Bone Joint Surg Am.* 1980;68:359.)

- Rupture common at the inferior pole of the patella
- Risk factors
  - □ Rheumatoid arthritis
  - □ Systemic lupus erythematosus
  - □ Diabetes
  - □ Chronic renal failure
  - □ Systemic corticosteroid therapy
  - □ Local steroid injection
  - □ Chronic patella tendinitis
- Anatomy of patellar tendon
  - □ Averages 4 mm thick but widens to 5 to 6 mm at the tibial tubercle
  - □ Merges with the medial and lateral retinaculum
  - □ **Composition:** 90% type I collagen
- Blood supply
  - □ Fat pad vessels supply the posterior aspect of the tendon via the inferior medial and lateral geniculate arteries.
  - □ Retinacular vessels supply anterior portion of tendon via the inferior medial geniculate and recurrent tibial arteries.
  - □ Proximal and distal insertion areas are relatively avascular and subsequently are a common site of rupture.

- Biomechanics
  - □ The greatest forces are at 60 degrees of knee flexion.
  - □ Forces through the patellar tendon are 3.2 times body weight while climbing stairs.
- History
  - □ Often a report of forceful quadriceps contraction against a flexed knee
  - □ Possible audible "pop"
  - □ Inability to bear weight or extend the knee against gravity
- Physical examination
  - □ Palpable defect
  - □ Hemarthrosis
  - □ Painful passive knee flexion
  - □ Partial or complete loss of active extension
  - □ Quadriceps atrophy with chronic injury
- Radiographic examination
  - □ AP and lateral x-rays
  - □ Patella alta visible on lateral view
    - Patella superior to Blumensaat line
    - Ultrasonography an effective means to determine continuity of the tendon
    - However, operator and reader dependent
  - □ MRI
    - Effective means to assess patella tendon, especially if other intra-articular or soft tissue injuries suspected
- Classification
  - □ No widely accepted means of classification
  - □ Can be categorized by
    - Location of tear
- Proximal insertion most common
  - □ Timing between injury and surgery
    - Most important factor for prognosis
    - **Acute:** within 2 weeks
- Treatment
  - □ Surgical treatment is required for restoration of the extensor mechanism.
  - □ Repairs are categorized as early or delayed.
- Nonoperative
  - □ Nonoperative treatment is reserved for partial tears in which patient able to extend the knee fully.
  - □ Treatment is immobilization in full knee extension for 3 to 6 weeks.
- Early repair
  - □ The overall outcome is better than for a delayed repair.

- □ Primary repair of the tendon is performed.
- □ Surgical approach is through a midline incision.
- □ Patellar tendon rupture and retinacular tears are exposed.
- □ Frayed edges and hematoma are debrided.
- □ Nonabsorbable sutures are used to repair the tendon to the patella.
- □ Sutures are passed through parallel, longitudinal bone tunnels and are tied proximally.
- □ Retinacular tears should be repaired.
- □ One can reinforce the repair with a cerclage wire, cable, or tape.
- □ One should assess the repair intraoperatively with knee flexion.
- ■ Postoperative management
  - □ Knee immobilizer or casting in extension.
  - □ Immediate isometric quadriceps exercises are prescribed.
  - □ Active flexion with passive extension may occur at 2 weeks; if allowed, start with 0 to 45 degrees and advance 30 degrees each week.
  - □ Active extension occurs at 6 weeks.
  - □ Initial full weight bearing in extension for 6 weeks.
  - □ All restrictions are lifted after full range of motion and 90% of the contralateral quadriceps strength are obtained, usually at 4 to 6 months.
- ■ Delayed repair
  - □ This occurs >6 weeks from the initial injury.
  - □ It often results in a poorer outcome.
  - □ Quadriceps contraction and patellar migration are commonly encountered.
  - □ Adhesions between the patella and femur may be present.
  - □ Options include hamstring and fascia lata autograft augmentation of primary repair or Achilles tendon allograft.
  - □ Postoperative management
    - • More conservative than with early repair.
    - • A bivalved cylinder cast is worn for 6 weeks.
    - • Active range of motion is started at 6 weeks.
- ■ Complications
  - □ Knee stiffness
  - □ Persistent quadriceps weakness
  - □ Rerupture
  - □ Infection
  - □ Patella baja

36 Tibial Plateau

EPIDEMIOLOGY

- Tibial plateau fractures constitute 1% of all fractures and 8% of fractures in the elderly.
- Isolated injuries to the lateral plateau account for 55% to 70% of tibial plateau fractures, as compared with 10% to 25% isolated medial plateau fractures and 10% to 30% bicondylar lesions.
- There is a wide spectrum of fracture patterns that involve the medial tibial plateau (10% to 23%), the lateral tibial plateau (55% to 70%), or both (11% to 31%).
- From 1% to 3% of these fractures are open injuries. *minority are open*

ANATOMY

- The tibial plateau is composed of the articular surfaces of the medial and lateral tibial plateaus, on which are the cartilaginous menisci. The medial plateau is larger and is concave in both the sagittal and coronal axes. The lateral plateau extends higher and is convex in both sagittal and coronal planes.
- The normal tibial plateau has a 10-degree posteroinferior slope.
- The two plateaus are separated from one another by the intercondylar eminence, which is nonarticular and serves as the tibial attachment of the cruciate ligaments. Three bony prominences exist 2 to 3 cm distal to the tibial plateau. Anteriorly is the tibial tubercle on which the patellar ligament inserts. Medially, the pes anserinus serves as attachment for the medial hamstrings. Laterally, the Gerdy tubercle is the insertion site of the iliotibial band.
- The medial articular surface and its supporting medial condyle are stronger than their lateral counterparts. As a result, fractures of the lateral plateau are more common.
- Medial plateau fractures are associated with higher energy injury and more commonly have associated soft tissue injuries, such as disruptions of the lateral collateral ligament complex, lesions of the peroneal nerve, and damage to the popliteal vessels.

MECHANISM OF INJURY

- Fractures of the tibial plateau occur in the setting of varus or valgus forces coupled with axial loading. Motor vehicle accidents account for the majority of these fractures in younger individuals, but elderly patients with osteopenic bone may experience these after a simple fall.

- The direction and magnitude of the generated force, age of the patient, bone quality, and amount of knee flexion at the moment of impact determine fracture fragment size, location, and displacement.
  - □ Young adults with strong, rigid bone typically develop split fractures and have a higher rate of associated ligamentous disruption.
  - □ Older adults with decreased bone strength and rigidity sustain depression and split-depression fractures and have a lower rate of ligamentous injury.
  - □ A bicondylar split fracture results from a severe axial force exerted on a fully extended knee.

CLINICAL EVALUATION

- Neurovascular examination is essential, especially with high-energy trauma. The trifurcation of the popliteal artery is tethered posteriorly between the adductor hiatus proximally and the soleus complex distally. The peroneal nerve is tethered laterally as it courses around the fibular neck.
- Hemarthrosis frequently occurs in the setting of a markedly swollen, painful knee on which the patient is unable to bear weight. Knee aspiration may reveal marrow fat.
- Direct trauma is usually evident on examination of the overlying soft tissues, and open injuries must be ruled out. Intra-articular instillation of more than 120 cc's saline may be necessary to evaluate possible communication with overlying lacerations.
- Compartment syndrome must be ruled out, particularly with higher-energy injuries and or fracture dislocations.
- Assessment for ligament injury is essential.

ASSOCIATED INJURIES

- Soft tissue injury is seen in approximately 90% of these fractures.
- Meniscal tears occur in up to 50% of tibial plateau fractures. Medial meniscus tears highly associated with medial plateau fractures and lateral meniscus tears associated with lateral tibial plateau fractures.
- Associated ligamentous injury to the cruciate or collateral ligaments occurs in up to 30% of tibial plateau fractures.
- Young adults, whose strong subchondral bone resists depression, are at the highest risk of collateral or cruciate ligament rupture.

- Fractures involving the medial tibial plateau may be associated with higher incidences of peroneal nerve or popliteal neurovascular lesions owing to higher-energy mechanisms; it is postulated that many of these represent knee dislocations that spontaneously reduced.
- Peroneal nerve injuries are caused by stretching (neurapraxia); these will usually resolve over time; however, these are rare.
- Arterial injuries frequently represent traction-induced intimal injuries presenting as thrombosis; only rarely do they present as transection injuries secondary to laceration or avulsion.

RADIOGRAPHIC EVALUATION

- Anteroposterior and lateral views supplemented by 40-degree internal (lateral plateau) and external rotation (medial plateau) oblique projections should be obtained.
- A 10- to 5-degree caudally tilted plateau view can be used to assess articular step-off.
- Avulsion of the fibular head, the Segond sign (lateral capsular avulsion) and Pellegrini–Steata lesion (calcification along the insertion of the medial collateral ligament) are all signs of associated ligamentous injury.
- A physician-assisted traction view is often helpful in higher-energy injuries with severe impaction and metadiaphyseal fragmentation to delineate the fracture pattern better and to determine the efficacy of ligamentotaxis for fracture reduction.
- Stress views, preferably with the patient under sedation or anesthesia and with fluoroscopic image intensification, are occasionally useful for the detection of collateral ligament ruptures.
- Computed tomography with two-dimensional or three-dimensional reconstruction is useful for delineating the degree of fragmentation or depression of the articular surface, as well as for preoperative planning.
- Magnetic resonance imaging is useful for evaluating injuries to the menisci, the cruciate and collateral ligaments, and the soft tissue envelope.
- Arteriography should be performed if there is a question of vascular compromise.

CLASSIFICATION

Schatzker (Fig. 36.1)

Type I: Lateral plateau, split fracture
Type II: Lateral plateau, split depression fracture (most common)

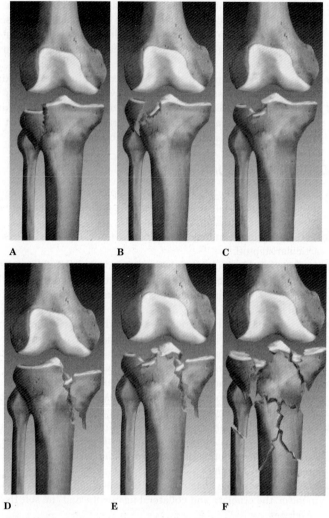

A   B   C

D   E   F

FIGURE 36.1 Schatzker classification. (From Bucholz RW, Heckman JD, Court-Brown C, et al., eds. *Rockwood and Green's Fractures in Adults.* 6th ed. Philadelphia: Lippincott Williams & Wilkins; 2006.)

Type III:	Lateral plateau, depression fracture
Type IV:	Medial plateau fracture
Type V:	Bicondylar plateau fracture
Type VI:	Plateau fracture with separation of the metaphysis from the diaphysis

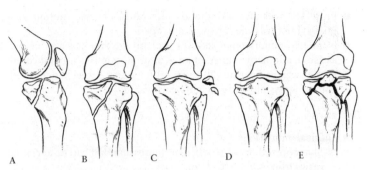

FIGURE 36.2 Moore classification.

- Types I to III are low-energy injuries.
- Types IV to VI are high-energy injuries.
- Type I usually occurs in younger individuals and is associated with medial collateral ligament injuries.
- Type III usually is extremely rare and will only occur in older individuals or those with osteopenia (Fig. 36.1).

Moore (Fig. 36.2)

- Type 1 is a split fracture of the medial tibial plateau in the coronal plane.
- Type 2 is an entire condyle fracture with the fracture line beginning in the opposite compartment and extending across the tibial eminence.
- Type 3 is a rim avulsion fracture; these fractures are associated with a high rate of associated neurovascular injury.
- Type 4 is another type of rim fracture, a rim compression injury usually associated with some types of contralateral ligamentous injury.
- Type 5 is a four-part fracture with the tibial eminence separated from the tibial condyles and the shaft.

OTA Classification of Tibial Plateau Fractures (Type 43)

See Fracture and Dislocation Classification Compendium at http://www.ota.org/compendium/compendium.html.

TREATMENT

Nonoperative

- Indicated for nondisplaced or minimally displaced fractures and in patients with advanced osteoporosis.

- Protected weight bearing and early range of knee motion in a hinged fracture brace are recommended.
- Isometric quadriceps exercises and progressive passive, active-assisted, and active range-of-knee motion exercises are indicated.
- Partial weight bearing (30 to 50 lb) for 8 to 12 weeks is allowed, with progression to full weight bearing.

Operative

- Surgical indications
  - □ The reported range of articular depression that can be accepted varies from <2 mm to 1 cm.
  - □ Instability >10 degrees of the nearly extended knee compared to the contralateral side is an accepted surgical indication. Split fractures are more likely to be unstable than pure depression fractures in which the rim is intact. (Fig. 36.3)
  - □ Open fractures.
  - □ Associated compartment syndrome.
  - □ Associated vascular injury.
- Operative treatment principles
  - □ Reconstruction of the articular surface, followed by reestablishment of tibial alignment, is the goal.

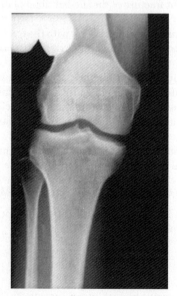

FIGURE 36.3 Stress exam demonstrating MCL incompetence in conjunction with a lateral tibial plateau fracture.

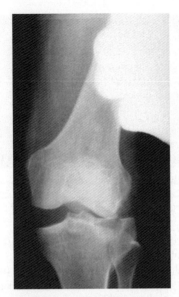

FIGURE 36.3 (Continued)

- ☐ Treatment involves reducing and buttressing of elevated articular segments with bone graft or bone graft substitute.
- ☐ Fracture fixation can involve use of plates and screws, screws alone, or external fixation.
- ☐ The choice of implant is related to the fracture patterns, the degree of displacement, and familiarity of the surgeon with the procedure.
- ☐ Adequate soft tissue reconstruction including preservation and/or repair of the meniscus as well as intra-articular and extra-articular ligamentous structures should be addressed.
- ■ Spanning external fixation across the knee may be used as a temporizing measure in patients with higher-energy injuries and limb shortening or significant soft tissue injury. The external fixator is used to keep the soft tissues out to length and provides some degree of fracture reduction until definitive surgery.
- ■ Arthroscopy may be used to evaluate the articular surfaces, the menisci, and the cruciate ligaments. It may also be used for evacuation of hemarthrosis and particulate debris, for meniscal procedures, and for arthroscopic-assisted reduction and fixation. Its role in the evaluation of rim disorders and its utility in the management of complicated fractures are limited. (Fig. 36.4)
- ■ An avulsed anterior cruciate ligament with a large bony fragment may be repaired. If the fragment is minimal or the ligament has an

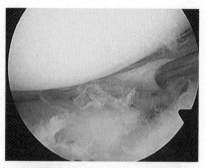

FIGURE 36.4 Arthroscopic evaluation of a Schatzker II tibial plateau fracture demonstrating articular incongruence.

intrasubstance tear, reconstruction should be delayed. Instability is generally not a problem.

■ Surgery in isolated injuries may proceed after a full appreciation of the personality of the fracture. This delay will also allow swelling to subside and local skin conditions to improve.

■ Schatzker type I to IV fractures can be fixed with percutaneous screws or lateral placed periarticular plate. If satisfactory closed reduction (<1-mm articular step-off) cannot be achieved with closed techniques, open reduction and internal fixation are indicated.

■ The menisci should never be excised to facilitate exposure.

■ Depressed fragments can be elevated from below en masse by using a bone tamp working through the split component or a cortical window. The metaphyseal defect should be filled with some type of osteoconductive material.

■ Type V and VI fractures can be managed using plate and screws, a ring fixator, or a hybrid fixator. Limited internal fixation can be added to restore the articular surface.

■ Percutaneous inserted plating, which is a more biologic approach, has been described. In this technique, the plate is slid subcutaneously without soft tissue stripping.

■ Use of locked plates has diminished the need for double plating bicondylar tibial plateau fractures.

■ Fractures of the posterior medial plateau may require a posteromedial incision for fracture reduction and plate stabilization.

■ **Postoperative care:** Patients are kept non–weight bearing with or without continuous passive motion and active range of motion are encouraged.

■ Weight bearing is allowed at 8 to 12 weeks.

COMPLICATIONS

- **Arthrofibrosis:** This is common, related to trauma from injury and surgical dissection, extensor retinacular injury, scarring, and postoperative immobility. More common in higher energy injuries.
- **Infection:** This is often related to ill-timed incisions through compromised soft tissues with extensive dissection for implant placement.
- **Compartment syndrome:** This uncommon but devastating complication involves the tight fascial compartments of the leg. It emphasizes the need for high clinical suspicion, serial neurovascular examinations, particularly in the unconscious or obtunded patient, aggressive evaluation, including compartment pressure measuring if necessary, and expedient treatment consisting of emergency fasciotomies of all compartments of the leg.
- **Malunion or nonunion:** This is most common in Schatzker VI fractures at the metaphyseal–diaphyseal junction, related to comminution, unstable fixation, implant failure, or infection.
- **Posttraumatic osteoarthritis:** This may result from residual articular incongruity, chondral damage at the time of injury, or malalignment of the mechanical axis.
- **Peroneal nerve injury:** This is most common with trauma to the lateral aspect of the leg where the peroneal nerve courses in proximity to the fibular head and lateral tibial plateau. Can be iatrogenic.
- **Popliteal artery laceration (rare).**
- **Avascular necrosis of small articular fragments:** This may result in loose bodies within the knee.

37 Tibia/Fibula Shaft

EPIDEMIOLOGY

- Fractures of the tibia and fibula shaft are the most common long bone fractures.
- In an average population, there are about 26 tibial diaphyseal fractures per 100,000 population per year.
- The highest incidence of adult tibia diaphyseal fractures seen in young males is between 15 and 19 years of age, with an incidence of 109 per 100,000 population per year.
- The highest incidence of adult tibia diaphyseal fractures seen in women is between 90 and 99 years of age, with an incidence of 49 per 100,000 population per year.
- The average age of a patient sustaining a tibia shaft fracture is 37 years, with men having an average age of 31 years and women 54 years.
- Diaphyseal tibia fractures have the highest rate of nonunion for all long bones.

ANATOMY

- The tibia is a long tubular bone with a triangular cross section. It has a subcutaneous anteromedial border and is bounded by four tight fascial compartments (anterior, lateral, posterior, and deep posterior) (Figs. 37.1 and 37.2).
- Blood supply
  - □ The nutrient artery arises from the posterior tibial artery, entering the posterolateral cortex distal to the origination of the soleus muscle. Once the vessel enters the intramedullary (IM) canal, it gives off three ascending branches and one descending branch. These give rise to the endosteal vascular tree, which anastomose with periosteal vessels arising from the anterior tibial artery.
  - □ The anterior tibial artery is particularly vulnerable to injury as it passes through a hiatus in the interosseus membrane.
  - □ The peroneal artery has an anterior communicating branch to the dorsalis pedis artery. It may therefore be occluded despite an intact dorsalis pedis pulse.

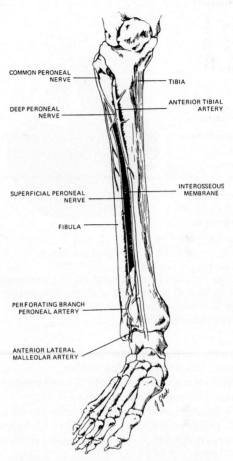

FIGURE 37.1 The anatomy of the tibial and fibular shaft. (From Rockwood CA Jr, Green DP, Bucholz RW, Heckman JD, eds. *Rockwood and Green's Fractures in Adults.* Vol 2. 4th ed. Philadelphia: Lippincott-Raven; 1996:2124.)

The distal third is supplied by periosteal anastomoses around the ankle with branches entering the tibia through ligamentous attachments.

☐ There may be a watershed area at the junction of the middle and distal thirds (controversial).

☐ If the nutrient artery is disrupted, there is reversal of flow through the cortex, and the periosteal blood supply becomes

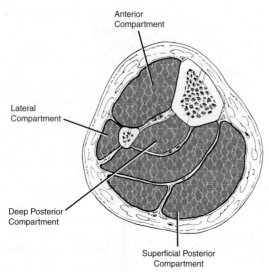

FIGURE 37.2 The four compartments of the leg. (From Bucholz RW, Heckman JD, Court-Brown C, et al., eds. *Rockwood and Green's Fractures in Adults*. 6th ed. Philadelphia: Lippincott Williams & Wilkins; 2006.)

more important. This emphasizes the importance of preserving periosteal attachments during fixation.

□ The fibula is responsible for 6% to 17% of a weight-bearing load. Its major function is for muscle attachment.

□ The common peroneal nerve courses around the neck of the fibula, which is nearly subcutaneous in this region; it is therefore especially vulnerable to direct blows or traction injuries at this level.

MECHANISM OF INJURY

■ Direct

□ **High-energy bending:** Motor vehicle accident

• Transverse, comminuted, displaced fractures commonly occur.

• Highly comminuted or segmental patterns are associated with extensive soft tissue compromise.

• Must rule out compartment syndrome and open fractures.

□ **Penetrating:** Gunshot

• The injury pattern is variable, but usually comminuted.

• Low-velocity missiles (handguns) do not pose the same degree of problem from bone or soft tissue damage that high-energy (motor vehicle accident) or high-velocity (shotguns, assault weapons) mechanisms may cause.

☐ **Low-energy bending:** Three- or four-point
  - Short oblique or transverse fractures occur, with a possible butterfly fragment.
  - May be comminuted and associated with extensive soft tissue compromise.
  - Compartment syndrome and open fractures may occur.

☐ **Fibula shaft fractures:** These typically result from direct trauma to the lateral aspect of the leg. Spiral fractures are seen proximally with rotational ankle fractures or low-energy twisting tibial injuries.

■ Indirect
  ☐ Torsional mechanisms
  - Twisting with the foot fixed and falls from low heights are causes.
  - These spiral, nondisplaced fractures have minimal comminution associated with little soft tissue damage.
  - Type 1 open fractures seen.

  ☐ Stress fractures
  - In military recruits, these injuries most commonly occur at the metaphyseal–diaphyseal junction, with sclerosis being most marked at the posteromedial cortex.
  - In ballet dancers, these fractures most commonly occur in the middle third; they are insidious in onset and are overuse injuries. "Dreaded black line" is pathognomonic (Fig. 37.3).
  - Plain radiographic findings may be delayed several weeks. Magnetic resonance imaging (MRI) is very sensitive for detecting these injuries.

CLINICAL EVALUATION

■ Evaluation of neurovascular status is critical. Dorsalis pedis and posterior tibial artery pulses must be evaluated and documented, especially in open fractures in which vascular flaps may be necessary. Common peroneal and tibial nerve integrity must be documented.

■ Assess soft tissue injury. Fracture blisters may contraindicate early open reduction of periarticular fractures.

■ Monitor for compartment syndrome. Pain out of proportion to the injury is the most reliable sign of compartment syndrome. Compartment pressure measurements that have been used as an indication for four-compartment fasciotomy have been a pressure within 30 mm Hg of diastolic pressure ($\Delta P < 30$ mm Hg). Deep

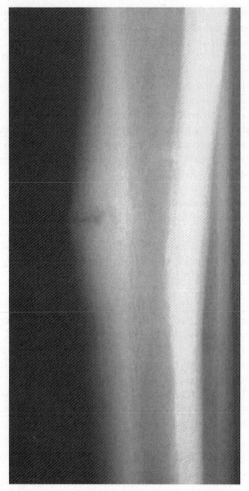

FIGURE 37.3 Example of anterior tibial stress fracture in ballet dancer. (From Schepsis AA, Busconi BD. *Sports Medicine*. Baltimore: Lippincott Williams & Wilkins; 2006.)

posterior compartment pressures may be elevated in the presence of a soft superficial posterior compartment.
■ Tibial fractures are associated with a high incidence of knee ligament injuries.
■ About 5% of all tibial fractures are bifocal, with two separate fractures of the tibia.

RADIOGRAPHIC EVALUATION

- Radiographic evaluation must include the entire tibia (anteroposterior [AP] and lateral views) with visualization of the ankle and knee joints.
- Oblique views may be helpful to further characterize the fracture pattern.
- Postreduction radiographs should include the knee and ankle for alignment and preoperative planning.
- A surgeon should look for the following features on the AP and lateral radiographs:
  □ **The presence of comminution:** This signifies a higher-energy injury.
  □ **The distance that bone fragments have displaced from their anatomic location:** Widely displaced fragments suggest that the soft tissue attachments have been damaged and the fragments may be avascular.
  □ **Osseous defects:** These may suggest missing bone or open wounds.
  □ Fracture lines may extend proximally to the knee or distally to the ankle joints.
  □ **The quality of the bone:** Is there evidence of osteopenia, metastases, or a previous fracture?
  □ **Osteoarthritis or the presence of a knee arthroplasty:** Either may change the treatment method selected by the surgeon.
  □ **Air in the soft tissues:** These are usually secondary to open fracture but may also signify the presence of gas gangrene, necrotizing fasciitis, or other anaerobic infections.
- Computed tomography and MRI usually are generally not necessary. CT may be useful in metaphyseal fractures if articular extension is suspected.
- Technetium bone scanning and MRI scanning may be useful in diagnosing stress fractures before these injuries become obvious on plain radiographs.
- Angiography is indicated if an arterial injury is suspected, based on anckle-branchial indexes (ABIs) or diminished pulses.

CLASSIFICATION

Poor sensitivity, reproducibility, and interobserver reliability have been reported for most classification schemes.

Descriptive

- **Open versus closed**
- **Anatomic location:** proximal, middle, or distal third
- **Fragment number and position:** comminution, butterfly fragments
- **Configuration:** transverse, spiral, oblique

- **Angulation:** varus/valgus, anterior/posterior
- Shortening
- **Displacement:** percentage of cortical contact
- Rotation
- Associated injuries

OTA Classification of Tibial Fractures

See Fracture and Dislocation Classification Compendium at http://www.ota.org/compendium/compendium.html.

Gustilo and Anderson Classification of Open Fractures

Type I: Clean skin opening of <1 cm, usually from inside to outside; minimal muscle contusion; simple transverse or short oblique fractures

Type II: Laceration >1-cm long, with extensive soft tissue damage; minimal to moderate crushing component; simple transverse or short oblique fractures with minimal comminution

Type III: Extensive soft tissue damage, including muscles, skin, and neurovascular structures; often a high-energy injury with a severe crushing component

  IIIA: Extensive soft tissue laceration, adequate bone coverage; segmental fractures, gunshot injuries, minimal periosteal stripping

  IIIB: Extensive soft tissue injury with periosteal stripping and bone exposure requiring soft tissue flap closure; usually associated with massive contamination

  IIIC: Vascular injury requiring repair

Tscherne Classification of Closed Fractures

- This classifies soft tissue injury in closed fractures and takes into account indirect versus direct injury mechanisms.

Grade 0: Injury from indirect forces with negligible soft tissue damage

Grade I: Closed fracture caused by low-moderate energy mechanisms, with superficial abrasions or contusions of soft tissues overlying the fracture

Grade II: Closed fracture with significant muscle contusion, with possible deep, contaminated skin abrasions associated with moderate to severe energy mechanisms and skeletal injury; high risk for compartment syndrome

Grade III: Extensive crushing of soft tissues, with subcutaneous degloving or avulsion, with arterial disruption or established compartment syndrome

TREATMENT

Nonoperative

Fracture reduction followed by application of a long leg cast with progressive weight bearing can be used for isolated, closed, low-energy fractures with minimal displacement and comminution.

- Cast with the knee in 0 to 5 degrees of flexion to allow for weight bearing with crutches as soon as tolerated by patient, with advancement to full weight bearing by the second to fourth week.
- After 3 to 6 weeks, the long leg cast may be exchanged for a patella-bearing cast or fracture brace.
- Union rates as high as 97% are reported, although with delayed weight bearing related to delayed union or nonunion. Hindfoot stiffness is the major limitation seen.

Acceptable Fracture Reduction

- Less than 5 degrees of varus/valgus angulation is recommended.
- Less than 10 degrees of anterior/posterior angulation is recommended (<5 degrees preferred).
- Less than 10 degrees of rotational deformity is recommended, with external rotation better tolerated than internal rotation.
- Less than 1 cm of shortening; 5 mm of distraction may delay healing 8 to 12 months.
- More than 50% cortical contact is recommended.
- Roughly, the anterior superior iliac spine, center of the patella, and base of the second proximal phalanx should be colinear.

Time to Union

- **The average time is 16 ± 4 weeks:** This is highly variable, depending on fracture pattern and soft tissue injury.
- Delayed union is defined as >20 weeks.
- **Nonunion:** This occurs when clinical and radiographic signs demonstrate that the potential for union is lost, including sclerotic ends at the fracture site and a persistent gap unchanged for several weeks. Nonunion has also been defined as lack of healing 9 months after fracture.

Tibia Stress Fracture

- Treatment consists of cessation of the offending activity.
- A short leg cast may be necessary, with partial-weight-bearing ambulation.

■ Surgery is reserved for those refractory to non-operative treatment or those that displace.

Fibula Shaft Fracture

■ Treatment consists of weight bearing as tolerated.
■ Although not required for healing, a short period of immobilization may be used to minimize pain.
■ Nonunion is uncommon because of the extensive muscular attachments.

Operative

Intramedullary Nailing

■ IM nailing carries the advantages of preservation of periosteal blood supply and limited soft tissue damage. In addition, it carries the biomechanical advantages of being able to control alignment, translation, and rotation. It is therefore recommended for most fracture patterns.
■ Locked versus unlocked nail
  □ **Locked nail:** This provides rotational control; it is effective in preventing shortening in comminuted fractures and those with significant bone loss. Interlocking screws can be removed at a later time to dynamize the fracture site, if needed, for healing.
  □ **Nonlocked nail:** This allows impaction at the fracture site with weight bearing, but it is difficult to control rotation. Nonlocked nails are rarely used.
■ Reamed versus unreamed nail
  □ **Reamed nail:** This is indicated for most closed and open fractures. It allows excellent IM splinting of the fracture and use of a larger-diameter, stronger nail.
  □ **Unreamed nail:** This is thought to preserve the IM blood supply in open fractures where the periosteal supply has been destroyed. It is currently reserved for higher-grade open fractures; its disadvantage is that it is significantly weaker than the larger reamed nail and has a higher risk of implant fatigue failure. Recent studies have shown this to be acceptable in closed tibial fractures.

Flexible Nails (Enders, Rush Rods)

■ Multiple curved IM pins exert a spring force to resist angulation and rotation, with minimal damage to the medullary circulation.

- These are rarely used in the United States because of the predominance of unstable fracture patterns and success with interlocking nails.
- They are recommended only in children or adolescents with open physes.

External Fixation

- Primarily used to treat severe open fractures, it can also be indicated in closed fractures complicated by compartment syndrome, concomitant head injury, or burns.
- Its popularity in the United States has waned with the increased use of reamed nails for most open fractures.
- **Union rates:** Up to 90%, with an average of 3.6 months to union.
- The incidence of pin tract infections is 10% to 15%.

Plates and Screws

- These are generally reserved for fractures extending into the metaphysis or epiphysis.
- Reported success rates as high as 97%.
- Complication rates of infection, wound breakdown, and malunion or nonunion increase with higher-energy injury patterns.

Proximal Tibia Fractures

- These account for about 7% of all tibia diaphyseal fractures.
- These fractures are notoriously difficult to nail because they frequently become malaligned, the commonest deformities being valgus and apex anterior angulation.
- Nailing may require use of special techniques such as blocking screws, unicortical plating, intraoperative external fixation or a lateral starting point.
- Use of a percutaneously inserted plate has had recent popularity.

Distal Tibia Fractures

- The risk for malalignment also exists with the use of an IM nail.
- With IM nailing, fibula plating or use of blocking screws may help to prevent malalignment.
- Use of a percutaneously inserted plate has had recent popularity.

Tibia Fracture with an Intact Fibula

- If the tibia fracture is nondisplaced, treatment consists of long leg casting with early weight bearing. Close observation is indicated to recognize any varus tendency.

- Some authors recommend IM nailing even if tibia fracture is nondisplaced.
- A potential risk of varus malunion exists (25%), particularly in patients >20 years.

Fasciotomy

- Evidence of compartment syndrome is an indication for emergent fasciotomy of all four-muscle compartments of the leg (anterior, lateral, superficial, and deep posterior) through one or multiple incision techniques. Following operative fracture fixation, the fascial openings should not be reapproximated.

COMPLICATIONS

- **Malunion:** This includes any deformity outside the acceptable range. Seen with nonoperative treatments and metaphyseal fractures.
- **Nonunion:** This is associated with high-velocity injuries, open fractures (especially Gustilo grade III), infection, intact fibula, inadequate fixation, and initial fracture displacement.
- Infection (more common following open fracture).
- **Soft tissue loss:** Delaying wound coverage for greater than 7 to 10 days in open fractures has been associated with higher rates of infection. Local rotational flaps or free flaps may be needed for adequate coverage.
- Stiffness at the knee and/or ankle may occur with nonoperative care.
- **Knee pain:** This is the most common complication associated with IM tibial nailing.
- **Hardware breakage:** Nail and locking screw breakage rates depend on the size of the nail used and the type of metal from which it is made. Larger reamed nails have larger cross screws; the incidence of nail and screw breakage is greater with unreamed nails that utilize smaller-diameter locking screws.
- Thermal necrosis of the tibial diaphysis following reaming is theoretical complication. Recent basic science work has discounted use of a tourniquet as a cause.
- **Reflex sympathetic dystrophy:** This is most common in patients unable to bear weight early and with prolonged cast immobilization. It is characterized by initial pain and swelling followed by atrophy of limb. Radiographic signs are spotty demineralization of foot and distal tibia and equinovarus ankle. It is treated by elastic compression stockings, weight bearing, sympathetic blocks, and foot orthoses, accompanied by aggressive physical therapy.

■ **Compartment syndrome:** Involvement of the anterior compa_
most common. Highest pressures occur at the time of o͏
closed reduction. It may require fasciotomy. Muscle death occ_
after 6 to 8 hours. Deep posterior compartment syndrome may b͏
missed because of uninvolved overlying superficial compartment,
and results in claw toes.

■ **Neurovascular injury:** Vascular compromise is uncommon except
with high-velocity, markedly displaced, often open fractures.
It most commonly occurs as the anterior tibial artery traverses the
interosseous membrane of the proximal leg. It may require saphenous vein interposition graft. The common peroneal nerve is vulnerable to direct injuries to the proximal fibula as well as fractures
with significant varus angulation. Overzealous traction can result
in distraction injuries to the nerve, and inadequate cast mold-
ing/padding may result in neurapraxia.

■ Fat embolism.

■ **Claw toe deformity:** This is associated with scarring of extensor
tendons or ischemia of posterior compartment muscles.

Injuries about the Ankle

ROTATIONAL ANKLE FRACTURES

Epidemiology

- Population-based studies suggest that the incidence of ankle fractures has increased dramatically since the early 1960s.
- The highest incidence of ankle fractures occurs in elderly women, although fractures of the ankle are generally not considered to be "fragility" fractures.
- Most ankle fractures are isolated malleolar fractures, accounting for two-thirds of fractures, with bimalleolar fractures occurring in one-fourth of patients and trimalleolar fractures occurring in the remaining 5% to 10%.
- The incidence of ankle fractures is approximately 187 fractures per 100,000 people each year.
- Open fractures are rare, accounting for just 2% of all ankle fractures.
- Increased body mass index is considered a risk factor for sustaining an ankle fracture.

Anatomy

- The ankle is a complex hinge joint composed of articulations among the fibula, tibia, and talus in close association with a complex ligamentous system (Fig. 38.1).
- The distal tibial articular surface is referred to as the "plafond," which, together with the medial and lateral malleoli, forms the mortise, a constrained articulation with the talar dome.
- The plafond is concave in the anteroposterior (AP) plane but convex in the lateral plane. It is wider anteriorly to allow for congruency with the wedge-shaped talus. This provides for intrinsic stability, especially in weight bearing.
- The talar dome is trapezoidal, with the anterior aspect 2.5 mm wider than the posterior talus. The body of the talus is almost entirely covered by articular cartilage.
- The medial malleolus articulates with the medial facet of the talus and divides into an anterior colliculus and a posterior colliculus, which serve as attachments for the superficial and deep deltoid ligaments, respectively.

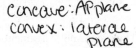

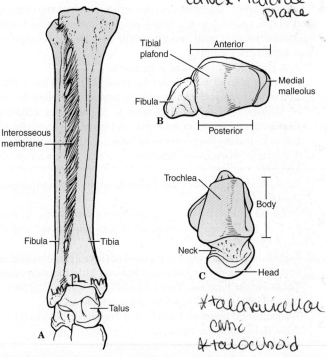

FIGURE 38.1 Bony anatomy of the ankle. Mortise view **(A)**, inferior superior view of the tibiofibular side of the joint **(B)**, and superior inferior view of the talus **(C)**. The ankle joint is a three-bone joint with a larger talar articular surface than matching tibiofibular articular surface. The lateral circumference of the talar dome is larger than the medial circumference. The dome is wider anteriorly than posteriorly. The syndesmotic ligaments allow widening of the joint with dorsiflexion of the ankle into a stable, close-packed position. (From Bucholz RW, Heckman JD, Court-Brown C, et al., eds. *Rockwood and Green's Fractures in Adults*. 6th ed. Philadelphia: Lippincott Williams & Wilkins; 2006.)

- The lateral malleolus represents the distal aspect of the fibula and provides lateral support to the ankle. No articular surface exists between the distal tibia and fibula, although there is some motion between the two. Some intrinsic stability is provided between the distal tibia and fibula just proximal to the ankle where the fibula sits between a broad anterior tubercle and a smaller posterior tubercle of the tibia. The distal fibula has articular cartilage on its medial aspect extending from the level of the plafond distally to a point halfway down its remaining length.

- The syndesmotic ligament complex exists between the distal tibia and fibula, resisting axial, rotational, and translational forces to maintain the structural integrity of the mortise. It is composed of four ligaments, including
  □ Anterior inferior tibiofibular ligament.
  □ Posterior inferior tibiofibular ligament (PITFL). This is thicker and stronger than the anterior counterpart. Therefore, torsional or translational forces that rupture the anterior tibiofibular ligament may cause an avulsion fracture of the posterior tibial tubercle, leaving the posterior tibiofibular ligament intact.
  □ Transverse tibiofibular ligament (inferior to posterior tibiofibular).
  □ Interosseous ligament (distal continuation of the interosseous membrane) (Fig. 38.2).
- The deltoid ligament provides ligamentous support to the medial aspect of the ankle. It is separated into superficial and deep components (Fig. 38.3).
  □ **Superficial portion:** This is composed of three ligaments that originate on the anterior colliculus but add little to ankle stability. **Tibionavicular ligament:** This suspends the spring ligament and prevents inward displacement of the talar head.
  Tibiocalcaneal ligament: This prevents valgus displacement.
  Superficial tibiotalar ligament.
  Talotibial Ligament: Most prominent of the 3.
  □ **Deep portion:** This intra-articular ligament (deep tibiotalar) originates on the intercollicular grove and the posterior colliculus of the distal tibia and inserts on the entire nonarticular medial surface of the talus. Its fibers are transversely oriented; it is the primary medial stabilizer against lateral displacement of the talus.
- The fibular collateral ligament is made up of three ligaments that, together with the distal fibula, provide lateral support to the ankle. The lateral ligamentous complex is not as strong as the medial complex (Fig. 38.4).
  □ **Anterior talofibular ligament:** This is the weakest of the lateral ligaments; it prevents anterior subluxation of the talus primarily in plantar flexion.
  □ **Posterior talofibular ligament:** This is the strongest of the lateral ligaments; it prevents posterior and rotatory subluxation of the talus.
  □ **Calcaneofibular ligament:** This is lax in neutral dorsiflexion owing to relative valgus orientation of calcaneus; it stabilizes the subtalar joint and limits inversion; rupture of this ligament will cause a positive talar tilt test.

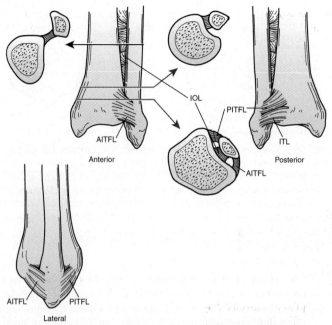

FIGURE 38.2 Three views of the tibiofibular syndesmotic ligaments. Anteriorly, the anterior inferior tibiofibular ligament (*AITFL*) spans from the anterior tubercle and anterolateral surface of the tibia to the anterior fibula. Posteriorly, the tibiofibular ligament has two components: the superficial posterior inferior tibiofibular ligament (*PITFL*), which is attached from the fibula across to the posterior tibia, and the thick, strong inferior transverse ligament (*ITL*), which constitutes the posterior labrum of the ankle. Between the anterior and posterior inferior talofibular ligaments resides the stout interosseous ligament (*IOL*). (Adapted from Browner B, Jupiter J, Levine A, eds. *Skeletal Trauma: Fractures, Dislocations, and Ligamentous Injuries.* 2nd ed. Philadelphia: WB Saunders; 1997.)

- Biomechanics
  - The normal range of motion (ROM) of the ankle in dorsiflexion is 30 degrees, and in plantar flexion it is 45 degrees; motion analysis studies reveal that a minimum of 10 degrees of dorsiflexion and 20 degrees of plantar flexion are required for normal gait.
  - The axis of flexion of the ankle runs between the distal aspect of the two malleoli, which is externally rotated 20 degrees compared with the knee axis.
  - A lateral talar shift of 1 mm will decrease surface contact by 40%; a 3-mm shift results in >60% decrease.

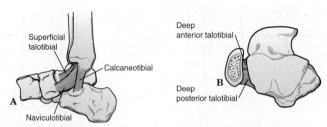

FIGURE 38.3 Medial collateral ligaments of the ankle. Sagittal plane **(A)** and transverse plane **(B)** views. The deltoid ligament includes a superficial component and a deep component. Superficial fibers mostly arise from the anterior colliculus and attach broadly from the navicular across the talus and into the medial border of the sustentaculum tali and the posterior medial talar tubercle. The deep layer of the deltoid ligament originates from the anterior and posterior colliculi and inserts on the medial surface of the talus. (Adapted from Browner B, Jupiter J, Levine A, eds. *Skeletal Trauma: Fractures, Dislocations, and Ligamentous Injuries*. 2nd ed. Philadelphia: WB Saunders; 1997.)

☐ Disruption of the syndesmotic ligaments may result in decreased tibiofibular overlap. Syndesmotic disruption associated with fibula fracture may be associated with a 2- to 3-mm lateral talar shift even with an intact deep deltoid ligament. Further lateral talar shift implies medial compromise.

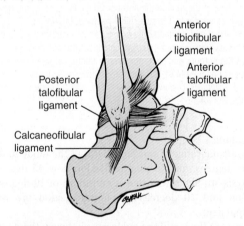

FIGURE 38.4 Lateral collateral ligaments of the ankle and the anterior syndesmotic ligament. (From Bucholz RW, Heckman JD, Court-Brown C, et al., eds. *Rockwood and Green's Fractures in Adults*. 6th ed. Philadelphia: Lippincott Williams & Wilkins; 2006.)

Mechanism of Injury

The pattern of ankle injury depends on many factors, including mechanism (axial versus rotational loading), chronicity (recurrent ankle instability may result in chronic ligamentous laxity and distorted ankle biomechanics), patient age, bone quality, position of the foot at time of injury, and the magnitude, direction, and rate of loading. Specific mechanisms and injuries are discussed in the section on classification.

Clinical Evaluation

- Patients may have a variable presentation, ranging from a limp to nonambulatory in significant pain and discomfort, with swelling, tenderness, and variable deformity.
- Neurovascular status should be carefully documented and compared with the contralateral side.
- The extent of soft tissue injury should be evaluated, with particular attention to possible open injuries and blistering. The quality of surrounding tissues should also be noted.
- The entire length of the fibula should be palpated for tenderness because associated fibular fractures may be found proximally as high as the proximal tibiofibular articulation. A "squeeze test" may be performed approximately 5 cm proximal to the intermalleolar axis to assess possible syndesmotic injury.
- A dislocated ankle should be reduced and splinted immediately (before radiographs if clinically evident) to prevent pressure or impaction injuries to the talar dome and to preserve neurovascular integrity.

Radiographic Evaluation

- AP, lateral, and mortise views of the ankle should be obtained.
- AP view
  □ Tibiofibula overlap of <10 mm is abnormal and implies syndesmotic injury.
  □ Tibiofibula clear space of >5 mm is abnormal and implies syndesmotic injury.
  □ **Talar tilt:** A difference in width of the medial and lateral aspects of the superior joint space of >2 mm is abnormal and indicates medial or lateral disruption.
- Lateral view
  □ The dome of the talus should be centered under the tibia and congruous with the tibial plafond.
  □ Posterior tibial tuberosity fractures can be identified, as well as direction of fibular injury.

□ Avulsion fractures of the talus by the anterior capsule may be identified.
■ Mortise view (Fig. 38.5)
   □ This is taken with the foot in 15 to 20 degrees of internal rotation to offset the intermalleolar axis.

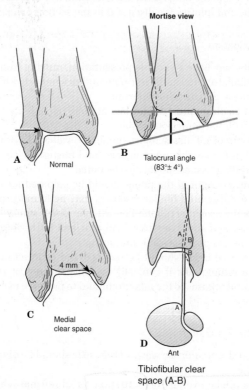

FIGURE 38.5 X-ray appearance of the normal ankle on mortise view. **(A)** The condensed subchondral bone should form a continuous line around the talus. **(B)** The talocrural angle should be approximately 83 degrees. When the opposite side can be used as a control, the talocrural angle of the injured side should be within a few degrees of the noninjured side. **(C)** The medial clear space should be equal to the superior clear space between the talus and the distal tibia and less than or equal to 4 mm on standard x-rays. **(D)** The distance between the medial wall of the fibula and the incisural surface of the tibia, the tibiofibular clear space, should be less than 6 mm. (**A–C,** Adapted from Browner B, Jupiter J, Levine A, eds. *Skeletal Trauma: Fractures, Dislocations, and Ligamentous Injuries.* 2nd ed. Philadelphia: WB Saunders; 1997; **D,** from Bucholz RW, Heckman JD, Court-Brown C, et al., eds. *Rockwood and Green's Fractures in Adults.* 6th ed. Philadelphia: Lippincott Williams & Wilkins; 2006.)

□ A medial clear space >4 to 5 mm is abnormal and indicates lateral talar shift.

□ **Talocrural angle:** The angle subtended between the intermalleolar line and a line parallel to the distal tibial articular surface should be between 8 and 15 degrees. The angle should be within 2 to 3 degrees of the uninjured ankle.

□ Tibiofibular overlap <1 cm indicates syndesmotic disruption.

□ Talar shift >1 mm is abnormal.

■ A physician-assisted stress view with the ankle dorsiflexed and the foot stressed in external rotation can be used to identify medial injury with an isolated fibula fracture. A gravity stress view is an alternative with similar sensitivity.

■ Computed tomography (CT) scans help to delineate bony anatomy, especially in patients with plafond injuries.

■ Magnetic resonance imaging (MRI) may be used for assessing occult cartilaginous, ligamentous, or tendinous injuries.

Classification

Lauge-Hansen (Rotational Ankle Fractures)

■ Four patterns are recognized, based on "pure" injury sequences, each subdivided into stages of increasing severity (figs 38.6 and 38.7).

■ This system is based on cadaveric studies.

■ Patterns may not always reflect clinical reality.

■ The system takes into account (1) the position of the foot at the time of injury and (2) the direction of the deforming force.

Supination–Adduction (SA)

■ This accounts for 10% to 20% of malleolar fractures.

■ This is the only type associated with medial displacement of the talus.

Stage I: Produces either a transverse avulsion-type fracture of the fibula distal to the level of the joint or a rupture of the lateral collateral ligaments

Stage II: Results in a vertical medial malleolus fracture

Supination–External Rotation (SER)

■ This accounts for 40% to 75% of malleolar fractures.

Stage I: Produces disruption of the anterior tibiofibular ligament with or without an associated avulsion fracture at its tibial or fibular attachment

Stage II: Results in the typical spiral fracture of the distal fibula, which runs from anteroinferior to posterosuperior

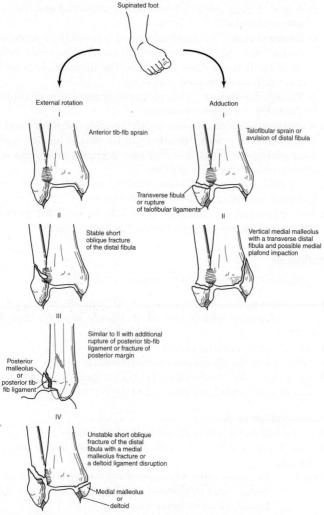

FIGURE 38.6 Schematic diagram and case examples of Lauge-Hansen supination–external rotation and supination–adduction ankle fractures. A supinated foot sustains either an external rotation or adduction force and creates the successive stages of injury shown in the diagram. The supination–external rotation mechanism has four stages of injury, and the supination–adduction mechanism has two stages. (From Bucholz RW, Heckman JD, Court-Brown C, et al., eds. *Rockwood and Green's Fractures in Adults.* 6th ed. Philadelphia: Lippincott Williams & Wilkins; 2006.)

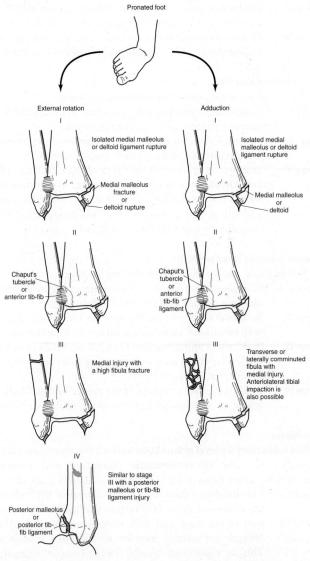

FIGURE 38.7 Schematic diagram and case examples of Lauge-Hansen pronation–external rotation and pronation–abduction ankle fractures. A pronated foot sustains either an external rotation or abduction force and creates the successive stages of injury shown in the diagram. The pronation–external rotation mechanism has four stages of injury, and the pronation–abduction mechanism has three stages. (From Bucholz RW, Heckman JD, Court-Brown C, et al., eds. *Rockwood and Green's Fractures in Adults.* 6th ed. Philadelphia: Lippincott Williams & Wilkins; 2006.)

Stage III: Produces either a disruption of the posterior tibiofibular ligament or a fracture of the posterior malleolus

Stage IV: Produces either a transverse avulsion-type fracture of the medial malleolus or a rupture of the deltoid ligament

Pronation–Abduction (PA)

■ This accounts for 5% to 20% of malleolar fractures.

Stage I: Results in either a transverse fracture of the medial malleolus or a rupture of the deltoid ligament

Stage II: Produces either a rupture of the syndesmotic ligaments or an avulsion fracture at their insertion sites

Stage III: Produces a transverse or short oblique fracture of the distal fibula at or above the level of the syndesmosis; this results from a bending force that causes medial tension and lateral compression of the fibula, producing lateral comminution or a butterfly fragment

Pronation–External Rotation (PER)

■ This accounts for 5% to 20% of malleolus fractures.

Stage I: Produces either a transverse fracture of the medial malleolus or a rupture of the deltoid ligament

Stage II: Results in disruption of the anterior tibiofibular ligament with or without avulsion fracture at its insertion sites

Stage III: Results in a spiral fracture of the distal fibula at or above the level of the syndesmosis running from anterosuperior to posteroinferior

Stage IV: Produces either a rupture of the posterior tibiofibular ligament or an avulsion fracture of the posterolateral tibia

Danis–Weber

■ **This is based on the level of the fibular fracture:** the more proximal, the greater the risk of syndesmotic disruption and associated instability. Three types of fractures are described (Fig. 38.8):

Type A: This involves a fracture of the fibula below the level of the tibial plafond, an avulsion injury that results from supination of the foot and that may be associated with an oblique or vertical fracture of the medial malleolus. This is equivalent to the Lauge-Hansen supination–adduction injury.

Type B: This oblique or spiral fracture of the fibula is caused by external rotation occurring at or near the level of the syndesmosis; 50% have an associated disruption of the anterior syndesmotic ligament, whereas the posterior syndesmotic ligament remains intact and attached to the

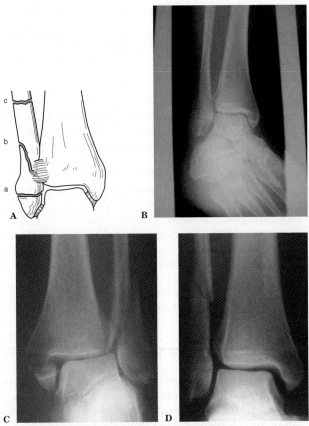

FIGURE 38.8 (A) Schematic diagram of the Danis–Weber classification of ankle fractures. **(B)** Weber A fracture, **(C)** Weber B fracture, **(D)** Weber C fracture. (From Bucholz RW, Heckman JD, Court-Brown C, et al., eds. *Rockwood and Green's Fractures in Adults.* 6th ed. Philadelphia: Lippincott Williams & Wilkins; 2006.)

distal fibular fragment. There may be an associated injury to the medial structures or the posterior malleolus. This is equivalent to the Lauge-Hansen supination–eversion injury.

Type C: This involves a fracture of the fibula above the level of the syndesmosis causing disruption of the syndesmosis almost always with associated medial injury. This category includes Maisonneuve-type injuries and corresponds to Lauge-Hansen pronation–eversion or pronation–abduction Stage III injuries.

OTA Classification of Ankle Fractures

See Fracture and Dislocation Classification Compendium at http://www.ota.org/compendium/compendium.html.

Fracture Variants

- Maisonneuve fracture
  - □ Originally described as an ankle injury with a fracture of the proximal third of the fibula, this is a pronation-external rotation type injury; it is important to distinguish it from direct trauma to the fibula.
- Curbstone fracture
  - □ This avulsion fracture off the posterior tibia is produced by a tripping mechanism.
- LeForte–Wagstaffe fracture
  - □ This anterior fibular tubercle avulsion fracture by the anterior tibiofibular ligament is usually associated with Lauge-Hansen SER-type fracture patterns.
- Tillaux–Chaput fracture
  - □ This avulsion of anterior tibial margin by the anterior tibiofibular ligament is the tibial counterpart of the LeForte–Wagstaffe fracture.
- Collicular fractures
  - □ **Anterior colliculus fracture:** The deep portion of the deltoid may remain intact.
  - □ **Posterior colliculus fracture:** The fragment is usually nondisplaced because of stabilization by the posterior tibial and the flexor digitorum longus tendons; classically, one sees a "supramalleolar spike" very clearly on an external rotation view.
- Pronation–dorsiflexion fracture
  - □ This displaced fracture off the anterior articular surface is considered a pilon variant when there is a significant articular fragment.

Treatment

The goal of treatment is anatomic restoration of the ankle joint. Fibular length and rotation must be restored.

Emergency Room

- Closed reduction should be performed for displaced fractures. Fracture reduction helps to minimize postinjury swelling, reduces

pressure on the articular cartilage, lessens the risk of skin break-down, and minimizes pressure on the neurovascular structures.
- Dislocated ankles should be reduced before radiographic evaluation if possible.
- Open wounds and abrasions should be cleansed and dressed in a sterile fashion as dictated by the degree of injury. Fracture blisters should be left intact and dressed with a well-padded sterile dressing.
- Following fracture reduction, a well-padded posterior splint with a U-shaped component should be placed to provide fracture stability and patient comfort.
- Postreduction radiographs should be obtained for fracture reassessment. The limb should be aggressively elevated with or without the use of ice.

Nonoperative

- Indications for nonoperative treatment include
  - □ Nondisplaced, stable fracture patterns with an intact syndesmosis.
  - □ Displaced fractures for which stable anatomic reduction of the ankle mortise is achieved.
  - □ An unstable or multiple trauma patient in whom operative treatment is contraindicated because of the condition of the patient or the limb.
- Patients with stable fracture patterns can be placed in a short leg cast or a removable boot or stirrup and allowed to bear weight as tolerated.
- For displaced fractures, if anatomic reduction is achieved with closed manipulation, a bulky dressing and a posterior splint with a U-shaped component may be used for the first few days while swelling subsides. The patient may then be placed in a long leg cast to maintain rotational control for 4 to 6 weeks with serial radiographic evaluation to ensure maintenance of reduction and healing. If adequate healing is demonstrated, the patient can be placed in a short leg cast or fracture brace. Weight bearing is restricted until fracture healing is demonstrated. The majority of unstable patterns are best treated operatively.

Operative

- Open reduction and internal fixation (ORIF) is indicated for
  - □ Failure to achieve or maintain closed reduction with amenable soft tissues

- ☐ Unstable fractures that may result in talar displacement or widening of the ankle mortise
- ☐ Fractures that require abnormal foot positioning to maintain reduction (e.g., extreme plantar flexion)
- ☐ Open fractures

- ■ ORIF should be performed once the patient's general medical condition, swelling about the ankle, and soft tissue status allow. Swelling, blisters, and soft tissue issues usually stabilize within 5 to 10 days after injury with elevation, ice, and compressive dressings. Occasionally, a closed fracture with severe soft tissue injury or massive swelling may require reduction and stabilization with use of external fixation to allow soft tissue management before definitive fixation.

- ■ Lateral malleolar fractures distal to the syndesmosis may be stabilized using a lag screw or Kirschner wires with tension banding. With fractures at or above the syndesmosis, restoration of fibular length and rotation is essential to obtain an accurate reduction. This is most often accomplished using a combination of lag screws and plate.

- ■ Management of medial malleolar fractures is controversial. In general, with a deltoid rupture the talus follows the fibula. Indications for operative fixation of the medial malleolus include concomitant syndesmotic injury, persistent widening of the medial clear space following fibula reduction, inability to obtain adequate fibular reduction, or persistent medial fracture displacement after fibular fixation. Medial malleolar fractures can usually be stabilized with cancellous screws or a figure-of-eight tension band.

- ■ Indications for fixation of posterior malleolus fractures include involvement of >25% of the articular surface, >2-mm displacement, or persistent posterior subluxation of the talus. Posterior malleolar fixation may be an alternative to syndesmotic fixation as the PITFL remains attached to the fragment. Fixation may be achieved by indirect reduction and placement of an anterior to posterior lag screw, or a posteriorly placed plate and/or screws through a separate incision.

- ■ Fibula fractures above the plafond may require syndesmotic stabilization. After fixation of the medial and lateral malleoli is achieved, the syndesmosis should be stressed intraoperatively by lateral pull on the fibula with a bone hook or by stressing the ankle in external rotation. Syndesmotic instability can then be recognized clinically and under image intensification. Distal tibia–fibula joint reduction is held with a large pointed reduction clamp. A syndesmotic screw is placed 1.5 to 2.0 cm above the plafond from the fibula to the tibia. Controversy exists as to the number of purchased cortices (three or four) and the size of the screw (3.5 or 4.5 mm). The need for ankle dorsiflexion during syndesmotic screw placement is also controversial. An anatomically reduced syndesmosis cannot be overtightened. Fixation o a posterior malleolar fracture fragment may obviate the need for syndesmotic fixation.

■ Very proximal fibula fractures with syndesmosis disruption can usually be treated with syndesmosis fixation without direct fibula reduction and stabilization. One must, however, ascertain correct fibula length and rotation before placing syndesmotic fixation.

■ Following fracture fixation, the limb is placed in a bulky dressing incorporating a plaster splint. Progression to weight bearing is based on the fracture pattern, stability of fixation, patient compliance, and philosophy of the surgeon.

Open Fractures

■ These fractures require emergent irrigation and debridement in the operating room.

■ External fixation may be used to temporize patients until soft tissue conditions allow for definitive fixation.

■ Stable fixation is important prophylaxis against infection and helps soft tissue healing. It is permissible to leave plates and screws exposed, but efforts should be made to cover hardware, if possible.

■ Tourniquet use is usually unnecessary in the cases and lead to post surgical swelling and reperfusion injury.

■ Antibiotic prophylaxis should be continued postoperatively.

■ Serial debridements may be required for removal of necrotic, infected, or compromised tissues.

Complications

■ **Nonunion:** Nonunions about the ankle are rare. When one develops it and usually involves the medial malleolus. These are associated with closed treatment, residual fracture displacement, interposed soft tissue, or associated lateral instability resulting in shear stresses across the deltoid ligament. If symptomatic, it may be treated with ORIF or electrical stimulation. Excision of the fragment may be necessary if it is not amenable to internal fixation and the patient is symptomatic.

■ **Malunion:** The lateral malleolus is usually shortened and malrotated; a widened medial clear space and a large posterior malleolar fragment are most predictive of poor outcome. The medial malleolus may heal in an elongated position resulting in residual instability.

■ **Wound problems:** Skin edge necrosis (3%) may occur; there is decreased risk with minimal swelling, no tourniquet, and good soft tissue technique. Fractures that are operated on in the presence of fracture blisters or abrasions have more than twice the complication rate.

- **Infection:** Occurs in <2% of closed fractures; leave implants in situ if stable, even with deep infection. One can remove the implant after the fracture unites. The patient may require serial debridements with possible arthrodesis as a salvage procedure.
- **Posttraumatic arthritis:** Secondary to damage at the time of injury, from altered mechanics, or as a result of inadequate reduction. It is rare in anatomically reduced fractures, with increasing incidence with articular incongruity.
- **Reflex sympathetic dystrophy:** Rare and may be minimized by anatomic restoration of the ankle and early return to function.
- **Compartment syndrome of the leg or foot:** Rare.
- **Tibiofibular synostosis:** This is associated with the use of a syndesmotic screw and is usually asymptomatic.
- **Loss of reduction:** Reported in 25% of unstable ankle injuries treated nonoperatively (Fig. 38.9).
- Loss of ankle ROM may occur.

Plafond (Pilon) Fractures

Epidemiology

- Pilon fractures account for 7% to 10% of all tibia fractures.
- Most pilon fractures are a result of high-energy mechanisms; thus, concomitant injuries are common and should be ruled out.
- Most common in men of 30 to 40 years old.

Mechanism of Injury

- **Axial compression (High energy):** Fall from a height, MVC
  - □ The force is axially directed through the talus into the tibial plafond, causing impaction of the articular surface; it may be associated with significant comminution. If the fibula remains intact, the ankle is forced into varus with impaction of the medial plafond. Plantar flexion or dorsiflexion of the ankle at the time of injury results in primarily posterior or anterior plafond injury, respectively.
- **Rotational (Low energy):** Sporting accident
  - □ Mechanism is primarily torsion combined with a varus or valgus stress. It produces two or more large fragments and minimal articular comminution. There is usually an associated fibula fracture, which is usually transverse or short oblique.
- Combined compression and shear

- ☐ These fracture patterns demonstrate components of both compression and shear. The vector of these two forces determines the fracture pattern.
- ■ Because of their high-energy nature, these fractures can be expected to have specific associated injuries: Calcaneus, tibial plateau, pelvis, and vertebral fractures.

Clinical Evaluation

- ■ Most pilon fractures are associated with high-energy trauma; full trauma evaluation and secondary survey is usually necessary.
- ■ Patients typically present nonambulatory with variable gross deformity of the involved distal leg.
- ■ Evaluation includes assessment of neurovascular status and evaluation of any associated injuries.
- ■ The tibia is nearly subcutaneous in this region; therefore, fracture displacement or excess skin pressure may convert a closed injury into an open one.
- ■ Swelling is often massive and rapid, necessitating serial neurovascular examinations as well as assessment of skin integrity, necrosis, and fracture blisters.
- ■ Meticulous assessment of soft tissue damage is of paramount importance. Significant damage occurs to the thin soft tissue envelope surrounding the distal tibia as the forces of impact are dissipated. This may result in inadequate healing of surgical incisions with wound necrosis and skin slough if not treated appropriately. Some advise waiting 7 to 10 days for soft tissue healing to occur before planning surgery.

Radiographic Evaluation

- ■ AP, lateral, and mortise radiographs should be obtained.
- ■ CT with coronal and sagittal reconstruction is helpful to evaluate the fracture pattern and articular surface.
- ■ Careful preoperative planning is essential with a strategically planned sequence of reconstruction; radiographs of the contralateral side may be useful as a template for preoperative planning.

Classification

Rüedi And Allgöwer

- ■ Based on the severity of comminution and the displacement of the articular surface (Fig. 38.10).
- ■ It has been the most commonly used classification. Its relevance today is minimal.
- ■ Prognosis correlates with increasing grade.

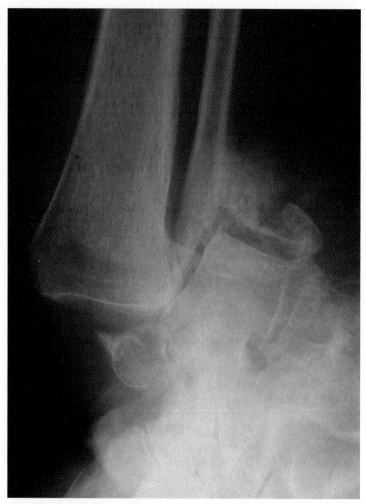

FIGURE 38.9 Example of a chronically dislocated ankle secondary to failure to properly immobilize a bimalleolar ankle fracture.

Type 1:   Nondisplaced cleavage fracture of the ankle joint
Type 2:   Displaced fracture with minimal impaction or comminution
Type 3:   Displaced fracture with significant articular comminution and metaphyseal impaction

OTA Classification of Distal Tibia Fractures

See Fracture and Dislocation Classification Compendium at http://www.ota.org/compendium/compendium.html.

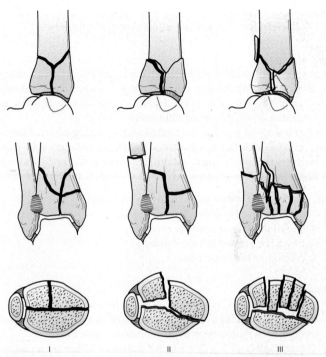

FIGURE 38.10 The Rüedi and Allgöwer classification. (Adapted from Müller M, Allgöwer M, Schneider R, et al. *Manual of Internal Fixation.* 2nd ed. New York: Springer-Verlag; 1979.)

Treatment

This is based on many factors, including patient age and functional status, severity of injury to bone, cartilage, and soft tissue envelope, degree of comminution and osteoporosis, and the capabilities of the surgeon.

Nonoperative

Treatment involves a long leg cast for 6 weeks followed by fracture brace and ROM exercises or early ROM exercises.

- This is used primarily for nondisplaced fracture patterns or severely debilitated patients.
- Manipulation of displaced fractures is unlikely to result in reduction of intra-articular fragments.
- Loss of reduction is common.
- Inability to monitor soft tissue status and swelling is a major disadvantage.

Operative
- Displaced pilon fractures are usually treated surgically.

Timing of Surgery
- Surgery may be delayed for several days (7 to 14 days on average) to allow for optimization of soft tissue status, including a diminution of swelling about the ankle, resolution of fracture blisters, and sloughing of compromised soft tissues.
- High-energy injuries can be treated with spanning external fixation to provide skeletal stabilization, restoration of length and partial fracture reduction while awaiting definitive surgery. Associated fibula fractures may undergo ORIF at the time of fixator application.

GOALS. The goals of operative fixation of pilon fractures include
- Maintenance of fibula length and stability.
- Restoration of tibial articular surface.
- Bone grafting of metaphyseal defects.
- Stabilizing of the distal tibia.

Surgical Tactic
- Articular fracture reduction can be achieved percutaneously or through small limited approaches assisted by a variety of reduction forceps, with fluoroscopy to judge fracture reduction.
- The metaphyseal fracture can be stabilized either with plates or with a nonspanning or spanning external fixator.
- Grafting of metaphyseal defects with some type of osteoconductive material is indicated.
- **Internal fixation:** Open fracture reduction and plate fixation may be the best way to achieve a precisely reduced articular surface. To minimize the complications of plating, the following techniques have been recommended:
  - ☐ Surgical delay until definitive surgical treatment using initial spanning external fixation for high-energy injuries
  - ☐ Use of small, precontoured, low-profile implants and mini-fragment screws
  - ☐ Avoidance of incisions over the anteromedial tibia
  - ☐ Use of indirect reduction techniques to minimize soft tissue stripping
  - ☐ Use of percutaneous techniques for plate insertion
- **Joint spanning external fixation:** This may be used in patients with significant soft tissue compromise or open fractures. Reduction is maintained via distraction and ligamentotaxis. If adequate reduction is obtained, external fixation may be used as definitive treatment.

□ **Articulating versus nonarticulating spanning external fixation:** Non-articulating (rigid) external fixation are most commonly used, theoretically allowing no ankle motion. Articulating external fixation allows motion in the sagittal plane, thus preventing ankle varus and shortening; application is limited, but theoretically it results in improved chondral lubrication and nutrition owing to ankle motion, and it may be used when soft tissue integrity is the primary indication for external fixation.

■ **Hybrid external fixation:** This is a type of nonspanning external fixator. Fracture reduction is enhanced using thin wires with or without olives to restore the articular surface and maintain bony stability. It is especially useful when internal fixation of any kind is contraindicated. There is a reported 3% incidence of deep wound infection.

ARTHRODESIS. Few advocate performing this procedure acutely. It is best done after fracture comminution has consolidated and soft tissues have recovered. It is generally performed as a salvage procedure after other treatments have failed and posttraumatic arthritis has ensued.

Postoperative Management

■ Initial splint placement in neutral dorsiflexion with careful monitoring of soft tissues.

■ Early ankle and foot motion when wounds and fixation allow.

■ Non–weight bearing for 12 to 16 weeks, then progression to full weight bearing once there is radiographic evidence of healing.

Complications

■ Even when accurate reduction is obtained, predictably excellent outcomes are not always achieved, and less than anatomic reduction can lead to satisfactory outcomes.

■ **Soft tissue slough, necrosis, and hematoma:** These result from initial trauma combined with improper handling of soft tissues. One must avoid excessive stripping and skin closure under tension. Secondary closure, skin grafts, or muscle flaps may be required for adequate closure. These complications have been minimized since recognition of the initial soft tissue insult and the strategies to minimize the effects (spanning external fixation, minimally invasive surgery, etc.)

■ **Nonunion:** Results from significant comminution and bone loss, as well as hypovascularity and infection. It has a reported incidence of 5% regardless of treatment method.

■ **Malunion:** Common with nonanatomic reduction, inadequate buttressing (early fixator removal) followed by collapse, or premature weight bearing. The reported incidence is up to 25% with use of external fixation.

■ **Infection:** Associated with open injuries and soft tissue devitalization. It has a high incidence with early surgery under unfavorable soft tissue conditions. Late infectious complications may manifest as osteomyelitis, malunion, or nonunion.

■ **Posttraumatic arthritis:** More frequent with increasing severity of intra-articular comminution; it emphasizes the need for anatomic restoration of the articular surface.

■ **Tibial shortening:** Caused by fracture comminution, metaphyseal impaction, or initial failure to restore length by fibula fixation.

■ **Decreased ankle ROM:** Patients usually average <10 degrees of dorsiflexion and <30 degrees of plantar flexion.

Lateral Ankle Ligament Injuries

■ Sprains of the lateral ligaments of the ankle are the most common musculoskeletal injury in sports.

■ In the United States, it is estimated that one ankle inversion injury occurs each day per 10,000 people.

■ One year after injury, occasional intermittent pain is present in up to 40% of patients.

Mechanism of Injury

■ Most ankle sprains are caused by a twisting or turning event to the ankle. This can result from either internal or external rotation.

■ Mechanism of injury and the exact ligaments injured depend on the position of the foot and the direction of the stress.
   □ With ankle plantar flexion, inversion injuries first strain the anterior talofibular ligament and then the calcaneofibular ligament.
   □ With the ankle dorsiflexion and inversion, the injury is usually isolated to the calcaneofibular ligament. With ankle dorsiflexion and external rotation, the injury more likely will involve the syndesmotic ligaments. The syndesmotic ligaments, and in particular the posterior and inferior tibiofibular ligament, can also be injured with the ankle dorsiflexed and the foot internally rotated.

Classification

■ **Mild ankle sprain:** Patients have minimal functional loss, no limp, minimal or no swelling, point tenderness, and pain with reproduction of mechanism of injury.

- **Moderate sprain:** Patients have moderate functional loss, inability to hop or toe rise on the injured ankle, a limp with walking, and localized swelling with point tenderness.
- **Severe sprain:** This is indicated by diffuse tenderness, swelling, and a preference for non–weight bearing.
- This system does not delineate the specific ligaments involved.

Clinical Evaluation

- Patients often describe a popping or tearing sensation in the ankle, and they remember the immediate onset of pain.
- Some patients have an acute onset of swelling around the lateral ankle ligaments and difficulty with weight bearing secondary to pain.
- Significant physical examination findings may include swelling, ecchymosis, tenderness, instability, crepitus, sensory changes, vascular status, muscle dysfunction, and deformity.
- The location of the pain helps to delineate the involved ligaments, and it can include the lateral aspect of the ankle, the anterior aspect of the fibula, the medial aspect of the ankle, and the syndesmotic region.
- The value of stress testing of the lateral collateral ankle ligaments in the acute setting is controversial.
  - ☐ At the time of injury, before swelling and inflammation occur, the physician may be able to obtain valuable information by performing an anterior drawer and varus stress examination of the lateral collateral ankle ligaments.
  - ☐ In patients who present several hours after injury and who have powerful reflex inhibition, a stress test without anesthesia is unlikely to give valuable clinical information.
- Injury to the lateral collateral ankle ligaments should be differentiated from other periarticular ligamentous injuries on examination. Significant initial ecchymosis along the heel indicates possible subtalar ligamentous sprain. To evaluate potential syndesmotic injury, the squeeze test and external rotation stress tests are performed (see later).

Radiographic Evaluation

- Most patients should probably undergo radiographic examination to rule out occult foot and ankle injuries with an x-ray series of the foot and ankle.
  - ☐ The injuries that need to be ruled out include fracture of the base of the fifth metatarsal, navicular fracture, fracture of the anterior process of the calcaneus, fracture of the lateral

process of the talus, os trigonal fracture, talar dome fracture (osteochondritis dissecans), and posterior malleolar fracture.

- In the acute setting, there probably is little role for performing radiographic stress testing.

Treatment

- Nonsurgical approaches are preferred for initial treatment for acute ankle sprains.
- Initial treatment involves the use of rest, ice, compression (elastic wrap), elevation (RICE) and protected weight bearing.
  □ For mild sprains, one can start early mobilization, ROM, and isometric exercises.
  □ For moderate or severe sprains, one can immobilize the ankle in neutral position, or slight dorsiflexion, for the first 10 to 14 days, and then initiate mobilization, ROM, and isometric exercises. Crutches are discontinued once the patient can tolerate full weight on the ankle.
- Once the initial inflammatory phase has resolved, for the less severe ankle sprains (mild to moderate), one can initiate a home rehabilitation program consisting of eversion muscle group strengthening, proprioceptive retraining, and protective bracing while the patient gradually returns to sports and functional activities. Bracing or taping is usually discontinued 3 to 4 weeks after resuming sports. For more severe sprains, taping or bracing programs are continued during sports activities for 6 months, and a supervised rehabilitation program used.
- Patients who continue to have pain in the ankle that does not decrease with time should be reevaluated for an occult osseous or chondral injury.
- Patients with a history of recurrent ankle sprains who sustain an acute ankle sprain are treated in a manner similar to that described earlier.

Syndesmosis Sprains

- Syndesmotic sprains account for approximately 1% of all ankle sprains.
- Syndesmotic sprains may occur without a fracture or frank diastasis.
- Many of these injuries probably go undiagnosed and cause chronic ankle pain.
- Injuries to the syndesmotic ligaments are more likely to result in greater impairment than straightforward lateral ankle sprains. In athletes, syndesmotic sprains result in substantially greater lost time from sports activities.

Classification

Diastases of the distal tibiofibular syndesmosis were classified into four types by Edwards and DeLee.

1. Type I diastasis involves lateral subluxation without fracture.
2. Type II involved lateral subluxation with plastic deformation of the fibula.
3. Type III involves posterior subluxation/dislocation of the fibula.
4. Type IV involves superior subluxation/dislocation of the talus within the mortise.

Clinical Evaluation

- Immediately after a syndesmotic ankle sprain, the patient will have well-localized tenderness in the area of the sprain, but soon thereafter, with ensuing swelling and ecchymosis, the precise location of the sprain often becomes obscured.
- Patients ordinarily present to physicians several hours, if not days, after these injuries, with difficulty in weight bearing, ecchymosis extending up the leg, and marked swelling. The clue to chronic, subclinical syndesmotic sprains is the history of vague ankle pain with push-off and normal imaging studies.
- The clinical examination involves palpating the involved ligaments and bones. The fibula should be palpated in a proximal to distal direction. The proximal tibiofibular joint should be assessed for tenderness or associated injury.
- Two clinical tests can be used to isolate syndesmotic ligament injury.
  - □ The squeeze test: involves squeezing the fibula at the midcalf. If this maneuver reproduces distal tibiofibular pain, it is likely that the patient has sustained some injury to the syndesmotic region.
  - □ The external rotation stress test: The patient is seated, with the knee flexed at 90 degrees. The examiner stabilizes the patient's leg and externally rotates the foot. If this reproduces pain at the syndesmosis, the test is positive, and the physician should assume, in the absence of bony injuries, that a syndesmotic injury has occured.

Radiographic Evaluation

- The radiographic evaluation of a syndesmotic injury, in an acute setting, involves an attempt at weight-bearing radiographs of the ankle (AP, mortise, lateral) and, if negative, an external rotation stress view.

- Without injury, a weight-bearing mortise view should show:
  - □ No widening of the medial clear space between the medial malleolus and the medial border of the talus
  - □ A tibiofibular clear space (the interval between the medial border of the fibula and the lateral border of the posterior tibial malleolus) of 6 mm or less
- With acute sprains, on lateral radiographs, a small avulsion fragment may be apparent. Similarly, with more chronic problems, calcification of the syndesmosis or posterior tibia may suggest syndesmotic injury.
- When routine x-rays are negative, and the patient is still suspected of having a syndesmotic injury, stress radiographs can be considered. The examiner should inspect stress radiographs for widening of the medial joint space and tibiofibular clear space on the mortise view and for posterior displacement of the fibula relative to the tibia on the lateral view.
- In difficult-to-diagnose acute cases or latent presentations, an MRI evaluation of the syndesmosis may delineate injury to the syndesmotic ligaments.

Treatment

- Tibiofibular syndesmotic ligamentous injuries are slower to recover than other ankle ligamentous injuries and may benefit from a more restrictive approach to initial management.
- Patients are immobilized in a non–weight-bearing cast for 2 to 3 weeks after injury. This is followed by use of a protective, modified, articulated ankle-foot orthosis that eliminates external rotation stress on the ankle for a variable period, depending on the functional needs and sports activities of the patient.
- Operative treatment is considered for patients with irreducible diastasis. To hold the syndesmotic ligaments while healing, two screws usually placed at the superior margin of the syndesmosis in a nonlagged fashion, from the fibula into the tibia. The patients are maintained non–weight bearing for 6 weeks, and the screws are removed approximately 12 to 16 weeks after fixation.

Achilles Tendon Rupture

Epidemiology

- Most Achilles tendon problems are related to overuse injuries and are multifactorial.
- The principal factors include host susceptibility and mechanical overload.
- The spectrum of injury ranges from paratenonitis to tendinosis to acute rupture.

■ In a trauma setting, a true rupture is the most common presentation.

■ Delayed or missed diagnosis of Achilles tendon rupture by primary treating physicians is relatively common (up to 25%).

Anatomy

■ The Achilles tendon is the largest tendon in the body.

■ It lacks a true synovial sheath and instead has a paratenon with visceral and parietal layers permitting approximately 1.5 cm of tendon glide.

■ It receives its blood supply from three sources:

   1. The musculotendinous junction

   2. The osseous insertion

   3. Multiple mesosternal vessels on the anterior surface of the tendon

Clinical Evaluation

■ With either partial or complete Achilles tendon rupture, patients typically experience sharp pain, often described as feeling like being kicked in the leg.

■ With a partial rupture, physical examination may only reveal a localized tender area of swelling.

■ With complete rupture, examination normally reveals a palpable defect in the tendon.

   □ In this setting, the Thompson test is generally positive (i.e., squeezing the calf does not cause active plantar flexion), and the patient usually is incapable of performing a single heel raise (Fig. 38.11).

   □ The Thompson test can be falsely positive when the accessory ankle flexors (posterior tibialis, flexor digitorum longus, flexor hallucis longus muscles, or accessory soleus muscles) are squeezed together with the contents of the superficial posterior leg compartment.

Treatment

■ Goals are to restore normal musculotendinous length and tension and thereby to optimize ultimate strength and function of the gastrocnemius–soleus complex.

■ Whether operative or nonoperative treatment best achieves these goals remains a matter of controversy.

   □ Proponents of surgical repair point to lower recurrent rupture rates, improved strength, and a higher percentage of patients who return to sports activities.

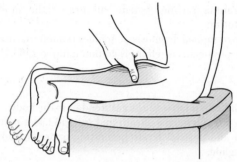

FIGURE 38.11 The Thompson test for continuity of the gastrocnemius–soleus complex. Without rupture of the Achilles tendon, squeezing the calf causes active plantar flexion of the foot. With rupture, squeezing the superficial posterior compartment of the leg does not induce plantar flexion of the foot. (Adapted from Browner B, Jupiter J, Levine A. *Skeletal Trauma: Fractures, Dislocations, and Ligamentous Injuries.* 2nd ed. Philadelphia: WB Saunders; 1997.)

- ☐ Proponents of nonoperative treatment stress the high surgical complication rates resulting from wound infection, skin necrosis, and nerve injuries.
- ☐ When major complications, including recurrent ruptures, are compared, both forms of treatment have similar complication rates.
- ☐ Most authors tend to treat active patients who are interested in continuing athletic endeavors with operative treatment and inactive patients or those with other complicating medical factors (e.g., immunosuppression, soft tissue injuries, history of recurrent lower extremity infections, vascular or neurologic impairment) with nonoperative approaches.
- ■ Nonoperative treatment begins with a period of immobilization.
  - ☐ Initially, the leg is placed in a splint for 2 weeks, with the foot in plantar flexion to allow hematoma consolidation.
  - ☐ Thereafter, a short or long leg cast is placed for 6 to 8 weeks, with less plantar flexion and progressive weight bearing generally permitted at 2 to 4 weeks after injury.
  - ☐ After removal of the cast, a heel lift is used while making the transition back to wearing normal shoes.
  - ☐ Progressive resistance exercises for the calf muscles are started at 8 to 10 weeks, with a return to athletic activities at 4 to 6 months.

- □ Patients are informed that attainment of maximal plantar flexion power may take 12 months or more and that some residual weakness is common.
- ■ Surgical treatment is often preferred when treating younger and more athletic patients.
  - □ Several different operative techniques have been described, including percutaneous and open approaches.
  - □ Percutaneous approaches have the advantage of decreased dissection but have historically carried the disadvantages of potential entrapment of the sural nerve and an increased chance of inadequate tendon capture.
  - □ Open approaches have the intrinsic advantages of permitting complete evaluation of the injury and inspection of final tendon end reapproximation; however, they carry the disadvantages of higher rates of wound dehiscence and skin adhesion problems.
    - The surgical technique uses a medial longitudinal approach to avoid injury to the sural nerve.
    - The paratenon is carefully dissected, and sutures are placed in each tendon end for tendon reapproximation. The paratenon is closed in a separate layer.
  - □ Postoperative management consists of a partial weight-bearing or weight bearing as tolerated in a short leg cast or boot for 6 to 8 weeks. As with nonoperatively treated patients, progressive resistance exercises are started at 8 to 10 weeks, with a return to sports at 4 to 6 months. Newer techniques and stronger sutures have led to more accelerated rehab protocols.
  - □ With distal ruptures or sleeve avulsions, an open technique and reattachment of the tendon to the calcaneus is performed. This is usually done with transosseous suture fixation.

Peroneal Tendon Subluxation

- ■ Subluxation and dislocation of the peroneal tendons are uncommon and usually result from sports activities.
- ■ They normally result from forced dorsiflexion or inversion and have been described principally in skiers when they dig the tips of the skis into the snow and create a sudden deceleration force with dorsiflexion of the ankle within the ski boot.
- ■ The injury is easily misdiagnosed as an ankle sprain, and it can result in recurrent or chronic dislocation.
- ■ Presentation is similar to that of a lateral ankle sprain with lateral ankle swelling, tenderness, and ecchymosis.

Clinical Evaluation

- Patients with peroneal tendon subluxation or dislocation demonstrate tenderness posterior to the lateral malleolus.
- The anterior drawer test is negative, and the patient has discomfort and apprehension with resisted eversion of the foot.
- Radiographic evaluation of a patient with peroneal tendon subluxation or dislocation may reveal a small fleck of bone off the posterior aspect of the lateral malleolus, which is best seen on the internal oblique or mortise view.
- If the diagnosis is unclear, as a result of swelling and diffuse ecchymosis, an MRI evaluation may help to delineate this soft tissue injury.

Treatment

- When the initial reduction of dislocated tendons is stable, nonoperative techniques can be successful.
  - □ Management consists of immobilization in a well-molded cast with the foot in slight plantar flexion and mild inversion in an attempt to relax the superior peroneal retinaculum and to maintain reduction in the retrofibular space. Non–weight-bearing immobilization is continued for 6 weeks to allow adequate time for retinacular and periosteal healing.
- When the diagnosis is made on a delayed basis or the patient presents with recurrent dislocations, operative treatment is considered because nonoperative measures are unlikely to work.
  - □ Surgical alternatives include transfer of the lateral Achilles tendon sheath, fibular osteotomy to create a deeper groove for the tendons, rerouting of the peroneal tendons under the fibulocalcaneal ligament, or simple reconstructive repair of the superior peroneal retinaculum with relocation of the tendons.
  - □ Postoperatively, the leg is splinted for 1 to 2 weeks in a slightly inverted and plantar flexed position; patients are then started on a passive motion exercise program to reduce scar formation in the peroneal groove and to increase the likelihood of good tendon nutrition and retinacular healing. Weight bearing is initiated 6 weeks postoperatively, and rehabilitation and focusing of strength and ROM are initiated soon thereafter.

Calcaneus Fractures

EPIDEMIOLOGY

- Calcaneus fractures account for approximately 2% of all fractures.
- The calcaneus, or os calcis, is the most frequently fractured tarsal bone.
- Displaced intra-articular fractures comprise 60% to 75% of calcaneus fractures.
- Ninety percent of calcaneus fractures occur in men between 21 and 45 years of age, with the majority being in industrial workers.
- Approximately 10% of calcaneus fractures are open injuries.

ANATOMY

- The anterior half of the superior articular surface contains three facets that articulate with the talus. The posterior facet is the largest and constitutes the major weight-bearing surface. The middle facet is located anteromedially on the sustentaculum tali. The anterior facet is often confluent with the middle facet.
- Between the middle and posterior facets lies the interosseous sulcus (calcaneal groove), which, with the talar sulcus, forms the sinus tarsi.
- The sustentaculum tali supports the neck of the talus medially; it is attached to the talus by the interosseus talocalcaneal and deltoid ligaments and contains the middle articular facet on its superior aspect. The flexor hallucis longus tendon passes beneath the sustentacular tali medially.
- The peroneal tendons pass between the calcaneus and the lateral malleolus laterally.
- The Achilles tendon attaches to the posterior tuberosity.

MECHANISM OF INJURY

- **Axial loading:** Falls from a height are responsible for most intra-articular fractures; they occur as the talus is driven down into the calcaneus, which is composed of a thin cortical shell surrounding cancellous bone. In motor vehicle accidents, calcaneus fractures may occur when the accelerator or brake pedal impacts the plantar aspect of the foot.

■ Twisting forces may be associated with extra-articular calcaneus fractures, in particular fractures of the anterior and medial processes or the sustentaculum. In diabetic patients, there is an increased incidence of tuberosity fractures from avulsion by the Achilles tendon.

CLINICAL EVALUATION

■ Patients typically present with moderate to severe heel pain, associated with tenderness, swelling, heel widening, and shortening. Ecchymosis around the heel extending to the arch is highly suggestive of calcaneus fracture. Blistering may be present and results from massive swelling usually within the first 36 hours after injury. Open fractures are rare, but when present they occur medially.

■ Careful evaluation of soft tissues and neurovascular status is essential. Compartment syndrome of the foot must be ruled out because this occurs in 10% of calcaneus fractures and may result in clawing of the lesser toes.

Associated Injuries

■ Up to 50% of patients with calcaneus fractures may have other associated injuries, including lumbar spine fractures (10%) or other fractures of the lower extremities (25%); intuitively, these injuries are more common in higher-energy injuries.

■ Bilateral calcaneus fractures are present in 5% to 10% of cases.

RADIOGRAPHIC EVALUATION

■ The initial radiographic evaluation of the patient with a suspected calcaneus fracture should include a lateral view of the hindfoot, an anteroposterior (AP) view of the foot, a Harris axial view, and an ankle series.

■ Lateral radiograph
  □ The "Böhler's" angle is composed of a line drawn from the highest point of the anterior process of the calcaneus to the highest point of the posterior facet and a line drawn tangential from the posterior facet to the superior edge of the tuberosity. The angle is normally between 20 and 40 degrees; a decrease in this angle indicates that the weight-bearing posterior facet of the calcaneus has collapsed, thereby shifting body weight anteriorly (Fig. 39.1).

  □ The Gissane (crucial) angle is formed by two strong cortical struts extending laterally, one along the lateral margin of the

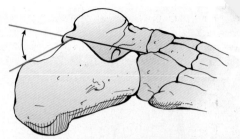

FIGURE 39.1 The Böhler angle. (From Bucholz RW, Heckman JD, Court-Brown C, et al., eds. *Rockwood and Green's Fractures in Adults.* 6th ed. Philadelphia: Lippincott Williams & Wilkins; 2006.)

posterior facet and the other extending anterior to the beak of the calcaneus. These cortical struts form an obtuse angle usually between 105 and 135 degrees and are visualized directly beneath the lateral process of the talus; an increase in this angle indicates collapse of the posterior facet (Fig. 39.2).

- **AP radiograph of the foot:** This may show extension of the fracture line into the calcaneocuboid joint.
- Harris axial view
  □ This is taken with the foot in dorsiflexion and the beam angled at 45 degrees cephalad.
  □ It allows visualization of the joint surface as well as loss of height, increase in width, and angulation of the tuberosity fragment (Fig. 39.3).
- Broden views have been replaced by computed tomography (CT) scanning. They are utilized intraoperatively to assess reduction.

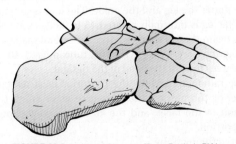

FIGURE 39.2 Angle of Gissane. (From Bucholz RW, Heckman JD, Court-Brown C, et al., eds. *Rockwood and Green's Fractures in Adults.* 6th ed. Philadelphia: Lippincott Williams & Wilkins; 2006.)

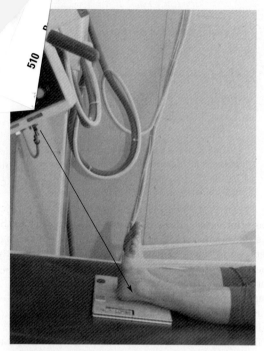

FIGURE 39.3 Photograph of the radiographic technique for obtaining the Harris or calcaneal radiographic view. Maximum dorsiflexion of the ankle was attempted to obtain an optimal view. (From Bucholz RW, Heckman JD, eds. *Rockwood and Green's Fractures in Adults.* 5th ed. Baltimore: Lippincott Williams & Wilkins; 2002.)

These are obtained with the patient supine and the x-ray cassette under the leg and the ankle. The foot is in neutral flexion, and the leg is internally rotated 15 to 20 degrees (Mortise). The x-ray beam then is centered over the lateral malleolus, and four radiographs are made with the tube angled 40, 30, 20, and 10 degrees toward the head of the patient.

☐ These radiographs show the posterior facet as it moves from posterior to anterior; the 10-degree view shows the posterior portion of the facet, and the 40-degree view shows the anterior portion.

■ Computed tomography
☐ CT images are obtained in the axial, 30-degree semicoronal, and sagittal planes.
☐ Three- to 5-mm slices are necessary for adequate analysis.

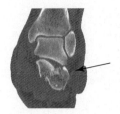

FIGURE 39.4 CT scan demonstrating involvement of the posterior facet.

☐ The coronal views provide information about the articular surface of the posterior facet, the sustentaculum, the overall shape of the heel, and the position of the peroneal and flexor hallucis tendons (Fig. 39.4).

☐ The axial views reveal information about the calcaneocuboid joint, the anteroinferior aspect of the posterior facet, and the sustentaculum.

☐ Sagittal reconstruction views provide additional information on the posterior facet, the calcaneal tuberosity, and the anterior process.

CLASSIFICATION

Extra-articular Fractures

These do not involve the posterior facet. They make up 25% to 30% of calcaneus fractures.

- **Anterior process fractures:** These may result from strong plantar flexion and inversion, which tighten the bifurcate and interosseous ligaments leading to avulsion fracture; alternatively, they may occur with forefoot abduction with calcaneocuboid compression. They are often confused with lateral ankle sprain and are seen on lateral or lateral oblique views.

- **Tuberosity fractures:** These may result from avulsion by the Achilles tendon, especially in diabetic patients or osteoporotic women, or rarely by direct trauma; they are seen on lateral radiographs.

- **Medial process fractures:** These vertical shear fractures are due to loading of heel in valgus; they are seen on axial radiographs.

- **Sustentacular fractures:** These occur with heel loading accompanied by severe foot inversion. They are often confused with medial ankle sprain and are seen on axial radiographs.

- **Body fractures not involving the subtalar articulation:** These are caused by axial loading. Significant comminution, widening, and loss of height may occur along with a reduction in the Böhler angle without posterior facet involvement.

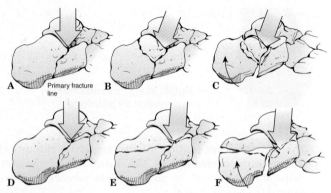

FIGURE 39.5 Mechanism of injury according to Essex-Lopresti. **(A–C)** Joint depression. **(D–F)** Tongue. (From Bucholz RW, Heckman JD, Court-Brown C, et al., eds. *Rockwood and Green's Fractures in Adults.* 6th ed. Baltimore: Lippincott Williams & Wilkins; 2005.)

Intra-articular Fractures

Essex-Lopresti Classification (Fig. 39.5)

Primary Fracture Line

The posterolateral edge of the talus splits the calcaneus obliquely through the posterior facet. The fracture line exits anterolaterally at the crucial angle or as far distally as the calcaneocuboid joint. Posteriorly, the fracture moves from plantar medial to dorsal lateral, producing two main fragments: the sustentacular (anteromedial) and tuberosity (posterolateral) fragments.

- The anteromedial fragment is rarely comminuted and remains attached to the talus by the deltoid and interosseous talocalcaneal ligaments.
- The posterolateral fragment usually displaces superolaterally with variable comminution, resulting in incongruity of the posterior facet as well as heel shortening and widening.

Secondary Fracture Line

With continued compressive forces, there is additional comminution, creating a free lateral piece of posterior facet separate from the tuberosity fragment.

- **Tongue-type fracture:** A secondary fracture line appears beneath the facet and exits posteriorly through the tuberosity.

- **Joint depression fracture:** A secondary fracture line exits just behind the posterior facet.
- Continued axial force causes the sustentacular fragment to slide medially, causing heel shortening and widening. As this occurs, the tuberosity fragment will rotate into varus. The posterolateral aspect of the talus will force the free lateral piece of the posterior facet down into the tuberosity fragment, rotating it as much as 90 degrees. This causes lateral wall blowout, which may extend as far anteriorly as the calcaneocuboid joint. As the lateral edge of the talus collapses further, there will be additional comminution of the articular surface.

Sanders Classification (Fig. 39.6)

- This is based on CT scan.
- This classification is based on the number and location of articular fragments; it is based on the coronal image, which shows the widest surface of the posterior facet of the talus.
- The posterior facet of the calcaneus is divided into three fracture lines (A, B, and C, corresponding to lateral, middle, and medial fracture lines on the coronal image).
- **Thus, there can be a total of four potential pieces:** lateral, central, medial, sustentaculum tali.

Type I:	All nondisplaced fractures regardless of the number of fracture lines
Type II:	Two-part fractures of the posterior facet; subtypes IIA, IIB, IIC, based on the location of the primary fracture line
Type III:	Three-part fractures with a centrally depressed fragment; subtypes IIIAB, IIIAC, IIIBC
Type IV:	Four-part articular fractures; highly comminuted

OTA Classification of Calcaneal Fractures

See Fracture and Dislocation Classification Compendium at http://www.ota.org/compendium/compendium.html.

TREATMENT

Despite adequate reduction and treatment, fractures of the os calcis may be severely disabling injuries, with variable prognoses and degrees of functional debilitation with chronic pain issues. Treatment remains controversial. Recent evidence has elucidated several factors associated with improved outcomes.

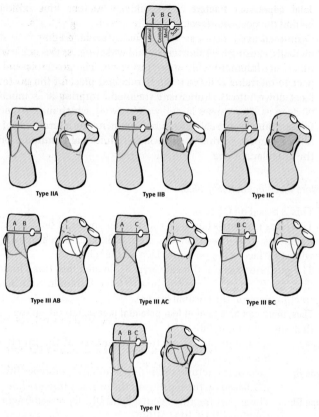

FIGURE 39.6 The Sanders computed tomography scan classification of calcaneal fractures. (Adapted from Sanders R. Current concepts review: displaced intra-articular fractures of the calcaneus. *J Bone Joint Surg Am.* 2000;82:233.)

Nonoperative

- Indications include
  - Nondisplaced or minimally displaced extra-articular fractures.
  - Nondisplaced intra-articular fractures.
  - Anterior process fractures with less than 25% involvement of the calcaneal-cuboid articulation.
  - Fractures in patients with severe peripheral vascular disease or insulin-dependent diabetes.
  - Fractures in patients with other medical comorbidities prohibiting surgery.

- □ Fractures associated with blistering and massive prolonged edema, large open wounds, or life-threatening injuries.
- ■ Initial treatment is placement of a bulky Jones dressing.
- ■ Nonoperative treatment consists of a supportive splint to allow dissipation of the initial fracture hematoma, followed by conversion to a prefabricated fracture boot locked in neutral flexion to prevent an equinus contracture and an elastic compression stocking to minimize dependent edema.
- ■ Early subtalar and ankle joint range-of-motion exercises are initiated, and non–weight-bearing restrictions are maintained for approximately 10 to 12 weeks, until radiographic union.

Operative

- ■ Indications
  - □ Displaced intra-articular fractures involving the posterior facet
  - □ Anterior process of the calcaneus fractures with >25% involvement of the calcaneal-cuboid articulation
  - □ Displaced fractures of the calcaneal tuberosity
  - □ Fracture-dislocations of the calcaneus
  - □ Selected open fractures of the calcaneus
- ■ Timing of surgery
  - □ Surgery should be performed within the initial 3 weeks of injury, before early fracture consolidation.
  - □ Surgery should not be attempted until swelling in the foot and ankle has adequately dissipated, as indicated by the reappearance of skin wrinkles.
  - □ Lateral "L" incision based on the blood supply of the lateral calcaneal artery.

Specific Fractures

Extra-articular Fractures

- ■ Anterior process fractures (Fig. 39.7)
  - □ Surgical management of anterior process fractures is performed for fractures involving >25% of the calcaneal-cuboid articulation on CT scan evaluation.
  - □ Definitive fixation involves small or minifragment screws.
  - □ The patient may ambulate in a hard-soled shoe, but regular shoes are discouraged for 10 to 12 weeks postoperatively.
- ■ Tuberosity (avulsion) fractures
  - □ These result from a violent pull of the gastrocnemius–soleus complex, such as with forced dorsiflexion secondary to a low-energy stumble and fall, producing an avulsed fragment of variable size.

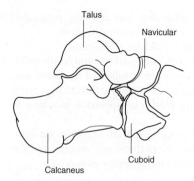

Talus

Navicular

Cuboid

Calcaneus

FIGURE 39.7 Anterior process fracture. Schematic lateral view. (From Bucholz RW, Heckman JD, eds. *Rockwood and Green's Fractures in Adults.* 5th ed. Baltimore: Lippincott Williams & Wilkins; 2002.)

- □ **Indications for surgery:** (1) the posterior skin is at risk from pressure from the displaced tuberosity, (2) the posterior portion of the bone is extremely prominent and will affect shoe wear, (3) the gastrocnemius–soleus complex is incompetent, or (4) the avulsion fragment involves the articular surface of the joint.
- □ Surgical treatment involves lag screw fixation with or without cerclage wire.
- ■ Calcaneus body fractures
  - □ True extra-articular fractures of the calcaneus, not involving the subtalar joint, probably account for 20% of all calcaneal fractures.
  - □ Minimally displaced fractures (<1 cm) are treated with early motion and non–weight bearing for 10 to 12 weeks.
  - □ Those with significant displacement resulting in varus/valgus deformity, lateral impingement, loss of heel height, or translation of the posterior tuberosity require open reduction and internal fixation.
- ■ Medial process fractures
  - □ Rare and usually nondisplaced.
  - □ The fracture is best seen on the axial radiographic view or on coronal CT scans.
  - □ Nondisplaced fractures can be treated with a short leg weight-bearing cast until the fracture heals at 8 to 10 weeks.
  - □ When fractures are displaced, closed manipulation may be considered.

Intra-articular Fractures

The Canadian Orthopaedic Trauma Society trial comparing operative to nonoperative treatment of displaced intra-articular calcaneal fractures found the following:

- Significantly better results occurred in patients with certain fracture groups undergoing operative treatment.
  - Women
  - Younger adults
  - Patients with a lighter workload
  - Patients not receiving Worker's Compensation
  - Patients with a higher initial Böhler angle (less severe initial injury)
  - Those with an anatomic reduction on postoperative CT evaluation
- Those having nonoperative treatment of their fracture were 5.5 times more likely to require a subtalar arthrodesis for posttraumatic arthritis than those undergoing operation.
- Operative goals include
  1. Restoration of congruity of the subtalar articulation.
  2. Restoration of the Böhler angle.
  3. Restoration of the normal width and height of the calcaneus.
  4. Maintenance of the normal calcaneocuboid articulation.
  5. Neutralization of the varus deformity of the fracture.
- Open reduction and internal fixation are generally performed through a lateral L-shaped incision, with care taken not to damage the sural nerve both proximally and distally.
- The posterior facet is reduced and stabilized with lag screws into the sustentaculum tali. The calcaneocuboid joint and the lateral wall are reduced. The length of the heel is regained with neutralization of varus. A thin plate is placed laterally and is used as a buttress. Bone void filling of the defect is not required but may be associated with earlier weight bearing.
- Good results have been reported for tongue-type fractures using percutaneous reduction (Essex-Lopresti maneuver) and lag screw fixation (Fig. 39.8).
- Primary subtalar or triple arthrodesis has had good reported results for select high-energy injuries (type 4).
- Postoperative management includes
  - Early supervised subtalar range-of-motion exercises.
  - Non–weight bearing for 8 to 12 weeks.
  - Full weight bearing by 3 months.

COMPLICATIONS

- **Wound dehiscence:** Most common at the angle of incision. Avoidance requires meticulous soft tissue technique and minimization of skin trauma during closure. It may be treated with wet to dry dressing changes, skin grafting, or muscle flap if necessary.

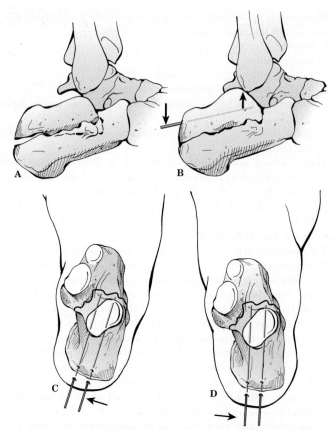

FIGURE 39.8 (A–D) Essex-Lopresti technique as modified by Tornetta. Once guide pins are correctly positioned, they are exchanged for 6.5- to 8.0-mm cannulated cancellous lag screws. (From Bucholz RW, Heckman JD, Court-Brown C, et al., eds. *Rockwood and Green's Fractures in Adults.* 6th ed. Philadelphia: Lippincott Williams & Wilkins; 2006.)

- **Calcaneal osteomyelitis:** The risk may be minimized by allowing soft tissue edema to resolve preoperatively.
- **Posttraumatic arthritis (subtalar or calcaneocuboid):** This reflects articular damage in addition to fracture displacement and comminution; thus, it may occur even in the presence of an anatomic reduction; it may be treated with injections or orthoses, or it may ultimately require subtalar or triple arthrodesis.
- **Increased heel width:** Some degree of heel widening is expected, even with open reduction and internal fixation. It may result in

lateral impingement on the peroneal tendons or the fibula. It is aggravated by increased residual lateral width and may be treated by wall resection or hardware removal.

■ **Loss of subtalar motion:** This is common with both operative and nonoperative treatment of intra-articular fractures.

■ **Peroneal tendonitis:** This is generally seen following nonoperative treatment and results from lateral impingement.

■ **Sural nerve injury:** This may occur in up to 15% of operative cases using a lateral approach.

■ **Chronic pain:** Despite nonoperative or operative treatment of calcaneal fractures, many patients have chronic heel pain that may be debilitating; many individuals are unable to return to gainful employment.

■ **Complex regional pain syndrome:** This may occur with operative or nonoperative management.

Talus

40

EPIDEMIOLOGY

- These are second in frequency among all tarsal fractures.
- The incidence of fractures of the talus ranges from 0.1% to 0.85% of all fractures and 5% to 7% of foot injuries.
- Approximately 14% to 26% of talar neck fractures had associated fracture of the medial malleolus.
- Lateral process of the talus fractures accounted for 2.3% of all snowboarding injuries and 15% of all ankle injuries.
- Fractures of the talar head are rare with an incidence of 3% to 5% of all fractures of the talus.

ANATOMY

- The body of the talus is covered superiorly by articular surface through which a person's body weight is transmitted. The anterior aspect is wider than the posterior aspect, which confers intrinsic stability to the ankle (Fig. 40.1).
- Medially and laterally, the articular cartilage extends plantar to articulate with the medial and lateral malleoli, respectively. The inferior surface of the body forms the articulation with the posterior facet of the calcaneus.

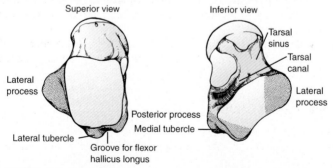

FIGURE 40.1 Superior and inferior views of the talus (*stippling* indicates the posterior and lateral processes). (From Bucholz RW, Heckman JD, Court-Brown C, et al., eds. *Rockwood and Green's Fractures in Adults.* 6th ed. Philadelphia: Lippincott Williams & Wilkins; 2006.)

- The neck of the talus is roughened by ligamentous attachments and vascular foramina. It deviates medially 15 to 25 degrees and is the most vulnerable to fracture.
- The talar head has continuous articular facets for the navicular anteriorly, the spring ligament inferiorly, the sustentaculum tali posteroinferiorly, and the deltoid ligament medially.
- There are two bony processes. The lateral process is wedge shaped and articulates with the posterior calcaneal facet inferomedially and the lateral malleolus superolaterally. The posterior process has a medial and lateral tubercle separated by a groove for the flexor hallucis longus tendon.
- An os trigonum is present in up to 50% of normal feet. It arises from a separate ossification center just posterior to the lateral tubercle of the posterior talar process.
- Sixty percent of the talus is covered by articular cartilage. No muscles originate from or insert onto the talus. The vascular supply is dependent on fascial structures to reach the talus; therefore, capsular disruptions may result in osteonecrosis.
- The vascular supply to the talus consists of
  - Arteries to the sinus tarsi (peroneal and dorsalis pedis arteries).
  - An artery of the tarsal canal (posterior tibial artery).
  - The deltoid artery (posterior tibial artery), which supplies the medial body.
  - Capsular and ligamentous vessels and intraosseous anastomoses.

MECHANISM OF INJURY

- Most commonly associated with a motor vehicle accident or a fall from a height with a component of hyperdorsiflexion of the ankle. The talar neck fractures as it impacts the anterior margin of the tibia.
- **"Aviator's astragalus"**: This historical term refers to the rudder bar of a crashing airplane impacting the plantar aspect of the foot, resulting in a talar neck fracture.

CLINICAL EVALUATION

- Patients typically present with ankle pain.
- Range of foot and ankle motion is typically painful and may elicit crepitus.
- Diffuse swelling of the hindfoot may be present, with tenderness to palpation of the talus and subtalar joint.
- Associated fractures of the foot and ankle are commonly seen with fractures of the talar neck and body.

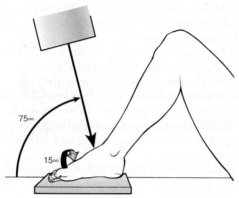

FIGURE 40.2 Canale and Kelly view of the foot. The correct position of the foot for x-ray evaluation is shown. (From Bucholz RW, Heckman JD, Court-Brown C, et al., eds. *Rockwood and Green's Fractures in Adults.* 6th ed. Philadelphia: Lippincott Williams & Wilkins; 2006.)

RADIOGRAPHIC EVALUATION

- Anteroposterior (AP), mortise, and lateral radiographs of the ankle, as well as AP, lateral, and oblique views of the foot are obtained.
- **Canale view:** This provides an optimum view of the talar neck. Taken with the ankle in maximum equinus, the foot is placed on a cassette, pronated 15 degrees, and the radiographic source is directed cephalad 15 degrees from the vertical (Fig. 40.2). This view was described for evaluation of posttraumatic deformity and is difficult to obtain in the acute setting.
- Computed tomography (CT) is helpful to characterize fracture pattern and displacement further and to assess articular involvement.
- Technetium bone scans or magnetic resonance imaging (MRI) may be useful in evaluating possible occult talar fractures.

CLASSIFICATION

Anatomic

- Lateral process fractures
- Posterior process fractures
- Talar head fractures
- Talar body fractures
- Talar neck fractures

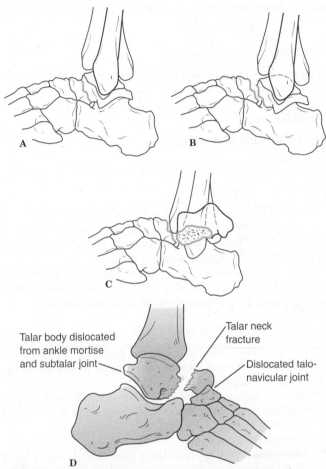

FIGURE 40.3 The three patterns of talar neck fractures as described by Hawkins. Note that type I fractures are nondisplaced. **(A)** Type I talar neck fractures with no displacement. **(B)** Type II talar neck fractures with displacement and subluxation of subtalar joint. **(C)** Type III talar neck fracture with displacement and dislocation of both ankle and subtalar joints. **(D)** Type IV talar neck fracture with dislocations of ankle, subtalar, and talo-navicular joints. (From Bucholz RW, Heckman JD, eds. *Rockwood and Green's Fractures in Adults.* 5th ed. Baltimore: Lippincott Williams & Wilkins; 2002.)

Hawkins Classification of Talar Neck Fractures (Fig. 40.3)

Type I:	Nondisplaced
Type II:	Associated subtalar subluxation or dislocation
Type III:	Associated subtalar and ankle dislocation

Type IV: **(Canale and Kelley):** Type III with associated talonavicular subluxation or dislocation

OTA Classification of Talar Fractures

See Fracture and Dislocation Classification Compendium at http://www.ota.org/compendium/compendium.html.

TREATMENT

Fractures of the Talar Neck and Body

These represent a continuum and are considered together.

Nondisplaced Fractures (Hawkins Type I)

- Fractures that appear nondisplaced on plain radiographs may show unrecognized comminution or articular step-off on CT scan. Fractures must truly be nondisplaced with no evidence of subtalar incongruity to be considered a type I fracture.
- Treatment consists of a short leg cast or boot for 8 to 12 weeks. The patient should remain non–weight bearing for 6 weeks until clinical and radiographic evidence of fracture healing is present.

Displaced Fractures (Hawkins Types II to IV)

- Immediate closed reduction (plantar flexion) is indicated, with urgent open reduction and internal fixation (ORIF) for all open or irreducible fractures (Fig. 40.4A).
- If anatomic reduction is obtained and confirmed by CT scan, the patient may be placed in a short leg splint, fracture fixation may be delayed (Fig. 40.4A).
- Surgical approaches include
  1. **Anteromedial:** This approach may be extended from a limited capsulotomy to a wide exposure with malleolar osteotomy (as the fracture progresses toward the body). The internal is just

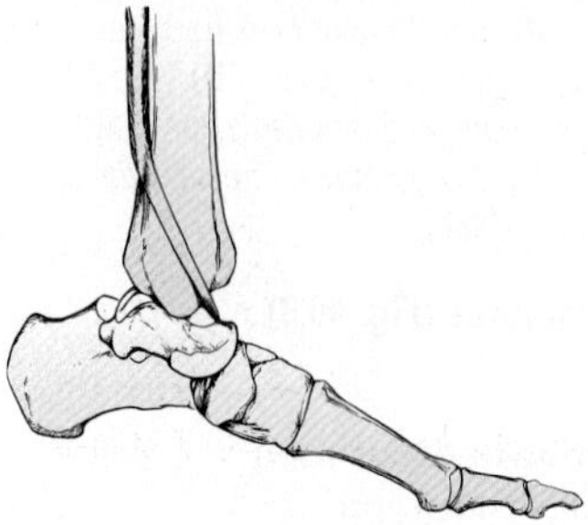

FIGURE 40.4 Hawkins 2 talar neck fracture **(A)** initial injury. Following closed reduction **(B)** note incongruity of subtalar joint.

medial to the anterior tibial tendon. This approach allows visualization of the talar neck and body. Care must be taken to preserve the saphenous vein and nerve and, more importantly, the deltoid artery.

2. **Posterolateral:** This approach provides access to posterior process and talar body. The interval is between the peroneus brevis and the flexor hallucis longus. The sural nerve must be protected. It is usually necessary to displace the flexor hallucis longus from its groove in the posterior process to facilitate exposure.

3. **Anterolateral:** This approach allows visualization of the sinus tarsi, lateral talar neck, and subtalar joint. Inadvertent damage to the artery of the tarsal sinus can occur through this approach.

4. **Combined anteromedial–anterolateral:** This is often used to allow maximum visualization of the talar neck.

■ **Internal fixation:** Two interfragmentary lag screws or headless screws are placed perpendicular to the fracture line. The screws can be inserted in antegrade or retrograde fashion. Posterior-to-anterior–directed screws have been demonstrated to be biomechanically stronger in a cadaver model, but clinically more difficult to place. Retrograde screw placement requires the use of headless screws or screws that are buried beneath the articular surface of the talar head.

■ Use of titanium screws allows better visualization with MRI for evaluation of subsequent osteonecrosis.

■ Areas of significant comminution and bone loss should be grafted.

■ Mini-fragment plates have been used more recently in cases of significant comminution to avoid shortening of the neck (Fig. 40.5A,B).

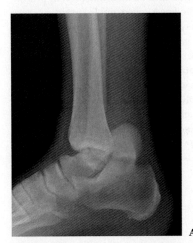
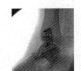

A   B

FIGURE 40.5 Hawkins 3 talar neck fracture **(A)** initial injury. Following ORIF of talus and of medial malleolar fracture **(B)**. Egol

- A short leg cast or removable boot should be placed postoperatively for 8 to 12 weeks, and the patient should be kept non–weight bearing.
- **Hawkins sign:** Subchondral osteopenia (seen on the Mortise ankle radiograph) in the talus at 6 to 8 weeks tends to indicate talar viability. However, the presence of this sign does not rule out osteonecrosis; its absence is also not diagnostic for osteonecrosis.

TALAR BODY FRACTURES

Classification

- Shear type I (A, B) (Fig. 40.6)
- Shear type II (C)
- Crush (D)

Treatment

- Non/Minimally displaced–Nonoperative
- Displaced-ORIF (may require medial malleolar osteotomy)

Lateral Process Fractures

These are intra-articular fractures of the subtalar or ankle joint that occur most frequently when the foot is dorsiflexed and inverted. There has been an increase in incidence with the rise in popularity of snowboarding.

- Lateral process fractures are often missed on initial patient presentation. Fracture is misinterpreted as a severe ankle sprain.
- Because of the difficulty in detecting and defining the extent of a lateral process fracture, a CT scan is frequently necessary to fully appreciate the extent of injury.
- **Less than 2-mm displacement:** Patients should have a short leg cast or boot for 6 weeks and be non–weight bearing for at least 4 weeks.
- **More than 2-mm displacement:** ORIF is performed using lag screws or wires through a lateral approach.
- **Comminuted fractures:** Nonviable fragments are excised.

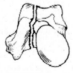

FIGURE 40.6 Talus body fractures

Posterior Process Fractures

These involve the posterior 25% of the articular surface and include the medial and lateral tubercles. Fractures may occur in a severe ankle inversion injury whereby the posterior talofibular ligament avulses the lateral tubercle or by forced equinus and direct compression.

- Diagnosis of fractures of the posterior process of the talus can be difficult, in part relating to the presence of an os trigonum.
- **Nondisplaced or minimally displaced:** Patients should have a short leg cast for 6 weeks and be non–weight bearing for at least 4 weeks.
- **Displaced:** ORIF is recommended if the fragment is large; primary excision is performed if the fragment is small; a posterolateral approach may be used.

Talar Head Fractures

These fractures result from plantarflexion and longitudinal compression along the axis of the forefoot. Comminution is common; one must also suspect navicular injury and talonavicular disruption.

- **Nondisplaced fractures:** Patients should be placed in a short leg cast molded to preserve the longitudinal arch and should be partially weight bearing for 6 weeks. An arch support is worn in the shoe to splint the talonavicular articulation for 3 to 6 months.
- **Displaced fractures:** ORIF is indicated, with primary excision of small fragments through an anterior or anteromedial approach.

COMPLICATIONS

- **Infection:** The risk may be minimized by early ORIF with soft tissue coverage for open injuries or waiting until swelling has decreased.
- **Osteonecrosis:** The rate of osteonecrosis is related to initial fracture displacement:
  Hawkins I: 0% to 15%
  Hawkins II: 20% to 50%
  Hawkins III: 50% to 100%
  Hawkins IV: Up to 100%
- **Posttraumatic arthritis:** This occurs in 40% to 90% of cases, typically related to articular incongruity or chondral injury at the time of fracture. This may be evident in either the ankle or subtalar joints. The rates of arthritis in the subtalar joint, ankle joint, or both joints are 50%, 30%, and 25%, respectively.
- **Delayed union and nonunion:** Delayed union (>6 months) may occur in up to 15% of cases. It may be treated by repeat fixation

and bone grafting or placement of some type of osteoinductive material.

- **Malunion:** Commonly varus (following talar neck fractures), this is related to initial fracture reduction associated with dorsomedial comminution. Malunion results in subtalar stiffness and excessive weight bearing on the lateral side of the foot; malunion is frequently painful.

- **Open fracture:** This complicates up to 15% to 25% of injuries and reflects the often high-energy mechanism that produces these fractures. Copious irrigation and meticulous debridement are necessary to prevent infectious complications. The reported infection rate for open talus fractures is 35% to 40%. The "extruded" talus is an extreme situation. Several reports have documented fair outcomes with replantation.

- **Skin slough:** This may occur secondary to prolonged dislocation, with pressure necrosis on the overlying soft tissues. When severe, it may result in pressure erosion, compromising soft tissue integrity and resulting in possible infection.

- **Interposition of long flexor tendons:** This may prevent adequate closed reduction and necessitate ORIF.

- **Foot compartment syndrome:** Rare. However, pain on passive extension of the toes must raise clinical suspicion of possible evolving or present compartment syndrome of the foot, particularly in a patient in whom symptoms are out of proportion to the apparent injury. Urgent fasciotomy is controversial. Some authors feel that the sequelae of foot compartment syndrome (claw toes) are less morbid than the fasciotomies required to release all foot compartments.

Subtalar Dislocation

- Subtalar dislocation, also known as peritalar dislocation, refers to the simultaneous dislocation of the distal articulations of the talus at the talocalcaneal and talonavicular joints.
- It most commonly occurs in young men.
- Inversion of the foot results in a medial subtalar dislocation, whereas eversion produces a lateral subtalar dislocation.
  - □ Up to 85% of dislocations are medial.
  - □ Lateral dislocations are often associated with a higher-energy mechanism and a worse long-term prognosis compared with medial subtalar dislocations.
- All subtalar dislocations require gentle and timely reduction.
- Reduction involves sufficient analgesia with knee flexion and longitudinal foot traction. Accentuation of the deformity is often necessary to "unlock" the calcaneus. Once the calcaneus is unlocked,

reversal of the deformity can be applied. Reduction is usually accompanied by a satisfying clunk.

- In many cases, a subtalar dislocation is stable following closed reduction.
- CT scan is useful after closed reduction to determine whether associated fractures are present and to detect possible talocalcaneal subluxation.
- A variety of bone and soft tissue structures may become entrapped, resulting in a block to closed reduction. With medial dislocations, the talar head can become trapped by the capsule of the talonavicular joint, the extensor retinaculum or extensor tendons, or the extensor digitorum brevis muscle. With a lateral dislocation, the posterior tibial tendon when entrapped may present a substantial barrier even to open reduction (Fig. 40.5).
- Open reduction, when necessary, is usually performed through a longitudinal anteromedial incision for medial dislocations and a sustentaculum tali approach for lateral dislocations.
- Following a short period of immobilization, physical therapy is instituted to regain subtalar and midtarsal mobility.

Total Dislocation of the Talus

- Total dislocation of the talus is a rare injury, resulting from an extension of the forces causing a subtalar dislocation.
- Most injuries are open (extrusion) (Fig. 40.7).
- Initial treatment is directed to the soft tissues.
- In general, open reduction of the completely dislocated talus is recommended.
- Results may be complicated by infection, osteonecrosis, and posttraumatic arthritis.

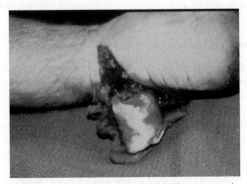

FIGURE 40.7 40 year old male involved in a motorcycle accident with an open extruded talus. (Courtesy Toni McLaurin M.D.)

41

Fractures of the Midfoot and Forefoot

MIDTARSAL (CHOPART) JOINT

Epidemiology

- Injuries to the midfoot are relatively rare.
- The annual incidence of midfoot fractures is 3.6 per 100,000 population per year.
- The most commonly fractured bone was the cuboid (50%), followed by the navicular (44%) and the cuneiform (6%).
- The male-to-female ratio is 1:1.2

Anatomy

- The midfoot is the section of the foot distal to Chopart joint line and proximal to Lisfranc joint line (Fig. 41.1).
- **Five tarsal bones comprise the midfoot:** The navicular, cuboid, and the medial, middle, and lateral cuneiforms.
- The midtarsal joint consists of the calcaneocuboid and talonavicular joints, which act in concert with the subtalar joint during inversion and eversion of the foot.
- The cuboid acts as a linkage across the three naviculocuneiform joints, allowing only minimal motion.
- Ligamentous attachments include the plantar calcaneonavicular (spring) ligament, bifurcate ligament, dorsal talonavicular ligament, dorsal calcaneocuboid ligament, dorsal cuboidonavicular ligament, and long plantar ligament (Fig. 41.2).

Mechanism of Injury

- **High-energy trauma:** This is most common and may result from direct impact from a motor vehicle accident or a combination of axial loading and torsion, such as during impact from a fall or jump from a height.
- **Low-energy injuries:** This may result in a sprain during athletic or dance activities.

Clinical Evaluation

- Patient presentation is variable, ranging from a limp with swelling and tenderness on the dorsum of the midfoot to nonambulatory

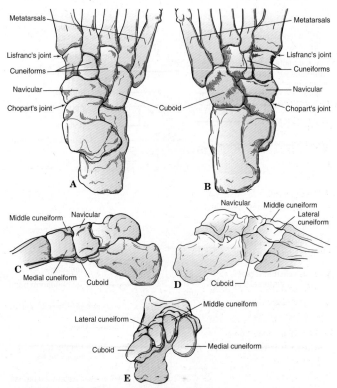

FIGURE 41.1 Bony anatomy of the midfoot. **(A)** Dorsal view. **(B)** Plantar view. **(C)** Medial view. **(D)** Lateral view. **(E)** Coronal view. (From Bucholz RW, Heckman JD, Court-Brown C, et al., eds. *Rockwood and Green's Fractures in Adults.* 6th ed. Philadelphia: Lippincott Williams & Wilkins; 2006.)

status with significant pain, gross swelling, ecchymosis, and variable deformity.

■ Stress maneuvers consist of forefoot abduction, adduction, flexion, and extension, and may result in reproduction of pain and instability.

■ A careful neurovascular examination should be performed. In cases of extreme pain and swelling, serial examinations may be warranted to evaluate the possibility of foot compartment syndrome.

Radiographic Evaluation

■ Anteroposterior (AP), lateral, and oblique radiographs of the foot should be obtained.

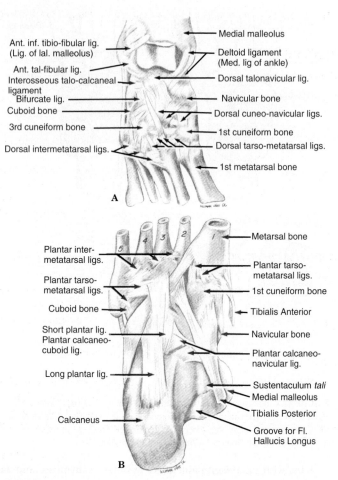

FIGURE 41.2 Ligamentous structure of the midfoot. **(A)** The dorsal view shows extensive overlap of the interosseous ligaments. **(B)** The plantar ligaments are thicker than their dorsal counterparts and are dynamically reinforced by the tibialis anterior, tibialis posterior, and peroneus longus tendons. Note the extensive attachments of the tibialis posterior throughout the midfoot bones. (From Bucholz RW, Heckman JD, Court-Brown C, et al., eds. *Rockwood and Green's Fractures in Adults.* 6th ed. Philadelphia: Lippincott Williams & Wilkins; 2006.)

- Stress views or weight-bearing x-rays may help to delineate subtle injuries.
- Computed tomography (CT) may be helpful in characterizing fracture-dislocation injuries with articular comminution.

■ Magnetic resonance imaging (MRI) may be used to evaluate ligamentous injury and/or more subtle injuries.

Classification

Medial Stress Injury

■ Inversion injury occurs with adduction of the midfoot on the hindfoot.
■ Flake fractures of the dorsal margin of the talus or navicular and of the lateral margin of the calcaneus or the cuboid may indicate a sprain.
■ In more severe injuries, the midfoot may be completely dislocated, or there may be an isolated talonavicular dislocation. A medial swivel dislocation is one in which the talonavicular joint is dislocated, the subtalar joint is subluxed, and the calcaneocuboid joint is intact.

Longitudinal Stress Injury

■ Force is transmitted through the metatarsal heads proximally along the rays with resultant compression of the midfoot between the metatarsals and the talus with the foot plantar flexed.
■ Longitudinal forces pass between the cuneiforms and fracture the navicular typically in a vertical pattern.

Lateral Stress Injury

■ **"Nutcracker fracture"**: This is the characteristic fracture of the cuboid as the forefoot driven laterally, crushing the cuboid between the calcaneus and the fourth and fifth metatarsal bases.
■ Most commonly, this is an avulsion fracture of the navicular with a comminuted compression fracture of the cuboid.
■ In more severe trauma, the talonavicular joint subluxes laterally, and the lateral column of the foot collapses because of comminution of the calcaneocuboid joint.

Plantar Stress Injury

■ Forces directed at the plantar region may result in sprains to the midtarsal region with avulsion fractures of the dorsal lip of the navicular, talus, or anterior process of the calcaneus.

Treatment

Nonoperative

■ **Sprains:** Nonrigid dressings are used with protected weight bearing for 4 to 6 weeks; prognosis is excellent. For severe sprains, midfoot immobilization may be indicated.

- Nondisplaced fractures may be treated with a short leg cast or fracture brace with initial non–weight bearing for 6 weeks.

Operative

- High-energy mechanisms resulting in displaced fracture patterns often require open reduction and internal fixation (ORIF; e.g., with Kirschner wires or lag screws) and/or external fixation.
- Prognosis guarded, depending on the degree of articular incongruity.
- Bone grafting of the cuboid may be necessary following reduction of lateral stress injuries.
- Severe crush injuries with extensive comminution may require arthrodesis to restore the longitudinal arch of the foot.

Complications

- Posttraumatic osteoarthritis may occur as a result of residual articular incongruity or chondral injury at the time of trauma. If severe and debilitating, it may require arthrodesis for adequate relief of symptoms.

TARSAL NAVICULAR

Epidemiology

- Isolated fractures of the navicular are rare and should be diagnosed only after ruling out concomitant injuries to the midtarsal joint complex.

Anatomy

- The navicular is the keystone of the medial longitudinal arch of the foot.
- It is wider on its dorsal and medial aspect than on its plantar and lateral aspect.
- The medial prominence known as the navicular tuberosity provides the attachment point for the posterior tibialis on its medial inferior surface.
- An accessory navicular may be present in 4% to 12% of patients and should not be confused with an acute fracture.
- Proximally, the articular surface is concave and articulates with the talus. This joint enjoys a significant arc of motion and transmits the motion of the subtalar joint to the forefoot. It is the point from which forefoot inversion and eversion are initiated.
- The distal articular surface of the navicular has three separate broad facets that articulate with each of the three cuneiforms.

These joints provide little motion; they mainly dissipate loading stresses.

- Laterally, the navicular rests on the dorsal medial aspect of the cuboid with a variable articular surface.
- Thick ligaments on its plantar and dorsal aspect support the navicular cuneiform joints. The spring ligament and superficial deltoid provide strong support to the plantar and medial aspects of the talonavicular joint.
- Anatomic variants to be aware of when viewing the navicular involve the shape of the tuberosity and the presence of an accessory navicular (os tibiale externum). They are present up to 15% of the time, and bilateral 70% to 90%.

Mechanism of Injury

- Direct blow, although uncommon, can cause avulsions to the periphery or crush injury in the dorsal plantar plane.
- More often, indirect forces of axial loading either directly along the long axis of the foot or obliquely cause navicular injury.
- Injury may result from a fall from a height or a motor vehicle accident. Stress fractures may occur in running and jumping athletes, with increased risk in patients with a cavus foot or calcaneal navicular coalition.

Clinical Evaluation

- Patients typically present with a painful foot and dorsomedial swelling and tenderness.
- Physical examination should include assessment of the ipsilateral ankle and foot, with careful palpation of all bony structures to rule out associated injuries.

Radiographic Evaluation

- AP, lateral, medial oblique, and lateral oblique views should be obtained to ascertain the extent of injury to the navicular as well as to detect associated injuries.
- If possible, the initial films should be weight bearing to detect ligamentous instability.
- Medial and lateral oblique x-rays of the midfoot will aid in assessing the lateral pole of the navicular as well as the medial tuberosity.
- CT may be obtained to better characterize the fracture.
- MRI or technetium scan may be obtained if a fracture is suspected but not apparent by plain radiography.

Classification

■ The most commonly used classification of navicular fractures is composed of three basic types with a subclassification for body fractures (Sangeorzan) (Fig. 41.3).

  □ Avulsion-type fracture can involve either the talonavicular or naviculocuneiform ligaments.

  □ Tuberosity fractures are usually traction-type injuries with disruption of the tibialis posterior insertion without joint surface disruption.

  □ Type I body fracture splits the navicular into dorsal and plantar segments.

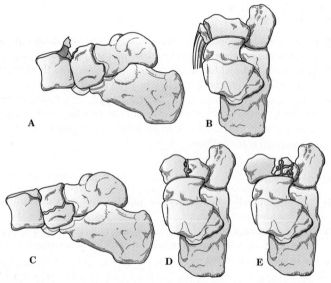

FIGURE 41.3 The present popular classification of navicular fractures is composed of three basic types with a subclassification for body fractures suggested by Sangeorzan. **(A)** Avulsion-type fracture can involve either the talonavicular or naviculocuneiform ligaments. **(B)** Tuberosity fractures are usually traction-type injuries with disruption of the tibialis posterior insertion without joint surface disruption. **(C)** A type I body fracture splits the navicular into dorsal and plantar segments. **(D)** A type II body fracture cleaves into medial and lateral segments. The location of the split usually follows either of the two intercuneiform joint lines. Stress fractures are usually included in this group. **(E)** A type III body fracture is distinguished by comminution of the fragments and significant displacement of the medial and lateral poles. (From Bucholz RW, Heckman JD, Court-Brown C, et al., eds. *Rockwood and Green's Fractures in Adults.* 6th ed. Philadelphia: Lippincott Williams & Wilkins; 2006.)

- □ Type II body fractures cleave into medial and lateral segments. The location of the split usually follows either of the two intercuneiform joint lines. Stress fractures can usually be included in this group.
- □ Type III body fractures are distinguished by comminution of the fragments and significant displacement of the medial and lateral poles.

OTA Classification of Navicular Fractures

See Fracture and Dislocation Classification Compendium at http://www.ota.org/compendium/compendium.html.

Anatomic Classification

Cortical Avulsion Fractures (Up To 50%)

- Excessive flexion or eversion of midfoot results in a dorsal lip avulsion of the navicular by the talonavicular capsule and the anterior fibers of the deltoid ligament.
- Symptomatic, small, nonarticular fragments may be excised. Large fragments (>25% articular surface) may be reattached with a lag screw.

Body Fractures (30%)
Tuberosity Fractures (20% to 25%)

- Forced eversion injury causes avulsion of the tuberosity by the posterior tibial tendon insertion or deltoid ligament.
- This is often part of the "nutcracker fracture," so concomitant midtarsal injury must be excluded.
- One must rule out the presence of an accessory navicular, which is bilateral in 70% to 90% of cases.
- If symptomatic, small fragments can be excised and the posterior tibial tendon reattached; larger fragments require ORIF with lag screw fixation, especially if posterior tibial tendon function is compromised.

Stress Fractures

- These occur primarily in young athletes.
- They frequently require bone scan or MRI for diagnosis.
- The fracture line is usually sagittally oriented in the middle third and may be complete or incomplete.
- Owing to increased incidence of persistent problems with pain and healing, screw fixation with autologous bone grafting should be used with comminuted fractures.

Treatment

The two most important criteria in obtaining a satisfactory outcome are maintenance or restoration of the medial column length and articular congruity of the talonavicular joint.

Nonoperative

- Nondisplaced fractures of the navicular should be treated in a short leg cast or fracture brace with restricted weight bearing for 6 to 8 weeks.
- Repeat radiographs should be obtained at 10 to 14 days after the initial injury to confirm the absence of bony or soft tissue instability. If instability appears or other injuries become apparent, appropriate surgical intervention should be considered.

Operative

- Surgical indications
  - Any unstable injury or fracture resulting in loss of position or articular congruity should be treated surgically.
  - Because the joint is concave, a 2-mm separation in any plane is considered incongruent. Most authors agree these injuries need to be managed aggressively with operative reduction.
  - Cortical avulsion fractures found to involve a significant portion of the dorsal anterior surface should be considered for operative treatment.
- Surgical management
  - Individual fragments are stabilized using K-wires or mini-fragment screws.
  - Bone graft should be considered for crushed areas requiring elevation.
  - If anatomic restoration of 60% or more of the talonavicular surface can be achieved, an effort should be made to salvage the joint.
  - If more than 40% of the articular surface cannot be reconstructed, an acute talonavicular fusion should be considered.
- Postoperative management
  - Cast or brace immobilization with non–weight bearing is recommended for 12 weeks.

Complications

- These include nonunion, arthritic degeneration, late instability, loss of normal foot alignment through bony resorption or collapse, and osteonecrosis.

- **Osteonecrosis:** The risk is increased with significantly displaced, markedly comminuted fractures. It may result in collapse of the navicular, with need for bone grafting and internal fixation.
- Posttraumatic osteoarthritis may occur as a result of articular incongruity, chondral damage, or free osteochondral fragments.

NAVICULAR DISLOCATION

- Isolated dislocation or subluxation of the navicular is rare.
- The mechanism is hyperplantar flexion of the forefoot with subsequent axial loading.
- Open reduction is usually necessary to restore both navicular position and articular congruity.

CUBOID FRACTURES

Epidemiology

- Injury to the cuboid can occur as an isolated entity but is usually seen in association with injuries to the talonavicular joint or other midfoot structures or in conjunction with Lisfranc injuries.

Anatomy

- The cuboid is part of the lateral support column of the foot.
- The cuboid articulates with the calcaneus proximally, the navicular and lateral cuneiform medially, and the lateral two metatarsals distally.
- Its plantar aspect forms a portion of the roof of the peroneal groove through which the peroneus longus tendon runs; scarring and irregularity of the peroneal groove caused by cuboid fracture may compromise function of peroneus longus tendon.

Mechanism of Injury

- **Direct:** This is uncommon; trauma to the dorsolateral aspect of the foot may result in fractures of the cuboid.
- **Indirect:** This accounts for most cuboid fractures.
  - "**Nutcracker injury**": Torsional stress or forefoot abduction may result in impaction of the cuboid between the calcaneus and the lateral metatarsals.
  - Extreme plantar flexion may cause isolated sprain or dislocation of calcaneocuboid joint in high-velocity trauma, dance injuries, or patients with Ehlers–Danlos syndrome.
- Stress fractures may occur in athletic individuals.

Clinical Evaluation

- Patients typically present with pain, swelling, and tenderness to palpation at the dorsolateral aspect of the foot.
- Palpation of all bony structures of the foot should be performed to rule out associated injuries.
- Pain on the lateral aspect of the foot may be confused with symptoms of peroneal tendonitis in cases of stress fractures of the cuboid.

Radiographic Evaluation

- AP, lateral, and oblique views of the foot should be obtained.
- Multiple medial oblique radiographic views may be needed to see the articular outlines of both the calcaneocuboid and cuboid metatarsal joints.
- As with other potential midfoot problems, weight-bearing or stress views should be obtained to rule out interosseus instability of surrounding structures.
- A small medial or dorsal avulsion fracture of the navicular is considered a sign of possible cuboid injury.
- CT scan may be necessary to assess the extent of injury and instability.
- MRI or bone scan may be used for diagnosing a stress fracture.

Classification

OTA Classification

See Fracture and Dislocation Classification Compendium at http://www.ota.org/compendium/compendium.html.

Treatment

Nonoperative

- Isolated fractures of the cuboid with no evidence of loss of osseous length or interosseus instability can be treated in a cast or removable boot.
- Non–weight bearing for 4 to 6 weeks is recommended.

Operative

- ORIF is indicated if there is more than 2 mm of joint surface disruption or any evidence of longitudinal compression.
- Severe comminution and residual articular displacement may necessitate calcaneocuboid arthrodesis for proper foot alignment and to minimize late complications.

Complications

- **Osteonecrosis:** This may complicate severely displaced fractures or those with significant comminution.
- **Posttraumatic osteoarthritis:** This may result from articular incongruity, chondral damage, or free osteochondral fragments.
- **Nonunion:** This may occur with significant displacement and inadequate immobilization or fixation. If severely symptomatic, it may necessitate ORIF with bone grafting.

CUNEIFORM FRACTURES

- These usually occur in conjunction with tarsometatarsal injuries.
- The usual mechanism is indirect axial loading of the bone.
- Localized tenderness over the cuneiform region, pain in the midfoot with weight bearing, or discomfort with motion through the tarsometatarsal joints can signify injury to these bones.
- AP, lateral, and oblique views should be obtained. These should be weight bearing if possible.
- Coronal and longitudinal CT scan of the midfoot can be used to better define the extent of the injury.

OTA Classification of Cuneiform Fractures

See Fracture and Dislocation Classification Compendium at http://www.ota.org/compendium/compendium.html.

TARSOMETATARSAL (LISFRANC) JOINT

Epidemiology

- These are generally considered rare.
- Approximately 20% of Lisfranc injuries may be initially overlooked (especially in polytraumatized patients).

Anatomy

- In the AP plane, the base of the second metatarsal is recessed between the medial and lateral cuneiforms. This limits translation of the metatarsals in the frontal plane.
- In the coronal plane, the middle three metatarsal bases are trapezoidal, forming a transverse arch that prevents plantar displacement of the metatarsal bases. The second metatarsal base is the keystone in the transverse arch of the foot (Fig. 41.4).
- There is only slight motion across the tarsometatarsal joints, with 10 to 20 degrees of dorsal plantar motion at the fifth metatarsocuboid joint and progressively less motion medially except for

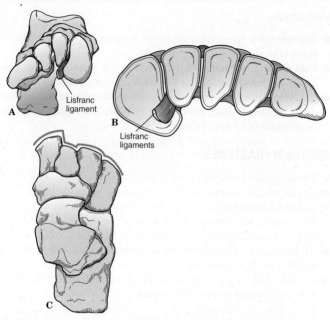

FIGURE 41.4 The anatomy of the tarsometatarsal joints. **(A)** Proximal view of the cuneiform and cuboid articular surfaces. **(B)** Distal view of the corresponding articular surfaces of the metatarsals. **(C)** Schematic representation of the contour of the tarsometatarsal joint line. Note the keying in place of the base of the second metatarsal. (From Bucholz RW, Heckman JD, Court-Brown C, et al., eds. *Rockwood and Green's Fractures in Adults.* 6th ed. Philadelphia: Lippincott Williams & Wilkins; 2006.)

the first metatarsocuneiform (20 degrees of plantar flexion from neutral).

- The ligamentous support begins with the strong ligaments linking the bases of the second through fifth metatarsals. The most important ligament is Lisfranc ligament, which attaches the medial cuneiform to the base of the second metatarsal.
- Ligamentous, bony, and soft tissue support provides for intrinsic stability across the plantar aspect of Lisfranc joint; conversely, the dorsal aspect of this articulation is not reinforced by structures of similar strength.
- There is no ligamentous connection between the base of the first and second metatarsals.
- The dorsalis pedis artery dives between the first and second metatarsals at Lisfranc joint and may be damaged during injury, approach or reduction.

Mechanism of Injury

Three most common mechanisms include

- **Twisting:** Forceful abduction of the forefoot on the tarsus results in fracture of the base of the second metatarsal and shear or crush fracture of the cuboid. Historically, this was seen in equestrian accidents when a rider fell from a horse with a foot engaged in a stirrup. It is commonly seen today in motor vehicle accidents.
- Axial loading of a fixed foot may be seen with (1) extrinsic axial compression applied to the heel, such as a heavy object striking the heel of a kneeling patient, or (2) extreme ankle equinus with axial loading of the body weight, such as a missed step off a curb or landing from a jump during a dance maneuver.
- Crushing mechanisms are common in industrial-type injuries to Lisfranc joint, often with sagittal plane displacement, soft tissue compromise, and compartment syndrome.

Clinical Evaluation

- Patients present with variable foot deformity, pain, swelling, and tenderness on the dorsum of the foot. Plantar ecchymosis is pathognomonic for a Lisfranc injury.
- Diagnosis requires a high degree of clinical suspicion.
  □ Twenty percent are misdiagnosed.
  □ Forty percent have no treatment in the first week.
- Be wary of the diagnosis of "midfoot sprain."
- A careful neurovascular examination is essential because dislocation of Lisfranc joint may be associated with impingement on or partial or complete laceration of the dorsalis pedis artery. In addition, dramatic swelling of the foot is common with high-energy mechanisms; compartment syndrome of the foot must be ruled out on the basis of serial neurovascular examination or compartment pressure monitoring if necessary.
- Stress testing may be performed by gentle, passive forefoot abduction and pronation, with the hindfoot firmly stabilized in the examiner's other hand. Alternatively, pain can typically be reproduced by gentle supination and pronation of the forefoot.

Radiographic Evaluation

Standard AP, lateral, and oblique films are usually diagnostic.

- The medial border of the second metatarsal should be colinear with the medial border of the middle cuneiform on the AP view (Fig. 41.5).

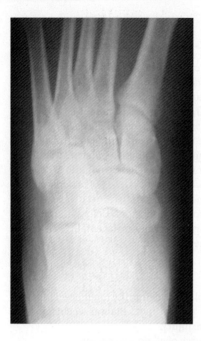

FIGURE 41.5 Anteroposterior view of the tarsometatarsal joint. Normal joint alignment on weight bearing. (From Bucholz RW, Heckman JD, Court-Brown C, et al., eds. *Rockwood and Green's Fractures in Adults.* 6th ed. Philadelphia: Lippincott Williams & Wilkins; 2006.)

- The medial border of the fourth metatarsal should be colinear with the medial border of the cuboid on the oblique view (Fig. 41.6).
- Dorsal displacement of the metatarsals on the lateral view is indicative of ligamentous compromise.
- Flake fractures around the base of the second metatarsal are indicative of disruption of Lisfranc joint.
- Weight-bearing radiographs provide a stress film of the joint complex.
- If clinically indicated, physician-directed stress views should be obtained. The forefoot is held in abduction for the AP view and in plantar flexion for the lateral view.
- A CT scan can be used to assess the plantar osseous structures as well as the amount of intra-articular comminution.
- MRI scanning is useful for suspected Lisfranc sprains.

Associated Injuries

- Fractures of the cuneiforms, cuboid (nutcracker), and/or metatarsals are common.
- The second metatarsal is the most frequent associated fracture.

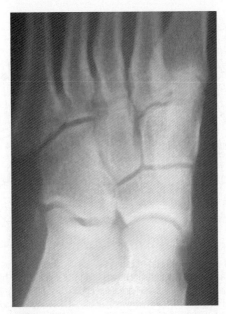

FIGURE 41.6 Medial oblique view of the tarsometatarsal joint. Normal joint alignment on weight bearing. (From Bucholz RW, Heckman JD, Court-Brown C, et al., eds. *Rockwood and Green's Fractures in Adults*. 6th ed. Philadelphia: Lippincott Williams & Wilkins; 2006.)

Classification

Classification schemes for Lisfranc injuries guide the clinician in defining the extent and pattern of injury, although they are of little prognostic value.

Quenu and Kuss (Fig. 41.7)

This classification is based on commonly observed patterns of injury.

Homolateral:	All five metatarsals displaced in the same direction
Isolated:	One or two metatarsals displaced from the others
Divergent:	Displacement of the metatarsals in both the sagittal and coronal planes

Myerson (Fig. 41.8)

This is based on commonly observed patterns of injury with regard to treatment.

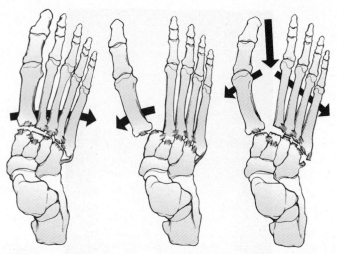

FIGURE 41.7 The common classification devised by Quenu and Kuss. Further subdivisions are used to identify the direction of dislocation in the homolateral pattern (medial or lateral) and the partial disruption (first or lesser). (From Bucholz RW, Heckman JD, Court-Brown C, et al., eds. *Rockwood and Green's Fractures in Adults.* 6th ed. Philadelphia: Lippincott Williams & Wilkins; 2006.)

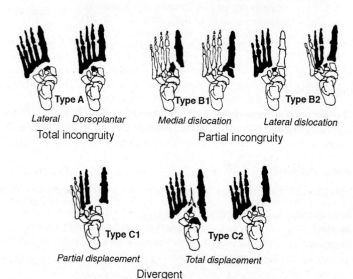

FIGURE 41.8 Myerson classification of Lisfranc fracture-dislocations. (From Myerson MS, Fisher RT, Burgess AR, et al. Fracture-dislocations of the tarsometatarsal joints: end results correlated with pathology and treatment. *Foot Ankle.* 1986;6:225–242.)

Total incongruity: Lateral and dorsoplantar
Partial incongruity: Medial and lateral
Divergent: Partial and total

Treatment

Nonoperative

- Injuries that present with painful weight bearing, pain with metatarsal motion, and tenderness to palpation but fail to exhibit any instability should be considered a sprain.
- Patients with nondisplaced ligamentous injuries with or without small plantar avulsion fractures of the metatarsal or tarsal bones should be placed in a well-molded short leg cast or removable boot.
- Initially, the patient is kept non–weight bearing with crutches and is permitted to bear weight as comfort allows.
- Repeat x-rays are necessary once swelling decreases, to detect osseous displacement.

Operative

- This should be considered when displacement of the tarsometatarsal joint is >2 mm.
- The best results are obtained through anatomic reduction and stable fixation.
- The most common approach is using two longitudinal incisions. The first is centered over the first/second intermetatarsal space, allowing identification of the neurovascular bundle and access to the medial two tarsometatarsal joints. A second longitudinal incision is made over the fourth metatarsal.
- The key to reduction is correction of the fracture-dislocation of the second metatarsal base. Clinical results suggest that accuracy and maintenance of reduction are of utmost importance and correlate directly with the overall outcome.
- Once reduction is accomplished, screw fixation is advocated for the medial column.
- The lateral metatarsals frequently reduce with the medial column, and Kirschner wire fixation is acceptable.
- If intercuneiform instability exists, one should use an intercuneiform screw.
- Stiffness from ORIF is not of significant concern because of the already limited motion of the tarsometatarsal joints.

Postoperative Management

- The foot is immobilized in a non–weight-bearing cast or boot for 6 to 8 weeks.

- Progressive weight bearing is then permitted as comfort allows.
- Advancement out of cast immobilization is done once pain-free, full weight bearing is achieved.
- Lateral column stabilization can be removed at 6 to 12 weeks.
- Medial fixation should not be removed for 4 to 6 months.
- Some advocate leaving screws indefinitely unless symptomatic.

Complications

- Posttraumatic arthritis
  - □ Present in most, but may not be symptomatic
  - □ Related to initial injury and adequacy of reduction
  - □ Treated with orthotics initially and arthrodesis late for the medial column
  - □ Possibly treated with interpositional arthroplasty for the lateral column
- Compartment syndrome
- Infection
- Complex mediated regional pain syndrome (RSD)
- Neurovascular injury
- Hardware failure

FRACTURES OF THE FOREFOOT

- The forefoot serves two purposes during gait.
  1. As a unit, it provides a broad plantar surface for load sharing. Weight-bearing studies show that the two sesamoids and the four lesser metatarsal heads share an equal amount of the forefoot load in normal gait.
  2. The forefoot is mobile in the sagittal plane. This enables the forefoot to alter the position of the individual metatarsal heads to accommodate uneven ground.

Metatarsals

Epidemiology

- This is a common injury; however, the true incidence of metatarsal shaft fractures is unknown, owing to the variety of physicians treating such injuries.

Anatomy

- Displaced fractures of the metatarsals result in the disruption of the major weight-bearing complex of the forefoot.

- Disruptions produce an alteration in the normal distribution of weight in the forefoot and lead to problems of metatarsalgia and transfer lesions (intractable plantar keratoses).

Mechanism of Injury

- **Direct:** This most commonly occurs when a heavy object is dropped on the forefoot.
- **Twisting:** This occurs with body torque when the toes are fixed, such as when a person catches the toes in a narrow opening with continued ambulation.
- **Avulsion:** This occurs particularly at the base of the fifth metatarsal.
- **Stress fractures:** These occur especially at the necks of the second and third metatarsals and the proximal fifth metatarsal.

Clinical Evaluation

- Patients typically present with pain, swelling, and tenderness over the site of fracture.
- Neurovascular evaluation is important, as well as assessment of soft tissue injury and ambulatory capacity.

Radiographic Evaluation

- In isolated injuries to the foot, weight-bearing films should be obtained in the AP and lateral planes.
- The lateral radiographic view of the metatarsals is important for judging sagittal plane displacement of the metatarsal heads.
- Oblique views can be helpful to detect minimally displaced fractures.
- Except in the case of an isolated direct blow, initial films should include the whole foot to rule out other potential collateral injuries that may also require attention.
- MRI and technetium bone scan may aid in the diagnosis of an occult stress fracture.

Classification

OTA Classification
See Fracture and Dislocation Classification Compendium at http://www.ota.org/compendium/compendium.html.

Specific Metatarsal Injuries

First Metatarsal Injuries
- This bone is larger and stronger than the lesser metatarsals and is less frequently injured.

- The lack of interconnecting ligaments between the first and second metatarsal bones allows independent motion.
- The first metatarsal head supports two sesamoid bones, which provide two of the six contact points of the forefoot.
- Injuries usually relate to direct trauma (often open and/or comminuted).
- Anatomic reduction and stable fixation are important.
- The best way to determine operative or nonoperative treatment is with stress radiographs. Manual displacement of the position of the first metatarsal through the joint or fracture site represents instability that requires fixation.
- If no evidence of instability can be seen on stress films, and no other injury of the midfoot or metatarsals is evident, isolated first metatarsal fractures can be adequately treated with a short leg cast or removable boot with weight bearing as tolerated for 4 to 6 weeks.
- Malunion, nonunion, and arthritic degeneration of the tarsometatarsal and metatarsophalangeal (MTP) joints are all possible complications of first metatarsal fractures. Transfer metatarsalgia to the lesser toes can occur with shortening of the metatarsal length.

Second, Third, and Fourth Metatarsal Injuries

- The four lesser metatarsals provide only one contact point each on the plantar weight-bearing surface.
- Significant ligamentous structures link each of the bones to their adjacent neighbors.
- Fractures of the central metatarsals are much more common than isolated first metatarsal fractures. Central metatarsal fractures may be isolated injuries or part of a more significant injury pattern.
- Indirect twisting mechanisms may result in a spiral pattern. One must be wary of Lisfranc injury with involvement of base of second metatarsal.
- Most isolated individual central metatarsal fractures can be treated closed with hard-soled shoes and progressive weight bearing as tolerated.
- The surgical criterion most often mentioned is any fracture displaying more than 10 degrees of deviation in the dorsal plantar plane or 3 to 4 mm translation in any plane.
- Complications of treating central metatarsal fractures usually stem from incomplete restoration of plantar anatomy.

Fifth Metatarsal Injuries

- These usually result from direct trauma.

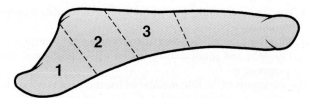

FIGURE 41.9 Three zones of proximal fifth metatarsal fracture. Zone *1*: Avulsion fracture. Zone *2*: Fracture at the metaphyseal–diaphyseal junction. Zone *3*: Proximal shaft stress fracture. (From Bucholz RW, Heckman JD, Court-Brown C, et al., eds. *Rockwood and Green's Fractures in Adults*. 6th ed. Philadelphia: Lippincott Williams & Wilkins; 2006.)

- Fractures are separated roughly into two groups, proximal base fractures and distal spiral fractures.
- Proximal fifth metatarsal fractures are further divided by the location of the fracture and the presence of prodromal symptoms (Fig. 41.9).
  - **Zone 1:** Cancellous tuberosity (93%)
    - Insertion of the peroneal brevis and plantar fascia
    - Involvement of the metatarsocuboid joint
  - **Zone 2:** Distal to the tuberosity (4%)
  - **Zone 3:** Distal to the proximal ligaments (3%)
    - Extension to the diaphysis for 1.5 cm
    - Usually stress fractures
- Zone 1 injury (pseudo-Jones)
  - This results from avulsion from lateral plantar aponeurosis.
  - Treatment is symptomatic, with a hard-soled shoe.
  - Healing is usually uneventful.
- Zone 2 injuries are true Jones fractures.
  - They result from adduction or inversion of the forefoot.
  - The fracture is caused by tensile stress along the lateral border of the metatarsal.
  - **Treatment is controversial:** Advocates recommend both weight bearing and non–weight bearing in a short leg cast as well as ORIF.
  - Union is frequently a concern.
- Zone 3 injuries are now referred to as proximal diaphyseal stress fractures.
  - These are relatively rare and seen mainly in athletes.
  - They occur in the proximal 1.5 cm of the diaphyseal shaft of the metatarsal.
  - Patients usually present with prodromal symptoms before complete fracture.

- □ This particular entity poses problems because of its tendency to nonunion.
- □ Initial treatment is between casted non–weight bearing for up to 3 months and surgical intervention with grafting and internal compression.
- The remainder of the fifth metatarsal fractures not resulting from a direct blow have been termed dancer's fractures.
  - □ The usual pattern is a spiral, oblique fracture progressing from distal-lateral to proximal-medial.
  - □ The mechanism of injury is a rotational force being applied to the foot while axially loaded in a plantar flexed position.
  - □ Treatment is symptomatic, with a hard-soled shoe.

Metatarsophalangeal Joints

- Mobility of the MTP joints is essential for forefoot comfort in normal gait; attempts should thus be made to salvage any motion at this level.

First Metatarsophalangeal Joint

Epidemiology

- Injuries to the first MTP joint are relatively common, especially in athletic activities or ballet.
- The incidence in US football and soccer has risen because of the use of artificial playing surfaces as well as lighter, more flexible shoes that permit enhanced motion at the MTP joint.

Anatomy

- The MTP joint is composed of a cam-shaped metatarsal head and a matched concave articulation on the proximal phalanx. These contours contribute little to the overall stability of the joint.
- Ligamentous constraints includes dorsal capsule reinforced by the extensor hallucis longus tendon, plantar plate (capsular ligament) reinforced by the flexor hallucis longus tendon, flexor hallucis brevis tendon, and medial and lateral collateral ligaments.
- The plantar capsule is a thick, weight-bearing structure with strong attachments to the base of the proximal phalanx. There is a thinner, more flexible attachment to the plantar aspect of the metatarsal head proximally. Imbedded in this plantar structure are the two sesamoids.

Mechanism of Injury

- **"Turf toe"**: This is a sprain of the first MTP joint. It reflects hyperextension injury to the first MTP joint as the ankle is in equinus, causing temporary subluxation with stretching on plantar capsule and plate.

■ In ballet dancers, injury may occur as a dancer "falls over" the maximally extended first MTP joint, injuring the dorsal capsule. Forced abduction may result in lateral capsular injury with possible avulsion from the base of the proximal phalanx.

■ Dislocation of the first MTP joint is usually the result of high-energy trauma, such as a motor vehicle accident, in which forced hyperextension of the joint occurs with gross disruption of the plantar capsule and plate.

Clinical Evaluation

■ Patients typically present with pain, swelling, and tenderness of the first MTP joint.

■ Pain may be reproduced with range of motion of the first MTP joint, especially at terminal dorsiflexion or plantar flexion.

■ Chronic injuries may present with decreased range of motion.

■ Most dislocations are dorsal with the proximal phalanx cocked up and displaced dorsally and proximally, producing a dorsal prominence and shortening of the toe.

Radiographic Evaluation

■ AP, lateral, and oblique views of the foot may demonstrate capsular avulsion or chronic degenerative changes indicative of longstanding injury.

Classification
Bowers and Martin

Grade I: Strain at the proximal attachment of the volar plate from the first metatarsal head

Grade II: Avulsion of the volar plate from the metatarsal head

Grade III: Impaction injury to the dorsal surface of the metatarsal head with or without an avulsion or chip fracture

Jahss Classification of First Metatarsophalangeal Dislocations

This is based on the integrity of the sesamoid complex.

Type I: Volar plate avulsed off the first metatarsal head, proximal phalanx displaced dorsally; intersesamoid ligament remaining intact and lying over the dorsum of the metatarsal head

Type IIA: Rupture of the intersesamoid ligament

Type IIB: Longitudinal fracture of either sesamoid

Treatment

■ First MTP sprains

 □ Rest, ice, compression, and elevation (RICE) and nonsteroidal anti-inflammatory medication are used.

- □ Protective taping with gradual return to activity is recommended; the patient may temporarily wear a hard-soled shoe with a rocker bottom for comfort.
- □ Pain usually subsides after 3 weeks of treatment, but an additional 3 weeks are usually necessary to regain strength and motion for return to competitive activity.
- □ Operative intervention is rarely indicated except in cases of intra-articular fractures or significant discrete instability. The presence of avulsion fragments and significant valgus instability may need to be addressed by ORIF or debridement and ligamentous repair.
- □ Displaced intra-articular fractures or osteochondral lesions should be fixed or debrided depending on their size.
- Dislocations
  - □ **Jahss Type I fracture:** Closed reduction may be initially attempted. However, if irreducible by closed means, it will require open reduction.
  - □ **Jahss Type IIA and Type IIB fractures:** These are easily reduced by closed means (longitudinal traction with or without hyperextension of the first MTP joint).
  - □ After reduction, the patient should be placed in a short leg walking cast with a toe extension for 3 to 4 weeks to allow capsular healing.
  - □ Displaced avulsion fractures of the base of the proximal phalanx should be fixed with either lag screws or a tension band technique. Small osteochondral fractures may be excised; larger fragments require reduction with Kirschner wires, compression screws, or headless screws.

Complications

- Hallux rigidus and degenerative arthritis complicate chronic injuries and may prevent return to competitive activity.
- **Posttraumatic osteoarthritis:** This may reflect chondral damage at the time of injury or may result from abnormal resultant laxity with subsequent degenerative changes.
- **Recurrent dislocation:** Uncommon, although it may occur in patients with connective tissue disorders.

Fractures and Dislocations of the Lesser Metatarsophalangeal Joints

Epidemiology

- "Stubbing" injuries are very common.
- The incidence is higher for the fifth MTP joint because its lateral position renders it more vulnerable to injury.

Anatomy

- Stability of the MTP joints is conferred by the articular congruity between the metatarsal head and the base of the proximal phalanx, the plantar capsule, the transverse metatarsal ligament, the flexor and extensor tendons, and the intervening lumbrical muscles.

Mechanism of Injury

- Dislocations are usually the result of low-energy stubbing injuries and are most commonly displaced dorsally.
- Avulsion or chip fractures may occur by the same mechanism.
- Comminuted intra-articular fractures may occur by direct trauma, usually from a heavy object dropped onto the dorsum of the foot.

Clinical Evaluation

- Patients typically present with pain, swelling, tenderness, and variable deformity of the involved digit.
- Dislocation of the MTP joint typically manifests as dorsal prominence of the base of the proximal phalanx.

Classification

Descriptive
- Location
- Angulation
- Displacement
- Comminution
- Intra-articular involvement
- Presence of fracture-dislocation

Treatment

Nonoperative
- Simple dislocations or nondisplaced fractures may be managed by gentle reduction with longitudinal traction and buddy taping for 4 weeks, with a rigid shoe orthosis to limit MTP joint motion, if necessary.

Operative
- Intra-articular fractures of the metatarsal head or the base of the proximal phalanx may be treated by excision of a small fragment, by benign neglect of severely comminuted fractures, or by ORIF with Kirschner wires or screw fixation for fractures with a large fragment.

Complications

- **Posttraumatic arthritis:** May result from articular incongruity or chondral damage at the time of injury.
- **Recurrent subluxation:** Uncommon and may be addressed by capsular imbrication, tendon transfer, cheilectomy, or osteotomy, if symptomatic.

Sesamoids

Epidemiology

- The incidence is highest with repetitive hyperextension at the MTP joints, such as in ballet dancers and runners.
- The medial sesamoid is more frequently fractured than the lateral owing to increased weight bearing on the medial side of the foot.

Anatomy

- The sesamoids are an integral part of the capsuloligamentous structure of the first MTP joint.
- They function within the joint complex as both shock absorbers and fulcrums in supporting the weight-bearing function of the first toe.
- Their position on either side of the flexor hallucis longus forms a bony tunnel to protect the tendon.
- Bipartite sesamoids are common (10% to 30% incidence in the general population) and must not be mistaken for acute fractures.
  - □ They are bilateral in 85% of cases.
  - □ They exhibit smooth, sclerotic, rounded borders.
  - □ They do not show callus formation after 2 to 3 weeks of immobilization.

Mechanism of Injury

- Direct blows such as a fall from a height or a simple landing from a jump as in ballet can cause acute fracture.
- Acute fractures can also occur with hyperpronation and axial loading seen with joint dislocations.
- Repetitive loading from improper running usually gives rise to the more insidious stress fracture.

Clinical Evaluation

- Patients typically present with pain well localized on the plantar aspect of the "ball" of the foot.

■ Local tenderness is present over the injured sesamoid, with accentuation of symptoms with passive extension or active flexion of the MTP joint.

Radiographic Evaluation

■ AP, lateral, and oblique views of the forefoot are usually sufficient to demonstrate transverse fractures of the sesamoids.
■ Occasionally, a tangential view of the sesamoids is necessary to visualize a small osteochondral or avulsion fracture.
■ Technetium bone scanning or MRI may be used to identify stress fractures not apparent by plain radiography.

Classification

Descriptive
■ Transverse versus longitudinal
■ Displacement
■ **Location:** Medial versus lateral

Treatment

■ Nonoperative management should initially be attempted, with soft padding combined with a short leg walking cast for 4 weeks followed by a bunion last shoe with a metatarsal pad for 4 to 8 weeks.
■ Sesamoidectomy is reserved for cases of failed conservative treatment. The patient is maintained postoperatively in a short leg walking cast for 3 to 4 weeks.

Complications

■ Sesamoid excision may result in problems of hallux valgus (medial sesamoid excision) or transfer pain to the remaining sesamoid owing to overload.

Phalanges and Interphalangeal Joints

Epidemiology

■ Phalangeal fractures are the most common injury to the forefoot.
■ The proximal phalanx of the fifth toe is the most often involved.

Anatomy

■ The first and fifth digits are in especially vulnerable positions for injury because they form the medial and lateral borders of the distal foot.

Mechanism of Injury

- A direct blow such as a heavy object dropped onto the foot usually causes a transverse or comminuted fracture.
- A stubbing injury is the result of axial loading with secondary varus or valgus force resulting in a spiral or oblique fracture pattern.

Clinical Evaluation

- Patients typically present with pain, swelling, and variable deformity of the affected digit.
- Tenderness can typically be elicited over the site of injury.

Radiographic Evaluation

- AP, lateral, and oblique views of the foot should be obtained.
- If possible, isolation of the digit of interest for the lateral radiograph may aid in visualization of the injury. Alternatively, the use of small dental radiographs placed between the toes has been described.
- Technetium bone scanning or MRI may aid in the diagnosis of stress fracture when the injury is not apparent on plain radiographs.

Classification

Descriptive
- **Location:** Proximal, middle, distal phalanx
- Angulation
- Displacement
- Comminution
- Intra-articular involvement
- Presence of fracture-dislocation

Treatment

- Nondisplaced fractures irrespective of articular involvement can be treated with a stiff-soled shoe and protected weight bearing with advancement as tolerated.
- Use of buddy taping between adjacent toes may provide pain relief and help to stabilize potentially unstable fracture patterns.
- Fractures with clinical deformity require reduction. Closed reduction is usually adequate and stable (Fig. 41.10).
- Operative reduction is reserved for those rare fractures with gross instability or persistent intra-articular discontinuity. This problem usually arises with an intra-articular fracture of the proximal phalanx of the great toe or multiple fractures of lesser toes.

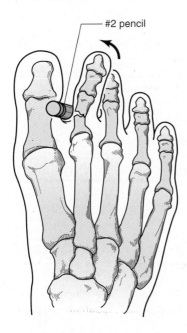

— #2 pencil

FIGURE 41.10 A method of closed reduction for displaced proximal phalanx fractures. A hard object, such as a pencil, is placed in the adjacent web space and is used as a fulcrum for reduction. (From Bucholz RW, Heckman JD, Court-Brown C, et al., eds. *Rockwood and Green's Fractures in Adults.* 6th ed. Philadelphia: Lippincott Williams & Wilkins; 2006.)

- A grossly unstable fracture of the proximal phalanx of the first toe should be reduced and stabilized with percutaneous Kirschner wires or mini-fragment screws.
- Unstable intra-articular fractures of any joint despite adequate reduction should be reduced and percutaneously pinned in place to avoid late malalignment.

Complications

- **Nonunion:** Uncommon.
- **Posttraumatic osteoarthritis:** May complicate fractures with intra-articular injury, with resultant incongruity. It may be disabling if it involves the great toe.

Dislocation of the Interphalangeal Joint

- Usually due to an axial load applied at the terminal end of the digit.
- Most such injuries occur in the proximal joint, are dorsal in direction, and occur in exposed, unprotected toes.
- Closed reduction under digital block and longitudinal traction comprise the treatment of choice for these injuries.
- Once reduced, the interphalangeal joint is usually stable and can be adequately treated with buddy taping and progressive activity as tolerated.

PART V

Pediatric Fractures and Dislocations

42

Pediatric Orthopaedic Surgery: General Principles

OVERVIEW

- The development and growth of the skeletal system from gestation to skeletal maturity create interrelated fibrous, tendinous, cartilaginous, and osseous changes resulting in patterns of susceptibility and reparative response that distinguish the pediatric patient from the adult.
- As a rule, the younger the patient, the greater the remodeling potential; thus, absolute anatomic reduction in a child is less important than in a comparable injury in an adult.

EPIDEMIOLOGY

- The overall mortality rate of children has fallen from 1 in 250 per year in 1900 to 1 in 4000 per year in 1986; this has been attributed to improved public education, preventive devices, and medical care.
- The leading cause of death in children age 1 to 14 is accidental trauma.
- Skeletal trauma accounts for 10% to 15% of all childhood injuries, with approximately 15% to 30% of these representing physeal injuries (phalanx fractures are the most common physeal injury).
- Over the past 50 years, the increasing fracture incidence in children has been mainly attributed to increased sports participation.
- From the ages of 0 to 16 years, 42% of boys will sustain at least one fracture compared with 27% of girls.
- The overall ratio of boys to girls who sustain a single, isolated fracture is 2.7:1. The peak incidence of fractures in boys occurs at age 16 years, with an incidence of 450 per 10,000 per year; the peak incidence in girls occurs at age 12 years, with an incidence of 250 per 10,000 per year.
- Open fractures in this population are rare (<5%).

ANATOMY

- Pediatric bone has a higher water content and lower mineral content per unit volume than adult bone. Therefore, pediatric bone has a lower modulus of elasticity (less brittle) and a higher ultimate strain to failure than adult bone. It is relatively stronger in tension than compression as compared to adult bone.

■ The physis (growth plate) is a unique cartilaginous structure that varies in thickness depending on age and location. It is frequently weaker than bone in torsion, shear, and bending, predisposing the child to injury through this delicate area.

■ **The physis is traditionally divided into four zones:** reserve (resting/germinal), proliferative, hypertrophic, and provisional calcification (or endochondral ossification) (Fig. 42.1).

■ The periosteum in a child is a thick fibrous structure (up to several millimeters) that encompasses the entire bone except the articular ends. The periosteum thickens and is continuous with the physis at the perichondral ring (ring of LaCroix), offering additional resistance to shear force.

■ As a general rule, ligaments in children are functionally stronger than bone. Therefore, a higher proportion of injuries that produce sprains in adults result in fractures in children.

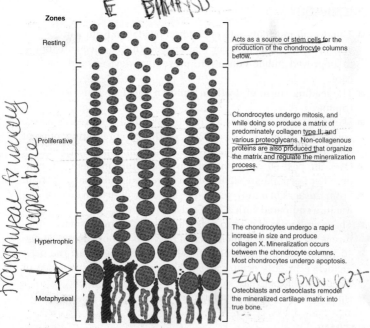

Zones

Resting — Acts as a source of stem cells for the production of the chondrocyte columns below.

Proliferative — Chondrocytes undergo mitosis, and while doing so produce a matrix of predominately collagen type II, and various proteoglycans. Non-collagenous proteins are also produced that organize the matrix and regulate the mineralization process.

Hypertrophic — The chondrocytes undergo a rapid increase in size and produce collagen X. Mineralization occurs between the chondrocyte columns. Most chondrocytes undergo apoptosis.

Metaphyseal — Osteoblasts and osteoclasts remodel the mineralized cartilage matrix into true bone.

FIGURE 42.1 The figure shows the process of endochondral ossification within the physis. Although not as organized, endochondral ossification follows a similar pattern during fracture repair. (From Bucholz RW, Heckman JD, Court-Brown C, et al., eds. *Rockwood and Green's Fractures in Adults.* 6th ed. Philadelphia: Lippincott Williams & Wilkins; 2006.)

■ The blood supply to the growing bone includes a rich metaphyseal circulation with fine capillary loops ending at the physis (in the neonate, small vessels may traverse the physis, ending in the epiphysis). *[handwritten: *cap loops ending at physis]*

MECHANISM OF INJURY

■ Because of structural differences, pediatric fractures tend to occur at lower energy than adult fractures. Most are a result of compression, torsion, or bending moments. *[handwritten: → TORUS FX stable]*
■ Compression fractures are found most commonly at the metaphyseal–diaphyseal junction and are referred to as "buckle fractures" or "torus fractures." Torus fractures rarely cause physeal injury, but they may result in acute angular deformity. Because torus fractures are impacted, they are stable and rarely require manipulative reduction. If manipulated, they usually regain the original fracture deformity as swelling subsides.
■ Torsional injuries result in two distinct patterns of fracture, depending on the maturity of the physis.
  □ In the very young child with a thick periosteum, the diaphyseal bone fails before the physis, resulting in a long spiral fracture.
  □ In the older child, similar torsional injury results in a physeal fracture. *[handwritten: → physeal angle fx]*
■ Bending moments in the young child cause "greenstick fractures" in which the bone is incompletely fractured, resulting in a plastic deformity on the concave side of the fracture. The fracture may need to be completed to obtain an adequate reduction.
■ Bending moments can also result in microscopic fractures that create plastic deformation of the bone with no visible fracture lines on plain radiographs; permanent deformity can result.
■ In the older child, bending moments result in transverse or short oblique fractures. Occasionally, a small butterfly fragment may be seen; however, because pediatric bone fails more easily in compression, there may only be a buckle of the cortex. *[handwritten: *pediatric fx fail more easily in compression]*

CLINICAL EVALUATION

■ Pediatric trauma patients should undergo full trauma evaluation with attention to airway, breathing, circulation, disability, and exposure. This should ideally be performed under the direction of a general surgical trauma team or pediatric emergency specialist (see Chapter 2).
■ Children are not good historians; therefore, keen diagnostic skills may be required for even the simplest problems. Parents may not be present at the time of injury and cannot always provide an

accurate history. It is important to evaluate the entire extremity because young children cannot always localize the site of injury.

- As a general rule, children will tolerate more pain and hardship than adults, especially if they understand what you are about to do, and trust you. It is therefore important to explain everything to children, listen to their suggestions whenever possible, and stop when they ask you to do so.
- Neurovascular evaluation is mandatory, both before and after manipulation.
- Periodic evaluation for compartment syndrome should be performed, particularly in a nonverbal patient who is irritable and who has a crush-type mechanism of injury. A high index of suspicion should be followed by compartment pressure monitoring.
- Intracompartmental blood loss from long bone fractures of the lower extremities can be a serious problem for the young child.
- Child abuse must be suspected in the following scenarios:
  □ Transverse femur fracture in a child <1 year old or a transverse humerus fracture in a child ≤3 years old.
  □ Metaphyseal corner fractures (caused by a traction/rotation mechanism).
  □ A history (mechanism of injury) that is inconsistent with the fracture pattern.
  □ An unwitnessed injury that results in fracture.
  □ Multiple fractures in various stages of healing.
  □ **Skin stigmata suggestive of abuse:** Multiple bruises in various stages of resolution, cigarette burns, etc.
- It is the obligation of the physician to ensure that the child is in a safe environment. If there is any question of abuse, the child should be admitted to the hospital and social services notified.

RADIOGRAPHIC EVALUATION

- Radiographs should include appropriate orthogonal views of the involved bone as well as the joint proximal and distal to the suspected area of injury. Should there be uncertainty as to the location of a suspected injury, the entire extremity may be placed on the radiographic plate.
- A thorough understanding of normal ossification patterns is necessary to adequately evaluate plain radiographs.
- Comparison views of the opposite extremity may aid in appreciating subtle deformities or in localizing a minimally displaced fracture. These should be obtained only when there is a question about the presence of a fracture seen on a radiograph of an injured extremity and not as a routine.

↗ posterior/anterior fat pad squirin
SC
Hun.
fx

- "Soft signs" such as the posterior fat pad sign in the elbow should be closely evaluated.
- A skeletal survey may be helpful in searching for other fractures in cases of suspected child abuse or multiple trauma.
- Computed tomography may be useful in evaluating complicated intra-articular fractures in the older child.
- Magnetic resonance imaging can be valuable in the preoperative evaluation of a complicated fracture; it may also help evaluate a fracture not clearly identifiable on plain films due to lack of ossification.
- Arthrograms are valuable in the intraoperative assessment of intra-articular fractures because radiolucent cartilaginous structures will not be apparent on fluoroscopic or plain radiographic evaluation.
- Bone scans may be used in the evaluation of osteomyelitis or tumor. *→ bone scan for spondylolisthesis /pars fx*
- Ultrasound can be useful for identifying epiphyseal separation in infants.

CLASSIFICATION

Salter–Harris Classification (Ogden Modification)

Pediatric physeal fractures have traditionally been described by the five-part Salter–Harris classification. The Ogden classification has extended the Salter–Harris classification to include periphyseal fractures, which do not radiographically appear to involve the physis but may interfere with the physeal blood supply and result in growth disturbance (Fig. 42.2). *→ as physeal blood supply is NOT in the physis*

Salter–Harris Types I to V

Type I: Transphyseal fracture involving the hypertrophic and calcified zones. Prognosis is usually excellent because of the preservation of the reserve and proliferative zones, although complete or partial growth arrest may occur in displaced fractures.

Type II: Transphyseal fracture that exits through the metaphysis. The metaphyseal fragment is known as the Thurston-Holland fragment. The periosteal hinge is intact on the side with the metaphyseal fragment. Prognosis is excellent, although complete or partial growth arrest may occur in displaced fractures.

Thurston-Holland Fragment

Type III: Transphyseal fracture that exits the epiphysis, causing intra-articular disruption as well as disrupting the reserve

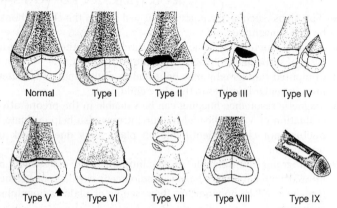

FIGURE 42.2 Salter–Harris (types I to V) and Ogden (Types VI to IX) classification of physeal injuries in children. (From Ogden JA. *Pocket Guide to Pediatric Fractures.* Baltimore: Williams & Wilkins; 1987:2542.)

and proliferative zones. Anatomic reduction and fixation without violating the physis are essential. Prognosis is guarded because partial growth arrest and resultant angular deformity are common problems.

Type IV: Fracture that traverses the epiphysis and the physis, exiting the metaphysis and disrupting all four zones of the physis. Anatomic reduction and fixation without violating the physis are essential. Prognosis is guarded because partial growth arrest and resultant angular deformity are common.

Type V: Crush injury to the physis. Diagnosis is generally made retrospectively. Prognosis is poor because growth arrest and partial physeal closure are common.

Ogden Types VI to IX

Type VI: Injury to the perichondral ring at the periphery of the physis. Usually, this is the result of an open injury. Close follow-up may allow early identification of a peripheral physeal bar that is amenable to excision. Prognosis is guarded because peripheral physeal bridges are common.

Type VII: Fracture involving the epiphysis only. This includes osteochondral fractures and epiphyseal avulsions. Prognosis is variable and depends on the location of the fracture and the amount of displacement.

Type VIII: Metaphyseal fracture. Primary circulation to the remodeling region of the cartilage cell columns is disrupted. Hypervascularity may cause angular overgrowth.

Type IX: Diaphyseal fracture. The mechanism for appositional growth (the periosteum) is interrupted. Prognosis is generally good if reduction is maintained. Cross-union between the tibia and fibula and between the radius and ulna may occur if there is intermingling of the respective periosteums.

TREATMENT

- Fracture management in the child differs from that in an adult owing to the presence of a thick periosteum in the case of a diaphyseal fracture or open physis in metaphyseal fractures.
  - □ The tough periosteum can be an aid to reduction because the periosteum on the concave side of the deformity is usually intact and can be made to serve as a hinge, preventing overreduction. Longitudinal traction will not reliably unlock the fragments when the periosteum is intact. Controlled recreation and exaggeration of the fracture deformity are effective means of disengaging the fragments to obtain reduction.
  - □ A periosteal flap entrapped in the fracture site or buttonholing of a sharp fracture end through the periosteum can prevent an adequate reduction.
  - □ Remanipulation of physeal injuries should not be attempted after 5 to 7 days.
- Unlike in the adult, considerable fracture deformity may be permitted, because the remodeling potential of the young child is great.
  - □ In general, the closer the fracture is to the joint (physis), the better the deformity is tolerated (e.g., 45 to 60 degrees of angulation in a proximal humeral fracture in a young child is permissible, whereas the midshaft fracture of the radius or tibia should be brought to within 10 degrees of normal alignment).
  - □ Rotational deformity does not spontaneously correct or remodel to an acceptable extent even in the young child and should be avoided.
- Severely comminuted or shortened fractures may require skin or skeletal traction. Traction pins should be placed proximal to the nearest distal physis (e.g., distal femur). Care should be taken not to place the traction pin through the physis.
- Fracture reduction should be performed under conscious sedation, followed by immobilization in either a splint or bivalved cast. Univalving, particularly with a fiberglass cast, does not provide adequate cast flexibility to accommodate extremity swelling.
- In children, casts or splints should encompass the joint proximal and distal to the site of injury because postimmobilization stiffness

is not a common problem for children. Only in rare fractures should short arm or short leg casts be applied initially as opposed to longer immobilization techniques (e.g., stable torus fractures of the distal radius).

☐ In some cases as soon as 2 days after cast application, children will run on short leg casts or climb monkey bars in short arm casts.

■ All fractures should be elevated at heart level, iced, and frequently monitored by responsible individuals, with attention to extremity warmth, color, capillary refill, and sensation. Patients in whom pronounced swelling is an issue or for whom the reliability of the guardian is in question should be admitted to the hospital for observation.

■ Fractures in which a reduction cannot be achieved or maintained should be splinted and the child prepared for general anesthesia, with which complete relaxation may be achieved.

■ Intra-articular fractures, Salter–Harris types III and IV, require anatomic reduction (<1 to 2 mm of displacement both vertically and horizontally) to restore articular congruity and to minimize physeal bar formation.

■ Indications for open reduction include:

☐ Most open fractures.

☐ Displaced intra-articular fractures (Salter–Harris types III and IV).

☐ Fractures with vascular injury.

☐ Fractures with an associated compartment syndrome.

☐ Unstable fractures that require abnormal positioning to maintain closed reduction.

COMPLICATIONS

Complications unique to pediatric fractures include the following:

■ **Complete growth arrest:** This may occur with physeal injuries in Salter–Harris fractures. It may result in limb length inequalities necessitating the use of orthotics, prosthetics, or operative procedures including epiphysiodesis or limb lengthening.

■ Overgrowth may be seen in certain pediatric fractures such as femoral diaphysis.

■ **Progressive angular or rotational deformities:** They may result from physeal injuries with partial growth arrest or malunion. They may occur in certain metaphyseal fractures such as the proximal tibia. If these result in significant functional disabilities or cosmetic deformity, they may require operative intervention, such as osteotomy, for correction.

■ **Osteonecrosis:** This may result from disruption of tenuous vascular supply in skeletally immature patients in whom vascular development is not complete (e.g., osteonecrosis of the femoral head in cases of slipped capital femoral epiphysis).

43

Pediatric Shoulder

PROXIMAL HUMERUS FRACTURES

Epidemiology

- These account for <5% of fractures in children.
- Incidence ranges from 1.2 to 4.4 per 10,000 per year.
- They are most common in adolescents owing to increased sports participation and are often metaphyseal, physeal, or both.
- Neonates may sustain birth trauma to the proximal humeral physis, representing 1.9% to 6.7% of physeal injuries (Fig. 43.1).

Anatomy

- Eighty percent of humeral growth occurs at the proximal physis, giving this region great remodeling potential.
- There are three centers of ossification in the proximal humerus:
  1. **Humeral head:** This ossifies at 6 months.
  2. **Greater tuberosity:** This ossifies at 1 to 3 years.
  3. **Lesser tuberosity:** This ossifies at 4 to 5 years.
     The greater and lesser tuberosities coalesce at 6 to 7 years and then fuse with the humeral head between 7 and 13 years of age.
- The joint capsule extends to the metaphysis, rendering some fractures of the metaphysis intracapsular (Fig. 43.2).

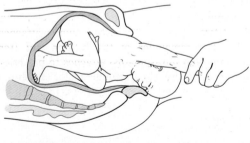

FIGURE 43.1 Hyperextension or rotation of the ipsilateral arm may result in a proximal humeral or physeal injury during birth. (From Bucholz RW, Heckman JD, Court-Brown C, et al., eds. *Rockwood and Green's Fractures in Adults.* 6th ed. Philadelphia: Lippincott Williams & Wilkins; 2006.)

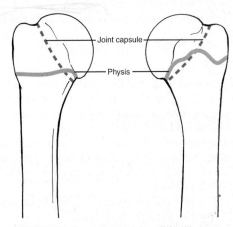

FIGURE 43.2 The anatomy of the proximal humerus.
(From Bucholz RW, Heckman JD, Court-Brown C,
et al., eds. *Rockwood and Green's Fractures in Adults.*
6th ed. Philadelphia: Lippincott Williams & Wilkins;
2006.)

- The primary vascular supply is via the anterolateral ascending branch of the anterior circumflex artery, with a small portion of the greater tuberosity and inferior humeral head supplied by branches from the posterior circumflex artery.
- The physis closes at age 14 to 17 years in girls and at age 16 to 18 years in boys.
- The physeal apex is posteromedial and is associated with a strong, thick periosteum.
- Type I physeal fractures occur through the hypertrophic zone adjacent to the zone of provisional calcification. The layer of embryonal cartilage is preserved, leading to normal growth.
- **Muscular deforming forces:** The subscapularis attaches to lesser tuberosity. The remainder of the rotator cuff (teres minor, supraspinatus, and infraspinatus) attaches to posterior epiphysis and greater tuberosity. The pectoralis major attaches to anterior medial metaphysis, and the deltoid connects to the lateral shaft.

Mechanism of Injury

- **Indirect:** This results from a fall backward onto an outstretched hand with the elbow extended and the wrist dorsiflexed. Birth injuries may occur as the arm is hyperextended or rotated as the infant is being delivered. Shoulder dystocia is strongly associated with macrosomia from maternal diabetes.

■ **Direct:** Direct trauma to the posterolateral aspect of the shoulder can occur.

Clinical Evaluation

■ Newborns present with pseudoparalysis with the arm held in extension. A history of birth trauma may be elicited. A fever is variably present. Infection, clavicle fracture, shoulder dislocation, and brachial plexus injury must be ruled out.

■ Older children present with pain, dysfunction, swelling, and ecchymosis, and the humeral shaft fragment may be palpable anteriorly. The shoulder is tender to palpation, with a painful range of motion that may reveal crepitus.

■ Typically, the arm is held in internal rotation to prevent pull of the pectoralis major on the distal fragment.

■ A careful neurovascular examination is required, including the axillary, musculocutaneous, radial, ulnar, and median nerves.

Radiographic Evaluation

■ Anteroposterior (AP), lateral (in the plane of the scapula; "Y" view), and axillary views should be obtained, with comparison views of the opposite side if necessary.

■ **Ultrasound:** This may be necessary in the newborn because the epiphysis is not yet ossified.

■ Computed tomography may be useful to help diagnose and classify posterior dislocations and complex fractures.

■ Magnetic resonance imaging is more useful than bone scan to detect occult fractures because the physis normally has increased radionuclide uptake, making a bone scan difficult to interpret.

Classification

Salter–Harris (Fig. 43.3)

Type I: Separation through the physis; usually a birth injury
Type II: Usually occurring in adolescents (>12 years); metaphyseal fragment always posteromedial
Type III: Intra-articular fracture; uncommon; associated with dislocations
Type IV: Rare; intra-articular transmetaphyseal fracture; associated with open fractures

Neer–Horowitz Classification of Proximal Humeral Plate Fractures

Grade I: <5-mm displacement
Grade II: Displacement less than one-third the width of the shaft

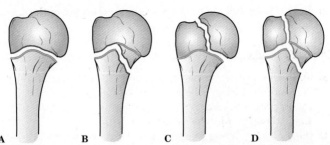

FIGURE 43.3 Physeal fractures of the proximal humerus. **(A)** Salter–Harris type I. **(B)** Salter–Harris type II. **(C)** Salter–Harris type III. **(D)** Salter–Harris type IV. (From Bucholz RW, Heckman JD, Court-Brown C, et al., eds. *Rockwood and Green's Fractures in Adults.* 6th ed. Philadelphia: Lippincott Williams & Wilkins; 2006.)

Grade III: Displacement one-third to two-thirds the width of the shaft

Grade IV: Displacement greater than two-thirds the width of the shaft, including total displacement

Treatment

Treatment depends on the age of the patient as well as the fracture pattern.

Newborns

- Most fractures are Salter–Harris type I. The prognosis is excellent.
- Ultrasound can be used to guide reduction.
- **Closed reduction:** This is the treatment of choice and is achieved by applying gentle traction, 90 degrees of flexion, then 90 degrees of abduction and external rotation.
- **Stable fracture:** The arm is immobilized against the chest for 5 to 10 days.
- **Unstable fracture:** The arm is held abducted and is externally rotated for 3 to 4 days to allow early callus formation.

Age 1 to 4 Years

- These are typically Salter–Harris type I or, less frequently, type II.
- Treatment is by closed reduction.
- The arm is held in a sling for 10 days followed by progressive activity.
- Extensive remodeling is possible.

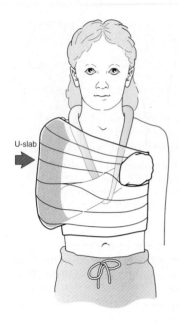

U-slab

FIGURE 43.4 Sling and swathe for immobilization of proximal humeral fracture. (From Bucholz RW, Heckman JD, Court-Brown C, et al., eds. *Rockwood and Green's Fractures in Adults*. 6th ed. Philadelphia: Lippincott Williams & Wilkins; 2006.)

Age 5 to 12 Years

- The metaphyseal fracture (type II) is the most common in this age group because this area is undergoing the most rapid remodeling and is therefore structurally vulnerable.
- Treatment is by closed reduction. Most are stable following reduction.
- **Stable fracture:** A sling and swathe is used (Fig. 43.4).
- **Unstable fracture:** The arm is placed in a shoulder spica cast with the arm in the salute position for 2 to 3 weeks, after which the patient may be placed in a sling, with progressive activity.

Age 12 Years to Maturity

- These are either Salter–Harris type II or, less frequently, type I.
- Treatment is typically by closed reduction.
- There is less remodeling potential than in younger children.
- **Stable fracture:** A sling and swathe is used for 2 to 3 weeks followed by progressive range-of-motion exercises.
- **Unstable fracture and Salter–Harris type IV:** Immobilization is maintained in a shoulder spica cast with the arm in the salute position for 2 to 3 weeks, after which the patient may be placed in a sling, with progressive activity.

■ One should consider surgical stabilization for displaced fractures in adolescents.

Acceptable Deformity

Age 1 to 4 years:	70 degrees of angulation with any amount of displacement
Age 5 to 12 years:	40 to 45 degrees of angulation and displacement of one-half the width of the shaft
Age 12 years to maturity:	15 to 20 degrees of angulation and displacement of <30% the width of the shaft

Open Treatment

■ Indications for open reduction and internal fixation include
  □ Open fractures.
  □ Fractures with associated neurovascular compromise.
  □ Salter–Harris type III and IV fractures with displacement.
  □ Irreducible fractures with soft tissue interposition (biceps tendon).
■ In children, fixation is most often achieved with percutaneous, smooth Kirschner wires or Steinmann pins.

Prognosis

■ Neer–Horowitz grade I and II fractures do well because of the remodeling potential of the proximal humeral physis.
■ Neer–Horowitz grade III and IV fractures may be left with up to 3 mm of shortening or residual angulation. This is well tolerated by the patient and is often clinically insignificant.
■ As a rule, the younger the patient, the higher the potential for remodeling and the greater the acceptable initial deformity.

Complications

■ **Proximal humerus varus:** Rare, usually affecting patients less than 1 year of age, but it may complicate fractures in patients as old as 5 years of age. It may result in a decrease of the neck-shaft angle to 90 degrees with humeral shortening and mild to moderate loss of glenohumeral abduction. Remodeling potential is great in this age group, however, so observation alone may result in improvement. Proximal humeral osteotomy may be performed in cases of extreme functional limitation.
■ **Limb length inequality:** Rarely significant and tends to occur more commonly in surgically treated patients as opposed to those treated nonoperatively.

- **Loss of motion:** Rare and tends to occur more commonly in surgically treated patients. Older children tend to have more postfracture difficulties with shoulder stiffness than younger children.
- **Inferior glenohumeral subluxation:** May complicate patients with Salter–Harris type II fractures of the proximal humerus secondary to a loss of deltoid and rotator cuff tone. It may be addressed by a period of immobilization followed by rotator cuff strengthening exercises.
- **Osteonecrosis:** May occur with associated disruption of the anterolateral ascending branch of the anterior circumflex artery, especially in fractures or dislocations that are not acutely reduced. This is almost never seen in closed fractures.
- **Nerve injury:** Most commonly axillary nerve injury in fracture-dislocations. Lesions that do not show signs of recovery in 4 months should be explored.
- **Growth arrest:** May occur when the physis is crushed or significantly displaced or when a physeal bar forms. It may require excision of the physeal bar. Limb lengthening may be required for functional deficits or severe cosmetic deformity.

CLAVICLE FRACTURES

Epidemiology

- Most frequent fracture in children (8% to 15% of all pediatric fractures).
- It occurs in 0.5% of normal deliveries and in 1.6% of breech deliveries (accounts for 90% of obstetric fractures). The incidence of birth fractures involving the clavicle ranges from 2.8 to 7.2 per 1000 term deliveries, and clavicular fractures account for 84% to 92% of all obstetric fractures.
- In macrosomic infants (>4000 g), the incidence is 13%.
- Eighty percent of clavicle fractures occur in the midshaft, most frequently just lateral to the insertion of the subclavius muscle, which protects the underlying neurovascular structures.
- Ten percent to 15% of clavicle fractures involve the lateral aspect, with the remainder (5%) representing medial fractures.

Anatomy

- The clavicle is the first bone to ossify; this occurs by intramembranous ossification.
- The secondary centers develop via endochondral ossification.
  - □ The medial epiphysis, where 80% of growth occurs, ossifies at age 12 to 19 years and fuses by age 22 to 25 years (last bone to fuse).
  - □ The lateral epiphysis does not ossify until it fuses at age 19 years.

- Clavicular range of motion involves rotation about its long axis (approximately 50 degrees) accompanied by elevation of 30 degrees with full shoulder abduction and 35 degrees of anterior–posterior angulation with shoulder protraction and retraction.
- The periosteal sleeve always remains in the anatomic position. Therefore, remodeling is ensured.

Mechanism of Injury

- **Indirect:** Fall onto an outstretched hand.
- **Direct:** This is the most common mechanism, resulting from direct trauma to the clavicle or acromion; it carries the highest incidence of injury to the underlying neurovascular and pulmonary structures.
- **Birth injury:** Occurs during delivery of the shoulders through a narrow pelvis with direct pressure from the symphysis pubis or from obstetric pressure directly applied to the clavicle during delivery.
- Medial clavicle fractures or dislocations usually represent Salter–Harris type I or II fractures. True sternoclavicular joint dislocations are rare. The inferomedial periosteal sleeve remains intact and provides a scaffold for remodeling. Because 80% of the growth occurs at the medial physis, there is great potential for remodeling.
- Lateral clavicle fractures occur as a result of direct trauma to the acromion. The coracoclavicular ligaments always remain intact and are attached to the inferior periosteal tube. The acromioclavicular ligament is always intact and is attached to the distal fragment.

Clinical Evaluation

- Birth fractures of the clavicle are usually obvious, with an asymmetric, palpable mass overlying the fractured clavicle. An asymmetric Moro reflex is usually present. Nonobvious injuries may be misdiagnosed as congenital muscular torticollis because the patient will often turn his or her head toward the fracture to relax the sternocleidomastoid muscle.
- Children with clavicle fractures typically present with a painful, palpable mass along the clavicle. Tenderness is usually discrete over the site of injury, but it may be diffuse in cases of plastic bowing. There may be tenting of the skin, crepitus, and ecchymosis.
- Neurovascular status must be carefully evaluated because injuries to the brachial plexus and upper extremity vasculature may result. R/O Erb palsy.

- Pulmonary status must be assessed, especially if direct trauma is the mechanism of injury. Medial clavicular fractures may be associated with tracheal compression, especially with severe posterior displacement.
- Differential diagnosis
  - □ **Cleidocranial dysostosis:** This defect in intramembranous ossification, most commonly affecting the clavicle, is characterized by absence of the distal end of the clavicle, a central defect, or complete absence of the clavicle. Treatment is symptomatic only.
  - □ **Congenital puseudarthrosis:** This most commonly occurs at the junction of the middle and distal thirds of the right clavicle, with smooth, pointed bone ends. Puseudarthrosis of the left clavicle is found only in patients with dextrocardia. Patients present with no antecedent history of trauma, only a palpable bump. Treatment is supportive only, with bone grafting and intramedullary fixation reserved for symptomatic cases.

Radiographic Evaluation

- Ultrasound evaluation may be used in the diagnosis of clavicular fracture in neonates.
- Because of the S shape of the clavicle, an AP view is usually sufficient for diagnostic purposes; however, special views have been described in cases in which a fracture is suspected but not well visualized on a standard AP view (Fig. 43.5).
  - □ **Cephalic tilt view (cephalic tilt of 35 to 40 degrees):** This minimizes overlapping structures to better show degree of displacement.
  - □ **Apical oblique view (injured side rotated 45 degrees toward tube with a cephalic tilt of 20 degrees):** This is best for visualizing nondisplaced middle third fractures.
- Patients with difficulty breathing should have an AP radiograph of the chest to evaluate possible pneumothorax or associated rib fractures.
- Computed tomography may be useful for the evaluation of medial clavicular fractures or suspected dislocation because most represent Salter–Harris type I or II fractures rather than true dislocations.

Classification

Descriptive

- Location
- Open versus closed

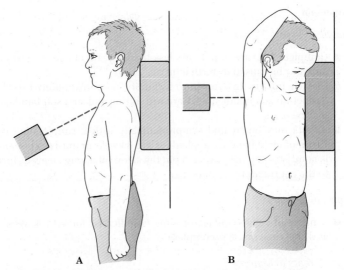

FIGURE 43.5 (A) Cephalic tilt views. **(B)** Apical lordotic view. (From Bucholz RW, Heckman JD, Court-Brown C, et al., eds. *Rockwood and Green's Fractures in Adults*. 6th ed. Philadelphia: Lippincott Williams & Wilkins; 2006.)

- Displacement
- Angulation
- **Fracture type:** segmental, comminuted, greenstick, etc.

Allman (Fig. 43.6)

Type I: Middle third (most common)
Type II: Distal to the coracoclavicular ligaments (lateral third)
Type III: Proximal (medial) third

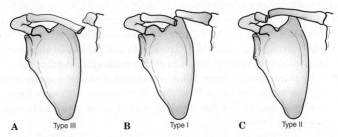

A   Type III   **B**   Type I   **C**   Type II

FIGURE 43.6 (A) Fracture of the medial third of the clavicle. **(B)** Fracture of the middle third of the clavicle. **(C)** Fracture of the lateral third of the clavicle. (From Bucholz RW, Heckman JD, Court-Brown C, et al., eds. *Rockwood and Green's Fractures in Adults*. 6th ed. Philadelphia: Lippincott Williams & Wilkins; 2006.)

Treatment

Newborn to Age 2 Years

- Complete fracture in patients less than 2 years of age is unusual and may be caused by birth injury.
- Clavicle fracture in a newborn will unite in approximately 1 week. Reduction is not indicated. Care with lifting and/or a soft bandage may be used.
- Infants may be treated symptomatically with a simple sling or figure-of-eight bandage applied for 2 to 3 weeks or until the patient is comfortable. One may also pin the sleeve of a long-sleeved shirt to the contralateral shoulder.

Age 2 to 12 Years

- A figure-of-eight bandage or sling is indicated for 2 to 4 weeks, at which time union is complete.

Age 12 Years to Maturity

- The incidence of complete fracture is higher.
- A figure-of-eight bandage or sling is used for 3 to 4 weeks. However, figure-of-eight bandages are often poorly tolerated and have been associated with ecchymosis, compression of axillary vessels, and brachial plexopathy.
- If the fracture is grossly displaced with tenting of the skin, one should consider closed or open reduction with internal fixation. Significant shortening and displacement are relative indications in older adolescents.

Open Treatment

- Operative treatment is indicated in open fractures and those with neurovascular compromise.
- Comminuted fragments that tent the skin may be manipulated and the dermis released from the bone ends with a towel clip. Typically, bony fragments are placed in the periosteal sleeve and the soft tissue repaired. One can also consider internal fixation.
- Bony prominences from callus will usually remodel; exostectomy may be performed at a later date if necessary, although from a cosmetic standpoint the surgical scar is often more noticeable than the prominence.

Complications

- **Neurovascular compromise:** Rare in children because of the thick periosteum that protects the underlying structures, although brachial plexus and vascular injury (subclavian vessels) may occur with severe displacement.

■ **Malunion:** Rare because of the high remodeling potential; it is well tolerated when present, and cosmetic issues of the bony prominence are the only long-term issue.

■ **Nonunion:** Rare (1% to 3%); it is probably associated with a congenital puseudarthrosis; it never occurs at <12 years of age.

■ **Pulmonary injury:** Rare injuries to the apical pulmonary parenchyma with pneumothorax may occur, especially with severe, direct trauma in an anterosuperior to posteroinferior direction.

ACROMIOCLAVICULAR JOINT INJURIES

Epidemiology

■ Rare in children less than 16 years of age.

■ The true incidence is unknown because many of these injuries actually represent pseudodislocation of the acromioclavicular joint.

Anatomy

■ The acromioclavicular joint is a diarthrodial joint; in mature individuals, an intra-articular disc is present.

■ The distal clavicle is surrounded by a thick periosteal sleeve that extends to the acromioclavicular joint.

Mechanism of Injury

■ Athletic injuries and falls comprise the majority of acromioclavicular injuries, with direct trauma to the acromion.

■ Unlike acromioclavicular injuries in adults, in children the coraco-clavicular (conoid and trapezoid) ligaments remain intact. Because of the tight approximation of the coracoclavicular ligaments to the periosteum of the distal clavicle, true dislocation of the acromioclavicular joint is rare.

■ The defect is a longitudinal split in the superior portion of the periosteal sleeve through which the clavicle is delivered, much like a banana being peeled from its skin.

Clinical Evaluation

■ The patient should be examined while in the standing or sitting position to allow the upper extremity to be dependent, thus stressing the acromioclavicular joint and emphasizing deformity.

■ A thorough shoulder examination should be performed, including assessment of neurovascular status and possible associated upper extremity injuries. Inspection may reveal an apparent step-off deformity of the injured acromioclavicular joint, with possible tenting of the skin overlying the distal clavicle. Range of motion may be limited by pain. Tenderness may be elicited over the acromioclavicular joint.

Radiographic Evaluation

- A standard trauma series of the shoulder (AP, scapular-Y, and axillary views) is usually sufficient for the recognition of acromioclavicular injury, although closer evaluation includes targeted views of the AC joint, which requires one-third to one-half the radiation to avoid overpenetration.
- Ligamentous injury may be assessed via stress radiographs in which weights (5 to 10 lb) are strapped to the wrists and an AP radiograph is taken of both shoulders for comparison.

Classification (Dameron and Rockwood) (Fig. 43.7)

Type I: Mild sprain of the acromioclavicular ligaments without periosteal tube disruption; distal clavicle stable to examination and no radiographic abnormalities

Type II: Partial disruption of the periosteal tube with mild distal clavicle instability; slight widening of the acromioclavicular space appreciated on radiographs

Type III: Longitudinal split of the periosteal tube with gross instability of the distal clavicle to examination; superior displacement of 25% to >100% present on radiographs as compared with the normal, contralateral shoulder

Type IV: Posterior displacement of the distal clavicle through a periosteal sleeve disruption with buttonholing through the trapezius; AP radiographs demonstrating superior displacement similar to type II injuries, but axillary radiographs demonstrating posterior displacement

Type V: Type III injury with 100% displacement; distal clavicle may be subcutaneous to palpation, with possible disruption of deltoid or trapezial attachments

Type VI: Infracoracoid displacement of the distal clavicle as a result of a superior-to-inferior force vector

Treatment

- For types I to III, nonoperative treatment is indicated, with sling immobilization, ice, and early range-of-motion exercises as pain subsides. Remodeling is expected. Complete healing generally takes place in 4 to 6 weeks.

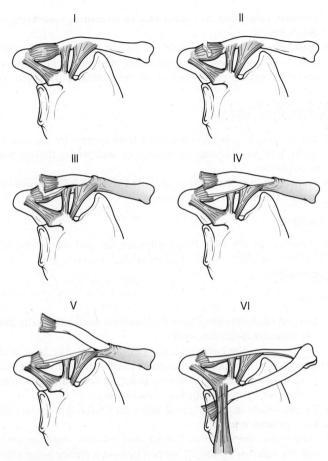

FIGURE 43.7 Dameron and Rockwood classification of distal/lateral fractures. (From Bucholz RW, Heckman JD, Court-Brown C, et al., eds. *Rockwood and Green's Fractures in Adults.* 6th ed. Philadelphia: Lippincott Williams & Wilkins; 2006.)

- Treatment for types IV to VI is operative, with reduction of the clavicle and repair of the periosteal sleeve. Internal fixation may be needed.

Complications

- **Neurovascular injury:** This is rare and is associated with posteroinferior displacement. The intact periosteal sleeve is thick and usually provides protection to neurovascular structures underlying the distal clavicle.

- **Open lesion:** Severe displacement of the distal clavicle, such as with type V acromioclavicular dislocation, may result in tenting of the skin, with possible laceration necessitating irrigation and debridement.

SCAPULA FRACTURES

- The scapula is relatively protected from trauma by the thoracic cavity and the rib cage anteriorly as well as by the encasing musculature.
- Scapular fractures are often associated with other life-threatening injuries that have greater priority.

Epidemiology

- These constitute only 1% of all fractures and 5% of shoulder fractures in the general population and are even less common in children.

Anatomy

- The scapula forms from intramembranous ossification. The body and spine are ossified at birth.
- The center of the coracoid is ossified at 1 year. The base of the coracoid and the upper one-fourth of the glenoid ossify by 10 years. A third center at the tip of the coracoid ossifies at a variable time. All three structures fuse by age 15 to 16 years.
- The acromion fuses by age 22 years via two to five centers that begin to form at puberty.
- Centers for the vertebral border and inferior angle appear at puberty and fuse by age 22 years. The center for the lower three-fourths of the glenoid appears at puberty and fuses by age 22 years.
- The suprascapular nerve traverses the suprascapular notch on the superior aspect of the scapula, medial to the base of the coracoid process, thus rendering it vulnerable to fractures in this region.
- The superior shoulder suspensory complex (SSSC) is a circular group of both bony and ligamentous attachments (acromion, glenoid, coracoid, coracoclavicular ligament, and distal clavicle). The integrity of the ring is breached only after more than one violation. This can dictate the treatment approach (Fig. 43.8).

Mechanism of Injury

- In children, most scapula fractures represent avulsion fractures associated with glenohumeral joint injuries. Other fractures are usually the result of high-energy trauma.

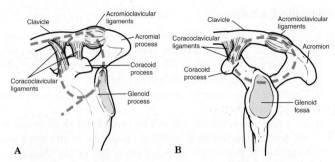

FIGURE 43.8 Superior shoulder suspensory complex. **(A)** Anteroposterior view of the bonesoft tissue ring and superior and inferior bone struts. **(B)** Lateral view of the bone and soft tissue ring. (From Bucholz RW, Heckman JD, Court-Brown C, et al., eds. *Rockwood and Green's Fractures in Adults*. 6th ed. Philadelphia: Lippincott Williams & Wilkins; 2006.)

- Isolated scapula fractures are extremely uncommon, particularly in children; child abuse should be suspected unless a clear and consistent mechanism of injury exists.
- The presence of a scapula fracture should raise suspicion of associated injuries because 35% to 98% of scapula fractures occur in the presence of other injuries including
  □ **Ipsilateral upper torso injuries:** fractured ribs, clavicle, sternum, shoulder trauma.
  □ **Pneumothorax:** seen in 11% to 55% of scapular fractures.
  □ **Pulmonary contusion:** present in 11% to 54% of scapula fractures.
  □ **Injuries to neurovascular structures:** brachial plexus injuries, vascular avulsions.
  □ **Spinal column injuries:** 20% lower cervical spine, 76% thoracic spine, 4% lumbar spine.
  □ **Others:** concomitant skull fractures, blunt abdominal trauma, pelvic fracture, and lower extremity injuries, which are all seen with higher incidences in the presence of a scapula fracture.
- Rate of mortality in setting of scapula fractures may approach 14%.

Clinical Evaluation

- Full trauma evaluation, with attention to airway, breathing, circulation, disability, and exposure should be performed, if indicated.
- Patients typically present with the upper extremity supported by the contralateral hand in an adducted and immobile positions, with painful range of shoulder motion, especially with abduction.
- A careful examination for associated injures should be pursued, with a comprehensive assessment of neurovascular status and an evaluation of breath sounds.

Radiographic Evaluation

- Initial radiographs should include a trauma series of the shoulder, consisting of true AP, axillary, and scapular-Y (true scapular lateral) views; these generally are able to demonstrate most glenoid, neck, body, and acromion fractures.
  - □ The axillary view may be used to delineate acromial and glenoid rim fractures further.
  - □ An acromial fracture should not be confused with an *os acromiale*, which is a rounded, unfused apophysis at the epiphyseal level and is present in approximately 3% of the population. When present, it is bilateral in 60% of cases. The os is typically in the anteroinferior aspect of distal acromion.
  - □ *Glenoid hypoplasia*, or *scapular neck dysplasia*, is an unusual abnormality that may resemble glenoid impaction and may be associated with humeral head or acromial abnormalities. It has a benign course and is usually noted incidentally.
- A 45-degree cephalic tilt (Stryker notch) radiograph is helpful to identify coracoid fractures.
- Computed tomography may be useful for further characterizing intra-articular glenoid fractures.
- Because of the high incidence of associated injuries, especially to thoracic structures, a chest radiograph is an essential part of the evaluation.

Classification

Classification by Location

Body (35%) and Neck (27%) Fractures
I.   Isolated versus associated disruption of the clavicle
II. Displaced versus nondisplaced

Glenoid Fractures (Ideberg and Goss) (Fig. 43.9)
Type IA: Anterior avulsion fracture
Type IB: Posterior rim avulsion
Type II: Transverse with inferior free fragment
Type III: Upper third including coracoid
Type IV Horizontal fracture extending through body
Type V: Combined II, III, and IV
Type VI: Extensively comminuted

- These can be associated with scapular neck fractures and shoulder dislocations.
- Treatment is nonoperative in most cases. Open reduction and internal fixation are indicated if a large anterior or posterior rim fragment is associated with glenohumeral instability.

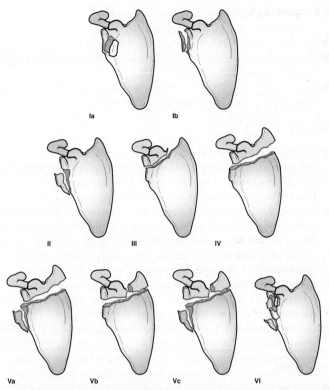

FIGURE 43.9 General classification of scapular/glenoid fractures. (From Bucholz RW, Heckman JD, Court-Brown C, et al., eds. *Rockwood and Green's Fractures in Adults.* 6th ed. Philadelphia: Lippincott Williams & Wilkins; 2006.)

Coracoid Fractures
These are isolated versus associated disruption of the acromioclavicular joint.

- These are avulsion-type injuries, usually occurring through the common physis of the base of the coracoid and the upper one-fourth of the glenoid.
- The coracoacromial ligament remains intact, but the acromioclavicular ligaments may be stretched.

Acromial Fractures
I: Nondisplaced
IA: Avulsion
IB: Direct trauma

II: Displaced without subacromial narrowing
III: Displaced with subacromial narrowing

- These are rare, usually the result of a direct blow.
- The os acromiale, which is an unfused ossification center, should not be mistaken for a fracture.
- Conservative treatment is recommended unless there is severe displacement of the acromioclavicular joint.

Treatment

- Scapula body fractures in children are treated nonoperatively, with the surrounding musculature maintaining reasonable proximity of fracture fragments. Operative treatment is indicated for fractures that fail to unite, which may benefit from partial body excision.
- Scapula neck fractures that are nondisplaced and not associated with clavicle fractures may be treated nonoperatively. Significantly displaced fractures may be treated in a thoracobrachial cast. Associated clavicular disruption, either by fracture or ligamentous instability (i.e., multiple disruptions in the SSSC) are generally treated operatively with open reduction and internal fixation of the clavicle alone or include open reduction and internal fixation of the scapula fracture through a separate incision.
- Coracoid fractures that are nondisplaced may be treated with sling immobilization. Displaced fractures are usually accompanied by acromioclavicular dislocation or lateral clavicular injury and should be treated with open reduction and internal fixation.
- Acromial fractures that are nondisplaced may be treated with sling immobilization. Displaced acromial fractures with associated subacromial impingement should be reduced and stabilized with screw or plate fixation.
- Glenoid fractures in children, if not associated with glenohumeral instability, are rarely symptomatic when healed and can generally be treated nonoperatively if they are nondisplaced.

Type I: Fractures involving greater than one-fourth of the glenoid fossa that result in instability may be amenable to open reduction and lag screw fixation.

Type II: Inferior subluxation of the humeral head may result, necessitating open reduction, especially when associated with a greater than 5 mm articular step-off. An anterior approach usually provides adequate exposure.

Type III: Reduction may be difficult; fractures occur through the junction between the ossification centers of the glenoid and are often accompanied by a fractured acromion or clavicle, or an acromioclavicular separation. Open reduction and internal fixation followed by early range of motion are indicated.

Types IV, V, VI: These are difficult to reduce, with little bone stock for adequate fixation in pediatric patients. A posterior approach is generally utilized for open reduction and internal fixation with Kirschner wire, plate, suture, or screw fixation for displaced fractures.

Complications

- **Posttraumatic osteoarthritis:** This may result from a failure to restore articular congruity.
- **Associated injuries:** These account for most serious complications because of the high-energy nature of these injuries.
- **Decreased shoulder motion:** Secondary to subacromial impingement from acromial fracture.
- **Malunion:** Fractures of the scapula body generally unite with nonoperative treatment; when malunion occurs, it is generally well tolerated but may result in painful scapulothoracic crepitus.
- **Nonunion:** Extremely rare, but when present and symptomatic it may require open reduction and plate fixation for adequate relief.
- **Suprascapular nerve injury:** May occur in association with scapula body, scapula neck, or coracoid fractures that involve the suprascapular notch.

GLENOHUMERAL DISLOCATIONS

Epidemiology

- Rare in children; Rowe reported that only 1.6% of shoulder dislocations occurred in patients <10 years of age, whereas 10% occurred in patients 10 to 20 years of age.
- Ninety percent are anterior dislocations.

Anatomy

- The glenohumeral articulation, with its large convex humeral head and correspondingly flat glenoid, is ideally suited to accommodate a wide range of shoulder motion. The articular surface and radius of curvature of the humeral head are about three times those of the glenoid fossa.
- Numerous static and dynamic stabilizers of the shoulder exist; these are covered in detail in Chapter 14.
- The humeral attachment of the glenohumeral joint capsule is along the anatomic neck of the humerus except medially, where

the attachment is more distal along the shaft. The proximal humeral physis is therefore extra-articular except along its medial aspect.

■ As in most pediatric joint injuries, the capsular attachment to the epiphysis renders failure through the physis much more common than true capsuloligamentous injury; therefore, fracture through the physis is more common than a shoulder dislocation in a skeletally immature patient.

■ In neonates, an apparent dislocation may actually represent a physeal injury.

Mechanism of Injury

■ **Neonates:** Pseudodislocation may occur with traumatic epiphyseal separation of the proximal humerus. This is much more common than a true shoulder dislocation, which may occur in neonates with underlying birth trauma to the brachial plexus or central nervous system.

■ Anterior glenohumeral dislocation may occur as a result of trauma, either direct or indirect.

  □ **Direct:** An anteriorly directed impact to the posterior shoulder may produce an anterior dislocation.

  □ **Indirect:** Trauma to the upper extremity with the shoulder in abduction, extension, and external rotation is the most common mechanism for anterior shoulder dislocation.

■ Posterior glenohumeral dislocation (2% to 4%)

  □ **Direct trauma:** This results from force application to the anterior shoulder, forcing the humeral head posteriorly.

  □ **Indirect trauma:** This is the most common mechanism.

  • The shoulder typically is in the position of adduction, flexion, and internal rotation at the time of injury with axial loading.

  • Electric shock or convulsive mechanisms may produce posterior dislocation owing to the overwhelming of the external rotators of the shoulder (infraspinatus and teres minor muscles) by the internal rotators (latissimus dorsi, pectoralis major, and subscapularis muscles).

■ **Atraumatic dislocations:** Recurrent instability related to congenital or acquired laxity or volitional mechanisms may result in anterior dislocation with minimal trauma.

Clinical Evaluation

■ Patient presentation varies according to the type of dislocation encountered.

Anterior Dislocation

- The patient typically presents with the affected upper extremity held in slight abduction and external rotation. The acutely dislocated shoulder is painful, with muscular spasm in an attempt to stabilize the joint.

- Examination typically reveals squaring of the shoulder caused by a relative prominence of the acromion, a relative hollow beneath the acromion posteriorly, and a palpable mass anteriorly.

- A careful neurovascular examination is important with attention to axillary nerve integrity. Deltoid muscle testing is usually not possible, but sensation over the deltoid may be assessed. Deltoid atony may be present and should not be confused with axillary nerve injury. Musculocutaneous nerve integrity can be assessed by the presence of sensation on the anterolateral forearm.

- Patients may present after spontaneous reduction or reduction in the field. If the patient is not in acute pain, examination may reveal a positive *apprehension test* in which passive placement of the shoulder in the provocative position (abduction, extension, and external rotation) reproduces the patient's sense of instability and pain. Posteriorly directed counterpressure over the anterior shoulder may mitigate the sensation of instability.

Posterior Dislocation

- Clinically, a posterior glenohumeral dislocation does not present with striking deformity; moreover, the injured upper extremity is typically held in the traditional sling position of shoulder internal rotation and adduction.

- A careful neurovascular examination is important to rule out axillary nerve injury, although it is much less common than with anterior glenohumeral dislocations.

- On examination, limited external rotation (often <0 degrees) and limited anterior forward elevation (often <90 degrees) may be appreciated.

- A palpable mass posterior to the shoulder, flattening of the anterior shoulder, and coracoid prominence may be observed.

Atraumatic Dislocation

- Patients present with a history of recurrent dislocations with spontaneous reduction.

- Often the patient will report a history of minimal trauma or volitional dislocation, frequently without pain.

- Multidirectional instability may be present bilaterally, as may characteristics of multiple joint laxity, including hyperextensibility of the elbows, knees, and metacarpophalangeal joints. Striae may be present.
- **Sulcus sign:** This is dimpling of skin below the acromion with longitudinal traction.

Superior and Inferior (Luxatio Erecta) Dislocation

- This is extremely rare in children, although cases have been reported.
- It may be associated with hereditary conditions such as Ehlers–Danlos syndrome.

Radiographic Evaluation

- **A trauma series of the affected shoulder is indicated:** AP, scapular-Y, and axillary views.
- **Velpeau axillary view:** Compliance is frequently an issue in the irritable, injured child in pain. If a standard axillary view cannot be obtained, the patient may be left in a sling and leaned obliquely backward 45 degrees over the cassette. The beam is directed caudally, orthogonal to the cassette, resulting in an axillary view with magnification.
- Special views (see Chapter 14)
  - □ **West Point axillary view:** Taken with the patient prone with the beam-directed cephalad to the axilla 25 degrees from the horizontal and 25 degrees medially. It provides a tangential view of the anteroinferior glenoid rim.
  - □ **Hill–Sachs view:** An AP radiograph is taken with the shoulder in maximal internal rotation to visualize posterolateral defect (Hill–Sachs lesion) caused by an impression fracture on the glenoid rim.
  - □ **Stryker notch view:** The patient is supine with the ipsilateral palm on the crown of head and the elbow pointing straight upward. The x-ray beam is directed 10 degrees cephalad, aimed at coracoid. One is able to visualize 90% of posterolateral humeral head defects.
- Computed tomography may be useful in defining humeral head or glenoid impression fractures, loose bodies, and anterior labral bony injuries (bony Bankart lesion).
- Single- or double-contrast arthrography may be utilized in cases in which the diagnosis may be unclear; it may demonstrate

pseudosubluxation, or traumatic epiphyseal separation of the proximal humerus, in a neonate with an apparent glenohumeral dislocation.

■ Magnetic resonance imaging may be used to identify rotator cuff, capsular, and glenoid labral (Bankart lesion) pathology.

■ Atraumatic dislocations may demonstrate congenital aplasia or absence of the glenoid on radiographic evaluation.

Classification

Degree of stability:	Dislocation versus subluxation
Chronology:	Congenital
	Acute versus chronic
	Locked (fixed)
	Recurrent
	Acquired: generally from repeated minor injuries (swimming, gymnastics, weights); labrum often intact; capsular laxity; increased glenohumeral joint volume; subluxation common
Force:	**Atraumatic:** usually owing to congenital laxity; no injury; often asymptomatic; self-reducing
	Traumatic: usually caused by one major injury; the anteroinferior labrum may be detached (Bankart lesion); unidirectional; generally requires assistance for reduction
Patient contribution:	Voluntary versus involuntary
Direction:	Subcoracoid
	Subglenoid
	Intrathoracic

Treatment

■ Closed reduction should be performed after adequate clinical evaluation and administration of analgesics and or sedation. Described techniques include (see the figures in Chapter 14)

□ *Traction–countertraction:* With the patient in the supine position, a sheet is placed in the axilla of the affected shoulder with traction applied to counter axial traction placed on the affected upper extremity. Steady, continuous traction eventually results in fatigue of the shoulder musculature in spasm and allows reduction of the humeral head.

□ *Stimson technique:* The patient is placed prone on the stretcher with the affected upper extremity hanging free. Gentle, manual traction or 5 lb of weight is applied to the wrist, with reduction effected over 15 to 20 minutes.

☐ *Steel maneuver:* With the patient supine, the examiner supports the elbow in one hand while supporting the forearm and wrist with the other. The upper extremity is abducted to 90 degrees and is slowly externally rotated. Thumb pressure is applied by the physician to push the humeral head into place, followed by adduction and internal rotation of the shoulder as the extremity is placed across the chest. There is a higher incidence of iatrogenic fracture.

■ Following reduction, acute anterior dislocations are treated with sling immobilization. Total time in sling is controversial but may be up to 4 weeks, after which an aggressive program of rehabilitation for rotator cuff strengthening is instituted. Posterior dislocations are treated for 4 weeks in a commercial splint or shoulder spica cast with the shoulder in neutral rotation, followed by physical therapy.

■ Recurrent dislocation or associated glenoid rim avulsion fractures (bony Bankart lesion) may necessitate operative management, including reduction and internal fixation of the anterior glenoid margin, repair of a Bankart lesion (anterior labral tear), capsular shift, or capsulorrhaphy. Postoperatively, the child is placed in sling immobilization for 4 to 6 weeks with gradual increases in range-of-motion and strengthening exercises.

■ Atraumatic dislocations rarely require reduction maneuvers as spontaneous reduction is the rule. Only after an aggressive, supervised rehabilitation program for rotator cuff and deltoid strengthening has been completed should surgical intervention be considered. Vigorous rehabilitation may obviate the need for operative intervention in up to 85% of cases.

■ Psychiatric evaluation may be necessary in the management of voluntary dislocators.

Complications

■ **Recurrent dislocation:** The incidence is 50% to 90%, with decreasing rates of recurrence with increasing patient age (up to 100% in children less than 10 years old). It may necessitate operative intervention, with >90% success rate in preventing future dislocation.

■ **Shoulder stiffness:** Procedures aimed at tightening static and dynamic constraints (subscapularis tendon-shortening, capsular shift, etc.) may result in "overtightening," resulting in a loss of range of motion, as well as possible subluxation in the opposing direction with subsequent accelerated glenohumeral arthritis.

- **Neurologic injury:** Neurapraxic injury may occur to nerves in proximity to the glenohumeral articulation, especially the axillary nerve and less commonly the musculocutaneous nerve. These typically resolve with time; a lack of neurologic recovery by 3 months may warrant surgical exploration.
- **Vascular injury:** Traction injury to the axillary artery has been reported in conjunction with nerve injury to the brachial plexus.

Pediatric Elbow

EPIDEMIOLOGY

- Elbow fractures represent 8% to 9% of all upper extremity fractures in children.
- Of all elbow fractures, 85% occur at the distal humerus; 55% to 75% of these are supracondylar.
- Most occur in patients 5 to 10 years of age, more commonly in boys.
- There is a seasonal distribution for elbow fractures in children, with the most occurring during the summer and the fewest during the winter.

ANATOMY

- **The elbow consists of three joints:** the ulnohumeral, radiocapitellar, and proximal radioulnar.
- The vascularity to the elbow is a broad anastomotic network that forms the intraosseous and extraosseous blood supplies.
  - □ The capitellum is supplied by a posterior branch of the brachial artery that enters the lateral crista.
  - □ The trochlea is supplied by a medial branch that enters along the nonarticular medial crista and a lateral branch that crosses the physis.
  - □ There is no anastomotic connection between these two vessels.
- The articulating surface of the capitellum and trochlea projects distally and anteriorly at an angle of approximately 30 to 45 degrees. The center of rotation of the articular surface of each condyle lies on the same horizontal axis; thus, malalignment of the relationships of the condyles to each other changes their arcs of rotation, limiting flexion and extension.
- The carrying angle is influenced by the obliquity of the distal humeral physis; this averages 6 degrees in girls and 5 degrees in boys and is important in the assessment of angular growth disturbances.
- In addition to anterior distal humeral angulation, there is horizontal rotation of the humeral condyles in relation to the diaphysis, with the lateral condyle rotated 5 degrees medially. This medial rotation is often significantly increased with displaced supracondylar fractures.

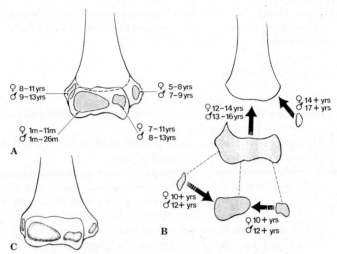

FIGURE 44.1 Ossification and fusion of the secondary centers of the distal humerus. **(A)** The average ages of the onset of ossification of the various ossification centers are shown for both boys and girls. **(B)** The ages at which these centers fuse with each other are shown for both boys and girls. **(C)** The contribution of each secondary center to the overall architecture of the distal humerus is represented by the *stippled areas.* (From Rockwood CA, Wilkins KE, Beaty JH. *Fractures and Dislocations in Children.* Philadelphia: Lippincott-Raven; 1999:662.)

- The elbow accounts for only 20% of the longitudinal growth of the upper extremity.
- **Ossification:** With the exception of the capitellum, ossification centers appear approximately 2 years earlier in girls compared with boys.
- **CRMTOL:** The following is a mnemonic for the appearance of the ossification centers around the elbow (Fig. 44.1):

Capitellum:	6 months to 2 years; includes the lateral crista of the trochlea
Radial head:	4 years
Medial epicondyle:	6 to 7 years
Trochlea:	8 years
Olecranon:	8 to 10 years; often multiple centers, which ultimately fuse
Lateral epicondyle:	12 years

MECHANISM OF INJURY

- **Indirect:** This is most commonly a result of a fall onto an outstretched upper extremity.

■ **Direct:** Direct trauma to the elbow may occur from a fall onto a flexed elbow or from an object striking the elbow (e.g., baseball bat, automobile).

CLINICAL EVALUATION

■ Patients typically present with varying degrees of gross deformity, usually accompanied by pain, swelling, tenderness, irritability, and refusal to use the injured extremity.

■ The ipsilateral shoulder, humeral shaft, forearm, wrist, and hand should be examined for associated injuries.

■ A careful neurovascular examination should be performed, with documentation of the integrity of the median, radial, and ulnar nerves, as well as distal pulses and capillary refill. Flexion of the elbow in the presence of antecubital swelling may cause neurovascular embarrassment; repeat evaluation of neurovascular integrity is essential following any manipulation or treatment.

■ All aspects of the elbow should be examined for possible open lesions; clinical suspicion may be followed with intra-articular injection of saline into the elbow to evaluate possible intra-articular communication of a laceration.

RADIOGRAPHIC EVALUATION

■ Standard anteroposterior (AP) and lateral views of the elbow should be obtained. On the AP view, the following angular relationships may be determined (Fig. 44.2):

  □ **Baumann angle:** This is the angulation of the lateral condylar physeal line with respect to the long axis of the humerus; normal is 15 to 20 degrees and equal to the opposite side.

  □ **Humeral–ulnar angle:** This angle is subtended by the intersection of the diaphyseal bisectors of the humerus and ulna; this best reflects the true carrying angle.

  □ **Metaphyseal–diaphyseal angle:** This angle is formed by a bisector of the humeral shaft with respect to a line delineated by the widest points of the distal humeral metaphysic.

■ On a true lateral radiograph of the elbow flexed to 90 degrees, the following landmarks should be observed (Fig. 44.3):

  □ **Teardrop:** This radiographic shadow is formed by the posterior margin of the coronoid fossa anteriorly, the anterior margin of the olecranon fossa posteriorly, and the superior margin of the capitellar ossification center inferiorly.

  □ **Diaphyseal–condylar angle:** This projects 30 to 45 degrees anteriorly; the posterior capitellar physis is typically wider than the anterior physis.

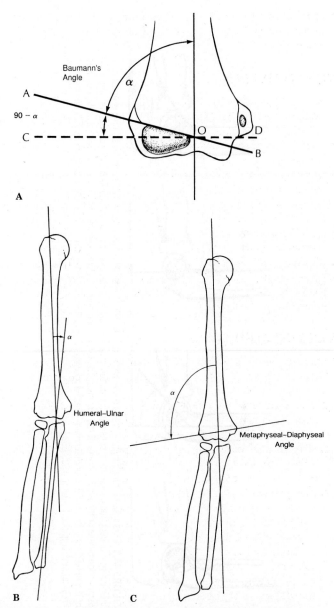

FIGURE 44.2 Anteroposterior x-ray angles for the elbow. **(A)** The Baumann angle (α). **(B)** The humeral–ulnar angle. **(C)** The metaphyseal–diaphyseal angle. (From O'Brien WR, Eilert RE, Chang FM, et al. The metaphyseal–diaphyseal angle as a guide to treating supracondylar fractures of the humerus in children. unpublished data, 1999.)

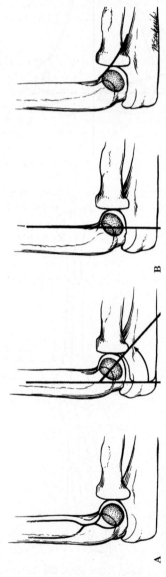

FIGURE 44.3 Intraosseous blood supply of the distal humerus. **(A)** The vessels supplying the lateral condylar epiphysis enter on the posterior aspect and course for a considerable distance before reaching the ossific nucleus. **(B)** Two definite vessels supply the ossification center of the medial crista of the trochlea. The lateral one enters by crossing the physis. The medial one enters by way of the nonarticular edge of the medial crista. (From Rockwood CA, Wilkins KE, Beaty JH. *Fractures and Dislocations in Children.* Philadelphia: Lippincott-Raven; 1999:663.)

- □ **Anterior humeral line:** When extended distally, this line should intersect the middle third of the capitellar ossification center.
- □ **Coronoid line:** A proximally directed line along the anterior border of the coronoid process should be tangent to the anterior aspect of the lateral condyle.
- ■ Special views
  - □ **Jones view:** Pain may limit an AP radiograph of the elbow in extension; in these cases, a radiograph may be taken with the elbow hyperflexed and the beam directed at the elbow through the overlying forearm with the arm flat on the cassette in neutral rotation.
  - □ Internal and external rotation views (column views) may be obtained in cases in which a fracture is suspected but not clearly demonstrated on routine views. These may be particularly useful in the identification of coronoid process or radial head fractures.
- ■ The contralateral elbow should be obtained for comparison as well as identification of ossification centers. A *pseudofracture* of an ossification center may exist in which apparent fragmentation of an ossification center may represent a developmental variant rather than a true fracture. This may be clarified with comparison views of the uninjured contralateral elbow.
- ■ **Fat pad signs:** Three fat pads overlie the major structures of the elbow (Fig. 44.4):

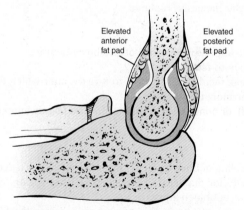

Elevated anterior fat pad

Elevated posterior fat pad

FIGURE 44.4 Elevated anterior and posterior fat pads. (Adapted from *The Journal of Bone and Joint Surgery*, in Bucholz RW, Heckman JD, Court-Brown C, et al., eds. *Rockwood and Green's Fractures in Adults.* 6th ed. Philadelphia: Lippincott Williams & Wilkins; 2006.)

□ **Anterior (coronoid) fat pad:** This triangular lucency seen anterior to the distal humerus may represent displacement of the fat pad owing to underlying joint effusion. The coronoid fossa is shallow; therefore, anterior displacement of the fat pad is sensitive to small effusions. However, an exuberant fat pad may be seen without associated trauma, diminishing the specificity of the anterior fat pad sign.

□ **Posterior (olecranon) fat pad:** The deep olecranon fossa normally completely contains the posterior fat pad. Thus, only moderate to large effusions cause posterior displacement, resulting in a high specificity of the posterior fat pad sign for intra-articular disorders (a fracture is present >70% of the time when the posterior fat pad is seen).

□ **Supinator fat pad:** This represents a layer of fat on the anterior aspect of the supinator muscle as it wraps around the proximal radius. Anterior displacement of this fat pad may represent a fracture of the radial neck; however, this sign has been reported to be positive in only 50% of cases.

□ Anterior and posterior fat pads may not be seen following elbow dislocation owing to disruption of the joint capsule, which decompresses the joint effusion.

SPECIFIC FRACTURES

Supracondylar Humerus Fractures

Epidemiology

- These comprise 55% to 75% of all elbow fractures.
- The male-to-female ratio is 3:2.
- The peak incidence is from 5 to 8 years, after which dislocations become more frequent.
- The left, or nondominant side, is most frequently injured.

Anatomy

- Remodeling of bone in the 5- to 8-year-old causes a decreased anteroposterior diameter in the supracondylar region, making this area susceptible to injury.
- Ligamentous laxity in this age range increases the likelihood of hyperextension injury.
- The anterior capsule is thickened and stronger than the posterior capsule. In extension, the fibers of the anterior capsule are taut, serving as a fulcrum by which the olecranon becomes firmly engaged in the olecranon fossa. With extreme force, hyperextension may cause

the olecranon process to impinge on the superior olecranon fossa and supracondylar region.

■ The periosteal hinge remains intact on the side of the displacement.

Mechanism of Injury

■ **Extension type:** Hyperextension occurs during fall onto an outstretched hand with or without varus/valgus force. If the hand is pronated, posteromedial displacement occurs. If the hand is supinated posterolateral displacement occurs. Posteromedial displacement is more common.

■ **Flexion type:** The cause is direct trauma or a fall onto a flexed elbow.

Clinical Evaluation

■ Patients typically present with a swollen, tender elbow with painful range of motion.

■ **S-shaped angulation at the elbow:** A complete (type III) fracture results in two points of angulation to give it an S shape.

■ **Pucker sign:** This is dimpling of the skin anteriorly secondary to penetration of the proximal fragment into the brachialis muscle; it should alert the examiner that reduction of the fracture may be difficult with simple manipulation.

■ **Neurovascular examination:** A careful neurovascular examination should be performed with documentation of the integrity of the median, radial, and ulnar nerves as well as their terminal branches. Capillary refill and distal pulses as well as warmth of the hand should be documented. The examination should be repeated following splinting or manipulation.

Classification

Extension Type
This represents 98% of supracondylar humerus fractures in children.

Gartland
This is based on the degree of displacement.

Type I: Nondisplaced

Type II: Displaced with intact posterior cortex; may be angulated or rotated

Type III: Complete displacement; posteromedial or posterolateral

Flexion Type
This comprises 2% of supracondylar humerus fractures in children.

Gartland

Type I:	Nondisplaced
Type II:	Displaced with intact anterior cortex
Type III:	Complete displacement; usually anterolateral

Treatment

Extension Type

Type I: Immobilization in a long arm cast or splint at 60 to 90 degrees of flexion is indicated for 2 to 3 weeks.

Type II: This is usually reducible by closed methods followed by casting; it may require pinning if unstable (crossed pins versus two lateral pins) or if reduction cannot be maintained without excessive flexion that may place neurovascular structures at risk.

Type III: Attempt closed reduction and pinning; traction (olecranon skeletal traction) may be needed for comminuted fractures with marked soft tissue swelling or damage.

Open reduction and internal fixation may be necessary for rotationally unstable fractures, open fractures, and those with neurovascular injury (crossed pins versus two lateral pins).

- Concepts involved in reduction
  - ☐ Displacement is corrected in the coronal and horizontal planes before the sagittal plane.
  - ☐ Hyperextension of the elbow with longitudinal traction is used to obtain apposition, which is only occasionally required.
  - ☐ Flexion of the elbow is done while applying a posterior force to the distal fragment.
  - ☐ Stabilization with control of displacement in the coronal, sagittal, and horizontal planes is recommended.
  - ☐ Lateral pins are placed first to obtain provisional stabilization, and if a medial pin is needed, the elbow can be extended before pin placement to help protect the ulnar nerve.

Flexion Type

Type I: Immobilization in a long arm cast in near extension is indicated for 2 to 3 weeks.

Type II: Closed reduction is followed by percutaneous pinning with two lateral pins or crossed pins.

Type III: Reduction is often difficult; most require open reduction and internal fixation with crossed pins.

- Immobilization in a long arm cast (or posterior splint if swelling is an issue) with the elbow flexed <90 degrees, depending on the extent of the swelling, and the forearm in neutral should be undertaken for 3 weeks postoperatively, at which time the cast may be discontinued and the pins removed. The patient should then be maintained in a sling when in danger of falling and given active range-of-motion exercises. Sports activity should be restricted for an additional 3 weeks.

Complications

- **Neurologic injury (7% to 10%):** This may be caused by a traction injury at the time of the fracture or very rarely at the time of reduction. The neurovascular structures may be tented or entrapped in the fracture site. Neurologic injury is also a component of Volkmann ischemic contracture. Most injuries seen from supracondylar humerus fractures are neurapraxias, requiring no treatment.
  □ Median nerve/anterior interosseous nerve (most common)
  □ Radial nerve
  □ **Ulnar nerve:** This is most common in flexion-type supracondylar fractures; early injury may result from tenting over the medial spike of the proximal fragment; late injury may represent progressive valgus deformity of the elbow. It is frequently iatrogenic in extension-type supracondylar fractures following medial pinning.
- **Vascular injury (0.5%):** This may represent direct injury to the brachial artery or may be secondary to antecubital swelling. This emphasizes the need for a careful neurovascular examination both on initial presentation and following manipulation or splinting, especially after elbow flexion is performed. Observation is warranted if the pulse is absent, yet the hand is still well perfused and warm.
- **Loss of motion:** A >5-degree loss of elbow motion occurs in 5% secondary to poor reduction or soft tissue contracture.
- **Myositis ossificans:** Rare and is seen after vigorous manipulation.
- **Angular deformity (varus more frequently than valgus):** Significant in 10% to 20%; the occurrence is decreased with percutaneous pinning (3%) compared with reduction and casting alone (14%).
- **Compartment syndrome (<1%):** This rare complication can be exacerbated by elbow hyperflexion when excessive swelling is present in the cubital fossa.

Lateral Condylar Physeal Fractures

Epidemiology

- These comprise 17% of all distal humerus fractures.
- Peak age is 6 years.
- Often result in less satisfactory outcomes than supracondylar fractures because

□ Diagnosis is less obvious and may be missed in subtle cases.

□ Loss of motion is more severe due to intra-articular nature.

□ The incidence of growth disturbance is higher.

Anatomy

■ The ossification center of the lateral condyle extends to the lateral crista of the trochlea.

■ Lateral condylar physeal fractures are typically accompanied by a soft tissue disruption between the origins of the extensor carpi radialis longus and the brachioradialis muscles; these origins remain attached to the free distal fragment, accounting for initial and late displacement of the fracture.

■ Disruption of the lateral crista of the trochlea (Milch type II fractures) results in posterolateral subluxation of the proximal radius and ulna with consequent cubitus valgus; severe posterolateral translocation may lead to the erroneous diagnosis of primary elbow dislocation.

Mechanism of Injury

■ **"Pull-off" theory:** Avulsion injury occurs by the common extensor origin owing to a varus stress exerted on the extended elbow.

■ **"Push-off" theory:** A fall onto an extended upper extremity results in axial load transmitted through the forearm, causing the radial head to impinge on the lateral condyle.

Clinical Evaluation

■ Unlike the patient with a supracondylar fracture of the elbow, patients with lateral condylar fractures typically present with little gross distortion of the elbow, other than mild swelling from fracture hematoma most prominent over the lateral aspect of the distal humerus.

■ Crepitus may be elicited, associated with supination–pronation motions of the elbow.

■ Pain, swelling, tenderness to palpation, painful range of motion, and pain on resisted wrist extension may be observed.

Radiographic Evaluation

■ AP, lateral, and oblique views of the elbow should be obtained.

■ Varus stress views may accentuate displacement of the fracture.

■ In a young child whose lateral condyle is not ossified, it may be difficult to distinguish between a lateral condylar physeal fracture and a complete distal humeral physeal fracture. In such cases, an

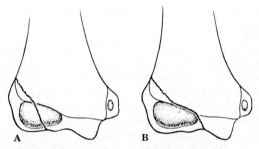

FIGURE 44.5 Physeal fractures of the lateral condyle.
(A) Salter–Harris type IV physeal injury (Milch type I).
(B) Salter–Harris type II physeal injury (Milch type II). (From Rockwood CA, Wilkins KE, Beaty JH. *Fractures and Dislocations in Children.* Philadelphia: Lippincott-Raven; 1999:753.)

arthrogram may be helpful, and the relationship of the lateral condyle to the proximal radius is critical.

☐ **Lateral condyle physeal fracture:** This disrupts the normal relationship with displacement of the proximal radius laterally owing to loss of stability provided by the lateral crista of the distal humerus.

☐ **Fracture of the entire distal humeral physis:** The relationship of the lateral condyle to the proximal radius is intact, often accompanied by posteromedial displacement of the proximal radius and ulna.

■ Magnetic resonance imaging (MRI) may help to appreciate the direction of the fracture line and the pattern of fracture.

Classification

Milch

Type I: The fracture line courses lateral to the trochlea and into the capitulotrochlear groove. It represents a Salter–Harris type IV fracture: the elbow is stable because the trochlea is intact; this is less common (Fig. 44.5).

Type II: The fracture line extends into the apex of the trochlea. It represents a Salter–Harris type II fracture: the elbow is unstable because the trochlea is disrupted; this is more common (Fig. 44.5).

Jakob

Stage I: Fracture nondisplaced with an intact articular surface
Stage II: Fracture with moderate displacement
Stage III: Complete displacement and rotation with elbow instability

Treatment

Nonoperative

- Nondisplaced or minimally displaced fractures (Jakob stage I; <2 mm) (40% of fractures) may be treated with simple immobilization in a posterior splint or long arm cast with the forearm in neutral position and the elbow flexed to 90 degrees. This is maintained for 3 to 6 weeks, until there is healing of the fracture, after which range-of-motion exercises are instituted.
- Closed reduction with a varus force as well as supination and extension may be attempted in Jakob type II fractures. If articular reduction is achieved, it should be held with percutaneous wires to prevent late displacement. An arthrogram can be performed to ensure a reduction was achieved.

Operative

- Open reduction is required for unstable Jakob stage II and III fractures (60%).
  - □ The fragment may be secured with two crossed, smooth Kirschner wires that diverge in the metaphysis.
  - □ The passage of smooth pins through the physis does not typically result in growth disturbance.
  - □ Care must be taken when dissecting near the posterior aspect of the lateral condylar fragment because the sole vascular supply is provided through soft tissues in this region.
  - □ Postoperatively, the elbow is maintained in a long arm cast at 60 to 90 degrees of flexion with the forearm in neutral rotation. The cast is discontinued 3 to 6 weeks postoperatively with pin removal. Active range-of-motion exercises are instituted.
- If treatment is delayed (>3 to 6 weeks), closed treatment should be strongly considered, regardless of displacement, owing to the high incidence of osteonecrosis of the condylar fragment and significant joint stiffness with late open reduction.

Complications

- **Lateral condylar overgrowth with spur formation:** This usually results from an ossified periosteal flap raised from the distal fragment at the time of injury or surgery. It may represent a cosmetic problem (cubitus pseudovarus) as the elbow gains the appearance of varus owing to a lateral prominence but is generally not a functional problem.
- **Delayed union or nonunion (>12 weeks):** This is caused by pull of extensors and poor metaphyseal circulation of the lateral condylar fragment, most commonly in patients treated nonoperatively.

It may result in cubitus valgus necessitating ulnar nerve transposition for tardy ulnar nerve palsy. Treatment ranges from benign neglect to osteotomy and compressive fixation late or at skeletal maturity.

- **Angular deformity:** Cubitus valgus occurs more frequently than varus owing to lateral physeal arrest. Tardy ulnar nerve palsy may develop necessitating transposition.
- **Neurologic compromise:** This is rare in the acute setting. Tardy ulnar nerve palsy may develop as a result of cubitus valgus.
- **Osteonecrosis:** This may be iatrogenic, especially when surgical intervention was delayed. It may result in a "fishtail" deformity with a persistent gap between the lateral physeal ossification center and the medial ossification of the trochlea. Osteonecrosis does not appear to have long-term clinical sequelae.

Medial Condylar Physeal Fractures

Epidemiology

- Represent <1% of distal humerus fractures.
- Typical age range is 8 to 14 years.

Anatomy

- Medial condylar fractures are Salter–Harris type IV fractures with an intra-articular component involving the trochlea and an extra-articular component involving the medial metaphysis and the medial epicondyle (common flexor origin).
- Only the medial crista is ossified by the secondary ossification centers of the medial condylar epiphysis.
- The vascular supply to the medial epicondyle and metaphysis is derived from the flexor muscle group. The vascular supply to the lateral aspect of the medial crista of the trochlea traverses the surface of the medial condylar physis, rendering it vulnerable in medial physeal disruptions with possible avascular complications and "fishtail" deformity.

Mechanism of Injury

- **Direct:** Trauma to the point of the elbow, such as a fall onto a flexed elbow, results in the semilunar notch of the olecranon traumatically impinging on the trochlea, splitting it with the fracture line extending proximally to metaphyseal region.
- **Indirect:** A fall onto an outstretched hand with valgus strain on the elbow results in an avulsion injury with the fracture line starting in the metaphysis and propagating distally through the articular surface.

- These are considered the mirror image of lateral condylar physeal fractures.
- Once dissociated from the elbow, the powerful forearm flexor muscles produce sagittal anterior rotation of the fragment.

Clinical Evaluation

- Patients typically present with pain, swelling, and tenderness to palpation over the medial aspect of the distal humerus. Range of motion is painful, especially with resisted flexion of the wrist.
- A careful neurovascular examination is important because ulnar nerve symptoms may be present.
- A common mistake is to diagnose a medial condylar physeal fracture erroneously as an isolated medial epicondylar fracture. This occurs based on tenderness and swelling medially in conjunction with radiographs demonstrating a medial epicondylar fracture only resulting from the absence of a medial condylar ossification center in younger patients.
- Medial epicondylar fractures are often associated with elbow dislocations, usually posterolateral; elbow dislocations are extremely rare before ossification of the medial condylar epiphysis begins. With medial condylar physeal fractures, subluxation of the elbow posteromedially is often observed. A positive fat pad sign indicates an intra-articular fracture, whereas a medial epicondyle fracture is typically extra-articular with no fat pad sign seen on radiographs.

Radiographic Evaluation

- AP, lateral, and oblique views of the elbow should be obtained.
- In young children whose medial condylar ossification center is not yet present, radiographs may demonstrate a fracture in the epicondylar region; in such cases, an arthrogram may delineate the course of the fracture through the articular surface, indicating a medial condylar physeal fracture.
- Stress views may help to distinguish epicondylar fractures (valgus laxity) from condylar fractures (both varus and valgus laxity).
- MRI may help to appreciate the direction of the fracture line and the pattern of fracture.

Classification

Milch (Fig. 44.6)

Type I: **Fracture line traversing through the apex of the trochlea:** Salter–Harris type II; more common presentation

Type II: **Fracture line through capitulotrochlear groove:** Salter–Harris type IV; infrequent presentation

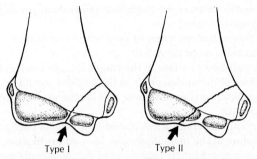

FIGURE 44.6 Fracture patterns. **Left:** In the Milch type I injury, the fracture line terminates in the trochlea notch (*arrow*). **Right:** In the Milch type II injury, the fracture line terminates in the capitulotrochlear groove (*arrow*). (From Rockwood CA, Wilkins KE, Beaty JH. *Fractures and Dislocations in Children.* Philadelphia: Lippincott-Raven; 1999:786.)

Kilfoyle

Stage I: Nondisplaced, articular surface intact

Stage II: Fracture line complete with minimal displacement

Stage III: Complete displacement with rotation of fragment from pull of flexor mass

Treatment

Nonoperative

- Nondisplaced or minimally displaced fractures (Kilfoyle stage I) may be treated with immobilization in a long arm cast or posterior splint with the forearm in neutral rotation and the elbow flexed to 90 degrees for 3 to 4 weeks, followed by range-of-motion and strengthening exercises.

- Closed reduction may be performed with the elbow extended and the forearm pronated to relieve tension on the flexor origin, with placement of a posterior splint or long arm cast. Unstable reductions require percutaneous pinning with two parallel metaphyseal pins.

- Closed reduction is often difficult because of medial soft tissue swelling, and open reduction is usually required for stage II and III fractures.

Operative

- Irreducible or unstable Kilfoyle stage II or III fractures of the medial condylar physis require open reduction and internal fixation. Rotation of the condylar fragment may preclude successful closed treatment.

☐ A medial approach may be used with identification and protection of the ulnar nerve.

☐ The posterior surface of the condylar fragment and the medial aspect of the medial crista of the trochlea should be avoided in the dissection because these provide the vascular supply to the trochlea.

☐ Smooth Kirschner wires placed in a parallel configuration extending to the metaphysis may be used for fixation, or cancellous screw fixation may be used in adolescents near skeletal maturity.

☐ Postoperative immobilization consists of long arm casting with the forearm in neutral rotation and the elbow flexed to 90 degrees for 3 to 4 weeks, at which time the pins and the cast may be discontinued and active range-of-motion exercises instituted.

■ If treatment is delayed (>3 to 6 weeks), closed treatment should be strongly considered, regardless of displacement, owing to the high incidence of osteonecrosis of the trochlea and significant joint stiffness from extensive dissection with late open reduction.

Complications

■ **Missed diagnosis:** The most common is a medial epicondylar fracture owing to the absence of ossification of the medial condylar ossification center. Late diagnosis of medial condylar physeal fracture should be treated nonoperatively.

■ **Nonunion:** Uncommon and usually represent untreated, displaced medial condylar physeal fractures secondary to pull of flexors with rotation. They tend to demonstrate varus deformity. After ossification, the lateral edge of the fragment may be observed to extend to the capitulotrochlear groove.

■ **Angular deformity:** Untreated or treated medial condylar physeal fractures may demonstrate angular deformity, usually varus, either secondary to angular displacement or from medial physeal arrest. Cubitus valgus may result from overgrowth of the medial condyle.

■ **Osteonecrosis:** This may result after open reduction and internal fixation, especially when extensive dissection is undertaken.

■ **Ulnar neuropathy:** This may be early, related to trauma, or more commonly, late, related to the development of angular deformities or scarring. Recalcitrant symptoms may be addressed with ulnar nerve transposition.

Transphyseal Fractures

Epidemiology

- Mostly occur in patients younger than age 6 to 7 years.
- These were originally thought to be extremely rare injuries. It now appears that with advanced imaging (e.g., MRI), they occur fairly frequently, although the exact incidence is not known owing to misdiagnoses.

Anatomy

- The epiphysis includes the medial epicondyle until age 6 to 7 years in girls and 8 to 9 years in boys, at which time ossification occurs. Fractures before this time thus include medial epicondyle.
- The younger the child, the greater the volume of the distal humerus that is occupied by the distal epiphysis; as the child matures, the physeal line progresses distally, with a V-shaped cleft forming between the medial and lateral condylar physes—this cleft protects the distal humeral epiphysis from fracture in the mature child because fracture lines tend to exit through the cleft.
- The joint surface is not involved in this injury, and the relationship between the radius and capitellum is maintained.
- The anteroposterior diameter of the bone in this region is wider than in the supracondylar region, and consequently there is not as much tilting or rotation.
- The vascular supply to the medial crista of the trochlea courses directly through the physis; in cases of fracture, this may lead to avascular changes.
- The physeal line is in a more proximal location in younger patients; therefore, hyperextension injuries to the elbow tend to result in physeal separations instead of supracondylar fractures through bone.

Mechanism of Injury

- **Birth injuries:** Rotatory forces coupled with hyperextension injury to the elbow during delivery may result in traumatic distal humeral physeal separation.
- **Child abuse:** Bright demonstrated that the physis fails most often in shear rather than pure bending or tension. Therefore, in young infants or children, child abuse must be suspected because a high incidence of transphyseal fracture is associated with abuse.
- **Trauma:** This may result from hyperextension injuries with posterior displacement, coupled with a rotation moment.

Clinical Evaluation

- Young infants or newborns may present with pseudoparalysis of the affected extremity, minimal swelling, and "muffled crepitus" because the fracture involves softer cartilage rather than firm, osseous tissue.
- Older children may present with pronounced swelling, refusal to use the affected extremity, and pain that precludes a useful clinical examination or palpation of bony landmarks. In general, because of the large, wide fracture surface there is less tendency for tilting or rotation of the distal fragment, resulting in less deformity than seen in supracondylar fractures. The bony relationship between the humeral epicondyles and the olecranon is maintained.
- A careful neurovascular examination should be performed because swelling in the cubital fossa may result in neurovascular compromise.

Radiographic Evaluation

- AP, lateral, and oblique radiographs should be obtained.
- The proximal radius and ulna maintain normal, anatomic relationships to each other, but they are displaced posteromedially with respect to the distal humerus. This is considered diagnostic of transphyseal fracture.
- Comparison views of the contralateral elbow may be used to identify posteromedial displacement.
- In the child whose lateral condylar epiphysis is ossified, the diagnosis is much more obvious. There is maintenance of the lateral condylar epiphysis to radial head relationship and posteromedial displacement of the distal humeral epiphysis with respect to the humeral shaft.
- Transphyseal fractures with large metaphyseal components may be mistaken for a low supracondylar fracture or a fracture of the lateral condylar physis. These may be differentiated by the presence of a smooth outline of the distal metaphysis in fractures involving the entire distal physis as compared with the irregular border of the distal aspect of the distal fragment seen in supracondylar fractures.
- Elbow dislocations in children are rare, but they may be differentiated from transphyseal fractures by primarily posterolateral displacement and a disrupted relationship between the lateral condylar epiphysis and the proximal radius.
- An arthrogram may be useful for clarification of the fracture pattern and differentiation from an intra-articular fracture.

- MRI may be helpful in appreciating the direction of the fracture line and the pattern of fracture.
- Ultrasound may be useful in evaluating neonates and infants in whom ossification has not yet begun.

Classification

DeLee

This is based on ossification of the lateral condyle.

Group A: Infant, before the appearance of the lateral condylar ossification center (birth to 7 months); diagnosis easily missed; Salter–Harris type I

Group B: Lateral condyle ossified (7 months to 3 years); Salter–Harris type I or II (fleck of metaphysis)

Group C: Large metaphyseal fragment, usually exiting laterally (3 to 7 years)

Treatment

Because many of these injuries in infants and toddlers represent child abuse injuries, it is not uncommon for parents to delay seeking treatment.

Nonoperative

- Closed reduction with immobilization is performed with the forearm pronated and the elbow in 90 degrees of flexion if the injury is recognized early (within 4 to 5 days). This is maintained for 3 weeks, at which time the patient is allowed to resume active range of motion.
- When treatment is delayed beyond 6 to 7 days of injury, the fracture should not be manipulated regardless of displacement because the epiphyseal fragment is no longer mobile and other injuries may be precipitated; rather, splinting for comfort should be undertaken. Most fractures eventually completely remodel by maturity.

Operative

- DeLee type C fracture patterns or unstable injuries necessitate percutaneous pinning for fixation. An arthrogram is usually performed to determine the adequacy of reduction.
- Angulation and rotational deformities that cannot be reduced by closed methods may require open reduction and internal fixation with pinning for fixation.

- Postoperatively, the patient may be immobilized with the forearm in pronation and the elbow flexed to 90 degrees. The pins and cast are discontinued at 3 weeks, at which time active range of motion is permitted.

Complications

- **Malunion:** Cubitus varus is most common, although the incidence is lower than with supracondylar fractures of the humerus because of the wider fracture surface of transphyseal fractures that do not allow as much angulation compared with supracondylar fractures.
- **Neurovascular injury:** Extremely rare because the fracture surfaces are covered with cartilage. Closed reduction and immobilization should be followed by repeat neurovascular assessment, given that swelling in the antecubital fossa may result in neurovascular compromise.
- **Nonunion:** Extremely rare because the vascular supply to this region is good.
- **Osteonecrosis:** May be related to severe displacement of the distal fragment or iatrogenic injury, especially with late exploration.

Medial Epicondylar Apophyseal Fractures

Epidemiology

- Comprise 14% of distal humerus fractures.
- Fifty percent are associated with elbow dislocations.
- The peak age is 11 to 12 years.
- The male-to-female ratio is 4:1.

Anatomy

- The medial epicondyle is a traction apophysis for the medial collateral ligament and wrist flexors. It does not contribute to humeral length. The forces across this physis are tensile rather than compressive.
- Ossification begins at 4 to 6 years of age; it is the last ossification center to fuse with the metaphysis (15 years) and does so independently of the other ossification centers.
- The fragment is usually displaced distally and may be incarcerated in the joint 15% to 18% of the time.
- It is often associated with fractures of the proximal radius, olecranon and coronoid.
- In younger children, a medial epicondylar apophyseal fracture may have an intracapsular component because the elbow capsule may

attach as proximally as the physeal line of the epicondyle. In the older child, these fractures are generally extracapsular given that the capsular attachment is more distal to the medial crista of the trochlea.

Mechanism of Injury

- **Direct:** Trauma to the posterior or posteromedial aspect of the medial epicondyle may result in fracture, although these are rare and tend to produce fragmentation of the medial epicondylar fragment.
- **Indirect:**
  - □ **Secondary to elbow dislocation:** The ulnar collateral ligament provides avulsion force.
  - □ Avulsion injury by flexor muscles results from valgus and extension force during a fall onto an outstretched hand or secondary to an isolated muscle avulsion from throwing a ball or arm wrestling, for example.
- **Chronic:** Related to overuse injuries from repetitive throwing, as seen in skeletally immature baseball pitchers.

Clinical Evaluation

- Patients typically present with pain, tenderness, and swelling medially.
- Symptoms may be exacerbated by resisted wrist flexion.
- A careful neurovascular examination is essential because the injury occurs in proximity to the ulnar nerve, which can be injured during the index trauma or from swelling about the elbow.
- Decreased range of motion is usually elicited and may be secondary to pain. Occasionally, a mechanical block to range of motion may result from incarceration of the epicondylar fragment within the elbow joint.
- Valgus instability can be appreciated on stress testing with the elbow flexed to 15 degrees to eliminate the stabilizing effect of the olecranon.

Radiographic Evaluation

- AP, lateral, and oblique radiographs of the elbow should be obtained.
- Because of the posteromedial location of the medial epicondylar apophysis, the ossification center may be difficult to visualize on the AP radiograph if it is even slightly oblique.
- The medial epicondylar apophysis is frequently confused with fracture because of the occasionally fragmented appearance of the

ossification center as well as the superimposition on the distal medial metaphysis. Better visualization may be obtained by a slight oblique of the lateral radiograph, which demonstrates the posteromedial location of the apophysis.

■ A gravity stress test may be performed, demonstrating medial opening on stress radiographs.

■ Complete absence of the apophysis on standard elbow views should prompt a search for the displaced fragment after comparison views of the contralateral, normal elbow are obtained. Specifically, incarceration within the joint must be sought because the epicondylar fragment may be obscured by the distal humerus.

■ Fat pad signs are unreliable, given that epicondylar fractures are extracapsular in older children and capsular rupture associated with elbow dislocation may compromise its ability to confine the hemarthrosis.

■ It is important to differentiate this fracture from a medial condylar physeal fracture; MRI or arthrogram may delineate the fracture pattern, especially when the medial condylar ossification center is not yet present.

Classification

■ Acute
  □ Nondisplaced
  □ Minimally displaced
  □ Significantly displaced (>5 mm) with a fragment proximal to the joint
  □ Incarcerated fragment within the olecranon–trochlea articulation
  □ Fracture through or fragmentation of the epicondylar apophysis, typically from direct trauma
■ Chronic
  □ Tension stress injuries (Little League elbow)

Treatment

Nonoperative

■ Most medial epicondylar fractures may be managed nonoperatively with immobilization. Studies demonstrate that although 60% may establish only fibrous union, 96% have good or excellent functional results.

■ Nonoperative treatment is indicated for nondisplaced or minimally displaced fractures and for significantly displaced fractures in older or low-demand patients.

- The patient is initially placed in a posterior splint with the elbow flexed to 90 degrees with the forearm in neutral or pronation.
- The splint is discontinued 3 to 4 days after injury and early active range of motion is instituted. A sling is worn for comfort.
- Aggressive physical therapy is generally not necessary unless the patient is unable to perform active range-of-motion exercises.

Operative

- An absolute indication for operative intervention is an irreducible, incarcerated fragment within the elbow joint. Closed manipulation may be used to attempt to extract the incarcerated fragment from the joint as described by Roberts. The forearm is supinated, and valgus stress is applied to the elbow, followed by dorsiflexion of the wrist and fingers to put the flexors on stretch. This maneuver is successful approximately 40% of the time.
- Relative indications for surgery include ulnar nerve dysfunction owing to scar or callus formation, valgus instability in an athlete, or significantly displaced fractures in younger or high-demand patients.
- Acute fractures of the medial epicondyle may be approached through a longitudinal incision just anterior to the medial epicondyle. Ulnar nerve identification is important, but extensive dissection or transposition is generally unnecessary. After reduction and provisional fixation with Kirschner wires, fixation may be achieved with a lag-screw technique. A washer may be used in cases of poor bone stock or fragmentation.
- Postoperatively, the patient is placed in a posterior splint or long arm cast with the elbow flexed to 90 degrees and the forearm pronated. This may be converted to a removable posterior splint or sling at 7 to 10 days postoperatively, at which time active range-of-motion exercises are instituted. Formal physical therapy is generally unnecessary if the patient is able to perform active exercises.

Complications

- **Unrecognized intra-articular incarceration:** An incarcerated fragment tends to adhere and form a fibrous union to the coronoid process, resulting in significant loss of elbow range of motion. Although earlier recommendations were to manage this nonoperatively, recent recommendations are to explore the joint with excision of the fragment.
- **Ulnar nerve dysfunction:** The incidence is 10% to 16%, although cases associated with fragment incarceration may have up to a 50% incidence of ulnar nerve dysfunction. Tardy ulnar neuritis may develop

in cases involving reduction of the elbow or manipulation in which scar tissue may be exuberant. Surgical exploration and release may be warranted for symptomatic relief.

- **Nonunion:** May occur in up to 60% of cases with significant displacement treated nonoperatively, although it rarely represents a functional problem.
- **Loss of extension:** A 5% to 10% loss of extension is seen in up to 20% of cases, although this rarely represents a functional problem. This emphasizes the need for early active range-of-motion exercises.
- **Myositis ossificans:** Rare, related to repeated and vigorous manipulation of the fracture. It may result in functional block to motion and must be differentiated from ectopic calcification of the collateral ligaments related to microtrauma, which does not result in functional limitation.

Lateral Epicondylar Apophyseal Fractures

Epidemiology

- Extremely rare in children.

Anatomy

- The lateral epicondylar ossification center appears at 10 to 11 years of age; however, ossification is not completed until the second decade of life.
- The lateral epicondyle represents the origin of many of the wrist and forearm extensors; therefore, avulsion injuries account for a proportion of the fractures, as well as displacement once the fracture has occurred.

Mechanism of Injury

- Direct trauma to the lateral epicondyle may result in fracture; these may be comminuted.
- Indirect trauma may occur with forced volar flexion of an extended wrist, causing avulsion of the extensor origin, often with significant displacement as the fragment is pulled distally by the extensor musculature.

Clinical Evaluation

- Patients typically present with lateral swelling and painful range of motion of the elbow and wrist, with tenderness to palpation of the lateral epicondyle.
- Loss of extensor strength may be appreciated.

Radiographic Evaluation

- The diagnosis is typically made on the AP radiograph, although a lateral view should be obtained to rule out associated injuries.
- The lateral epicondylar physis represents a linear radiolucency on the lateral aspect of the distal humerus and is commonly mistaken for a fracture. Overlying soft tissue swelling, cortical discontinuity, and clinical examination should assist the examiner in the diagnosis of lateral epicondylar apophyseal injury.

Classification

Descriptive

- Avulsion
- Comminution
- Displacement

Treatment

Nonoperative

- With the exception of an incarcerated fragment within the joint, almost all lateral epicondylar apophyseal fractures may be treated with immobilization with the elbow in the flexed, supinated position until comfortable, usually by 2 to 3 weeks.

Operative

- Incarcerated fragments within the elbow joint may be simply excised. Large fragments with associated tendinous origins may be reattached with screws or Kirschner wire fixation and postoperative immobilization for 2 to 3 weeks until comfortable.

Complications

- **Nonunion:** Commonly occurs with established fibrous union of the lateral epicondylar fragment, although it rarely represents a functional or symptomatic problem.
- **Incarcerated fragments:** May result in limited range of motion, most commonly in the radiocapitellar articulation, although free fragments may migrate to the olecranon fossa and limit terminal extension.

Capitellum Fractures

Epidemiology

- Of these fractures, 31% are associated with injuries to the proximal radius.
- Rare in children, representing 1:2000 fractures about the elbow.

■ No verified, isolated fractures of the capitellum have ever been described in children younger than 12 years of age.

Anatomy

■ The fracture fragment is composed mainly of pure articular surface from the capitellum and essentially nonossified cartilage from the secondary ossification center of the lateral condyle.

Mechanism of Injury

■ Indirect force from axial load transmission from the hand through the radial head causes the radial head to strike the capitellum.
■ The presence of recurvatum or cubitus valgus predisposes the elbow to this fracture pattern.

Clinical Evaluation

■ Patients typically present with minimal swelling with painful range of motion. Flexion is often limited by the fragment.
■ Valgus stress tends to reproduce the pain over the lateral aspect of the elbow.
■ Supination and pronation may accentuate the pain.

Radiographic Evaluation

■ AP and lateral views of the elbow should be obtained.
■ Radiographs of the normal, contralateral elbow may be obtained for comparison.
■ If the fragment is large and encompasses ossified portions of the capitellum, it is most readily appreciated on the lateral radiograph.
■ Oblique views of the elbow may be obtained if radiographic abnormality is not appreciated on standard AP and lateral views, especially because a small fragment may be obscured by the density of the overlying distal metaphysis on the AP view.
■ Arthrography or MRI may be helpful when a fracture is not apparent but is suspected to involve purely cartilaginous portions of the capitellum.

Classification

Type I: **Hahn–Steinthal fragment:** Large osseous component of capitellum, often involving the lateral crista of the trochlea

Type II: **Kocher–Lorenz fragment:** Articular cartilage with minimal subchondral bone attached; "uncapping of the condyle"

Treatment

Nonoperative
- Nondisplaced or minimally displaced fractures may be treated with casting with the elbow in hyperflexion.
- Immobilization should be maintained until 2 to 4 weeks or evidence of radiographic healing, at which time active exercises should be instituted.

Operative
- Adequate reduction of displaced fractures is difficult with closed manipulation. Modified closed reduction involving placement of a Steinmann pin into the fracture fragment with manipulation into the reduced position may be undertaken, with postoperative immobilization consisting of casting with the elbow in hyperflexion.
- Excision of the fragment is indicated for fractures in which the fragment is small, comminuted, old (>2 weeks), or not amenable to anatomic reduction without significant dissection of the elbow.
- Open reduction and internal fixation may be achieved by the use of two lag screws, headless screws, or Kirschner wires placed posterior to anterior or anterior to posterior. The heads of the screws must be countersunk to avoid intra-articular impingement.
- Postoperative immobilization should consist of casting with the elbow in hyperflexion for 2 to 4 weeks depending on stability, with serial radiographic evaluation.

Complications

- **Osteonecrosis of the capitellar fragment:** This is uncommon; synovial fluid can typically sustain the fragment until healing occurs.
- **Posttraumatic osteoarthritis:** This may occur with secondary incongruity from malunion or particularly after a large fragment is excised.
- **Stiffness:** Loss of extension is most common, especially with healing of the fragment in a flexed position. This is typically not significant because it usually represents the last several degrees of extension.

T-Condylar Fractures

Epidemiology

- Rare, especially in young children, although this rarity may represent misdiagnosis because purely cartilaginous fractures would not be demonstrated on routine radiographs.
- Peak incidence is in patients 12 to 13 years of age.

Anatomy

- Because of the muscular origin of the flexor and extensor muscles of the forearm, fragment displacement is related not only to the inciting trauma but also to the tendinous attachments. Displacement therefore includes rotational deformities in both the sagittal and coronal planes.
- Fractures in the young child may have a relatively intact distal humeral articular surface despite osseous displacement of the overlying condylar fragments because of the elasticity of the cartilage in the skeletally immature patient.

Mechanism of Injury

- **Flexion:** Most represent wedge-type fractures as the anterior margin of the semilunar notch is driven into the trochlea by a fall onto the posterior aspect of the elbow in >90 degrees of flexion. The condylar fragments are usually anteriorly displaced with respect to the humeral shaft.
- **Extension:** In this uncommon mechanism, a fall onto an outstretched upper extremity results in a wedge-type fracture as the coronoid process of the ulna is driven into the trochlea. The condylar fragments are typically posteriorly displaced with respect to the humeral shaft.

Clinical Evaluation

- The diagnosis is most often confused with extension-type supracondylar fractures because the patient typically presents with the elbow extended, with pain, limited range of motion, variable gross deformity, and massive swelling about the elbow.
- The ipsilateral shoulder, humeral shaft, forearm, wrist, and hand should be examined for associated injuries.
- A careful neurovascular examination is essential, with documentation of the integrity of the median, radial, and ulnar nerves, as well as distal pulses and capillary refill. Massive swelling in the antecubital fossa should alert the examiner to evaluate for compartment syndrome of the forearm. Flexion of the elbow in the presence of antecubital swelling may cause neurovascular embarrassment; repeat evaluation of neurovascular integrity is thus essential following any manipulation or treatment.
- All aspects of the elbow should be examined for possible open lesions; clinical suspicion may be followed with intra-articular injection of saline into the elbow to evaluate possible intra-articular communication of a laceration.

Radiographic Evaluation

- Standard AP and lateral views of the injured elbow should be obtained.
- Comparison views of the normal, contralateral elbow may be obtained in which the diagnosis is not readily apparent. Oblique views may aid in further fracture definition.
- In younger patients, the vertical, intercondylar component may involve only cartilaginous elements of the distal humerus; the fracture may thus appear to be purely supracondylar, although differentiation of the two fracture patterns is important because of the potential for articular disruption and incongruency with T-type fractures. An arthrogram should be obtained when intra-articular extension is suspected.
- Computed tomography and MRI are of limited value and are not typically used in the acute diagnosis of T-type fractures. In younger patients, these modalities often require heavy sedation or anesthesia outside of the operating room, in which case an arthrogram is preferred because it allows for evaluation of the articular involvement as well as treatment in the operating room setting.

Classification

Type I: Nondisplaced or minimally displaced
Type II: Displaced, with no metaphyseal comminution
Type III: Displaced, with metaphyseal comminution

Treatment

Nonoperative

- This is reserved only for truly nondisplaced type I fractures. Thick periosteum may provide sufficient intrinsic stability such that the elbow may be immobilized in flexion with a posterior splint. Mobilization is continued for 1 to 4 weeks after injury.
- Skeletal olecranon traction with the elbow flexed to 90 degrees may be used for patients with extreme swelling, soft tissue compromise, or delayed cases with extensive skin injury that precludes immediate operative intervention. If used as definitive treatment, skeletal traction is usually continued for 2 to 3 weeks, at which time sufficient stability exists for the patient to be converted to a hinged brace for an additional 2 to 3 weeks.

Operative

- Closed reduction and percutaneous pinning are used with increasing frequency for minimally displaced type I injuries in accord with the current philosophy that the articular damage, which cannot be appreciated on standard radiography, may be worse than the apparent osseous involvement.

- ☐ Rotational displacement is corrected using a percutaneous joy-stick in the fracture fragment, with placement of multiple, oblique Kirschner wires for definitive fixation.
- ☐ The elbow is then protected in a posterior splint, with removal of pins at 3 to 4 weeks postoperatively.

■ Open reduction and internal fixation are undertaken for type II and III fractures using either a posterior, triceps-splitting approach, or the triceps-sparing approach as described by Bryan and Morrey. Olecranon osteotomy is generally not necessary for exposure and should be avoided.

- ☐ The articular surface is first anatomically reduced and provisionally stabilized with Kirschner wires, followed by metaphyseal reconstruction with definitive fixation using a combination of Kirschner wires, compression screws, and plates.
- ☐ In the pediatric subset, newer, smaller 2.4-, 2.7-, and 3.5- mm precontoured plates have been introduced and fit the smaller anatomy. Each column may be supported with a plate. Sometimes as with adults, bicolumnar plating is performed with the two plates placed 90 degrees offset from one another.
- ☐ Postoperatively, the elbow is placed in a flexed position for 5 to 7 days, at which time active range of motion is initiated and a removable cast brace is provided.

Complications

■ **Loss of range of motion:** T-type condylar fractures are invariably associated with residual stiffness, especially to elbow extension, owing to the often significant soft tissue injury as well as articular disruption. This can be minimized by ensuring anatomic reduction of the articular surface, employing arthrographic visualization if necessary, as well as stable internal fixation to decrease soft tissue scarring.

■ **Neurovascular injury:** Rare, but is related to significant antecubital soft tissue swelling. Nerve injury to the median, radial, or ulnar nerves may result from the initial fracture displacement or intraoperative traction, although these typically represent neurapraxias that resolve without intervention.

■ **Growth arrest:** Partial or total growth arrest may occur in the distal humeral physis, although it is rarely clinically significant because T-type fractures tend to occur in older children. Similarly, the degree of remodeling is limited, and anatomic reduction should be obtained at the time of initial treatment.

■ **Osteonecrosis of the trochlea:** This may occur especially in association with comminuted fracture patterns in which the vascular supply to the trochlea may be disrupted.

Radial Head and Neck Fractures

Epidemiology

■ Of these fractures, 90% involve either physis or neck; the radial head is rarely involved because of the thick cartilage cap.

■ Represent 5% to 8.5% of elbow fractures.

■ The peak age of incidence is 9 to 10 years.

■ Commonly associated fractures include the olecranon, coronoid, and medial epicondyle.

Anatomy

■ Ossification of the proximal radial epiphysis begins at 4 to 6 years of age as a small, flat nucleus. It may be spheric or may present as a bipartite structure; these anatomic variants may be appreciated by their smooth, rounded borders without cortical discontinuity.

■ Normal angulation of the radial head with respect to the neck ranges between 0 and 15 degrees laterally, and from 10 degrees anterior to 5 degrees posterior angulation.

■ Most of the radial neck is extracapsular; therefore, fractures in this region may not result in a significant effusion or a positive fat pad sign.

■ No ligaments attach directly to the radial head or neck; the radial collateral ligament attaches to the orbicular ligament, which originates from the radial aspect of the ulna.

Mechanism of Injury

■ Acute
   □ **Indirect:** This is most common, usually from a fall onto an outstretched hand with axial load transmission through the proximal radius with trauma against the capitellum.
   □ **Direct:** This is uncommon because of the overlying soft tissue mass.

■ Chronic
   □ Repetitive stress injuries may occur, most commonly from overhead throwing activities. Although most "Little League elbow" injuries represent tension injuries to the medial epicondyle, compressive injuries from valgus stress may result in an osteochondrotic-type disorder of the radial head or an angular deformity of the radial neck.

Clinical Evaluation

- Patients typically present with lateral swelling of the elbow, with pain exacerbated by range of motion, especially supination and pronation.
- Crepitus may be elicited on supination and pronation.
- In a young child, the primary complaint may be wrist pain; pressure over the proximal radius may accentuate the referred wrist pain.

Radiographic Evaluation

- AP and lateral views of the elbow should be obtained. Oblique views may aid in further definition of the fracture line.
- Special views
  - □ **Perpendicular views:** With an acutely painful, flexed elbow, AP evaluation of the elbow may be obtained by taking one radiograph perpendicular to the humeral shaft, and a second view perpendicular to the proximal radius.
  - □ **Radiocapitellar (Greenspan) view:** This oblique lateral radiograph is obtained with the beam directed 45 degrees in a proximal direction, resulting in a projection of the radial head anterior to the coronoid process of the anterior ulna (Fig. 20.1).
- A positive supinator fat pad sign may be present, indicating injury to the proximal radius.
- Comparison views of the contralateral elbow may help identify subtle abnormalities.
- When a fracture is suspected through nonossified regions of the radial head, an arthrogram may be performed to determine displacement.
- MRI may be helpful in appreciating the direction of the fracture line and the pattern of fracture.

Classification

O'Brien

- This is based on the degree of angulation.
- **Type I:** <30 degrees
- **Type II:** 30 to 60 degrees
- **Type III:** >60 degrees

Wilkins

- This is based on the mechanism of injury.
- Valgus injuries are caused by a fall onto an outstretched hand (compression); angular deformity of the head is usually seen (Fig. 44.7).

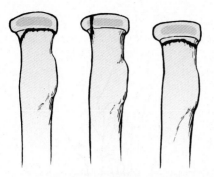

FIGURE 44.7 Types of valgus injuries. **Left:** Type A: Salter–Harris type I or II physeal injury. **Center:** Type B: Salter–Harris type IV injury. **Right:** Type C: Total metaphyseal fracture pattern. (From Bucholz RW, Heckman JD, Court-Brown C, et al., eds. *Rockwood and Green's Fractures in Adults.* 6th ed. Philadelphia: Lippincott Williams & Wilkins; 2006.)

Type A: Salter–Harris type I or II physeal injury
Type B: Salter–Harris type III or IV intra-articular injury
Type C: Fracture line completely within the metaphysis
■ Fracture associated with elbow dislocation
  □ Reduction injury
  □ Dislocation injury

Treatment

Nonoperative
■ Simple immobilization is indicated for O'Brien type I fractures with <30-degree angulation. This can be accomplished with the use of a collar and cuff, a posterior splint, or a long arm cast for 7 to 10 days with early range of motion.
■ Type II fractures with 30- to 60-degree angulation should be managed with manipulative closed reduction.
  □ This may be accomplished by distal traction with the elbow in extension and the forearm in supination; varus stress is applied to overcome the ulnar deviation of the distal fragment and open up the lateral aspect of the joint, allowing for disengagement of the fragments for manipulation (Patterson) (Fig. 44.8).
  □ Israeli described a technique in which the elbow is placed in flexion, and the surgeon's thumb is used to apply pressure over the radial head while the forearm is forced into a pronated position (Fig. 44.9).
  □ Chambers reported another technique for reduction in which an Esmarch wrap is applied distally to proximally, and the radius is reduced by the circumferential pressure.
  □ Following reduction, the elbow should be immobilized in a long arm cast in pronation with 90 degrees of flexion. This should be maintained for 10 to 14 days, at which time range-of-motion exercises should be initiated.

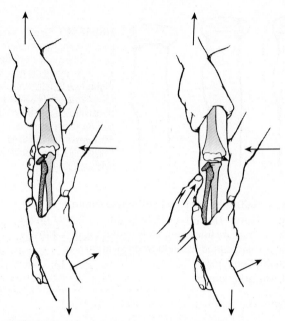

FIGURE 44.8 Patterson's manipulative technique. **Left:** An assistant grabs the patient's arm proximally with one hand placed medially against the distal humerus. The surgeon applies distal traction with the forearm supinated and pulls the forearm into varus. **Right:** Digital pressure applied directly over the tilted radial head completes the reduction. (Adapted from Patterson RF. Treatment of displaced transverse fractures of the neck of the radius in children. *J Bone Joint Surg.* 1934;16:696–698; in Bucholz RW, Heckman JD, Court-Brown C, et al., eds. *Rockwood and Green's Fractures in Adults.* 6th ed. Philadelphia: Lippincott Williams & Wilkins; 2006.)

Operative

- O'Brien type II fractures (30- to 60-degree angulation) that are unstable following closed reduction may require the use of percutaneous Kirschner wire fixation. This is best accomplished by the use of a Steinmann pin placed in the fracture fragment under image intensification for manipulation, followed by oblique Kirschner wire fixation after reduction is achieved. The patient is then placed in a long arm cast in pronation with 90-degree elbow flexion for 3 weeks, at which time the pins and cast are discontinued and active range of motion is initiated.
- Indications for open reduction and internal fixation include fractures that are irreducible by closed means, type III fractures

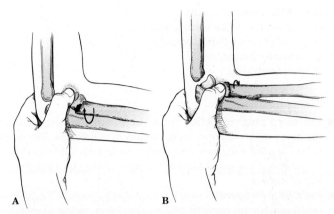

FIGURE 44.9 Flexion–pronation (Israeli) reduction technique. **(A)** With the elbow in 90 degrees of flexion, the thumb stabilizes the displaced radial head. Usually the distal radius is in a position of supination. The forearm is pronated to swing the shaft up into alignment with the neck (*arrow*). **(B)** Movement is continued to full pronation for reduction (*arrow*). (From Bucholz RW, Heckman JD, Court-Brown C, et al., eds. *Rockwood and Green's Fractures in Adults*. 6th ed. Philadelphia: Lippincott Williams & Wilkins; 2006.)

(>60-degree angulation), fractures with >4-mm translation, and medial displacement fractures (these are notoriously difficult to reduce by closed methods). Open reduction with oblique Kirschner wire fixation is recommended; transcapitellar pins are contraindicated because of a high rate of breakage as well as articular destruction from even slight postoperative motion.

- The results of open treatment are not significantly different from those of closed treatment; therefore, closed treatment should be performed when possible.
- Radial head excision gives poor results in children owing to the high incidence of cubitus valgus and radial deviation at the wrist due to the continued growth of the child.

Prognosis

- From 15% to 23% patients will have a poor result regardless of treatment.
- Predictors of a favorable prognosis include
  □ <10 years of age.
  □ Isolated injury.
  □ Minimal soft tissue injury.

☐ Good fracture reduction.
☐ <30-degree initial angulation.
☐ <3-mm initial displacement.
☐ Closed treatment.
☐ Early treatment.

Complications

- Decreased range of motion occurs in (in order of decreasing frequency) pronation, supination, extension, and flexion. The reason is loss of joint congruity and fibrous adhesions. Additionally, enlargement of the radial head following fracture may contribute to loss of motion.
- **Radial head overgrowth:** From 20% to 40% of patients will experience posttraumatic overgrowth of the radial head, owing to increased vascularity from the injury that stimulates epiphyseal growth.
- **Premature physeal closure:** Rarely results in shortening >5 mm, although it may accentuate cubitus valgus.
- **Osteonecrosis of the radial head:** Occurs in 10% to 20%, related to amount of displacement; 70% of cases of osteonecrosis are associated with open reduction.
- **Neurologic:** Usually posterior interosseous nerve neurapraxia; during surgical exposure, pronating the forearm causes the posterior interosseous nerve to move ulnarly, out of the surgical field.
- **Radioulnar synostosis:** This is the most serious complication, usually occurring following open reduction with extensive dissection, but it has been reported with closed manipulations and is associated with a delay in treatment of >5 days. It may require exostectomy to improve function.
- **Myositis ossificans:** May complicate up to 32% of cases, mostly involving the supinator.

Radial Head Subluxation

Epidemiology

- Referred to as "nursemaid's elbow" or "pulled elbow."
- Male-to-female ratio is 1:2.
- Occurs in the left elbow 70% of the time.
- Occurs at ages 6 months to 6 years, with a peak at ages 2 to 3 years.
- Recurrence rate is 5% to 30%.

Anatomy

- Primary stability of the proximal radioulnar joint is conferred by the annular ligament, which closely apposes the radial head within the radial notch of the proximal ulna.

- The annular ligament becomes taut in supination of the forearm owing to the shape of the radial head.
- The substance of the annular ligament is reinforced by the radial collateral ligament at the elbow joint.
- After age 5 years, the distal attachment of the annular ligament to the neck of the radius strengthens significantly to prevent tearing or subsequent displacement.

Mechanism of Injury

- Longitudinal traction force on extended elbow is the cause, although it remains controversial whether the lesion is produced in forearm supination or pronation (it is more widely accepted that the forearm must be in pronation for the injury to occur).

Clinical Evaluation

- Patients typically present with an appropriate history of sudden, longitudinal traction applied to the extended upper extremity (such as a child "jerked" back from crossing the street), often with an audible snap. The initial pain subsides rapidly, and the patient allows the upper extremity to hang in the dependent position with the forearm pronated and elbow slightly flexed and refuses to use the ipsilateral hand (pseudoparalysis).
- A history of a longitudinal pull may be absent in 33% to 50% of cases.
- Effusion is rare, although tenderness can usually be elicited over the anterior and lateral aspects of the elbow.
- A neurovascular examination should be performed, although the presence of neurovascular compromise should alert the physician to consider other diagnostic possibilities because neurovascular injury is not associated with simple radial head subluxation.

Radiographic Evaluation

- Radiographs are not necessary if there is a classic history, the child is 5 years old or younger, and the clinical examination is strongly supportive. Otherwise, standard AP and lateral views of the elbow should be obtained.
- Radiographic abnormalities are not typically appreciated, although some authors have suggested that on the AP radiograph >3-mm lateral displacement of the radial head with respect to the capitellum is indicative of radial head subluxation. However, disruption of the radiocapitellar axis is subtle and often obscured by even slight rotation; therefore, even with a high index of suspicion, appreciation of this sign is generally present in only 25% of cases.

■ Ultrasound is not routinely used in the evaluation of radial head subluxation, but it may demonstrate an increase in the echonegative area between the radial head and the capitellum (radiocapitellar distance typically about 7.2 mm; a difference of >3 mm between the normal and injured elbow suggests radial head subluxation).

Classification

■ A classification scheme for radial head subluxation does not exist.
■ It is important to rule out other diagnostic possibilities, such as early septic arthritis or proximal radius fracture, which may present in a similar fashion, especially if a history of a longitudinal pull is absent.

Treatment

■ Closed reduction
  □ The forearm is supinated with thumb pressure on the radial head.
  □ The elbow is then brought into maximum flexion with the forearm still in supination.
  □ Hyperpronation may also be used to reduce the subluxation.
■ A palpable "click" may be felt on reduction.
■ The child typically experiences a brief moment of pain with the reduction maneuver, followed by the absence of pain and normal use of the upper extremity 5 to 10 minutes later.
■ Postreduction films are generally unnecessary. A child who remains irritable may require further workup for other disorders or a repeat attempt at reduction. If the subluxation injury occurred 12 to 24 hours before evaluation, reactive synovitis may be present that may account for elbow tenderness and a reluctance to move the joint.
■ Sling immobilization is generally unnecessary if the child is able to use the upper extremity without complaint.

Complications

■ **Chronically unreduced subluxation:** Unrecognized subluxation of the radial head generally reduces spontaneously with relief of painful symptoms. In these cases, the subluxation is realized retrospectively.
■ **Recurrence:** Affects 5% to 39% of patients, but generally ceases after 4 to 5 years when the annular ligament strengthens, especially at its distal attachment to the radius.

■ **Irreducible subluxation:** Rare, owing to interposition of the annular ligament. Open reduction may be necessary with transection and repair of the annular ligament to obtain stable reduction.

Elbow Dislocations

Epidemiology

■ Represent 3% to 6% of all elbow injuries.
■ The peak age is 13 to 14 years, after physes are closed.
■ **There is a high incidence of associated fractures:** medial epicondyle, coronoid, and radial head and neck.

Anatomy

■ This is a "modified hinge" joint (ginglymoid) with a high degree of intrinsic stability owing to joint congruity, opposing tension of triceps and flexors, and ligamentous constraints. Of these, the anterior bundle of the medial collateral ligament is the most important.
■ Three separate articulations
  1. Ulnohumeral (hinge)
  2. Radiohumeral (rotation)
  3. Proximal radioulnar (rotation)
■ Stability
  □ **AP:** Trochlea/olecranon fossa (extension); coronoid fossa, radiocapitellar joint, biceps/triceps/brachialis (flexion)
  □ **Valgus:** Medial collateral ligament complex (anterior bundle the primary stabilizer [flexion and extension]) anterior capsule and radiocapitellar joint (extension)
  □ **Varus:** Ulnohumeral articulation, lateral ulnar collateral ligament (static); anconeus muscle (dynamic)
■ Range of motion is 0 to 150 degrees of flexion, 85 degrees of supination, and 80 degrees of pronation.
■ Functionally, range of motion requires 30 to 130 degrees of flexion, 50 degrees of supination, and 50 degrees of pronation.
■ Extension and pronation are the positions of relative instability.

Mechanism of Injury

■ Most commonly, the cause is a fall onto an outstretched hand or elbow, resulting in a levering force to unlock the olecranon from the trochlea combined with translation of the articular surfaces to produce the dislocation.

- **Posterior dislocation:** This is a combination of elbow hyperextension, valgus stress, arm abduction, and forearm supination with resultant soft tissue injuries to the capsule, collateral ligaments (especially medial), and musculature.
- **Anterior dislocation:** A direct force strikes the posterior aspect of the flexed elbow.

Clinical Evaluation

- Patients typically present guarding the injured upper extremity with variable gross instability and massive swelling.
- A careful neurovascular examination is crucial and should be performed before radiographs or manipulation. At significant risk of injury are the median, ulnar, radial, and anterior interosseous nerves and the brachial artery.
- Serial neurovascular examinations should be performed when massive antecubital swelling exists or the patient is believed to be at risk for compartment syndrome.
- Following manipulation or reduction, repeat neurovascular examinations should be performed to monitor neurovascular status.
- Angiography may be necessary to identify vascular compromise. The radial pulse may be present with brachial artery compromise as a result of collateral circulation.

Radiographic Evaluation

- Standard AP and lateral radiographs of the elbow should be obtained.
- Radiographs should be scrutinized for associated fractures about the elbow, most commonly disruption of the apophysis of the medial epicondyle, or fractures involving the coronoid process and radial neck.

Classification

- **Chronologic:** Acute, chronic (unreduced), or recurrent.
- **Descriptive:** Based on the relationship of the proximal radioulnar joint to the distal humerus.
- Posterior
  - □ **Posterolateral:** >90% dislocations
  - □ Posteromedial
- **Anterior:** Represents only 1% of pediatric elbow dislocations.
- **Divergent:** This is rare.
- **Medial and lateral dislocations:** These are not described in the pediatric population.

- **Fracture dislocation:** Most associated osseous injuries involve the coronoid process of the olecranon, the radial neck, or the medial epicondylar apophysis of the distal humerus. Rarely, shear fractures of the capitellum or trochlea may occur.

Treatment

Posterior Dislocation
Nonoperative

- Acute posterior elbow dislocations should be initially managed with closed reduction using sedation and analgesia. Alternatively, general or regional anesthesia may be used.
- **Young children (0 to 8 years old):** With the patient prone and the affected forearm hanging off the edge of the table, anteriorly directed pressure is applied to the olecranon tip, effecting reduction.
- **Older children (>8 years old):** With the patient supine, reduction should be performed with the forearm supinated and the elbow flexed while providing distal traction (Parvin method). Reduction with the elbow hyperextended is associated with median nerve entrapment and increased soft tissue trauma.
- Neurovascular status should be reassessed, followed by evaluation of stable range of motion.
- Postreduction radiographs are essential.
- Postreduction management should consist of a posterior splint at 90 degrees with loose circumferential wraps and elevation. Attention should be paid to antecubital and forearm swelling.
- Early, gentle, active range of motion 5 to 7 days after reduction is associated with better long-term results. Forced, passive range of motion should be avoided because redislocation may occur. Prolonged immobilization is associated with unsatisfactory results and greater flexion contractures.
- A hinged elbow brace through a stable arc of motion may be indicated in cases of instability without associated fractures.
- Full recovery of motion and strength requires 3 to 6 months.

Operative

- Indicated for cases of soft tissue and/or bony entrapment in which closed reduction is not possible.
- A large, displaced coronoid fragment requires open reduction and internal fixation to prevent recurrent instability. Medial epicondylar apophyseal disruptions with entrapped fragments must be addressed.
- Lateral ligamentous reconstruction in cases of recurrent instability and dislocation is usually unnecessary.

■ An external fixator for grossly unstable dislocations (with disruption of the medial collateral ligament) may be required as a salvage procedure.

Anterior Dislocation

■ Acute anterior dislocation of the elbow may be managed initially with closed reduction using sedation and analgesia.

■ Initial distal traction is applied to the flexed forearm to relax the forearm musculature, followed by dorsally directed pressure on the volar forearm coupled with anteriorly directed pressure on the distal humerus.

■ Triceps function should be assessed following reduction because stripping of the triceps tendon from its olecranon insertion may occur.

■ Associated olecranon fractures usually require open reduction and internal fixation.

Divergent Dislocation

■ This is a rare injury, with two types:

☐ **Anterior–posterior type (ulna posteriorly, radial head anteriorly):** This is more common; reduction is achieved in the same manner as for a posterior dislocation concomitant with posteriorly directed pressure over the anterior radial head prominence.

☐ **Mediolateral (transverse) type (distal humerus wedged between radius laterally and ulna medially):** This is extremely rare; reduction is by direct distal traction on extended elbow with pressure on the proximal radius and ulna converging them.

Complications

■ **Loss of motion (extension):** This is associated with prolonged immobilization with initially unstable injuries. Some authors recommend posterior splint immobilization for 3 to 4 weeks, although recent trends have been to begin early (1 week) supervised range of motion. Patients typically experience a loss of the terminal 10 to 15 degrees of extension, which is usually not functionally significant.

■ **Neurologic compromise:** Neurologic deficits occur in 10% of cases. Most complications occur with entrapment of the median nerve. Ulnar nerve injuries are most commonly associated with disruptions of the medial epicondylar apophysis. Radial nerve injuries occur rarely.

☐ Spontaneous recovery is usually expected; a decline in nerve function (especially after manipulation) or severe pain in nerve distribution is an indication for exploration and decompression.

☐ Exploration is recommended if no recovery is seen after 3 months following electromyography and serial clinical examinations.

- **Vascular injury (rare):** The brachial artery is most commonly disrupted during injury.
  - ☐ Prompt recognition of vascular injury is essential, with closed reduction to re-establish perfusion.
  - ☐ If, after reduction, perfusion is not re-established, angiography is indicated to identify the lesion, with arterial reconstruction with reverse saphenous vein graft when indicated.
- **Compartment syndrome (Volkmann contracture):** May result from massive swelling from soft tissue injury. Postreduction care must include aggressive elevation and avoidance of hyperflexion of the elbow. Serial neurovascular examinations and compartment pressure monitoring may be necessary, with forearm fasciotomy when indicated.
- **Instability/redislocation:** Rare (<1%) after isolated, traumatic posterior elbow dislocation; the incidence is increased in the presence of associated coronoid process and radial head fracture (combined with elbow dislocation, this completes the *terrible triad of the elbow*). It may necessitate hinged external fixation, capsuloligamentous reconstruction, internal fixation, or prosthetic replacement of the radial head.
- **Heterotopic bone/myositis ossificans:** This occurs in 3% of pure dislocations, 18% when associated with fractures, most commonly caused by vigorous attempts at reduction.
  - ☐ Anteriorly, it forms between the brachialis muscle and the capsule; posteriorly, it may form medially or laterally between the triceps and the capsule.
  - ☐ The risk is increased with a greater degree of soft tissue trauma or the presence of associated fractures.
  - ☐ It may result in significant loss of function.
  - ☐ Forcible manipulation or passive stretching increases soft tissue trauma and should be avoided.
  - ☐ Indomethacin or local radiation therapy is recommended for prophylaxis postoperatively and in the presence of significant soft tissue injury and/or associated fractures. Radiation therapy is contraindicated in the presence of open physes.
- **Osteochondral fractures:** Anterior shear fractures of the capitellum or trochlea may occur with anterior dislocations of the elbow. The presence of an unrecognized osteochondral fragment in the joint may be the cause of an unsatisfactory result of what initially appeared to be an uncomplicated elbow dislocation.
- **Radioulnar synostosis:** The incidence is increased with an associated radial neck fracture.
- **Cubitus recurvatum:** With significant disruption of the anterior capsule, hyperextension of the elbow may occur late, although this is rarely of any functional or symptomatic significance.

Olecranon Fractures

Epidemiology

- These account for 5% of all elbow fractures.
- The peak age is 5 to 10 years.
- Twenty percent of patients have an associated fracture or dislocation; the proximal radius is the most common.

Anatomy

- The olecranon is metaphyseal and has a relatively thin cortex, which may predispose the area to greenstick-type fractures.
- The periosteum is thick, which may prevent the degree of separation seen in adult olecranon fractures.
- The larger amount of epiphyseal cartilage may also serve as a cushion to lessen the effects of a direct blow.

Mechanism of Injury

- **Flexion injuries:** With the elbow in a semiflexed postion, the pull of the triceps and brachialis muscles places the posterior cortex in tension; this force alone, or in combination with a direct blow, may cause the olecranon to fail. The fracture is typically transverse.
- **Extension injuries:** With the arm extended, the olecranon becomes locked in the olecranon fossa; if a varus or valgus force is then applied, stress is concentrated in the distal aspect of the olecranon; resultant fractures are typically greenstick fractures that remain extra-articular and may extend proximal to the coronoid process.
- **Shear injuries:** A direct force is applied to the posterior olecranon, resulting in tension failure of the anterior cortex; the distal fragment is displaced anteriorly by the pull of the brachialis and biceps; this is differentiated from the flexion-type injury by an intact posterior periosteum.

Clinical Evaluation

- Soft tissue swelling is typically present over the olecranon.
- An abrasion or contusion directly over the olecranon may indicate a flexion-type injury.
- The patient may lack active extension, although this is frequently difficult to evaluate in an anxious child with a swollen elbow.

Radiographic Evaluation

- Standard AP and lateral x-rays of the elbow should be obtained.
- Fracture lines associated with a flexion injury are perpendicular to the long axis of the olecranon; these differentiate the fracture from

the residual physeal line, which is oblique and directed proximal and anterior.

- The longitudinal fracture lines associated with extension injuries may be difficult to appreciate.
- The radiographs should be scrutinized to detect associated fractures, especially proximal radius fractures.

Classification

- **Group A:** Flexion injuries
- **Group B:** Extension injuries
  1. Valgus pattern
  2. Varus pattern
- **Group C:** Shear injuries

Treatment

Nonoperative

- Nondisplaced flexion injuries are treated with splint immobilization in 5 to 10 degrees of flexion for 3 weeks; radiographs should be checked in 5 to 7 days to evaluate for early displacement.
- Extension injuries generally need correction of the varus or valgus deformity; this may be accomplished by locking the olecranon in the olecranon fossa with extension and applying a varus or valgus force to reverse the deformity; overcorrection may help to prevent recurrence of the deformity.
- Shear injuries can be treated with immobilization in a hyperflexed position if the posterior periosteum remains intact, with the posterior periosteum functioning as a tension band; operative intervention should be considered if excessive swelling is present that may result in neurovascular compromise in a hyperflexed position.

Operative

- Displaced or comminuted fractures may require surgical stabilization.
- Determining whether the posterior periosteum is intact is key to determining the stability of a fracture; if a palpable defect is present, or if the fragments separate with flexion of the elbow, internal fixation may be needed.
- Fixation may be achieved with Kirschner wires and a tension band, tension band alone, cancellous screws alone, or cancellous screws and tension band.
- Removal of hardware is frequently required and should be considered when deciding on a fixation technique (i.e., tension band with wire versus tension band with suture).

■ Postoperatively, the elbow is immobilized in a cast at 70 to 80 degrees of flexion for 3 weeks, after which active motion is initiated.

Complications

■ **Delayed union:** Rare (<1%) and is usually asymptomatic, even if it progresses to a nonunion.
■ **Nerve injury:** Rare at the time of injury; ulnar neurapraxia has been reported after development of a pseudarthrosis of the olecranon when inadequate fixation was used.
■ **Elongation:** Elongation of the tip of the olecranon may occur after fracture; the apophysis may elongate to the point that it limits elbow extension.
■ **Loss of reduction:** Associated with fractures treated nonoperatively that subsequently displace; it may result in significant loss of elbow function if it is not identified early in the course of treatment.

45 Pediatric Forearm

EPIDEMIOLOGY

- These injuries are very common. They make up 40% of all pediatric fractures (only 4% are diaphyseal fractures), with a 3:1 male predominance in distal radius fractures.
- Eighty percent occur in children >5 years of age.
- The peak incidence corresponds to the peak velocity of growth when the bone is weakest owing to a dissociation between bone growth and mineralization.
- Fifteen percent have ipsilateral supracondylar fractures.
- One percent have neurologic injuries, most commonly median nerve.
- Of pediatric forearm fractures, 60% occur in the distal metaphyses of the radius or ulna, 20% in the shaft, 14% in the distal physis, and <4% in the proximal third.

ANATOMY

- The radial and ulnar shafts ossify during the eighth week of gestation.
- The distal radial epiphysis appears at the age of 1 year (often from two centers); the distal ulnar epiphysis appears at the age of 5 years; the radial head appears at the age of 5 to 7 years; the olecranon appears at the age of 9 to 10 years. These all close between the ages of 16 and 18 years.
- The distal physis accounts for 80% of forearm growth.
- With advancing skeletal age, there is a tendency for fractures to occur in an increasingly distal location owing to the distal recession of the transition between the more vulnerable wider metaphysis and the more narrow and stronger diaphysis.
- Osteology
  - The radius is a curved bone, cylindric in the proximal third, triangular in the middle third, and flat distally with an apex lateral bow.
  - The ulna has a triangular shape throughout, with an apex posterior bow in the proximal third.
  - The proximal radioulnar joint is most stable in supination where the broadest part of the radial head contacts the radial notch of

the ulna and the interosseous membrane is most taut. The annular ligament is its major soft tissue stabilizer.

□ The distal radioulnar joint (DRUJ) is stabilized by the ulnar collateral ligament, the anterior and posterior radioulnar ligaments, and the pronator quadratus muscle. Three percent of distal radius fractures have concomitant DRUJ disruption.

□ The triangular fibrocartilage complex (TFCC) has an articular disc joined by volar and dorsal radiocarpal ligaments and by ulnar collateral ligament fibers. It attaches to the distal radius at its ulnar margin, with its apex attached to the base of the ulna styloid, extending distally to the base of the fifth metacarpal.

□ The periosteum is very strong and thick in the child. It is generally disrupted on the convex fracture side, whereas an intact hinge remains on the concave side. This is an important consideration when attempting closed reduction.

■ Biomechanics

□ The posterior distal radioulnar ligament is taut in pronation, whereas the anterior ligament is taut in supination.

□ The radius effectively shortens with pronation and lengthens with supination.

□ The interosseous space is narrowest in pronation and widest in neutral to 30 degrees of supination. Further supination or pronation relaxes the membrane.

□ The average range of pronation/supination is 90/90 degrees (50/50 degrees necessary for activities of daily living).

□ Middle third deformity has a greater effect on supination, with the distal third affecting pronation to a greater degree.

□ Malreduction of 10 degrees in the middle third limits rotation by 20 to 30 degrees.

□ Bayonet apposition (overlapping) does not reduce forearm rotation.

■ Deforming muscle forces (Fig. 45.1)

□ **Proximal third fractures:**

• **Biceps and supinator:** These function to flex and supinate the proximal fragment.

• **Pronator teres and pronator quadratus:** These pronate the distal fragment.

□ **Middle third fractures:**

• **Supinator, biceps, and pronator teres:** The proximal fragment is in neutral position.

• **Pronator quadratus:** Pronates the distal fragment.

□ **Distal third fractures:**

• **Brachioradialis:** Dorsiflexes and radially deviates the distal segment.

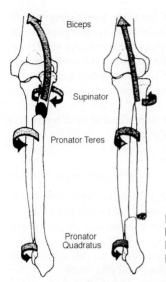

FIGURE 45.1 Deforming muscle forces in both bone forearm fractures. (Adapted from Cruess RL. Importance of soft tissue evaluation in both hand and wrist trauma: statistical evaluation. *Orthop Clin North Am.* 1973;4:969.)

Biceps

Supinator

Pronator Teres

Pronator Quadratus

- ● **Pronator quadratus, wrist flexors and extensors, and thumb abductors:** They also cause fracture deformity.

MECHANISM OF INJURY

- ■ **Indirect:** The mechanism of injury involves a fall onto an outstretched hand. Forearm rotation determines the direction of angulation:
  - □ **Pronation:** flexion injury (dorsal angulation)
  - □ **Supination:** extension injury (volar angulation)
- ■ **Direct:** Direct trauma to the radial or ulnar shaft.

CLINICAL EVALUATION

- ■ The patient typically presents with pain, swelling, variable gross deformity, and a refusal to use the injured upper extremity.
- ■ A careful neurovascular examination is essential. Injuries to the wrist may be accompanied by symptoms of carpal tunnel compression, and more proximal fractures may be associated with anterior interosseous nerve (AIN) or posterior interosseous nerve (PIN) injuries.
- ■ The ipsilateral hand, wrist, forearm, and arm should be palpated, with examination of the ipsilateral elbow and shoulder to rule out associated fractures or dislocations.
- ■ In cases of dramatic swelling of the forearm, compartment syndrome should be ruled out on the basis of serial neurovascular

examinations with compartment pressure monitoring if indicated. Pain on passive extension of the digits is most sensitive for recognition of a possible developing compartment syndrome; the presence of any of the "classic" signs of compartment syndrome (pain out of proportion to injury, pallor, paresthesias, pulselessness, paralysis) should be aggressively evaluated with possible forearm fasciotomy.

■ Examination of skin integrity must be performed, with removal of all bandages and splints placed in the field.

RADIOGRAPHIC EVALUATION

■ Anteroposterior and lateral views of forearm, wrist, and elbow should be obtained. The forearm should not be rotated to obtain these views; instead, the beam should be rotated to obtain a cross-table view.

■ The bicipital tuberosity is the landmark for identifying the rotational position of the proximal fragment (Fig. 45.2):
  □ **Ninety degrees of supination:** It is directed medially.
  □ **Neutral:** It is directed posteriorly.
  □ **Ninety degrees of pronation:** This is directed laterally.
  □ In the normal, uninjured radius, the bicipital tuberosity is 180 degrees to the radial styloid.

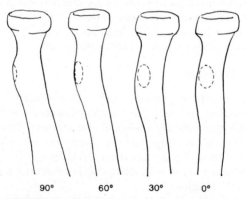

90°   60°   30°   0°

FIGURE 45.2 The normal bicipital tuberosity from full supination (90 degrees) to midposition (0 degrees). In children, these characteristics are less clearly defined. (From Rockwood CA Jr, Wilkins KE, Beaty JH, eds. *Rockwood and Green's Fractures in Children.* Vol 3. 4th ed. Philadelphia: Lippincott-Raven; 1996:515.)

RADIUS AND ULNA SHAFT FRACTURES

Classification

Descriptive

1. **Location:** proximal, middle, distal third
2. **Type:** plastic deformation, incomplete (greenstick), compression (torus or buckle), or complete
3. Displacement
4. Angulation

Nonoperative Treatment

■ Gross deformity should be corrected on presentation to limit injury to soft tissues. The extremity should be splinted for pain relief and prevention of further injury if closed reduction will be delayed (Fig. 45.3).

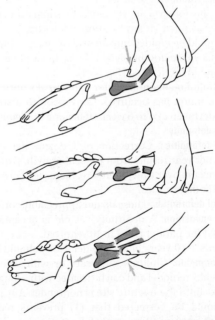

FIGURE 45.3 Top: Traction and counteraction of the thumb is used to increase the deformity. **Center:** With traction still maintained, the thumb slips farther distally to correct the angulation. It is best to avoid disrupting the periosteum, but on occasion this is necessary. **Bottom:** Ulnar or radial deviation can also be corrected by traction and thumb pressure. (Redrawn from Weber BG, Brunner C, Freuler F. *Treatment of Fractures in Children and Adolescents.* New York: Springer-Verlag; 1980.)

■ The extent and type of fracture and the child's age are the factors that determine whether reduction can be carried out with sedation, local anesthesia, or general anesthesia.

■ Finger traps may be applied with weights to aid in reduction.

■ Closed reduction and application of a well-molded (both three-point and interosseous molds) long arm cast or splint should be performed for most fractures, unless the fracture is open, unstable, irreducible, or associated with compartment syndrome.

  □ Reduction should be maintained with pressure on the side of the intact periosteum (concave side).

  □ Exaggeration of the deformity to disengage the fragment and to relieve tension of the periosteum is only performed for distal radius fractures, not shaft fractures.

■ Because of deforming muscle forces, the level of the fracture determines forearm rotation of immobilization:

  □ **Proximal third fractures:** supination

  □ **Middle third fractures:** neutral

  □ **Distal third fractures:** pronation

  □ Placing the forearm in extremes of supination or pronation should be avoided for any location of fracture.

■ The cast should be molded into an oval to increase the width of the interosseous space and bivalved if forearm swelling is a concern. The arm should be elevated (Fig. 45.4).

■ The cast should be maintained for 4 to 8 weeks until radiographic evidence of union has occurred. Conversion to a short arm cast may be undertaken at 4 to 6 weeks if healing is adequate.

■ **Acceptable deformity:**

  □ **Angular deformities:** Correction of 1 degree per month, or 10 degrees per year results from physeal growth. Exponential correction occurs over time; therefore, increased correction occurs for greater deformities.

  □ **Rotational deformities:** These do not appreciably correct.

  □ **Bayonet apposition:** A deformity ≤1 cm is acceptable and will remodel if the patient is <8 to 10 years old.

  □ In patients >10 years of age, no deformity should be accepted.

■ **Plastic deformation:** Children <4 years or with deformities <20 degrees usually remodel and can be treated with a long arm cast for 4 to 6 weeks until the fracture site is nontender. Any plastic deformation should be corrected that (1) prevents reduction of a concomitant fracture, (2) prevents full rotation in a child >4 years, or (3) exceeds 20 degrees.

  □ General anesthesia is typically necessary, because forces of 20 to 30 kg are usually required for correction.

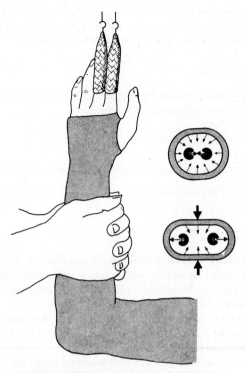

FIGURE 45.4 While the cast hardens, it is pressed together by both hands to form an oval. This increases the width of the interosseus space. Traction should be released gradually while this is done. (Redrawn from Weber BG, Brunner C, Freuler F. *Treatment of Fractures in Children and Adolescents.* New York: Springer-Verlag; 1980.)

☐ The apex of the bow should be placed over a well-padded wedge, with application of a constant force for 2 to 3 minutes, followed by application of a well-molded long arm cast.

☐ The correction should have less than 10 to 20 degrees of angulation.

■ **Greenstick fractures:** Nondisplaced or minimally displaced fractures may be immobilized in a well-molded long arm cast. They should be slightly overcorrected to prevent recurrence of deformity.

☐ Completing the fracture decreases the risk of recurrence of the deformity; however, reduction of the displaced fracture may be more difficult. Therefore, it may be beneficial to carefully fracture the intact cortex while preventing displacement. A well-molded long arm cast should then be applied.

Operative Indications

- Unstable/unacceptable fracture reduction after closed reduction
- Open fracture/compartment syndrome
- Floating elbow
- Refracture with displacement
- Segmental fracture
- Age (usually older than 10 years if significant angulation persists)

Surgical stabilization of pediatric forearm fractures is required in 1.5% to 31% of cases.

Operative Treatment

- **Intramedullary fixation:** Percutaneous insertion of intramedullary rods or wires may be used for fracture stabilization. Typically, flexible (elastic) rods or rods with inherent curvature to permit restoration of the radial bow are used.
  - □ The radius is reduced first, with insertion of the rod just proximal to the radial styloid after visualization of the two branches of the superficial radial nerve.
  - □ The ulna is then reduced, with insertion of the rod either antegrade through the olecranon or retrograde through the distal metaphysis, with protection of the ulnar nerve.
  - □ Postoperatively, a volar splint is placed for 4 weeks. The hardware is left in place for 6 to 9 months, at which time removal may take place, provided solid callus is present across the fracture site and the fracture line is obliterated.
- **Plate fixation:** Severely comminuted fractures or those associated with segmental bone loss are ideal indications for plate fixation, because in these patterns rotational stability is needed. Plate fixation is also used in cases of forearm fractures in skeletally mature individuals.
- **Ipsilateral supracondylar fractures:** When associated with forearm fractures, a "floating elbow" results. These may be managed by conventional pinning of the supracondylar fracture followed by cast immobilization of the forearm fracture. Stabilization of the forearm fracture may be required if there is gross instability or displacement and there is concern about a compartment syndrome.

Complications

- **Refracture:** This occurs in 5% of patients and is more common after greenstick fractures and after plate removal.
- **Malunion:** This is a possible complication.
- **Synostosis:** Rare complication in children. Risk factors include high-energy trauma, surgery, repeated manipulations, proximal fractures, and head injury.
- **Compartment syndrome:** One should always bivalve the cast after a reduction.
- **Nerve injury:** Median, ulnar, and PIN nerve injuries have all been reported. There is an 8.5% incidence of iatrogenic injury in fractures that are surgically stabilized.

MONTEGGIA FRACTURE

- This is a proximal ulna fracture or plastic deformation with associated dislocation of the radial head.
- Comprises 0.4% of all forearm fractures in children.
- The peak incidence is between 4 and 10 years of age.
- Ulna fracture is usually located at the junction of the proximal and middle thirds.
- **Bado classification of Monteggia fractures (Fig. 45.5):**

Type I: Anterior dislocation of the radial head with fracture of ulna diaphysis at any level with anterior angulation; 70% of cases; may occur from a direct blow, hyperpronation, or hyperextension

Type II: Posterior/posterolateral dislocation of the radial head with fracture of ulna diaphysis with posterior angulation; 3% to 6% of cases; a variant of posterior elbow dislocation when the anterior cortex of the ulna is weaker than the elbow ligaments

Type III: Lateral/anterolateral dislocation of the radial head with fracture of ulna metaphysis; 23% of cases (ulna fracture usually greenstick); occurs with varus stress on an outstretched hand planted firmly against a fixed surface

Type IV: Anterior dislocation of the radial head with fractures of both radius and ulna within proximal third at the same level; 1% to 11% of cases

MONTEGGIA FRACTURE EQUIVALENTS (FIG. 45.6)

Type I: Isolated radial head dislocation

Type II: Ulna and proximal radius (neck) fracture

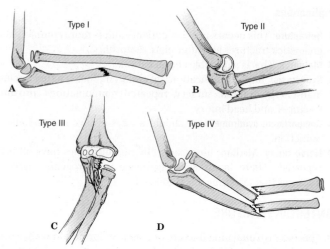

FIGURE 45.5 Bado classification. **(A)** Type I (anterior dislocation): The radial head is dislocated anteriorly and the ulna has a short oblique or greenstick fracture in the diaphyseal or proximal metaphyseal area. **(B)** Type II (posterior dislocation): The radial head is posteriorly and posterolaterally dislocated; the ulna is usually fractured in the metaphysis in children. **(C)** Type III (lateral dislocation): There is lateral dislocation of the radial head with a greenstick metaphyseal fracture of the ulna. **(D)** Type IV (anterior dislocation with radius shaft fracture): The pattern of injury is the same as with a Type I injury, with the inclusion of a radius shaft fracture below the level of the ulnar fracture. (From Bucholz RW, Heckman JD, Court-Brown C, et al., eds. *Rockwood and Green's Fractures in Adults.* 6th ed. Philadelphia: Lippincott Williams & Wilkins; 2006.)

Type III: Isolated radial neck fracture
Type IV: Elbow dislocation (ulnohumeral)
- **Treatment:** Based on the type of ulna fracture rather than on the Bado type. Plastic deformation is treated with reduction of ulnar bow. Incomplete fractures are treated with closed reduction and casting (types I and III are more stable with immobilization in 100 to 110 degrees of flexion and full supination). Complete fractures are treated with Kirschner wires or intramedullary fixation if one is unable to reduce or maintain to the reduction of the radial head.
- Ten degrees of angulation are acceptable in children <10 years old, provided reduction of radial head is adequate.
- **Complications:**
  - **Nerve injury:** There is a 10% to 20% incidence of PIN (most common in types I and III).
  - Myositis ossificans occurs in 7% of cases.

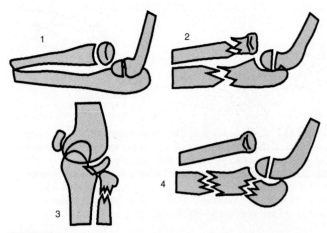

FIGURE 45.6 Type I Monteggia equivalents: **1,** isolated anterior radial head dislocation; **2,** ulnar fracture with fracture of the radial neck; **3,** isolated radial neck fractures; **4,** elbow (ulnohumeral) dislocation with or without fracture of the proximal radius. (From Bucholz RW, Heckman JD, Court-Brown C, et al., eds. *Rockwood and Green's Fractures in Adults.* 6th ed. Philadelphia: Lippincott Williams & Wilkins; 2006.)

GALEAZZI FRACTURE

- A middle to distal third radius fracture, with intact ulna, and disruption of the DRUJ. A Galeazzi equivalent is a distal radial fracture with a distal ulnar physeal fracture (more common).
- This injury is rare in children; 3% of distal radius fractures have concurrent DRUJ disruption.
- Peak incidence is between ages 9 and 12 years.
- Classified by position of radius (Fig. 45.7)

Type I: Dorsal displacement of distal radius, caused by supination force. Reduces with forced pronation and dorsal to volar force on the distal radius.

Type II: Volar displacement, caused by pronation. Reduces with supination and volar to dorsal force on the distal radius.

- The operative indication is a failure to maintain reduction. This is treated with cross-pinning, intramedullary pins, or plating.
- **Complications:**
  - **Malunion:** This results most frequently from persistent ulnar subluxation.

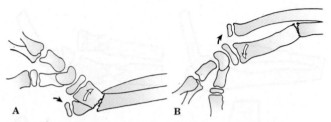

FIGURE 45.7 Walsh classification. **(A)** The most common pattern in which there is dorsal displacement with supination of the distal radius (*open arrow*). The distal ulna (*black arrow*) lies volar to the dorsally displaced distal radius. **(B)** The least common pronation pattern. There is volar or anterior displacement of the distal radius (*open arrow*), and the distal ulna lies dorsal (*black arrow*). (Adapted from Walsh HPJ, McLaren CANP. Galeazzi fractures in children. *J Bone Joint Surg Br.* 1987;69:730–733.)

  ☐ **Ulnar physeal arrest:** Occurs in 55% of Galeazzi equivalent fractures.

DISTAL RADIUS FRACTURES

Physeal Injuries

- **Salter-Harris types I and II:** Gentle closed reduction is followed by application of a long arm cast or sugar tong splint with the forearm pronated (Fig. 45.8); 50% apposition with no angular or rotational deformity is acceptable. Growth arrest can occur in 25% of patients if two or more manipulations are attempted. Open reduction is indicated if the fracture is irreducible (periosteum or pronator quadratus may be interposed).

- **Salter-Harris type III:** Anatomic reduction is necessary. Open reduction and internal fixation with smooth pins or screws parallel to the physis is recommended if the fracture is inadequately reduced.

- **Salter-Harris types IV and V:** Rare injuries. Open reduction and internal fixation is indicated if the fracture is displaced; growth disturbance is likely.

- Complications
  - ☐ Physeal arrest may occur from original injury, late reduction (>7 days after injury), or multiple reduction attempts. It may lead to radial deformity or ulnar positivity.
  - ☐ Ulnar styloid nonunion is often indicative of a TFCC tear. The styloid may be excised and the TFCC repaired.
  - ☐ **Carpal tunnel syndrome:** Decompression may be indicated.

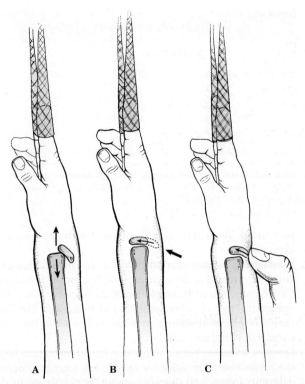

FIGURE 45.8 Acceptable method of closed reduction of distal physeal fractures of the radius. **(A)** Position of the fracture fragments as finger trap traction with countertraction is applied (*arrows*). **(B)** Often with traction alone, the fracture will reduce without external pressure (*arrows*). **(C)** If the reduction is incomplete, simply applying direct pressure over the fracture site in a distal and volar direction with the thumb often completes the reduction while maintaining traction. This technique theoretically decreases the shear forces across the physis during the reduction process. (From Bucholz RW, Heckman JD, Court-Brown C, et al., eds. *Rockwood and Green's Fractures in Adults.* 6th ed. Philadelphia: Lippincott Williams & Wilkins; 2006.)

Metaphyseal Injuries

- Classified by the direction of displacement, involvement of the ulna, and the biomechanical pattern (torus, incomplete, complete).
- Treatment
  - **Torus fractures:** If only one cortex is involved, then the injury is stable and may be treated with protected immobilization for

TABLE 45.1	Acceptable Angular Corrections in Degrees		
	Sagittal Plane		
Age (yr)	Boys	Girls	**Frontal Plane**
4–9	20	15	15
9–11	15	10	5
11–13	10	10	0
>13	5	0	0

Acceptable residual angulation is that which will result in total radiographic and functional correction. (Courtesy B. deCourtivron, MD. Centre Hospitalie Universitaire de Tours. Tours, France from Bucholz RW, Heckman JD, Court-Brown C, et al., eds. *Rockwood and Green's Fractures in Adults*. 6th ed. Philadelphia: Lippincott Williams & Wilkins; 2006.)

pain relief. Bicortical injuries should be treated in a long arm cast.

☐ **Incomplete (greenstick) fractures (Table 45.1):** These have a greater ability to remodel in the sagittal plane than in the frontal plane. Closed reduction with completion of the fracture is indicated to reduce the risk of subsequent loss of reduction. The patient should be placed in supination to reduce the pull of the brachioradialis in a long arm cast.

☐ **Complete fractures:** Finger traps may hinder reduction because the periosteum may tighten with traction. Exaggeration of the deformity (often >90 degrees) should be performed to disengage the fragments. The angulated distal fragment may then be apposed onto the end of the proximal fragment, with simultaneous correction of rotation The patient should be placed in a well-molded long arm cast for 3 to 4 weeks (Fig. 45.9). Indications for percutaneous pinning include loss of reduction, excessive local swelling preventing placement of a well-molded cast, floating elbow, and multiple manipulations. Open reduction is indicated if the fracture is irreducible (<1% of all distal radius fractures), if the fracture is open, or if the patient has compartment syndrome.

■ Complications

☐ **Malunion:** Loss of reduction may occur in up to 30% of metaphyseal fractures with bayonet opposition. Residual malangulation of more than 20% may result in loss of forearm rotation.

☐ **Nonunion:** This rare complication is usually indicative of an alternate pathologic state.

☐ **Refracture:** Usually results from an early return to activity (before 6 weeks).

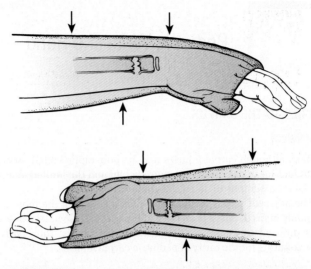

FIGURE 45.9 Three-point molding. **Top:** Three-point molding for dorsally angulated (apex volar) fractures, with the proximal and distal points on the dorsal aspect of the cast and the middle point on the volar aspect just proximal to the fracture site. **Bottom:** For volar angulated fractures, where the periosteum is intact volarly and is disrupted on the dorsal surface, three-point molding is performed with the proximal and distal points on the volar surface of the cast and the middle point just proximal to the fracture site on the dorsal aspect of the cast. (From Bucholz RW, Heckman JD, Court-Brown C, et al., eds. *Rockwood and Green's Fractures in Adults.* 6th ed. Philadelphia: Lippincott Williams & Wilkins; 2006.)

- ☐ **Growth disturbance:** The average disturbance of growth is 3 mm (either overgrowth or undergrowth) with maximal overgrowth in 9 to 12 year olds.
- ☐ **Neurovascular injuries:** One needs to avoid extreme positions of immobilization.

Pediatric Wrist and Hand

INJURIES TO THE CARPUS

Epidemiology

- Rare, although carpal injuries may be underappreciated owing to difficulties in examining an injured child and the limited ability of plain radiographs to detail the immature skeleton.
- The adjacent physis of the distal radius is among the most commonly injured; this is protective of the carpus as load transmission is diffused by injury to the distal radial physis, thus partially accounting for the rarity of pediatric carpal injuries.

Anatomy

- The cartilaginous anlage of the wrist begins as a single mass; by the 10th week, this transforms into eight distinct masses, each in the contour of its respective mature carpal bone.
- The appearance of ossification centers of the carpal bones ranges from 6 months for the capitate to 8 years of age for the pisiform. The order of appearance of the ossification centers is very consistent: capitate, hamate, triquetrum, lunate, scaphoid, trapezium, trapezoid, and pisiform (Fig. 46.1).
- The ossific nuclei of the carpal bones are uniquely protected by cartilaginous shells. As the child matures, a "critical bone-to-cartilage ratio" is reached, after which carpal fractures are increasingly common (adolescence).

Mechanism of Injury

- The most common mechanism of carpal injury in children is direct trauma to the wrist.
- Indirect injuries result from falls onto the outstretched hand, with consequent axial compressive force with the wrist in hyperextension. In children, injury by this mechanism occurs from higher-energy mechanisms, such as falling off a moving bicycle or fall from a height.

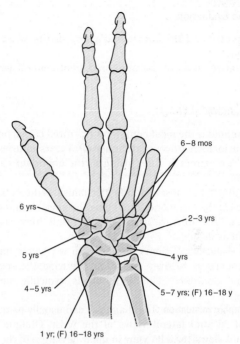

FIGURE 46.1 The age at the time of appearance of the ossific nucleus of the carpal bones and distal radius and ulna. The ossific nucleus of the pisiform (not shown) appears at about 6 to 8 years of age. (From Bucholz RW, Heckman JD, Court-Brown C, et al., eds. *Rockwood and Green's Fractures in Adults.* 6th ed. Philadelphia: Lippincott Williams & Wilkins; 2006.)

Clinical Evaluation

■ The clinical presentation of individual carpal injuries is variable, but in general, the most consistent sign of carpal injury is well-localized tenderness. In the agitated child, however, appreciation of localized tenderness may be difficult, because distal radial pain may be confused with carpal tenderness.

■ A neurovascular examination is important, with documentation of distal sensation in median, radial, and ulnar distributions, appreciation of movement of all digits, and assessment of distal capillary refill.

■ Gross deformity may be present, ranging from displacement of the carpus to prominence of individual carpal bones.

Radiographic Evaluation

■ Anteroposterior (AP) and lateral views of the wrist should be obtained.

■ Comparative views of the uninjured, contralateral wrist may be helpful.

Scaphoid Fracture

■ The scaphoid is the most commonly fractured carpal bone.

■ The peak incidence occurs at the age of 15 years; injuries in the first decade are extremely rare, owing to the abundant cartilaginous envelope.

■ Unlike adults, the most common mechanism is direct trauma, with fractures of the distal one-third being the most common. Proximal pole fractures are rare and typically result from scapholunate ligament avulsion.

■ **Clinical evaluation:** Patients present with wrist pain and swelling, with tenderness to deep palpation overlying the scaphoid and anatomic snuffbox. The snuffbox is typically obscured by swelling.

■ **Radiographic evaluation:** The diagnosis can usually be made on the basis of AP and lateral views of the wrist. Oblique views and "scaphoid views," or a PA view in ulnar deviation of the wrist, may aid in the diagnosis or assist in further fracture definition. Technetium bone scan has been replaced with magnetic resonance imaging. Alternatively, computed tomography and ultrasound evaluation may be used to diagnose occult scaphoid fractures.

Classification (Fig. 46.2)

Type A: Fractures of the distal pole
A1: Extraarticular distal pole fractures
A2: Intraarticular distal pole fractures
Type B: Fractures of the middle third (waist fractures)
Type C: Fractures of the proximal pole

Treatment

■ A fracture should be presumed if snuffbox tenderness is present, even if a fracture is not obvious on plain radiographs. Initial treatment in the emergency department should consist of a thumb spica splint or cast immobilization if swelling is not pronounced. In the pediatric population, a long arm cast or splint is typically necessary for adequate initial immobilization. This should be

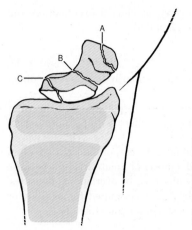

FIGURE 46.2 Three types of scaphoid fractures. **(A)** Distal third. **(B)** Middle third. **(C)** Proximal pole. (From Bucholz RW, Heckman JD, Court-Brown C, et al., eds. *Rockwood and Green's Fractures in Adults.* 6th ed. Philadelphia: Lippincott Williams & Wilkins; 2006.)

maintained for 2 weeks, at which time repeat evaluation should be undertaken.

■ For stable, nondisplaced fractures, a long arm cast should be placed with the wrist in neutral deviation and flexion/extension and maintained for 6 to 8 weeks or until radiographic evidence of healing has occurred.

■ Displaced fractures in the pediatric population may be initially addressed with closed reduction and percutaneous pinning. Distal pole fractures can generally be reduced by traction and ulnar deviation.

■ Residual displacement >1 mm, angulation >10 degrees, or scaphoid fractures in adolescents generally require open reduction and internal fixation. A headless compression screw or smooth Kirschner wires may be used for fracture fixation, with postoperative immobilization consisting of a long arm thumb spica cast for 6 weeks.

Complications

■ **Delayed union, nonunion, and malunion:** These are rare in the pediatric population and may necessitate operative fixation with bone grafting to achieve union.

■ **Osteonecrosis:** Extremely rare in the pediatric population and occurs with fractures of the proximal pole in skeletally mature individuals.

■ **Missed diagnosis:** Clinical suspicion should outweigh normal-appearing radiographs, and a brief period of immobilization

(2 weeks) can be followed by repeat clinical examination and further radiographic studies if warranted.

Lunate Fracture

- This extremely rare injury occurs primarily from severe, direct trauma (e.g., crush injury).
- Clinical evaluation reveals tenderness to palpation on the volar wrist overlying the distal radius and lunate, with painful range of motion.
- **Radiographic evaluation:** AP and lateral views of the wrist are often inadequate to establish the diagnosis of lunate fracture because osseous details are frequently obscured by overlapping densities.
  - □ Oblique views may be helpful, but computed tomography or technetium bone scanning best demonstrate fracture.
- Treatment
  - □ Nondisplaced fractures or unrecognized fractures generally heal uneventfully and may be recognized only in retrospect. When diagnosed, they should be treated in a short arm cast or splint for 2 to 4 weeks until radiographic and symptomatic healing occurs.
  - □ Displaced or comminuted fractures should be treated surgically to allow adequate apposition for formation of vascular anastomoses. This may be achieved with open reduction and internal fixation, although the severity of the injury mechanism typically results in concomitant injuries to the wrist that may result in growth arrest.
- Complications
  - □ **Osteonecrosis:** Referred to as "lunatomalacia" in the pediatric population, this occurs in children less than 10 years of age. Symptoms are rarely dramatic, and radiography reveals mildly increased density of the lunate with no change in morphology. Immobilization of up to 1 year may be necessary for treatment, but it usually results in good functional and symptomatic recovery.

Triquetrum Fracture

- Rare, but the true incidence unknown owing to the late ossification of the triquetrum, with potential injuries unrecognized.
- The mechanism of fracture is typically direct trauma to the ulnar wrist or avulsion by dorsal ligamentous structures.
- Clinical evaluation reveals tenderness to palpation on the dorsoulnar aspect of the wrist as well as painful range of motion.

- ■ **Radiographic evaluation:** Transverse fractures of the body can generally be identified on AP views in older children and adolescents. Distraction views may be helpful in these cases.
- ■ Treatment
  - ◻ Nondisplaced fractures of the triquetrum body or dorsal chip fractures may be treated in a short arm cast or ulnar gutter splint for 2 to 4 weeks when symptomatic improvement occurs.
  - ◻ Significantly displaced fractures may be amenable to open reduction and internal fixation.

Pisiform Fracture

- ■ No specific discussions of pisiform fractures in the pediatric population exist in the literature.
- ■ Direct trauma causing a comminuted fracture or a flexor carpi ulnaris avulsion may occur in late adolescence.
- ■ Radiographic evaluation is typically unrevealing, because ossification of the pisiform does not occur until the age of 8 years.
- ■ Treatment is symptomatic only, with immobilization in an ulnar gutter splint until the patient is comfortable.

Trapezium Fracture

- ■ Extremely rare in children and adults.
- ■ The mechanism of injury is axial loading of the adducted thumb, driving the base of the first metacarpal onto the articular surface of the trapezium with dorsal impaction. Avulsion fractures may occur with forceful deviation, traction, or rotation of the thumb. Direct trauma to the palmar arch may result in avulsion of the trapezial ridge by the transverse carpal ligament.
- ■ Clinical evaluation reveals tenderness to palpation of the radial wrist, accompanied by painful range of motion at the first carpometacarpal joint with stress testing.
- ■ **Radiographic evaluation:** Fractures are difficult to identify because of the late ossification of the trapezium. In older children and adolescents, identifiable fractures may be appreciated on standard AP and lateral views.
  - ◻ Superimposition of the first metacarpal base may be eliminated by obtaining a Robert view or a true AP view of the first carpometacarpal joint and trapezium.
- ■ **Treatment:**
  - ◻ Most fractures are amenable to thumb spica splinting or casting to immobilize the first carpometacarpal joint for 3 to 5 weeks.

    ☐ Rarely, severely displaced fractures may require open reduction and internal fixation to restore articular congruity and maintain carpometacarpal joint integrity.

Trapezoid Fracture

- Fractures of the trapezoid in children are extremely rare.
- Axial load transmitted through the second metacarpal may lead to dislocation, more often dorsal, with associated capsular ligament disruption. Direct trauma from blast or crush injuries may cause trapezoid fracture.
- Clinical evaluation demonstrates tenderness proximal to the base of the second metacarpal with painful range of motion of the second carpometacarpal joint.
- **Radiographic evaluation:** Fractures are difficult to identify secondary to late ossification. In older children and adolescents, they may be identified on the AP radiograph based on a loss of the normal relationship between the second metacarpal base and the trapezoid. Comparison with the contralateral, normal wrist may aid in the diagnosis. The trapezoid, or fracture fragments, may be superimposed over the trapezium or capitate, and the second metacarpal may be proximally displaced.
- **Treatment:**
  - ☐ Most fractures may be treated with a splint or short arm cast for 3 to 5 weeks.
  - ☐ Severely displaced fractures may require open reduction and internal fixation with Kirschner wires with attention to restoration of articular congruity.

Capitate Fracture

- Uncommon as an isolated injury owing to its relatively protected position.
- A fracture of the capitate is more commonly associated with greater arc injury pattern (transscaphoid, transcapitate perilunate fracture-dislocation). A variation of this is the "naviculocapitate syndrome," in which the capitate and scaphoid are fractured without associated dislocation.
- The mechanism of injury is typically direct trauma or a crushing force that results in associated carpal or metacarpal fracture. Hyperdorsiflexion may cause impaction of the capitate waist against the lunate or dorsal aspect of the radius.
- Clinical evaluation reveals point tenderness as well as variable painful dorsiflexion of the wrist as the capitate impinges on the dorsal rim of the radius.

■ **Radiographic evaluation:** Fracture can usually be identified on the AP radiograph, with identification of the head of the capitate on lateral views to determine rotation or displacement. Distraction views may aid in fracture definition as well as identification of associated greater arc injuries. Magnetic resonance imaging may assist in evaluating ligamentous disruption.

■ **Treatment:** Splint or cast immobilization for 6 to 8 weeks may be performed for minimally displaced capitate fractures. Open reduction is indicated for fractures with extreme displacement or rotation to avoid osteonecrosis. Fixation may be achieved with Kirschner wires or compression screws.

■ Complications
  □ **Midcarpal arthritis (late):** Caused by capitate collapse as a result of displacement of the proximal pole.
  □ **Osteonecrosis:** Rare and most often involves severe displacement of the proximal pole. It may result in functional impairment and emphasizes the need for accurate diagnosis and stable reduction.

Hamate Fracture

■ There are no specific discussions in the literature concerning hamate fractures in the pediatric population.

■ The mechanism of injury typically involves direct trauma to the volar aspect of the ulnar wrist. For example in racquet sports, softball, or golf.

■ **Clinical evaluation:** Patients typically present with pain and tenderness over the hamate. Ulnar and median neuropathy can also be seen, as well as rare injuries to the ulnar artery.

■ **Radiographic evaluation:** The diagnosis of hamate fracture can usually be made on the basis of the AP view of the wrist. Fracture of the hamate is best visualized on the carpal tunnel or 20-degree supination oblique view (oblique projection of the wrist in radial deviation and semisupination). A hamate fracture should not be confused with an os hamulus proprium, which represents a secondary ossification center.

■ **Treatment:** All hamate fractures should be initially treated with immobilization in a short arm splint or cast unless compromise of neurovascular structures warrants exploration. Excision of fragments is generally not necessary in the pediatric population.

■ Complications
  □ **Symptomatic nonunion:** May be treated with excision of the nonunited fragment.

Ulnar or median neuropathy: Related to the proximity of the hamate to these nerves and may require surgical exploration and release.

INJURIES TO THE HAND

Epidemiology

- **Biphasic distribution:** These injuries are seen in toddlers and adolescents. The injuries are typically crush injuries in toddlers and are typically related to sports participation in adolescents.
- The number of hand fractures in children is higher in boys and peaks at 13 years of age, which coincides with participation of boys in organized contact athletics.
- The annual incidence of pediatric hand fractures is 26.4 per 10,000 children, with the majority occurring about the metacarpophalangeal joint.
- Hand fractures account for up to 25% of all pediatric fractures.

Anatomy (Fig. 46.3)

- As a rule, extensor tendons of the hand insert onto epiphyses.
- At the level of the metacarpophalangeal joints, the collateral ligaments originate from the metacarpal epiphysis and insert almost exclusively onto the epiphysis of the proximal phalanx; this accounts for the high frequency of Salter–Harris type II and III injuries in this region.
- The periosteum of the bones of the pediatric hand is usually well developed and accounts for intrinsic fracture stability in seemingly unstable injuries; this often serves as an aid to achieving or maintaining fracture reduction. Conversely, the exuberant periosteum may become interposed in the fracture site, thus preventing effective closed reduction.

Mechanism of Injury

- The mechanism of hand injuries varies considerably. In general, fracture patterns emerge based on the nature of the traumatic force:
  - **Nonepiphyseal:** torque, angular force, compressive load, direct trauma
  - **Epiphyseal:** avulsion, shear, splitting
  - **Physeal:** shear, angular force, compressive load

Clinical Evaluation

- The child with a hand injury is typically uncooperative because of pain, unfamiliar surroundings, parent anxiety, and "white coat"

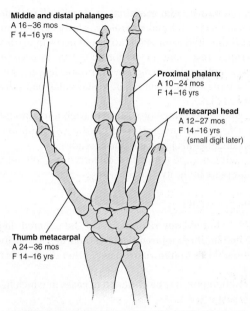

Middle and distal phalanges
A 16–36 mos
F 14–16 yrs

Proximal phalanx
A 10–24 mos
F 14–16 yrs

Metacarpal head
A 12–27 mos
F 14–16 yrs
(small digit later)

Thumb metacarpal
A 24–36 mos
F 14–16 yrs

FIGURE 46.3 Appearance of secondary ossification centers (A). Fusion of secondary centers to the primary centers (F). (From Bucholz RW, Heckman JD, Court-Brown C, et al., eds. *Rockwood and Green's Fractures in Adults.* 6th ed. Philadelphia: Lippincott Williams & Wilkins; 2006.)

fear. Simple observation of the child at play may provide useful information concerning the location and severity of injury. Game playing (e.g., "Simon says") with the child may be utilized for clinical evaluation.

- **History:** A careful history is essential because it may influence treatment. This should include
  - ☐ Patient age
  - ☐ Hand dominance
  - ☐ Refusal to use the injured extremity
  - ☐ **The exact nature of the injury:** crush, direct trauma, twist, tear, laceration, etc.
  - ☐ The exact time of the injury (for open fractures)
  - ☐ **Exposure to contamination:** barnyard, brackish water, animal/human bite
  - ☐ **Treatment provided:** cleansing, antiseptic, bandage, tourniquet
- **Physical examination:** The entire hand should be exposed and examined for open injuries. Swelling as well as the presence of gross deformity (rotational or angular) should be noted.

- A careful neurovascular examination is critical, with documentation of capillary refill and neurologic status (two-point discrimination). If the child is uncooperative and nerve injury is suspected, the "wrinkle test" may be performed. This is accomplished by immersion of the affected digit in warm, sterile water for 5 minutes and observing corrugation of the distal volar pad (absent in the denervated digit).
- Passive and active range of motion of each joint should be determined. Observing tenodesis with passive wrist motion is helpful for assessing digital alignment and cascade.
- Stress testing may be performed to determine collateral ligament and volar plate integrity

Radiographic Evaluation

- AP, lateral, and oblique radiographs of the affected digit or hand should be obtained. Injured digits should be viewed individually, when possible, to minimize overlap of other digits over the area of interest.
- Stress radiographs may be obtained in cases in which ligamentous injury is suspected.
- The examiner must be aware that cartilaginous injury may have occurred despite negative plain radiographs. Treatment must be guided by clinical as well as radiographic factors.

Treatment

General Principles

- **"Fight-bite"injuries:** Any short, curved laceration overlying a joint in the hand, particularly the metacarpal–phalangeal joint, must be suspected of having been caused by a tooth. These injuries must be assumed to be contaminated with oral flora and should be addressed with broad-spectrum antibiotics.
- Most pediatric hand fractures are treated nonoperatively, with closed reduction using conscious sedation or regional anesthesia (e.g., digital block). Hematoma blocks or fracture manipulation without anesthesia should be avoided in younger children.
- Finger traps may be utilized with older children or adolescents but are generally poorly tolerated in younger children.
- Immobilization may consist of short arm splints (volar, dorsal, ulnar gutter, etc.) or metal finger splints. With conscientious follow-up and cast changes as indicated, immobilization is rarely necessary beyond 4 weeks.
- Operative indications include unstable fracture patterns, in which the patient may benefit from percutaneous Kirschner wire fixation;

open fractures, which may require irrigation, debridement, and secondary wound closure; and fractures in which reduction is
unattainable by closed means—these may signify interposed
periosteum or soft tissue that requires open reduction.

■ Subungual hematomas that occupy >50% of the nailplate should
be evacuated with the use of a needle, cautery tip, or heated
paper clip. A higher incidence of late nail deformities associated with failure to decompress subungual hematomas has
been reported.

■ Nailbed injuries should be addressed with removal of the compromised nail, repair of the nailbed with 6-0 or 7-0 absorbable suture
or some type of "dermal glue," and retention of the nail under the
nailfold as a biologic dressing to protect the healing nailbed.
Alternatively, commercially made stents are available for use as
dressings.

Management of Specific Fracture Patterns

Metacarpals

■ Pediatric metacarpal fractures are classified as follows:

Type A: Epiphyseal and Physeal Fractures

■ Fractures include the following:
   □ Epiphyseal fractures
   □ **Physeal fractures:** Salter–Harris type II fractures of the fifth
     metacarpal most common
   □ Collateral ligament avulsion fractures
   □ Oblique, vertical, and horizontal head fractures
   □ Comminuted fractures
   □ Boxer's fractures with an intraarticular component
   □ Fractures associated with bone loss

■ Most require anatomic reduction (if possible) to reestablish joint
congruity and to minimize posttraumatic arthrosis.
   □ Stable fracture reductions may be splinted in the "protected po-
     sition," consisting of metacarpophalangeal flexion >70 degrees
     and interphalangeal joint extension to minimize joint
     stiffness.
   □ Percutaneous pinning may be necessary to obtain stable reduc-
     tion; if possible, the metaphyseal component (Thurston-
     Holland fragment) should be included in the fixation.

■ Early range of motion is essential.

Type B: Metacarpal Neck

■ Fractures of the fourth and fifth metacarpal necks are commonly
seen as pediatric analogs to boxer's fractures in adults.

- The degree of acceptable deformity varies according to the metacarpal injured, especially in adolescents:
  □ More than 15-degree angulation for the second and third metacarpals is unacceptable.
  □ More than 40- to 45-degree angulation for the fourth and fifth metacarpals is unacceptable.
- These are typically addressed by closed reduction using the Jahss maneuver by flexing the metacarpophalangeal joint to 90 degrees and placing an axial load through the proximal phalanx. This is followed by splinting in the "protected position."
- Unstable fractures require operative intervention with either percutaneous pins (may be intramedullary or transverse into the adjacent metacarpal) or plate fixation (adolescents).

Type C: Metacarpal Shaft

- Most of these fractures may be reduced by closed means and splinted in the protected position.
- Operative indications include unstable fractures, rotational deformity, dorsal angulation >10 degrees for second and third metacarpals, and >20 degrees for fourth and fifth metacarpals, especially for older children and adolescents in whom significant remodeling is not expected.
- Operative fixation may be achieved with closed reduction and percutaneous pinning (intramedullary or transverse into the adjacent metacarpal). Open reduction is rarely indicated, although the child presenting with multiple, adjacent, displaced metacarpal fractures may require reduction by open means.

Type D: Metacarpal Base

- The carpometacarpal joint is protected from frequent injury owing to its proximal location in the hand and the stability afforded by the bony congruence and soft tissue restraints.
- The fourth and fifth carpometacarpal joints are more mobile than the second and third; therefore, injury to these joints is uncommon and usually results from high-energy mechanisms.
- Axial loading from punching mechanisms typically results in stable buckle fractures in the metaphyseal region.
- Closed reduction using regional or conscious sedation and splinting with a short arm ulnar gutter splint may be performed for the majority of these fractures, leaving the proximal interphalangeal joint mobile.
- Fracture-dislocations in this region may result from crush mechanisms or falls from a height; these may initially be addressed with attempted closed reduction, although transverse metacarpal

pinning is usually necessary for stability. Open reduction may be necessary, especially in cases of multiple fracture-dislocations at the carpometacarpal level.

Thumb Metacarpal

■ Fractures are uncommon and are typically related to direct trauma.

■ Metaphyseal and physeal injuries are the most common fracture patterns.

■ Structures inserting on the thumb metacarpal constitute potential deforming forces:

□ **Opponens pollicis:** broad insertion over metacarpal shaft and base that displaces the distal fragment into relative adduction and flexion

□ **Abductor pollicis longus:** multiple sites of insertion including the metacarpal base, resulting in abduction moment in cases of fracture-dislocation

□ **Flexor pollicis brevis:** partial origin on the medial metacarpal base, resulting in flexion and apex dorsal angulation in metacarpal shaft fractures

□ **Adductor pollicis:** possible adduction of the distal fragment

Thumb Metacarpal Head and Shaft Fractures

■ These typically result from direct trauma.

■ Closed reduction is usually adequate for the treatment of most fractures, with postreduction immobilization consisting of a thumb spica splint or cast.

■ Anatomic reduction is essential for intraarticular fractures and may necessitate the use of percutaneous pinning with Kirschner wires.

Thumb Metacarpal Base Fractures

These are subclassified as follows (Fig. 46.4):

■ **Type A:** fractures distal to the physis

□ They are often transverse or oblique, with apex-lateral angulation and an element of medial impaction.

□ They are treated with closed reduction with extension applied to the metacarpal head and direct pressure on the apex of the fracture, then immobilized in a thumb spica splint or cast for 4 to 6 weeks.

□ Up to 30 degrees of residual angulation may be accepted in younger children.

□ Unstable fractures may require percutaneous Kirschner wire fixation, often with smooth pins to cross the physis.

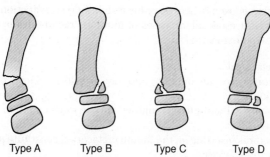

Type A   Type B   Type C   Type D

FIGURE 46.4 Classification of thumb metacarpal fractures.
(A) Metaphyseal fracture. **(B** and **C)** Salter–Harris type II physeal
fractures with lateral or medial angulation. **(D)** Salter–Harris
type III fracture (pediatric Bennett fracture). (From Bucholz RW,
Heckman JD, Court-Brown C, et al., eds.*Rockwood and Green's
Fractures in Adults.* 6th ed. Philadelphia: Lippincott Williams &
Wilkins; 2006.)

Transcarpometacarpal pinning may be performed but is usually
reserved for more proximal fracture patterns.

■ **Type B:** Salter–Harris type II fracture, metaphyseal medial
  □ The shaft fragment is typically angulated laterally and displaced
    proximally owing to the pull of the abductor pollicis longus;
    adduction of the distal fragment is common because of the pull
    of the adductor pollicis.
  □ Anatomic reduction is essential to avoid growth disturbance.
  □ Closed reduction followed by thumb spica splinting is initially
    indicated, with close serial follow-up. With maintenance of
    reduction, immobilization should be continued for 4 to 6 weeks.
  □ Percutaneous pinning is indicated for unstable fractures with
    capture of the metaphyseal fragment if possible. Alternatively,
    transmetacarpal pinning to the second metacarpal may be
    necessary. Open reduction may be required for anatomic
    restoration of the physis.
■ **Type C:** Salter–Harris type II fracture, metaphyseal lateral
  □ These are similar to type B fractures, but they are less common
    and typically result from more significant trauma, with conse-
    quent apex medial angulation.
  □ Periosteal buttonholing is common and may prevent anatomic
    reduction.
  □ Open reduction is frequently necessary for restoration of
    anatomic relationships.
■ **Type D:** intraarticular Salter–Harris type III or IV fractures
  □ These are the pediatric analogs to the adult Bennett fracture.

- □ They are rare, with deforming forces similar to type B fractures, with the addition of lateral subluxation at the level of the carpometacarpal articulation caused by the intraarticular component of the fracture.
- □ Nonoperative methods of treatment vary in results. The most consistent results are obtained with open reduction and percutaneous pinning or internal fixation in older children.
- □ Severe comminution or soft tissue injury may be initially addressed with oblique skeletal traction.
- □ External fixation may be used for contaminated open fractures with potential bone loss.

Phalanges (Fig. 46.5)

- ■ The physes are located at the proximal aspect of the phalanges.
- ■ The collateral ligaments of the proximal and distal interphalangeal joints originate from the collateral recesses of the proximal bone and insert onto both the epiphysis and metaphysis of the distal bone and volar plate.
- ■ The volar plate originates from the metaphyseal region of the phalangeal neck and inserts onto the epiphysis of the more distal phalanx.
- ■ The extensor tendons insert onto the dorsal aspect of the epiphysis of the middle and distal phalanges.
- ■ The periosteum is typically well developed and exuberant, often resisting displacement and aiding reduction, but occasionally interposing at the fracture site and preventing adequate reduction.

Proximal and Middle Phalanges

Pediatric fractures of the proximal and middle phalanges are subclassified as follows:

- ■ **Type A:** physeal
  - □ Of pediatric hand fractures, 41% involve the physis. The proximal phalanx is the most frequently injured bone in the pediatric population.
  - □ The collateral ligaments insert onto the epiphysis of the proximal phalanx; in addition to the relatively unprotected position of the physis at this level, this contributes to the high incidence of physeal injuries.
  - □ A pediatric "gamekeeper's" thumb is a Salter–Harris type III avulsion fracture, with the ulnar collateral ligament attached to an epiphyseal fragment of the proximal aspect of the proximal phalanx.
  - □ Treatment is initially by closed reduction and splinting in the protected position.

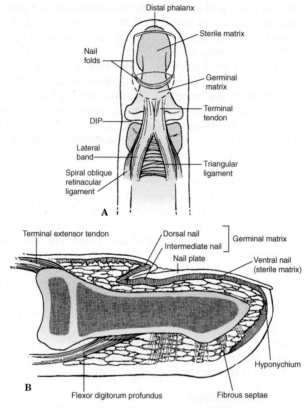

FIGURE 46.5 Anatomy about the distal phalanx. **(A)** The skin, nail, and extensor apparatus share a close relationship with the bone of the distal phalanx. Specific anatomic structures at the terminal aspect of the digit are labeled. **(B)** This lateral view of the nail demonstrates the tendon insertions and the anatomy of the specialized nail tissues. (From Bucholz RW, Heckman JD, Court-Brown C, et al., eds. *Rockwood and Green's Fractures in Adults*. 6th ed. Philadelphia: Lippincott Williams & Wilkins; 2006.)

- ☐ Unstable fractures may require percutaneous pinning. Fractures with >25% articular involvement or >1.5 mm displacement require open reduction with internal fixation with Kirschner wires or screws.
- ■ **Type B:** shaft
  - ☐ Shaft fractures are not as common as those surrounding the joints.

- □ Proximal phalangeal shaft fractures are typically associated with apex volar angulation and displacement, created by forces of the distally inserting central slip and lateral bands coursing dorsal to the apex of rotation, as well as the action of the intrinsics on the proximal fragment pulling it into flexion.
- □ Oblique fractures may be associated with shortening and rotational displacement. This must be recognized and taken into consideration for treatment.
- □ Closed reduction with immobilization in the protected position for 3 to 4 weeks is indicated for the majority of these fractures.
- □ Residual angulation >30 degrees in children <10 years of age, >20 degrees in children >10 years of age, or any malrotation requires operative intervention, consisting of closed reduction and percutaneous crossed pinning. Intramedullary pinning may allow rotational displacement.

■ **Type C:** neck (Fig. 46.6)

- □ Fractures through the metaphyseal region of the phalanx are commonly associated with door-slamming injuries.
- □ Rotational displacement and angulation of the distal fragment are common, because the collateral ligaments typically remain attached distal to the fracture site. This may allow interposition of the volar plate at the fracture.
- □ Closed reduction followed by splinting in the protected position for 3 to 4 weeks may be attempted initially, although closed reduction with percutaneous crossed pinning is usually required.

■ **Type D:** intraarticular (condylar)

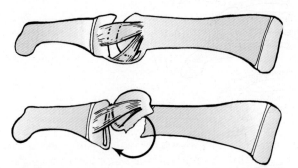

FIGURE 46.6 Phalangeal neck fractures are often unstable and rotated. These fractures are difficult to reduce and control by closed means because of the forces imparted by the volar plate and ligaments. (Adapted from Wood BE. Fractures of the hand in children. *Orthop Clin North Am.* 1976;7:527–534.)

- ☐ These arise from a variety of mechanisms, ranging from shear or avulsion resulting in simple fractures to combined axial and rotational forces that may result in comminuted, intraarticular T- or Y-type patterns.
- ☐ Open reduction and internal fixation are usually required for anatomic restoration of the articular surface. This operation is most often performed through a lateral or dorsal incision, with fixation using Kirschner wires or miniscrews.

Distal Phalanx

- These injuries are frequently associated with soft tissue or nail compromise and may require subungual hematoma evacuation, soft tissue reconstructive procedures, or nailbed repair.
- Pediatric distal phalangeal fractures are subclassified as follows:
  - ☐ Physeal
    - Dorsal mallet injuries (Fig. 46.7)
    - **Type A:** Salter–Harris type I or II injuries
    - **Type B:** Salter–Harris type III or IV injuries
    - **Type C:** Salter–Harris type I or II associated with joint dislocation

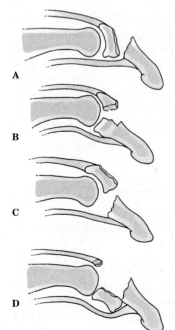

FIGURE 46.7 (A–D) Mallet-equivalent physeal fracture types. (From Bucholz RW, Heckman JD, Court-Brown C, et al., eds. *Rockwood and Green's Fractures in Adults.* 6th ed. Philadelphia: Lippincott Williams & Wilkins; 2006.)

Type D: Salter–Harris fracture associated with extensor tendon avulsion

- A mallet finger may result from a fracture of the dorsal lip with disruption of the extensor tendon. Alternatively, a mallet finger may result from a purely tendinous disruption and may therefore not be radiographically apparent.
- Treatment of type A and nondisplaced or minimally displaced type B injuries is full-time extension splinting for 4 to 6 weeks.
- Type C, D, and displaced type B injuries typically require operative management. Type B injuries are usually amenable to Kirschner wire fixation with smooth pins. Type C and D injuries generally require open reduction and internal fixation.

- Volar (reverse) mallet injuries
  - These are associated with flexor digitorum profundus rupture ("jersey finger:" seen in football and rugby players, most commonly involving the ring finger).
  - Treatment is primary repair using heavy suture, miniscrews, or Kirschner wires. Postoperative immobilization is continued for 3 weeks.

- Extraphyseal
  Type A: Transverse diaphyseal
  Type B: Longitudinal splitting
  Type C: Comminuted
  - The mechanism of injury is almost always direct trauma.
  - Nailbed injuries must be recognized and addressed.
  - Treatment is typically closed reduction and splinting for 3 to 4 weeks with attention to concomitant injuries. Unstable injuries may require percutaneous pinning, either longitudinally from the distal margin of the distal phalanx or across the distal interphalangeal joint (uncommon) for extremely unstable or comminuted fractures.

Complications

- **Impaired nail growth:** Failure to repair the nailbed adequately may result in germinal matrix disturbance that causes anomalous nail growth. This is frequently a cosmetic problem, but it may be addressed with reconstructive procedures if pain, infection, or hygiene is an issue.
- **Extensor lag:** Despite adequate treatment, extensor lag up to 10 degrees is common, although not typically of functional significance. This occurs most commonly at the level of the proximal interphalangeal joint secondary to tendon adherence. Exploration, release, and or reconstruction may result in further cosmetic or functional disturbance.

- **Malunion:** Apex dorsal angulation can disturb intrinsic balance and can also result in prominence of metacarpal heads in palm with pain on gripping. Rotational or angulatory deformities, especially of the second and third metacarpals, may produce functional and cosmetic disturbances, thus emphasizing the need to maintain as near an anatomic relationship as possible.
- **Nonunion:** Uncommon but may occur especially with extensive soft tissue injury and bone loss, as well as in open fractures with gross contamination and infection.
- **Infection, osteomyelitis:** Grossly contaminated wounds require meticulous debridement, appropriate antibiotic coverage, and possible delayed closure.
- **Metacarpophalangeal joint extension contracture:** This may result if splinting is not in the protected position (i.e., metacarpophalangeal joints at >70 degrees), owing to soft tissue contracture.

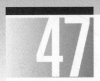

Pediatric Hip

PEDIATRIC HIP FRACTURES

Epidemiology

■ Hip fractures are rare in children, occurring less than 1% as often as in adults.

Anatomy

■ Ossification (Fig. 47.1)
  □ **Proximal femur:** week 7 in utero
  □ **Proximal femoral epiphysis:** age 4 to 8 months
  □ **Trochanter:** age 4 years
■ The proximal femoral epiphysis fuses by the age of 18 years, the trochanteric apophysis by the age of 16 to 18 years.
■ The proximal femoral physis contributes significantly to metaphyseal growth of the femoral neck and less to primary appositional growth of the femoral head. Thus, disruptions in this region may lead to architectural changes that may affect the overall anatomic development of the proximal femur.
■ The trochanteric apophysis contributes significantly to appositional growth of the greater trochanter and less to the metaphyseal growth of the femur.
■ Blood is supplied to the hip by the lateral femoral circumflex artery and, more importantly, the medial femoral circumflex artery. Anastomoses at the anterosuperior portion of the intertrochanteric groove form the extracapsular ring. Ascending retinacular vessels go to the epiphysis (Fig. 47.2).
■ By 3 or 4 years of age, the lateral posterosuperior vessels (branches of the medial femoral circumflex) predominate and supply the entire anterolateral portion of the capital femoral epiphysis.
■ Vessels of the ligamentum teres contribute little before the age of 8 years and approximately 20% in adulthood.
■ Capsulotomy does not damage the blood supply to the femoral head, but violation of the intertrochanteric notch or the lateral ascending cervical vessels can render the femoral head avascular.

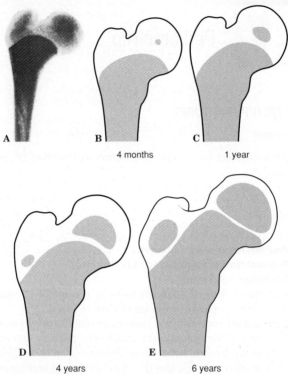

FIGURE 47.1 The transformation of the preplate to separate growth zones for the femoral head and greater trochanter. The diagram shows development of the epiphyseal nucleus in the proximal end of the femur. **(A)** X-ray of the proximal end of the femur of a stillborn girl, weight 325 g. **(B–E)** Drawings made on the basis of x-rays. (Adapted from Edgren W. Coxa plana: a clinical and radiological investigation with particular reference to the importance of the metaphyseal changes for the final shape of the proximal part of the femur. *Acta Orthop Scand.* 1965;84(suppl):24.)

Mechanism of Injury

- Axial loading, torsion, hyperabduction, or a direct blow can result in a hip fracture. Severe, direct trauma (e.g., motor vehicle accident) accounts for 75% to 80% of pediatric hip fractures.
- **Pathologic:** Fractures that occur through bone cysts, fibrous dysplasia, or tumor invaded bone account for the remainder.
- **Stress fractures:** These are uncommon in the pediatric population.

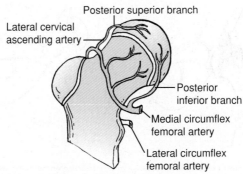

FIGURE 47.2 Arterial supply of the proximal femur. The capital femoral epiphysis and physis are supplied by the medial circumflex artery through two retinacular vessel systems: the posterosuperior and posteroinferior. The lateral circumflex artery supplies the greater trochanter and the lateral portion of the proximal femoral physis and a small area of the anteromedial metaphysis. (From Bucholz RW, Heckman JD, Court-Brown C, et al., eds. *Rockwood and Green's Fractures in Adults.* 6th ed. Philadelphia: Lippincott Williams & Wilkins; 2006.)

Clinical Evaluation

- The patient typically presents with a shortened and externally rotated lower extremity.
- Range of hip motion is painful with variable crepitus.
- Swelling, ecchymosis, and tenderness to palpation are generally present over the injured hip.
- A careful neurovascular examination should be performed.

Radiographic Evaluation

- Anteroposterior (AP) views of the pelvis and a cross-table lateral view of the affected hip should be obtained, with the leg extended and internally rotated as far as is tolerable by the patient.
- Developmental coxa vara should not be confused with hip fracture, especially in patients <5 years of age. Comparison with the contralateral hip may aid in the distinction.
- Computed tomography may aid in the diagnosis of nondisplaced fractures or stress fractures.
- A radioisotope bone scan obtained 48 hours after injury may demonstrate increased uptake at the occult fracture site.
- Magnetic resonance imaging may detect occult fractures within 24 hours of injury.

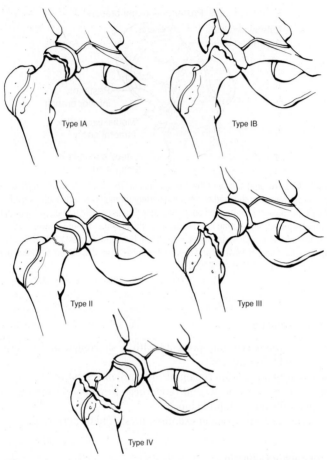

FIGURE 47.3 Delbet classification of hip fractures in children. Type I, transepiphyseal, with (type IB) or without (type IA) dislocation from the acetabulum; type II, transcervical; type III, cervicotrochanteric; and type IV, intertrochanteric. (From Bucholz RW, Heckman JD, Court-Brown C, et al., eds. *Rockwood and Green's Fractures in Adults*. 6th ed. Philadelphia: Lippincott Williams & Wilkins; 2006.)

Classification

Delbet Classification of Pediatric Hip Fractures (Fig. 47.3)

Type I: Transepiphyseal fracture
- 8% of pediatric hip fractures
- Incidence of osteonecrosis approaches 100%, especially if associated with a hip dislocation

- End of spectrum of slipped capital femoral epiphysis; consider hypothyroidism, hypogonadism, and renal disease
- In newborns, differential diagnosis includes CDH and septic arthritis

Type II: Transcervical fracture
- 45% of pediatric hip fractures (most common type)
- 80% are displaced
- Osteonecrosis in up to 50% of cases

Type III: Cervicotrochanteric fracture
- 30% of pediatric hip fractures
- More common in children than in adults
- Rate of osteonecrosis of 20% to 30%

Type IV: Intertrochanteric fracture
- 10% to 15% of pediatric hip fractures
- Fewer complications than in other hip fractures because vascular supply is more abundant

Treatment

Type I: Closed reduction with pin fixation is indicated, using partially threaded pins in an older child and smooth pins in a younger child. Open reduction and internal fixation may be necessary if the fracture is irreducible by closed methods.

Type II: **Nondisplaced:** The choice is abduction spica cast versus in situ pinning; these fractures may go on to coxa vara or nonunion.

Displaced: Closed reduction and pinning (open reduction if necessary) are indicated; transphyseal pinning should be avoided.

Type III: **Nondisplaced:** Traction is indicated initially, followed by spica cast versus immediate abduction spica versus in situ pinning.

Displaced: Open reduction and internal fixation are recommended, with avoidance of transphyseal pinning.

Type IV: Depends on age and size of patient. Two to 3 weeks of traction are indicated, then abduction spica for 6 to 12 weeks is indicated for nondisplaced fractures. Open reduction and internal fixation may be necessary for unstable fractures or if one is unable to achieve or maintain a closed reduction.

Complications

- **Osteonecrosis:** The overall incidence is 40% after pediatric hip fracture. This is directly related to initial fracture displacement and fracture location. Ratliff described three types (Fig. 47.4):

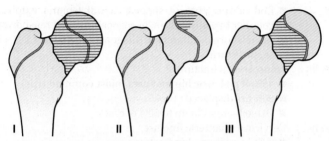

FIGURE 47.4 Three types of osteonecrosis. (Adapted from Ratliff AHC. Fractures of the neck of the femur in children. *J Bone Joint Surg Br.* 1962;44:528.)

Type I: Diffuse, complete head involvement, and collapse; poor prognosis (60%)

Type II: Localized head involvement only; minimal collapse (22%)

Type III: Femoral neck involved only; head sparing (18%)

- **Premature physeal closure:** The incidence is ≤60%, with increased incidence with pins penetrating the physis. It may result in femoral shortening, coxa vara, and short femoral neck. The proximal femoral epiphysis contributes to only 15% of growth of the entire lower extremity. The presence of premature physeal closure in association of osteonecrosis may result in significant leg length discrepancy.
- **Coxa vara:** The incidence is 20%, usually secondary to inadequate reduction. Open reduction and internal fixation are associated with a reduced incidence of coxa vara.
- **Nonunion:** The incidence is 10%, primarily owing to inadequate reduction or inadequate internal fixation. It may require valgus osteotomy with or without bone graft to achieve union.

TRAUMATIC DISLOCATION OF THE HIP

Epidemiology

- More common than hip fractures.
- **Bimodal distribution:** The incidence is greater between 2 and 5 years, owing to joint laxity and soft pliable cartilage, and between 11 and 15 years of age as athletic injuries and those associated with vehicular trauma become more common.
- **Posterior dislocations:** These occur 10 times more frequently than anterior dislocations.

Mechanism of Injury

- **Younger patients (age <5 years):** These injuries may occur as a result of relatively insignificant trauma such as a fall from a standing height.

■ **Older patients (>11 years):** These injuries tend to occur with athletic participation and vehicular accidents (bicycles, automobiles, etc.). In this age group, there is a higher association with acetabular fractures.

■ Posterior dislocations are usually the result of an axial load applied to a flexed and adducted hip; anterior dislocations occur with a combination of abduction and external rotation.

Clinical Evaluation

■ In cases of posterior hip dislocation, the patient typically presents with the affected hip flexed, adducted, and internally rotated. Anterior hip dislocation typically presents with extension, abduction, and external rotation of the affected hip.

■ A careful neurovascular examination is essential, with documentation of integrity of the sciatic nerve and its branches in posterior dislocations. Femoral nerve function and limb perfusion should be carefully assessed in anterior dislocations. This examination should be repeated after closed reduction.

■ Ipsilateral femur fracture often occurs and must be ruled out prior to hip manipulation.

Radiographic Evaluation

■ AP views of the pelvis and a lateral view of the affected hip should be obtained. Pain, swelling, or obvious deformity in the femoral region is an indication for femoral radiographs, to rule out associated fracture.

■ Fracture fragments from the femoral head or acetabulum are typically more readily appreciated on radiographs obtained after reduction of the hip dislocation because anatomic landmarks are more clearly delineated. Depending on patient age these fracture patterns may not be visible on plain radiographs or CT.

■ Following reduction, computed tomography should be obtained to delineate associated femoral head or acetabular fracture, as well as the presence of interposed soft tissue.

Classification

Descriptive

Direction: Anterior versus posterior
Fracture-dislocation: Fractures to the femoral head or acetabulum
Associated injuries: Presence of ipsilateral femur fracture, etc.

Treatment

Nonoperative

- Closed reduction using conscious sedation may be performed for patients presenting less than 12 hours after dislocation.
- Skeletal traction may be used for reduction of a chronic or neglected hip dislocation, with reduction taking place over a 3- to 6-day period and continued traction for an additional 2 to 3 weeks to achieve stability.

Operative

- Dislocations more than 12 hours old may require reduction with the patient under general anesthesia. Open reduction may be necessary, if irreducible, with surgical removal of interposing capsule, inverted limbus, or osteocartilaginous fragments.
- Open reduction is also indicated in cases of sciatic nerve compromise in which surgical exploration is necessary.
- Hip dislocations associated with ipsilateral femoral shaft fractures should be initially addressed with reduction of the dislocation under general anesthesia. If manipulative closed reduction is unsuccessful, skeletal traction may be applied to the trochanteric region to allow control of the proximal fragment. Internal or external fixation of the femoral shaft fracture may then be performed. Occasionally, operative fixation of the femoral shaft fracture is necessary to achieve stable reduction of the hip.
- Hip stability should be assessed intraoperatively. Isolated dislocations are usually stable.
- Postoperatively, the patient should be placed in skeletal traction or spica cast for 4 to 6 weeks if hip stability is in question.

Complications

- **Osteonecrosis (8% to 10%):** This has a decreased incidence with patient age <5 years and an increased incidence with severe displacement and delay in reduction.
- **Epiphyseal separation:** Traumatic physeal injury may occur at the time of dislocation and may result in osteonecrosis or growth arrest.
- **Recurrent dislocation:** In traumatic cases, it may result from absolute capsular tears or capsular attenuation. It is also associated with hyperlaxity or congenital syndromes (e.g., Down syndrome). It may be addressed with surgical "tightening" of the hip, with capsular repair, or with plication as well as spica casting for 4 to 6 weeks postoperatively.

- **Degenerative joint disease:** This may result from nonconcentric hip reduction secondary to trapped soft tissue or bony fragments or from the initial trauma. Articular incongruity secondary to associated femoral head or acetabular fracture, or entrapped osteochondral fragments, may exacerbate degenerative processes.
- **Nerve injury (2% to 13%):** Sciatic nerve injury can occur with posterior dislocation and is typically a neuropraxia. Treatment for a suspected neuropraxia is usually observation. Indications for exploration include laceration or incarceration of the nerve in the joint is suspected (rare).
- **Chondrolysis (6%):** Injury occurs at the time of hip dislocation. Management is symptomatic treatment with nonsteroidal antiinflammatory drugs and weight-relieving devices as needed. Distraction arthroplasty may be necessary at some point.

48 Pediatric Femoral Shaft

EPIDEMIOLOGY

- Represent 1.6% of all fractures in the pediatric population.
- Boys are more commonly affected at a ratio of 2.6:1.
- Bimodal distribution of incidence: The first peak is from 2 to 4 years of age, and the second is in mid-adolescence.
- There is also a seasonal distribution, with a higher incidence during the summer months.
- In children younger than walking age, 80% are caused by child abuse; this decreases to 30% in toddlers.
- In adolescence, >90% of femoral fractures are caused by motor vehicle accident.

ANATOMY

- During childhood, remodeling in the femur causes a change from primarily weaker woven bone to stronger lamellar bone.
- Up to age 16 years, there is a geometric increase in the femoral shaft diameter and relative cortical thickness of the femur, resulting in a markedly increased area moment of inertia and strength. This partially explains the bimodal distribution of injury pattern, in which younger patients experience fractures under load conditions reached in normal play or minor trauma, whereas in adolescence high-energy trauma is required to reach the stresses necessary for fracture (Fig. 48.1).

MECHANISM OF INJURY

- **Direct trauma:** Motor vehicle accident, pedestrian injury, fall, and child abuse are causes.
- **Indirect trauma:** Rotational injury.
- **Pathologic fractures:** Causes include osteogenesis imperfecta, nonossifying fibroma, bone cysts, and tumors. Severe involvement from myelomeningocele or cerebral palsy may result in generalized osteopenia and a predisposition to fracture with minor trauma.

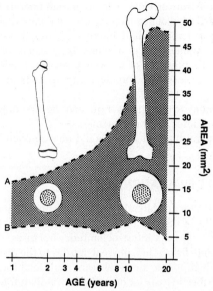

FIGURE 48.1 The *shaded area* represents cortical thickness by age group. This rapid increase in cortical thickness may contribute to the diminishing incidence of femoral fractures during late childhood. (Redrawn from Netter FH. *The Ciba Collection of Medical Illustrations.* Vol. 8. Musculoskeletal system. Part I. Anatomy, physiology, and metabolic disorders. Summit, NJ, Ciba-Geigy, 1987; in Bucholz RW, Heckman JD, eds. *Rockwood and Green's Fractures in Adults.* 5th ed. Baltimore: Lippincott Williams & Wilkins; 2002.)

CLINICAL EVALUATION

- Patients with a history of high-energy injury should undergo full trauma evaluation as indicated.
- The presence of a femoral shaft fracture results in an inability to ambulate, with extreme pain, variable swelling, and variable gross deformity. The diagnosis is more difficult in patients with multiple trauma or head injury or in nonambulatory, severely disabled children.
- A careful neurovascular examination is essential.
- Splints or bandages placed in the field must be removed with a careful examination of the overlying soft tissues to rule out the possibility of an open fracture.

- Hypotension from an isolated femoral shaft fracture is uncommon. The Waddell triad of head injury, intra-abdominal or intrathoracic trauma, and femoral shaft fracture is strongly associated with vehicular trauma and is a more likely cause of volume loss. However, the presence of a severely swollen thigh may indicate large volume loss into muscle compartments surrounding the fracture.
- Compartment syndrome is rare and occurs only with severe hemorrhage into thigh compartments.
- The ipsilateral hip and knee should be examined for associated injuries.

RADIOGRAPHIC EVALUATION

- Anteroposterior and lateral views of the femur should be obtained.
- Radiographs of the hip and knee should be obtained to rule out associated injuries; intertrochanteric fractures, femoral neck fractures, hip dislocation, physeal injuries to the distal femur, ligamentous disruptions, meniscal tears, and tibial fractures have all been described in association with femoral shaft fractures.
- MRI or CT scans are generally unnecessary but may aid in the diagnosis of otherwise occult nondisplaced, buckle, or stress fractures.

CLASSIFICATION

Descriptive

- Open versus closed
- **Level of fracture:** proximal, middle, distal third
- **Fracture pattern:** transverse, spiral, oblique, butterfly fragment
- Comminution
- Displacement
- Angulation

Anatomic

- Subtrochanteric
- Shaft
- Supracondylar

TREATMENT

Treatment is age dependent, with considerable overlap among age groups. The size of the child must be considered when choosing a treatment method, as well as the mechanism of the injury (i.e., iso-lated, low-energy versus high-energy polytrauma). The American Academy of Orthopaedic Surgeons has recently released an evidence based summary of recommendations for treatment of pediatric diaphy-seal femur fractures which can be found at http:/www.aaos.org/research/guidelines/PDFFguidelines.asp

Age <6 Months

- Pavlik harness or a posterior splint is indicated.
- Traction and spica casting are rarely needed in this age group.

Ages 6 Months to 4 Years

- Immediate spica casting is nearly always the treatment of choice (>95%).
- Skeletal traction followed by spica casting may be needed if one is unable to maintain length and acceptable alignment; a traction pin is preferably placed proximal to the distal femoral physis.
- External fixation may be considered for multiple injuries or open fracture.

Ages 4 to 12 Years

- Flexible or elastic intramedullary nails placed in a retrograde fashion are frequently used in this age group. (Flexible or elastic nails are generally contraindicated for larger children, >100 lb, and in fractures that are highly comminuted and may shorten.)
- External fixation or bridge plating may be considered for multiple injuries, some open fractures, and those fractures not amenable to elastic nailing.
- Some centers are using interlocked nails inserted through the greater trochanter or lateral to the greater trochanter (contro-versial).
- Spica casting may be used for the axially stable fractures in this age group.

Ages 12 to Maturity

- Intramedullary fixation with either flexible (if pattern and size permit) or interlocked nails that avoid the piriformis fossa has become the treatment of choice.
- Locked submuscular plates either placed open or in a percuta-neous manner may be considered for shaft, supracondylar, or subtrochanteric fractures.

| | | TABLE 48.1 Acceptable Angulation | | |

Age	Varus/Valgus (degrees)	Anterior/Posterior (degrees)	Shortening (mm)
Birth to 2 years	30	30	15
2–5 years	15	20	20
6–10 years	10	15	15
11 years to maturity	5	10	10

From Buckholz RW, Heckman JD, eds. *Rockwood and Green's Fractures in Adults.* 5th ed. Baltimore: Lippincott Williams & Wilkins; 2002:948.

- External fixation may still be considered for multiple injuries or open fracture. Complications such as pin site infection and refractures have led to the loss of popularity of this implant.

Reduction Criteria (Table 48.1)

- Length
  - □ **Ages 2 to 11 years:** Up to 2 cm overriding is acceptable.
  - □ **Age >11 years:** Up to 1 cm overriding is acceptable.
- Angulation
  - □ **Sagittal plane:** Up to 30 degrees of recurvatum/procurvatum is acceptable.
  - □ **Frontal plane:** Up to 10 degrees of varus/valgus angulation is acceptable (varus commonly seen with spica casting).
  - □ This varies with pattern, age, and location of fracture along the femur.
- Rotation
  - □ Up to 10 degrees is acceptable; external rotation is better tolerated than internal rotation.

Operative Indications

- Multiple trauma, including head trauma
- Open fracture
- Vascular injury
- Pathologic fracture
- Uncooperative patient
- Body habitus not amenable to spica casting

Operative Options

- Intramedullary nailing
  - □ **Flexible (elastic) nails:** These are inserted retrograde proximal to the distal femoral physis.

- □ **Reamed, locked intramedullary nails:** These are placed antegrade through the piriformis fossa, greater trochanter, or a portal lateral to the trochanter. The distal physis should not be traversed. A piriformis entry point is not recommended for patients with open physes, because of proximal femoral growth abnormalities and the risk of osteonecrosis of the femoral head owing to disruption of the vascular supply. A trochanteric entry point theoretically reduces the risk of osteonecrosis, but it may affect growth at the trochanteric apophysis.
- ■ External fixation
  - □ **Lateral, unilateral frame:** This spares the rectus femoris, but affects the vastus lateralis (knee stiffness is still a problem). Pin tract infection and refractures are other problems.
  - □ This approach is useful in multiple trauma, especially in those who are hemodynamically unstable, have open fractures or burn patients.
- ■ Plate fixation
  - □ This may be accomplished using a 3.5 or 4.5 mm compression plate, with or without interfragmentary compression of

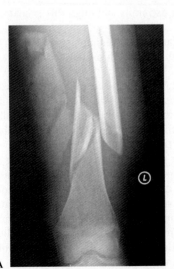
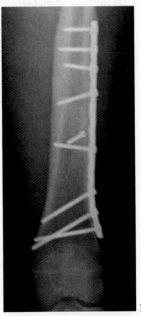

A   **B**

FIGURE 48.2 A 12-year-old male with distal left femur fracture **(A)** treated with open plate and screw fixation. The patient healed by 4 months and was followed until physeal closure **(B)**.

fragments; it is less desirable because of the long incision necessary, significant periosteal stripping, quadriceps scarring, frequent need for plate removal, and infection. (Fig. 48.2)

☐ Percutaneously placed, submuscular locking plates are useful for supracondylar, shaft, and subtrochanteric fractures in which intramedullary devices have limited fixation. Less soft tissue stripping is needed, but infection and plate removal concerns remain.

COMPLICATIONS

■ **Malunion:** Remodeling will not correct rotational deformities. An older child will not remodel as well as a younger child. Anteroposterior remodeling occurs much more rapidly and completely in the femur than varus/valgus angular deformity. For this reason, greater degrees of sagittal angulation are acceptable.

■ **Nonunion:** Rare; even with segmental fractures, children often have sufficient osteogenic potential to fill moderate defects. Children 5 to 10 years of age with established nonunion may require bone grafting and plate fixation, although the trend in older (>12 years) children is locked intramedullary nailing.

■ **Muscle weakness:** Many patients demonstrate weakness, typically in hip abductors, quadriceps, or hamstrings, with up to a 30% decrease in strength and 1 cm thigh atrophy as compared with the contralateral, uninjured lower extremity, although this is seldom clinically significant.

■ **Leg length discrepancy:** Secondary to shortening or overgrowth. It represents the most common complication after femoral shaft fracture.

☐ **Overgrowth:** Overgrowth of 1.5 to 2.0 cm is common in the 2- to 10-year age range in patients treated with spica casting. It is most common during the initial 2 years after fracture, especially with fractures of the distal third of the femur and those associated with greater degrees of trauma.

☐ **Shortening:** Up to 2.0 cm (age dependent) of initial shortening is acceptable because of the potential for overgrowth. For fractures with greater than 3.0 cm of shortening, skeletal traction may be employed before spica casting to obtain adequate length. If the shortening is unacceptable at 6 weeks after fracture, the decision must be made whether osteoclasis and distraction with external fixation are preferable to a later limb length equalization procedure.

■ **Osteonecrosis:** Proximal femoral osteonecrosis may result from antegrade placement of an intramedullary nail owing to the precarious vascular supply. This is of particular concern when the proximal femoral physis is not yet closed, because the major vascular supply to the femoral head is derived from the lateral ascending cervical artery, which crosses the capsule at the level of the trochanteric notch. Recently, intramedullary nails with a trochanteric or an extratrochanteric starting point have been advocated to reduce the risk of osteonecrosis. Radiographic changes may be seen as late as 15 months after antegrade intramedullary nailing.

49 Pediatric Knee

OVERVIEW

- **The knee is a ginglymoid (hinge) joint consisting of three articulations:** patellofemoral, tibiofemoral, and tibiofibular.
- Under normal cyclic loading, the knee may experience up to five times body weight per step.
- The normal range of motion is from 0 degrees of extension to 140 degrees of flexion, with 8 to 12 degrees of rotation through the flexion/extension arc (many children will hyperextend at the knee).
- The dynamic and static stability of the knee is conferred mainly by soft tissues (ligaments, muscles, tendons, menisci) in addition to the bony articulations.
- Because ligaments in the immature skeleton are more resistant to tensile stresses than are physeal plates and metaphyseal bone, trauma leads to physeal separation and avulsions not seen in the skeletally mature patient.
- There are three physeal plates with secondary ossification centers.
- Appearance of ossification centers is as follows:
  - **Distal femur:** 39th fetal week
  - **Proximal tibia:** by 2 months
  - **Tibial tubercle:** 9 years
- Physeal closure is as follows:
  - **Distal femur:** 16 to 19 years
  - **Proximal tibia:** 16 to 19 years
  - **Tibial tubercle:** 15 to 17 years
- The patella is a sesamoid bone, with its own ossification center, which appears at age 3 to 5 years.
- **Tibial spine:** This is the site of insertion of the anterior cruciate ligament (ACL).
- Two-thirds of longitudinal growth of the lower extremity is provided by the distal femoral (9 mm/year) and proximal tibial (6 mm/year) physes.

DISTAL FEMORAL PHYSEAL FRACTURES

Epidemiology

- The most commonly injured physis around the knee.

- Comprise 1% to 6% of all physeal injuries and less than 1% of all fractures in children.
- Most (two-thirds) are Salter–Harris type II fractures and occur in adolescents.
- 12% to 15% of all femur fractures occur in children.

Anatomy

- The distal femoral epiphysis is the largest and fastest growing physis in the body.
- There is no inherent protection of the physis. Ligamentous and tendinous structures insert on the epiphysis.
- The sciatic nerve divides at the level of the distal femur.
- The popliteal artery gives off the superior geniculate branches to the knee just posterior to the femoral metaphysis.

Mechanism of Injury

- Direct trauma to the distal femur may occur from vehicular trauma, falling onto a flexed knee, or during athletic activity, such as a lateral blow to the knee with a planted, cleated foot as in football. In infants, distal femoral fracture may be associated with child abuse.
- **Indirect injury:** Varus/valgus or hyperextension/hyperflexion force; results in simultaneous compression to one aspect of the physis with distraction to the other. Indirect force may result in epiphyseal separation from the metaphysis. Most typically, the physeal separation begins on the tension side and exits the metaphysis on the compression side (Salter–Harris type II).
- Birth injury secondary to breech presentation or arthrogryposis may cause this physeal separation injury.
- Minimal trauma in conditions that cause generalized weakening of the growth plate (osteomyelitis, leukemia, myelodysplasia) may also be causative.

Clinical Evaluation

- Patients are typically unable to bear weight on the injured lower extremity, although patients with a nondisplaced physeal injury from a low-energy mechanism (e.g., athletic injury) may ambulate with an antalgic gait.
- Older children and adolescents may relate a history of hearing or feeling a "pop"; along with associated knee effusion and soft tissue swelling, this may be confused with a ligamentous injury.
- The knee is typically in flexion owing to hamstring spasm.

- Gross shortening or angular deformity is variable, with potential compromise of the neurovascular structures resulting from traction injury, laceration or compression. A complete neurovascular assessment is thus critical.
- Point tenderness may be elicited over the physis; this is usually performed by palpating the distal femur at the level of the superior pole of the patella and adductor tubercle.
- Most commonly, epiphyseal displacement is in the coronal plane producing a varus or valgus deformity.

Radiographic Evaluation (Table 49.1)

- Anteroposterior (AP), lateral, and oblique views should be obtained. Radiographs of the contralateral lower extremity may be obtained for comparison if the diagnosis is in doubt.

TABLE 49.1	Imaging Studies in the Evaluation of Distal Femoral Physeal Fractures	
Study	**Indications**	**Limitations**
Plain films	First study, often sufficient	May miss nondisplaced Salter type I or III fractures or underestimate fracture displacement
Computed tomography scan	Best defines fracture pattern and amount of displacement; useful in deciding whether surgery is needed and for planning surgery	Poor cartilage visualization; less useful than magnetic resonance imaging in evaluating for occult Salter type I or III fracture
Magnetic resonance imaging	Evaluation of occult Salter I or III fracture possible; infants with little epiphyseal ossification	Availability, cost, insurance company authorizations; identifies associated soft tissue injuries; unclear that study changes initial treatment
Stress views	Differentiate occult Salter fracture from ligament injury	Painful, muscle spasm may not permit opening of fracture if patient is awake; unclear that study changes initial treatment
Contralateral x-rays	Infants, or to assess physeal width	Usually not needed

Modified from Bucholz RW, Heckman JD, Court-Brown C, et al., eds. *Rockwood and Green's Fractures in Adults.* 6th ed. Philadelphia: Lippincott Williams & Wilkins; 2006.

- Stress views may be obtained to diagnose nondisplaced separations in which the clinical examination is highly suggestive of physeal injury (knees with effusion and point tenderness over physis in the setting of a negative AP and lateral radiograph). Adequate analgesia is necessary to relax muscular spasm and to prevent both false-negative stress radiographs and physeal injury.
- The physeal line should be 3 to 5 mm thick until adolescence.
- Salter–Harris type III injuries usually have vertically oriented epiphyseal fracture components that are best appreciated on an AP view.
- Computed tomography may be useful to assess in fracture fragment definition.
- In infants, separation of the distal femoral physis may be difficult to assess unless there is gross displacement because only the center of the epiphysis is ossified at birth; this should be in line with the anatomic axis of the femur on both AP and lateral views. Magnetic resonance imaging, ultrasound, or arthrography may aid in the diagnosis of distal femoral injury in these patients.
- Arteriography of the lower extremity should be pursued if vascular injury is suspected.

Classification

Salter–Harris (Fig. 49.1)

Type I: Seen in newborns and adolescents; diagnosis easily missed; physeal widening may be apparent on comparison films and instability may be demonstrated on stress radiographs

Type II: Most common injury of the distal femoral physis; displacement usually medial or lateral, with metaphyseal fragment on compression side

Type III: Intra-articular fracture exiting the epiphysis (typically medial condyle from valgus stress)

Type IV: Intra-articular fracture exiting the metaphysis; high incidence of growth inhibition with bar formation; rare injury

Type V: Physeal crush injury; difficult diagnosis, made retrospectively after growth arrest; narrowing of physis possible

Displacement

Anterior: Results from hyperextension injury; high incidence of neurovascular injury from proximal metaphyseal spike driven posteriorly

Posterior: Rare injury caused by knee hyperflexion

Medial: Valgus force most common, usually Salter–Harris type II

Lateral: Varus force

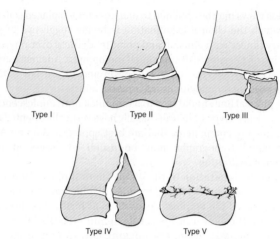

Type I   Type II   Type III

Type IV   Type V

FIGURE 49.1 The Salter–Harris classification of fractures involving the distal femoral physis. (From Bucholz RW, Heckman JD, Court-Brown C, et al., eds. *Rockwood and Green's Fractures in Adults*. 6th ed. Philadelphia: Lippincott Williams & Wilkins; 2006.)

Treatment

Nonoperative

- Indicated for nondisplaced fractures.
- A tense knee joint effusion may be relieved by sterile aspiration for symptomatic relief.
- Closed reduction using general anesthesia may be performed for displaced fractures in which a stable result can be obtained (Fig. 49.2).
- Sufficient traction should be applied during manipulation to minimize grinding of physeal cartilage (90% traction, 10% leverage). The position of immobilization varies with direction of displacement:
  - □ **Medial/lateral:** Immobilize in 15 to 20 degrees of knee flexion. Cast in valgus mold for medial metaphyseal fragment and varus mold for lateral metaphyseal fragment to tension intact periosteum.
  - □ **Anterior:** Immobilize initially at 90 degrees of knee flexion, then decrease flexion with time.
  - □ **Posterior:** Immobilize in extension.
- A residual varus/valgus deformity after reduction tends not to remodel.

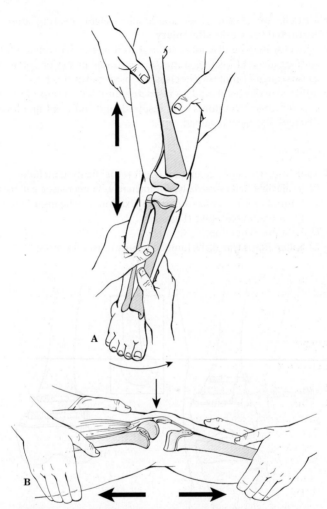

FIGURE 49.2 Closed reduction and stabilization of a Salter–Harris type I or II distal femur fracture. **(A)** With medial or lateral displacement, traction is applied longitudinally along the axis of the deformity to bring the fragments back to length. **(B)** For anterior displacement, the reduction can be done with the patient prone or supine. Length is gained first, then a flexion moment is added. (From Bucholz RW, Heckman JD, Court-Brown C, et al., eds. *Rockwood and Green's Fractures in Adults.* 6th ed. Philadelphia: Lippincott Williams & Wilkins; 2006.)

- Crutch ambulation with toe-touch weight bearing may be instituted at 3 weeks after injury.
- The cast may be discontinued at 4 to 8 weeks depending on the patient age and healing status. A removable posterior splint and active range-of-motion exercises are instituted at this time.
- Athletic activities should be restricted until knee range of motion has returned, symptoms have resolved, and sufficient quadriceps strength has been regained.

Operative

- Indications for open reduction and internal fixation include:
  - **Irreducible Salter–Harris type II fracture with interposed soft tissue:** Cannulated 4.0- or 6.5-mm screw fixation may be used to secure the metaphyseal spike (Fig. 49.3).
  - Unstable reduction.
  - **Salter–Harris type III, IV:** Joint congruity must be restored.

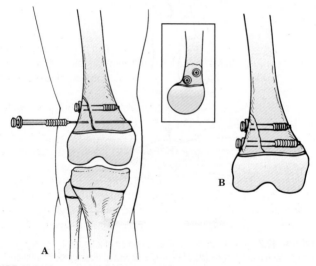

FIGURE 49.3 Screw fixation following closed or open reduction of a Salter–Harris type II fracture with a large metaphyseal fragment. **(A)** When using cannulated screws, place both guide wires before screw placement to avoid rotation of the fragment while drilling or inserting screw. Screw threads should be past the fracture site to enable compression. Washers help increase compression. Screws may be placed anterior and posterior to each other, which is particularly helpful when trying to fit multiple screws in a small metaphyseal fragment. **(B)** This form of fixation is locally "rigid," but it must be protected with long leg immobilization or long lever arm. (From Bucholz RW, Heckman JD, Court-Brown C, et al., eds. *Rockwood and Green's Fractures in Adults.* 6th ed. Philadelphia: Lippincott Williams & Wilkins; 2006.)

- To minimize residual deformity and growth disturbance, specific principles should be observed for internal fixation.
  - Avoid crossing the physis if possible.
  - If the physis must be crossed, use smooth pins as perpendicular as possible to the physis.
  - Remove fixation that crosses the physis as soon as possible.
- Postoperatively, the patient is maintained in a long leg cast in 10 degrees of knee flexion. The patient may be ambulatory with crutches in 1 to 2 days with non–weight bearing on the injured extremity. At 1 week, the patient may begin straight leg raises.
- If at 4 weeks evidence of osseous healing is demonstrated radiographically, the cast may be discontinued with a posterior splint in place for protection. The patient may be advanced to partial weight bearing with active range-of-motion exercises.
- The patient typically resumes a normal, active lifestyle at 4 to 6 months after injury.

Complications

Acute

- **Popliteal artery injury (<2%):** Associated with hyperextension or anterior epiphyseal displacement injuries in which a traction injury may be sustained or by direct laceration from the sharp metaphyseal spike.
  - A cool, pulseless foot that persists despite reduction should be worked up with angiography to rule out laceration.
  - Vascular embarrassment that resolves following reduction should be observed for 48 to 72 hours to rule out an intimal tear and subsequent thrombosis.
- **Peroneal nerve palsy (3%):** Caused by traction injury during fracture or reduction or secondary to initially anterior/medial displaced epiphysis. Persistent peroneal palsy over 3 to 6 months should be evaluated by electromyography, and by exploration as may be indicated.
- **Recurrent displacement:** Fractures of questionable stability following closed reduction should receive operative fixation (either percutaneous pins or internal fixation) to prevent late or recurrent displacement. Anterior and posterior displacements are particularly unstable.

Late

- **Knee instability (up to 37% of patients):** Knee instability may be present, indicating concomitant ligamentous compromise that was not appreciated at the time of index presentation. The patient may be treated with rehabilitation for lower extremity strengthening or may require operative treatment. Collateral ligaments may be acutely repaired if instability exists after fracture fixation.

- **Angular deformity (19%):** Results from the initial physeal injury (Salter–Harris types I and II), asymmetric physeal closure (bar formation, Salter–Harris types III and IV), or unrecognized physeal injury (Salter–Harris type V).
  - ☐ Observation, physeal bar excision (<30% of physis >2 years of remaining growth), hemiepiphysiodesis, epiphyseolysis, or wedge osteotomy may be indicated.
- Physeal Closure is usually the rule for distal femoral physeal fractures (nearly 100%). A resultant leg length discrepancy (24%) depends upon the amount of remaining growth: Usually clinically insignificant if <2 years of growth remain; otherwise, the discrepancy tends to progress at the rate of 1 cm per year.
  - ☐ Discrepancy <2.0 cm at skeletal maturity usually is of no functional or cosmetic significance.
  - ☐ Discrepancy of 2.5 to 5 cm may be treated with contralateral epiphysiodesis (femoral or tibial, or both) or femoral shortening depending on the projected length discrepancy.
  - ☐ Discrepancy >5 cm may be an indication for femoral lengthening combined with epiphysiodesis of the contralateral distal femur or proximal tibia.
- **Knee stiffness (16%):** Results from adhesions or capsular or muscular contracture following surgery. It is usually related to the duration of immobilization; therefore, early discontinuation of the cast with active range of motion is desirable.

PROXIMAL TIBIAL FRACTURES

Epidemiology

- Comprise 0.6% to 0.8% of all physeal injuries.
- Average age is 14 years.
- Most occur in adolescent boys.

ANATOMY

- The popliteal artery traverses the posterior aspect of the knee and is tethered to the knee capsule by connective tissue septa posterior to the proximal tibia. The vascular supply is derived from the anastomosis of the inferior geniculate arteries.
- The physis is well protected by osseous and soft tissue structures, which may account for the low incidence of injuries to this structure.

☐ **Lateral:** fibula
☐ **Anterior:** patellar tendon/ligament
☐ **Medial:** medial collateral ligament (MCL; inserts into metaphysis)
☐ **Posteromedial:** semimembranosus insertion

Mechanism of Injury

- **Direct:** Trauma to the proximal tibia (motor vehicle bumper, lawn-mower accident).
- **Indirect:** More common and involves hyperextension, abduction, or hyperflexion from athletic injury, motor vehicle accident, fall, or landing from a jump with a concurrent MCL tear.
- **Birth injury:** Results from hyperextension during breech delivery or arthrogryposis.
- **Pathologic condition:** Osteomyelitis of the proximal tibia and myelomeningocele are causes.

Clinical Evaluation

- Patients typically present with an inability to bear weight on the injured extremity. The knee may be tense with hemarthrosis, and extension is limited by hamstring spasm.
- Tenderness is present 1 to 1.5 cm distal to the joint line, and variable gross deformity may be present.
- Neurovascular status should be carefully assessed for popliteal artery or peroneal nerve compromise. The anterior, lateral, superficial posterior, and deep posterior compartments should be palpated for pain or turgor. Patients suspected of having elevated compartment pressures should receive serial neurovascular examinations with measurement of compartment pressures as indicated.
- Associated ligamentous injuries should be suspected, although it may be difficult to appreciate these injuries secondary to the dramatic presentation of the fracture.

Radiographic Evaluation

- AP, lateral, and oblique views of the affected knee should be obtained. Radiographs of the contralateral knee may be obtained for comparison.
- Stress radiographs in coronal and sagittal planes may be obtained, but hyperextension of the knee should be avoided because of potential injury to popliteal structures.
- Most patients with proximal tibial physeal injuries are adolescents in whom the secondary ossicle of the tibial tubercle has appeared. A smooth, horizontal radiolucency at the base of the tibial tubercle should not be confused with an epiphyseal fracture.

TABLE 49.2	Classifications and Implications of Proximal Tibial Physeal Fractures
Classification	**Implications**
Mechanism of injury	
I. Hyperextension	Risk of vascular disturbance
II. Varus/valgus	Usually results from jumping; very near maturity
III. Flexion	See tibial tubercle fractures, type IV, in the next section
Salter–Harris pattern	
I	50% nondisplaced
II	30% nondisplaced
III	Associated collateral ligament injury possible
IV	Rare
V	Has been reported; diagnosis usually late

Modified from Bucholz RW, Heckman JD, Court-Brown C, et al., eds. *Rockwood and Green's Fractures in Adults*. 6th ed. Philadelphia: Lippincott Williams & Wilkins; 2006.

- Magnetic resonance imaging may aid in identification of soft tissue interposition when reduction is difficult or impossible.
- Computed tomography may aid in fracture definition, especially with Salter–Harris type III or IV fractures.
- Arteriography may be indicated in patients in whom vascular compromise (popliteal artery) is suspected.

Classification (Table 49.2)

Salter–Harris

Type I: Transphyseal injury; diagnosis often missed; may require stress or comparison views; 50% initially nondisplaced.

Type II: Most common; transphyseal injury exiting the metaphysis; one-third nondisplaced; those that displace usually do so medially into valgus

Type III: Intra-articular fracture of the lateral plateau; MCL often torn

Type IV: Intra-articular fracture of the medial or lateral plateau; fracture line exiting the metaphysis

Type V: Crush injury; retrospective diagnosis common after growth arrest

Treatment

Nonoperative

- Nondisplaced fractures may be treated with a long leg cast with the knee flexed to 30 degrees. The patient should be followed closely with serial radiographs to detect displacement.

- Displaced fractures may be addressed with gentle closed reduction, with limited varus and hyperextension stress to minimize traction to the peroneal nerve and popliteal vasculature, respectively. The patient is placed in a long leg cast in flexion (typically 30 to 60 degrees, depending on the position of stability).
- The cast may be discontinued at 4 to 6 weeks after injury. If the patient is symptomatically improved and radiographic evidence of healing is documented, active range-of-motion and quadriceps strengthening exercises are initiated.

Operative

- Displaced Salter type I or II fractures in which stable reduction cannot be maintained may be treated with percutaneous smooth pins across the physis (type I) or parallel to the physis (metaphysis) in type II.
- Open reduction and internal fixation are indicated for displaced Salter–Harris types III and IV to restore articular congruity. This may be achieved with pin or screw fixation parallel to the physis; articular congruity is the goal.
- Postoperatively, the patient is immobilized in a long leg cast with the knee flexed to 30 degrees. This is continued for 6 to 8 weeks, at which time the cast may be removed with initiation of active range-of-motion exercises.

Complications

Acute

- **Recurrent displacement:** This may occur if closed reduction and casting without operative fixation is performed on an unstable injury. It is likely secondary to unrecognized soft tissue injury.
- **Popliteal artery injury (10%):** This occurs especially in hyperextension injuries; it is related to tethering of the popliteal artery to the knee capsule posterior to the proximal tibia (Fig. 49.4). Arteriography may be indicated when distal pulses do not return following prompt reduction of the injury.
- **Peroneal nerve palsy:** This traction injury results from displacement, either at the time of injury or during attempted closed reduction, especially with a varus moment applied to the injury site.

Late

- **Angular deformity:** Results from the physeal injury (Salter–Harris types I and II), resulting in asymmetric physeal closure (bar formation, Salter–Harris type III and IV), or an unrecognized physeal

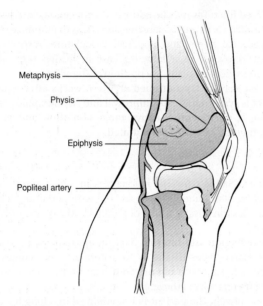

FIGURE 49.4 Posterior displacement of the epiphysis following fracture-separation at the time of injury can cause arterial injury. In addition, a posteriorly displaced fragment can cause persistent arterial occlusion by direct pressure. (From Bucholz RW, Heckman JD, Court-Brown C, et al., eds. *Rockwood and Green's Fractures in Adults.* 6th ed. Philadelphia: Lippincott Williams & Wilkins; 2006.)

injury (Salter–Harris type V). However, Salter–Harris classification has shown to be not useful in predicting growth disturbance in proximal tibial fracture types.

  □ Observation, physeal bar excision (<30% of physis, >2 years of remaining growth), hemiepiphysiodesis, epiphyseolysis, or wedge osteotomy may be indicated.

■ **Leg length discrepancy:** This is usually clinically insignificant if <2 years of growth remain; otherwise, discrepancy tends to progress at the rate of 1 cm per year. Treatment for leg length discrepancy remains similar to that for distal femur physeal injuries.

TIBIAL TUBERCLE FRACTURES

Epidemiology

■ Represent 0.4% to 2.7% of all physeal injuries.
■ They are seen most commonly in athletic boys 14 to 16 years old.

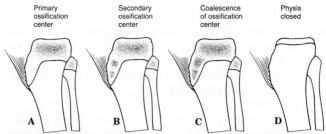

| Primary ossification center | Secondary ossification center | Coalescence of ossification center | Physis closed |

FIGURE 49.5 Development of the tibial tubercle. **(A)** In the cartilaginous stage, no ossification center is present in the cartilaginous anlage of the tibial tubercle. **(B)** In the *apophyseal stage,* the secondary ossification center forms in the cartilaginous anlage of the tibial tubercle. **(C)** In the *epiphyseal stage,* the primary and secondary ossification centers of the proximal tibial epiphysis have coalesced. **(D)** In the *bony stage,* the proximal tibial physis has closed. (From Rockwood CA Jr, Wilkins KE, Beaty JH, eds. *Rockwood and Green's Fractures in Children.* Vol 3. 4th ed. Philadelphia: Lippincott–Raven; 1996:1274.)

- It is important to differentiate these fractures from Osgood–Schlatter disease.

Anatomy (Fig. 49.5)

- The tibial tubercle physis, which is continuous with the tibial plateau, is most vulnerable between the ages of 13 and 16 years, when it closes from posterior to anterior.
- The insertion of the medial retinaculum extends beyond the proximal tibial physis into the metaphysic; therefore, after tibial tubercle fracture, limited active extension of the knee is still possible, although patella alta and extensor lag are present.
- The tubercle is located one to two fingerbreadths below the joint line. It is in line with the medial patella in flexion and the lateral patella in extension.

Mechanism of Injury

- The mechanism of injury is typically indirect, usually resulting from a sudden accelerating or decelerating force involving the quadriceps mechanism.
- Predisposing factors include:
  - Patella baja.
  - Tight hamstrings (increased flexion torque).
  - Pre-existing Osgood–Schlatter disease (uncertain whether mechanical vulnerability or overdevelopment of quadriceps mechanism).
  - Disorders with physeal anomalies.

Clinical Evaluation

■ Patients typically present with a limited ability to extend the knee as well as an extensor lag. The leg is held in 20 to 40 degrees of flexion by spastic hamstrings.

■ Swelling and tenderness over the tibial tubercle are typically present, often with a palpable defect.

■ Hemarthrosis is variable.

■ Patella alta may be observed if displacement is severe. The transverse retinaculum may be torn. Meniscal and cruciate ligaments may be found in severe injuries.

Radiographic Evaluation

■ AP and lateral views of the knee are sufficient for the diagnosis, although a slight internal rotation view best delineates the injury because the tibial tubercle lies just lateral to the tibial axis.

■ Patella alta may be noted.

Classification

Watson–Jones

Type I: Small fragment avulsed and displaced proximally; fracture through secondary ossification center

Type II: Secondary ossification center already coalesced with proximal tibial epiphysis; fracture at level of horizontal portion of tibial physis

Type III: Fracture line passing proximally through tibial epiphysis and into joint; possibly confused with Salter–Harris type III tibial physeal injury

Ogden

This modification of the Watson–Jones classification (see earlier) subdivides each type into A and B categories to account for the degree of displacement and comminution (Fig. 49.6).

Treatment

Nonoperative

■ Indicated for type IA fractures with intact extensor mechanism.

■ It consists of manual reduction and immobilization in a long leg cast with the knee extended, with patellar molding.

■ The cast is worn for 4 to 6 weeks, at which time the patient may be placed in a posterior splint for an additional 2 weeks. Gentle active

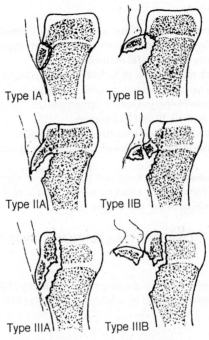

Type IA   Type IB

Type IIA   Type IIB

Type IIIA   Type IIIB

FIGURE 49.6 Ogden classification of tibial tuberosity fractures in children. (Adapted from Ogden JA. *Skeletal Injury in the Child.* 2nd ed. Philadelphia: WB Saunders; 1990:808.)

range-of-motion exercises and quadriceps strengthening exercises are instituted and advanced as symptoms abate.

Operative

- Indicated for types IB, II, III fractures or irreducible type IA fractures (periosteum may be interposed).
- A vertical midline approach is used; the fracture can be stabilized using smooth pins (>3 years from skeletal maturity), screws, threaded Steinmann pins, or a tension band.
- Postoperatively, the extremity is placed in a long leg cast in extension with patella molding for 4 to 6 weeks, at which time the patient may be placed in a posterior splint for an additional 2 weeks. Gentle active range-of-motion exercises and quadriceps strengthening exercises are instituted and advanced as symptoms abate.

Complications

- **Genu recurvatum:** This occurs secondary to premature closure of anterior physis; it is rare because injury occurs typically in adolescent patients near skeletal maturity.
- **Loss of knee motion:** Loss of flexion may be related to scarring or postoperative immobilization. Loss of extension may be related to nonanatomic reduction and emphasizes the need for operative fixation of type IB, II, and III fractures.
- **Patella alta:** May occur if reduction is insufficient.
- **Osteonecrosis of fracture fragment:** Rare because of soft tissue attachments.
- **Compartment syndrome:** Rare, but it may occur with concomitant tearing of the anterior tibial recurrent vessels that retract to the anterior compartment when torn.

TIBIAL SPINE (INTERCONDYLAR EMINENCE) FRACTURES

Epidemiology

- Relatively rare injury, occurring in 3 per 100,000 children per year.
- Most commonly caused by a fall from a bicycle (50%).

Anatomy

- **There are two tibial spines:** anterior and posterior. The ACL spans the medial aspect of the lateral femoral condyle to the anterior tibial spine.
- In the immature skeleton, ligaments are more resistant to tensile stresses than are physeal cartilage or cancellous bone; therefore, forces that would lead to an ACL tear in an adult cause avulsion of the incompletely ossified tibial spine in a child.

Mechanism of Injury

- **Indirect trauma:** The mechanism includes rotatory, hyperextension, and valgus forces.
- **Direct trauma:** Extremely rare, secondary to multiple trauma with significant knee injury.

Clinical Evaluation

- Patients are typically reluctant to bear weight on the affected extremity.
- Hemarthrosis is usually present, with painful range of motion and a variable bony block to full extension.

■ The MCL and lateral collateral ligament (LCL) should be stressed with varus/valgus pressure to rule out associated injury.

Radiographic Evaluation

■ AP and lateral views should be obtained. The AP view should be scrutinized for osseous fragments within the tibiofemoral articulation; these may be difficult to appreciate because only a thin, ossified sleeve may be avulsed.

■ Obtaining an AP radiograph to account for the 5 degrees of posterior slope of the proximal tibia may aid in visualization of an avulsed fragment.

■ Stress views may be useful in identification of associated ligamentous or physeal disruptions.

Classification

Meyers and McKeever (Fig. 49.7)

Type I: Minimal or no displacement of fragment
Type II: Angular elevation of anterior portion with intact posterior hinge
Type III: Complete displacement with or without rotation (15%)
Type IV: Comminuted (5%)

Types I and II account for 80% of tibial spine fractures.

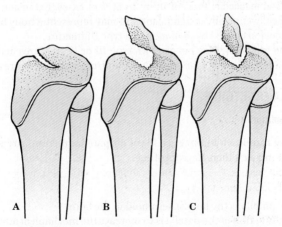

FIGURE 49.7 Classification of tibial spine fractures. **(A)** Type I, minimal displacement. **(B)** Type II, hinged posteriorly. **(C)** Type III, complete separation. (From Bucholz RW, Heckman JD, Court-Brown C, et al., eds. *Rockwood and Green's Fractures in Adults.* 6th ed. Philadelphia: Lippincott Williams & Wilkins; 2006.)

Treatment

Nonoperative

- Indicated for type I and II fractures of the tibial spine.
- The knee should be immobilized in extension; the fat pad may contact the spine in extension and thus help with reduction.
- After 4 to 6 weeks, the cast is removed with initiation of active range-of-motion and quadriceps and hamstrings strengthening.

Operative

- Indicated for type III and IV fractures of the tibial spine owing to historically uniformly poor results with nonoperative management. (Recent 2009 evidence may contradict this thinking)
- Debridement of fracture site is recommended with fixation using sutures, pins, or screws.
- The fracture may be repaired arthroscopically with an ACL guide, or by arthrotomy.
- Postoperatively, the patient is placed in a long leg cast with the knee in slight (10 to 20 degree) flexion. In 4 to 6 weeks, the cast is removed with initiation of active range-of-motion and quadriceps and hamstrings strengthening.

Complications

- **Loss of extension:** Present in up to 60% of cases. Extension loss is typically clinically insignificant and may represent a bony block to extension caused by malunion of a type III fracture.
- **Knee instability:** May persist with type III or IV fractures accompanied by collateral ligament injuries and/or physeal fractures.

PATELLA FRACTURES

Epidemiology

- Very rare in children; only 1% of all patella fractures are seen in patients less than 16 years of age.

Anatomy

- The patella is the largest sesamoid in the body.
- The function of the patella is to increase the mechanical advantage and leverage of the quadriceps tendon, aid in nourishment of the femoral articular surface, and protect the femoral condyles from direct trauma.
- Forces generated by the quadriceps in children are not as high as in adults owing to a smaller muscle mass and shorter moment arm.

- The blood supply to the patella derives from the anastomotic ring from the superior and inferior geniculate arteries. An additional supply through the distal pole is from the fat pad.
- The ossification center appears between 3 and 5 years. Ossification then proceeds peripherally and is complete by 10 to 13 years.
- Patella fracture must be differentiated from a bipartite patella (present in up to 8% of patients), which is located superolaterally. One should obtain contralateral films because bilateral bipartite patella is present in up to 50% of cases.

Mechanism of Injury

- **Direct:** Most common and involves trauma to the patella secondary to a fall or motor vehicle accident. Cartilage anlage acts as a cushion to a direct blow.
- **Indirect:** A sudden accelerating or decelerating force on the quadriceps.
- **Marginal fracture:** Usually medial owing to patellar subluxation or dislocation laterally.
- Predisposing factors include
  □ Previous trauma to the knee extensor mechanism.
  □ Spasticity or contracture of the extensor mechanism.

Clinical Evaluation

- Patients typically present with refusal to bear weight on the affected extremity.
- Swelling, tenderness, and hemarthrosis are usually present, often with limited or absent active extension of the knee.
- Patella alta may be present with avulsion or sleeve fractures, and a palpable osseous defect may be appreciated.
- An apprehension test may be positive and may indicate the presence of a spontaneously reduced patellar dislocation that resulted in a marginal fracture.

Radiographic Evaluation

- AP, lateral views of the knee should be obtained. A patellar (sunrise) view is often difficult to obtain in the acute setting, but may be of value if the AP and lateral are negative.
- Transverse fracture patterns are most often appreciated on lateral view of the knee. The extent of displacement may be better appreciated on a stress view with the knee flexed to 30 degrees (greater flexion may not be tolerated by the patient).
- Longitudinally oriented and marginal fractures may be best appreciated on AP or sunrise views. It is important to distinguish this

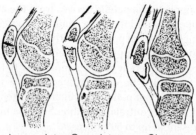

Incomplete Complete Sleeve

FIGURE 49.8 Patellar fractures in children. (Adapted from Ogden JA. *Skeletal Injury in the Child.* 2nd ed. Philadelphia: WB Saunders; 1990:761.)

from osteochondral fracture, which may involve a large amount of articular surface.

■ Stellate fractures and bipartite patella are best appreciated on AP radiographs. Comparison views of the opposite patella may aid in delineating a bipartite patella.

Classification

Based on Pattern (Fig. 49.8)

Transverse:	Complete versus incomplete
Marginal fractures:	Generally resulting from lateral subluxation or dislocation of the patella; may be either medial (avulsion) or lateral (direct trauma from condyle)
Sleeve fracture:	Unique to immature skeleton; consisting of an extensive sleeve of cartilage pulled from the osseous patella with or without an osseous fragment from the pole
Stellate:	Generally from direct trauma in the older child
Longitudinal avulsion	

Treatment

Nonoperative

■ Indicated for nondisplaced fractures (<3 mm) with an intact extensor mechanism.
■ Consists of a well-molded cylinder cast with the knee in extension.
■ Progressive weight bearing is permitted as tolerated. The cast is generally discontinued at 4 to 6 weeks.

Operative

- **Displaced fractures (>3 mm diastasis or >3 mm articular step-off):** Stabilization involves use of cerclage wire, tension band technique, sutures, or screws; the retinaculum must also be repaired.
- **Sleeve fracture:** Careful reduction of the involved pole and cartilaginous sleeve is performed with fixation and retinacular repair; if this is missed, the result is an elongated patella with extensor lag and quadriceps weakness.
- Postoperatively, the leg is maintained in a well-molded cylinder cast for 4 to 6 weeks. Quadriceps strengthening and active range-of-motion exercises are instituted as soon as possible.
- Partial patellectomy should be reserved for severe comminution.

Complications

- **Quadriceps weakness:** Compromised quadriceps function occurs secondary to missed diagnosis or inadequate treatment with functional elongation of the extensor mechanism and loss of mechanical advantage.
- **Patella alta:** Results from functional elongation of the extensor mechanism and is associated with quadriceps atrophy and weakness.
- **Posttraumatic osteoarthritis:** Degenerative changes occur secondary to chondral damage at the time of injury.

OSTEOCHONDRAL FRACTURES

Epidemiology

- Typically involve the medial or lateral femoral condyles or the patella.
- Often occur in association with patellar dislocation.

Anatomy

- As the knee flexes, the patella engages the condylar groove. At 90 to 135 degrees, the patella rides within the notch.

Mechanism of Injury

- **Exogenous:** A direct blow or a shearing force (patellar dislocation). This is the most common pathologic process.
- **Endogenous:** A flexion/rotation injury of the knee. Contact between the tibia and the femoral condyle results in osteochondral fracture of the condyle.

Clinical Evaluation

- The patient presents with knee effusion and tenderness over the site of fracture.
- The knee is held in a position of comfort, usually in 15 to 20 degrees of flexion.

Radiographic Evaluation

- Standard knee AP and lateral x-rays often establish the diagnosis.
- Schuss and Tunnel views may be helpful to localize the fragment near the notch.

Treatment

- Operative excision versus fixation of fragment depends on the size and location of the defect as well as on the timing of surgery.
- Small fragments or injuries to non–weight-bearing regions may be excised either open or arthroscopically.
- Large fragments may be fixed with subchondral or headless lag screws.
- If surgery is delayed more than 10 days after the injury, the piece should be excised because the cartilage is not typically viable.
- Postoperatively, in patients with internal fixation, a long leg cast with 30 degrees of flexion is applied. The patient is typically non–weight bearing for 6 weeks.
- If excision is performed, the patient may bear weight as tolerated and range the knee after soft tissues heal.

PATELLA DISLOCATION

Epidemiology

- Patella dislocation is more common in women. Dislocation is also associated with physiologic laxity, and in patients with hypermobility and connective tissue disorders (e.g., Ehlers–Danlos or Marfan syndrome).

Anatomy

- The "Q angle" is defined as the angle subtended by a line drawn from the anterior superior iliac spine through the center of the patella and a second line from the center of the patella to the tibial tubercle (Fig. 35.4). The Q angle ensures that the resultant vector of pull with quadriceps action is laterally directed; this lateral moment is normally counterbalanced by patellofemoral, patellotibial, and retinacular structures as well as patellar engagement within the trochlear groove. An increased Q angle predisposes to patella dislocation.

■ Dislocations are associated with patella alta, congenital abnormalities of the patella and trochlea, hypoplasia of the vastus medialis, and hypertrophic lateral retinaculum.

Mechanism of Injury

■ **Lateral dislocation:** The mechanism is forced internal rotation of the femur on an externally rotated and planted tibia with the knee in flexion. It is associated with a 5% risk of osteochondral fractures.

■ Medial instability is rare and usually iatrogenic, congenital, traumatic, or associated with atrophy of the quadriceps musculature.

■ **Intra-articular dislocation:** Uncommon, but it may occur following knee trauma in adolescent boys. The patella is avulsed from the quadriceps tendon and is rotated around the horizontal axis, with the proximal pole lodged in the intercondylar notch.

Clinical Evaluation

■ Patients with an unreduced patella dislocation will present with hemarthrosis, an inability to flex the knee, and a displaced patella on palpation.

■ Patients with a lateral dislocation may also present with medial retinacular pain.

■ Patients with reduced or chronic patella dislocation may demonstrate a positive "apprehension test," in which a laterally directed force applied to the patella with the knee in extension reproduces the sensation of impending dislocation, causing pain and quadriceps contraction to limit patellar mobility.

Radiographic Evaluation

■ AP and lateral views of the knee should be obtained. In addition, an axial (sunrise) view of both patellae should be obtained. Various axial views have been described by several authors (Fig. 49.9).
  □ **Hughston 55 degrees of knee flexion:** sulcus angle, patellar index
  □ **Merchant 45 degrees of knee flexion:** sulcus angle, congruence angle

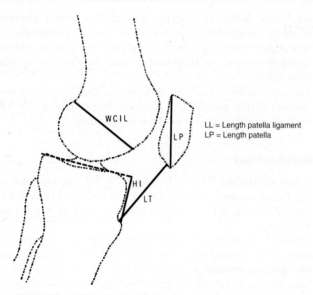

FIGURE 49.9 Insall–Salvati technique for measuring patellar height. (Adapted from Insall NJ. *Surgery.* New York: Churchill Livingstone; 1984.)

- □ **Laurin 20 degrees of knee flexion:** patellofemoral index, lateral patellofemoral angle
- ■ Assessment of patella alta or baja is based on the lateral radiograph of the knee.
  - □ **Blumensaat line:** The lower pole of the patella should lie on a line projected anteriorly from the intercondylar notch on the lateral radiograph with the patient's knee flexed to 30 degrees.
  - □ **Insall–Salvati ratio:** The ratio of the length of the patellar ligament (LL; from the inferior pole of the patella to the tibial tubercle) to the patellar length (LP; the greatest diagonal length of the patella) should be 1.0. A ratio of 1.2 indicates patella alta, whereas 0.8 indicates patella baja (Fig. 35.5).

Classification

Reduced versus unreduced
Congenital versus acquired
Acute (traumatic) versus chronic (recurrent)
Lateral, medial, intra-articular, superior

Treatment

Nonoperative

- Reduction and casting or bracing in knee extension may be undertaken with or without arthrocentesis for comfort.
- The patient may ambulate in locked extension for 3 weeks, at which time progressive flexion can be instituted with physical therapy for quadriceps strengthening. After a total of 6 to 8 weeks, the patient may be weaned from the brace.
- Surgical intervention for acute dislocations is rarely indicated except for displaced intra-articular fractures.
- Intra-articular dislocations may require reduction with patient under anesthesia.
- Functional taping with moderate success has been described in the physical therapy literature.

Operative

- Primarily used in cases of recurrent dislocations.
- No single procedure corrects all patella malalignment problems—the patient's age, diagnosis, level of activity, and condition of the patellofemoral articulation must be taken into consideration.
- Patellofemoral instability should be addressed by correction of all malalignment factors.
- Degenerative articular changes influence the selection of realignment procedure.
- Surgical interventions include
  - **Lateral release:** Indicated for patellofemoral pain with lateral tilt, lateral retinacular pain with lateral patellar position, and lateral patellar compression syndrome. It may be performed arthroscopically or as an open procedure.
  - **Medial plication:** May be performed at the time of lateral release to centralize the patella.
  - **Proximal patellar realignment:** Medialization of the proximal pull of the patella is indicated when a lateral release/medial plication fails to centralize the patella. The release of tight proximal lateral structures and reinforcement of the pull of medial supporting structures, especially the vastus medialis obliquus, are performed in an effort to decrease lateral patellar tracking and improve congruence of the patellofemoral articulation. Indications include recurrent patella dislocations after failed nonoperative therapy and acute dislocations in young, athletic patients, especially with medial patella avulsion fractures or radiographic lateral subluxation/tilt after closed reduction.

Distal patella realignment: Reorientation of the patella ligament and the tibial tubercle is indicated when an adult patient experiences recurrent dislocations and patellofemoral pain with malalignment of the extensor mechanism. This is contraindicated in patients with open physes (in children the gracillis tendon may be transferred into the patella) and normal Q angles. It is designed to advance and medialize tibial tubercle, thus correcting patella alta and normalizing the Q angle.

Complications

- **Redislocation:** A younger age at initial dislocation increases the risk of recurrent dislocation. Recurrent dislocation is an indication for surgical intervention.
- **Loss of knee motion:** May result from prolonged immobilization.
- **Patellofemoral pain:** May result from retinacular disruption at the time of dislocation or from chondral injury.

KNEE DISLOCATION

Epidemiology

- Infrequent in skeletally immature individuals, because physeal injuries to the distal femur or proximal tibia are more likely to result.

Anatomy

- Typically occurs with major ligamentous disruptions (both cruciates and equivalent spine injuries with disruption of either MCL and/or LCL) about the knee.
- Associated with major disruption of soft tissue and damage to neurovascular structures; vascular repair must take place within the first 6 to 8 hours to avoid permanent damage.
- Associated with other knee injuries, including tibial spine fractures, osteochondral injuries, and meniscal tears.

Mechanism of Injury

- Most dislocations occur as a result of multiple trauma from motor vehicle accidents or falls from a height.

Clinical Evaluation

- Patients almost always present with gross knee distortion. Immediate reduction should be undertaken without waiting for radiographs in the displaced position. Of paramount importance is the arterial supply, with secondary consideration given to neurologic status.

■ The extent of ligamentous injury is related to the degree of displacement, with injury occurring with displacement greater than 10% to 25% of the resting length of the ligament. Gross instability may be appreciated after reduction.

■ A careful neurovascular examination is critical both before and after reduction. The popliteal artery is at risk during traumatic dislocation of the knee owing to the bowstring effect across the popliteal fossa secondary to proximal and distal tethering. Peroneal nerve injuries are also common, mostly in the form of traction neurapraxias.

Radiographic Evaluation

■ Gross dislocation should be reduced first and not delayed for films.
■ AP and lateral views are sufficient to establish the diagnosis; the most common direction is anterior.
■ Radiographs should be scrutinized for associated injuries to the tibial spine, distal femoral physis, or proximal tibial physis. Stress views may be obtained to detect collateral ligament injury.
■ It remains controversial whether all patients should have an arteriogram. Some authors state that if pulses are present both before and after reduction, arteriography is not indicated. The patient must be monitored for 48 to 72 hours after reduction because late thrombus may develop as a result of intimal damage.

Classification

Descriptive

Based on displacement of the proximal tibia in relation to the distal femur. It also should include open versus closed and reducible versus irreducible. The injury may be classified as occult, indicating a knee dislocation with spontaneous reduction.

Anterior:	Forceful knee hyperextension beyond 30 degrees; most common; associated with PCL with or without ACL tear, with increasing incidence of popliteal artery disruption with increasing degree of hyperextension
Posterior:	Posteriorly directed force against proximal tibia of flexed knee; "dashboard" injury; accompanied by ACL/PCL disruption as well as popliteal artery compromise with increasing proximal tibial displacement
Lateral:	Valgus force; medial supporting structures disrupted, often with tears of both cruciate ligaments

Medial: Varus force; lateral and posterolateral structures disrupted

Rotational: Varus/valgus with rotatory component; usually result in buttonholing of femoral condyle through capsule

Treatment

- Treatment is based on prompt recognition and reduction of the knee dislocation, with recognition of vascular injury and operative intervention if necessary.
- No large series have been reported, but early ligamentous repair is indicated for young patients.

Complications

- **Vascular compromise:** Unrecognized and untreated vascular compromise to the leg, usually in the form of an unrecognized intimal injury with late thrombosis and ischemia, represents the most serious and potentially devastating complication from a knee dislocation. Careful, serial evaluation of neurovascular status is essential, up to 48 to 72 hours after injury, with aggressive use of arteriography as indicated.
- **Peroneal nerve injury:** Usually represents a traction neurapraxia that will resolve. Electromyography may be indicated if resolution does not occur within 3 to 6 months.

50 | Pediatric Tibia and Fibula

EPIDEMIOLOGY

- Tibia fractures represent the third most common pediatric long bone fracture, after femur and forearm fractures.
- They represent 15% of pediatric fractures.
- The average age of occurrence is 8 years of age.
- Of these fractures, 30% are associated with ipsilateral fibular fractures.
- Ratio of incidence in boys and girls is 2:1.
- The tibia is the second most commonly fractured bone in abused children; 26% of abused children with fractures have a tibia fracture.

ANATOMY (GENERAL)

- The anteromedial aspect of the tibia is subcutaneous, with no overlying musculature for protection.
- Three consistent ossification centers form the tibia:
  - **Diaphyseal:** Ossifies at 7 weeks of gestation.
  - **Proximal epiphysis:** The ossification center appears just after birth, with closure at age 16 years.
  - **Distal epiphysis:** The ossification center appears in second year, with closure at age 15 years.
- The medial malleolus and tibial tubercle may present as separate ossification centers and should not be confused with fracture.
- Fibular ossification centers:
  - **Diaphyseal:** Ossifies at 8 weeks of gestation.
  - **Distal epiphysis:** The ossification center appears at age 2 years, with closure at age 16 years.
  - **Proximal epiphysis:** The ossification center appears at age 4 years, with closure at age 16 to 18 years.

MECHANISM OF INJURY

- Of pediatric ipsilateral tibia and fibula fractures, 50% result from motor vehicle trauma.
- Of tibia fractures with an intact fibula, 81% are caused by indirect rotational forces.

- Children aged 1 to 4 years old are susceptible to bicycle spoke trauma, whereas children 4 to 14 years old most often sustain tibia fractures during athletic or motor vehicle accidents.
- Isolated fibula fractures are usually the result of a direct blow.

CLINICAL EVALUATION

- Full pediatric trauma protocol must be observed because >60% of tibial fractures are associated with motor vehicle or pedestrian-motor vehicle trauma.
- Patients typically present with the inability to bear weight on the injured lower extremity, as well as pain, variable gross deformity, and painful range of motion of the knee or ankle.
- Neurovascular evaluation is essential, with assessment of both the dorsalis pedis and posterior tibial artery pulses.
- Palpation of the anterior, lateral, and posterior (deep and superficial) muscle compartments should be performed to evaluate possible compartment syndrome. When suspected, compartment pressure measurement should be undertaken, with emergent fasciotomies performed in the case of compartment syndrome.
- Field dressings/splints should be removed with exposure of the entire leg to assess soft tissue compromise and to rule out open fracture.

RADIOGRAPHIC EVALUATION

- Anteroposterior (AP) and lateral views of the tibia and knee should be obtained. AP, lateral, and mortise views of the ankle should be obtained to rule out concomitant ankle injury.
- Comparison radiographs of the uninjured contralateral extremity are rarely necessary.
- MRI may be obtained to rule out occult fracture in the appropriate clinical setting. Clinical suspicion for an occult fracture is usually treated without confirmatory testing.

PROXIMAL TIBIAL METAPHYSEAL FRACTURES

Epidemiology

- Uncommon, representing <5% of pediatric fractures and 11% of pediatric tibia fractures.
- Peak incidence is at 3 to 6 years.

Anatomy

- The proximal tibial physis is generally structurally weaker than the metaphyseal region; this accounts for the lower incidence of fractures in the tibial metaphysis.

Mechanism of Injury

- Most common is force applied to lateral aspect of the extended knee that causes the cortex of the medial metaphysis to fail in tension, usually as nondisplaced greenstick fractures of the medial cortex.
- The fibula usually does not fracture, although plastic deformation may occur.

Clinical Evaluation

- The patient typically presents with pain, swelling, and tenderness in the region of the fracture.
- Motion of the knee is painful, and the child usually refuses to ambulate.
- Valgus deformity may be present.

Radiographic Evaluation

- See above.

Classification

Descriptive

Angulation
Displacement
Open versus closed
Pattern: transverse, oblique, spiral, greenstick, plastic deformation, torus
Comminution

Treatment

Nonoperative

- Nondisplaced fractures may be treated in a long leg cast with the knee in near full extension and with a varus mold.
- Displaced fractures should undergo closed reduction with the patient under general anesthesia, with application of a long leg cast with the knee in full extension and varus moment placed on the cast to prevent valgus collapse.
- The cast should be maintained for 6 to 8 weeks with frequent radiographic evaluation to rule out displacement.
- Normal activities may be resumed when normal knee and ankle motions are restored and the fracture site is nontender.

Operative

- Fractures that cannot be reduced by closed means should undergo open reduction with removal of interposed soft tissue.
- The pes anserinus insertion should be repaired if torn, with restoration of tension.
- A long leg cast with the knee in full extension should be placed and maintained for 6 to 8 weeks postoperatively with serial radiographs to monitor healing.
- Open fractures or grossly contaminated fractures with associated vascular compromise may be treated with debridement of compromised tissues and external fixation, particularly in older children. Regional or free flap or skin grafting may be required for skin closure.

Complications

- **Progressive valgus angulation:** May result from a combination of factors, including disruption of the lateral physis at the time of injury, exuberant medial callus formation that results in fracture overgrowth, entrapment of periosteum at the medial fracture site with consequent stimulation of the physis, or concomitant pes anserinus injury that results in a loss of inhibitory tethering effect on the physis, allowing overgrowth. The deformity is most prominent within 1 year of fracture; younger patients may experience spontaneous correction with remodeling, although older patients may require hemiepiphysiodesis or corrective osteotomy.
- **Premature proximal tibial physeal closure:** May occur with unrecognized crush injury (Salter V) to the proximal tibial physis, resulting in growth arrest. This most commonly affects the anterior physis and leads to a recurvatum deformity of the affected knee.

DIAPHYSEAL FRACTURES OF THE TIBIA AND FIBULA

Epidemiology

- Of pediatric tibial fractures, 39% occur in the middle third.
- Approximately 30% of pediatric diaphyseal fractures are associated with a fracture of the fibula. Occasionally, this is in the form of plastic deformation, producing valgus alignment of the tibia.
- Isolated fractures of the fibular shaft are rare and result from direct trauma to the lateral aspect of the leg.

Anatomy

- The nutrient artery arises from the posterior tibial artery, entering the posterolateral cortex distal to the origination of the soleus muscle, at the oblique line of the tibia. Once the vessel enters the intramedullary canal, it gives off three ascending branches and one descending branch. These give rise to the endosteal vascular tree, which anastomoses with periosteal vessels arising from the anterior tibial artery.

- The anterior tibial artery is particularly vulnerable to injury as it passes through a hiatus in the interosseus membrane.
- The peroneal artery has an anterior communicating branch to the dorsalis pedis artery.
- The fibula is responsible for 6% to 17% of weight-bearing load. The common peroneal nerve courses around the neck of the fibula, which is nearly subcutaneous in this region; it is therefore especially vulnerable to direct blows or traction injuries at this level.

Mechanism of Injury

- **Direct:** Trauma to the leg occurs, mostly in the form of vehicular trauma or pedestrian–motor vehicle accident.
- **Indirect:** In younger children, most tibial fractures result from torsional forces. These spiral and oblique fractures occur as the body mass rotates on a planted foot. The fibula prevents significant shortening when intact, but the fracture frequently falls into varus.

Clinical Evaluation

- The patient typically presents with pain, swelling, and tenderness in the region of the fracture.
- Motion of the knee is painful, and the child usually refuses to ambulate.
- Children with stress fractures of the tibia may complain of pain on weight bearing that is partially relieved by rest.
- Compartment syndrome: In pediatric tibia fractures, compartment syndrome is most common after severe injury in which the interosseous membrane surrounding the anterior compartment is disrupted. Patients with elevated compartment pressures 30 mm Hg or within 30 mm Hg of diastolic blood pressure should receive emergency fasciotomies of all four compartments of the leg to avoid neurologic and ischemic sequelae.

Radiographic Evaluation

- See above.

Classification

Descriptive

Angulation
Displacement

Open versus closed
Pattern: transverse, oblique, spiral, greenstick, plastic deformation, torus
Comminution

Treatment

Nonoperative

- Most pediatric fractures of the tibia and fibula are uncomplicated and may be treated by simple manipulation and casting, especially when they are nondisplaced or minimally displaced. However, isolated tibial diaphyseal fractures tend to fall into varus, whereas fractures of the tibia and fibula tend to fall into valgus with shortening and recurvatum (Fig. 50.1).
- Displaced fractures may be initially treated with closed reduction and casting with the patient under general anesthesia.
  - □ In children, acceptable reduction includes 50% apposition of the fracture ends, <1 cm of shortening, and <5- to 10-degree angulation in the sagittal and coronal planes with <5 degrees of rotation.
  - □ A long leg cast is applied with the ankle slightly plantar flexed (20 degrees for distal and middle third fractures, 10 degrees for proximal third fractures) to prevent posterior angulation of the fracture in the initial 2 to 3 weeks. The knee is flexed to 45 degrees to provide rotational control and to prevent weight bearing.
  - □ Fracture alignment must be carefully monitored, particularly during the initial 3 weeks. Atrophy and diminished swelling may result in loss of reduction. Some patients require repeat manipulation and cast application under general anesthesia 2 to 3 weeks after initial casting.
  - □ The cast may require wedging (opening or closing wedge) to provide correction of angulatory deformity. If the anticipated wedge is to be greater than 15 degrees, it is advisable to change the cast.
  - □ Time to healing varies according to patient age:
    - **Neonates:** 2 to 3 weeks
    - **Children:** 4 to 6 weeks
    - **Adolescents:** 8 to 12 weeks

Operative

- Operative management of tibial fractures in children is typically required in <5% of cases.

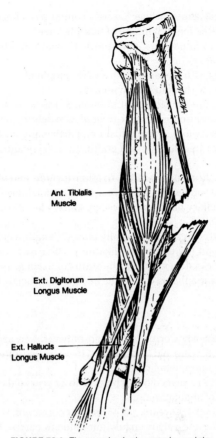

Ant. Tibialis
Muscle

Ext. Digitorum
Longus Muscle

Ext. Hallucis
Longus Muscle

FIGURE 50.1 The muscles in the anterior and the lateral compartments of the lower leg produce a valgus deformity in complete ipsilateral tibia and fibula fractures. (From Bucholz RW, Heckman JD, eds. *Rockwood and Green's Fractures in Adults.* 5th ed. Baltimore: Lippincott Williams & Wilkins; 2002.)

- Indications for operative management include
  - Open fracture
  - Fractures in which a stable reduction is unable to be achieved or maintained
  - Associated vascular injury
  - Fractures associated with compartment syndrome

- **Relative Indications include:** Severely comminuted fractures
  - ☐ Associated femoral fracture (floating knee)
  - ☐ Fractures in patients with spasticity syndromes (cerebral palsy, head injury)
  - ☐ Patients with bleeding diatheses (hemophilia)
  - ☐ Patients with multisystem injuries
- Open fractures or grossly contaminated fractures with associated vascular compromise may be treated with debridement of compromised tissues and external fixation, particularly in older children. Regional or free flaps or skin grafting may be required for skin closure.
- Other methods of operative fixation include percutaneous pins, plates and screws, flexible or "elastic" intramedullary nails or rigid intramedullary nails (in adolescents after closure of the proximal tibia physis).
- Postoperatively, a cast is usually placed (length depending on the location and the method of fixation). The cast is maintained for 4 to 16 weeks depending on the status of healing, as evidenced by serial radiographs, as well as the healing of associated injuries.

Complications

- **Angular deformity:** Correction of deformity varies by age and gender.
  - ☐ Girls <8 years old and boys <10 years old often experience significant remodeling.
  - ☐ Girls 9 to 12 years old and boys 11 to 12 years old can correct up to 50% of angulation.
  - ☐ In children >13 years, <25% angular correction is expected.
  - ☐ Posterior and valgus angulation tends to correct the least with remodeling.
- **Malrotation:** Rotational deformity of the tibia does not correct with remodeling and is poorly tolerated, often resulting in malpositioning of the foot with the development of associated ankle and foot problems. Supramalleolar osteotomy may be required for rotational correction.
- **Premature proximal tibial physeal closure:** This may occur with unrecognized crush injury (Salter-Harris type V) to the proximal tibial physis, resulting in growth arrest. This most commonly affects the anterior physis and leads to a recurvatum deformity of the affected knee.
- **Delayed union and nonunion:** Uncommon in children, but it may occur as a result of infection, the use of external fixation, or inadequate immobilization. Fibulectomy, bone grafting, reamed intramedullary nailing (adolescents), and plate fixation with bone

grafting have all been described as methods to treat tibial nonunions in the pediatric population.

FRACTURES OF THE DISTAL TIBIAL METAPHYSIS

Epidemiology

■ Fractures of the distal third of the tibia comprise approximately 50% of pediatric tibia fractures.
■ Most occur in patients younger than 14 years, with the peak range of incidence in children between ages 2 and 8 years.

Anatomy

■ Distally, the tibia flares out as the cortical diaphyseal bone changes to cancellous metaphyseal bone overlying the articular surface. This is similar to the tibial plateau in that there is primarily cancellous bone within a thin cortical shell.

Mechanism of Injury

■ **Indirect:** An axial load results from a jump or fall from a height.
■ **Direct:** Trauma to the lower leg occurs, such as in bicycle spoke injuries in which a child's foot is thrust forcibly between the spokes of a turning bicycle wheel, resulting in severe crush to the distal leg, ankle, and foot with variable soft tissue injury.

Clinical Evaluation

■ Patients typically are unable to ambulate or are ambulatory only with severe pain.
■ Although swelling may be present with variable abrasions or lacerations, the foot, ankle, and leg typically appear relatively normal without gross deformity.
■ The entire foot, ankle, and leg should be exposed to evaluate the extent of soft tissue injury and to assess for possible open fracture.
■ A careful neurovascular examination is important, and the presence of compartment syndrome must be excluded.
■ In cases of bicycle spoke injuries, palpation of all bony structures of the foot and ankle should be performed as well as assessment of ligamentous integrity and stability.

Radiographic Evaluation

■ See Above.
■ Computed tomography is usually unnecessary, but it may aid in fracture definition in comminuted or complex fractures.

Classification

Descriptive

Angulation
Displacement
Open versus closed
Pattern: transverse, oblique, spiral, greenstick, plastic deformation, torus
Comminution
Associated injuries: knee, ankle, foot

Treatment

Nonoperative

- Nondisplaced, minimally displaced, torus, or greenstick fractures should be treated with manipulation and placement of a long leg cast.
- In cases of recurvatum deformity of the tibial fracture, the foot should be placed in plantar flexion to prevent angulation into recurvatum.
- After 3 to 4 weeks of cast immobilization, if the fracture demonstrates radiographic evidence of healing, the long leg cast is discontinued and is changed to a short leg walking cast with the ankle in the neutral position.
- A child with a bicycle spoke injury should be admitted as an inpatient for observation, because the extent of soft tissue compromise may not be initially evident.
  - □ A long leg splint should be applied with the lower extremity elevated for 24 hours, with serial examination of the soft tissue envelope over the ensuing 48 hours.
  - □ If no open fracture exists and soft tissue compromise is minimal, a long leg cast may be placed before discharge, with immobilization as described previously.

Operative

- Surgical intervention is warranted for cases of open fracture or when stable reduction is not possible by closed means.
- Unstable distal tibial fractures can typically be managed with closed reduction and percutaneous pinning using Steinmann pins or Kirschner wire fixation. Rarely, a comminuted fracture may require open reduction and internal fixation using pins or plates and screws placed either open or in a percutaneous manner.

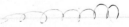

Flexible or elastic intramedullary nails may be utilized as well (Fig. 50.2).

☐ Postoperatively, the patient may be immobilized in a cast. The fracture should be monitored with serial radiographs to assess healing. At 3 to 4 weeks, the pins may be removed with replacement of the cast either with a long leg cast or a short leg walking cast, based on the extent of healing.

■ Open fractures may require external fixation to allow for wound management. Devitalized tissue should be debrided as necrosis becomes apparent. Aspiration of large hematomas should be undertaken to avoid compromise of overlying skin. Skin grafts or flaps (regional or free) may be necessary for wound closure.

Complications

■ **Recurvatum:** Inadequate reduction or fracture subsidence may result in a recurvatum deformity at the fracture. Younger patients tend to tolerate this better, because remodeling typically renders the deformity clinically insignificant. Older patients may require supramalleolar osteotomy for severe recurvatum deformity that compromises ankle function and gait.

■ **Premature distal tibial physeal closure:** May occur with unrecognized crush injury (Salter-Harris type V) to the distal tibial physis, resulting in growth arrest.

TODDLER'S FRACTURE

Epidemiology

■ A toddler's fracture is by definition a spiral fracture of the tibia in the appropriate age group.
■ Most of these fractures occur in children younger than 2.5 years.
■ The average age of incidence is 27 months.
■ This tends to occur in boys more often than in girls and in the right leg more frequently than the left.

Anatomy

■ The distal epiphysis appears at approximately 2 years of age; thus, physeal injuries of the distal tibia may not be readily apparent and must be suspected.

Mechanism of Injury

■ The classic description of the mechanism of a toddler's fracture is external rotation of the foot with the knee in fixed position,

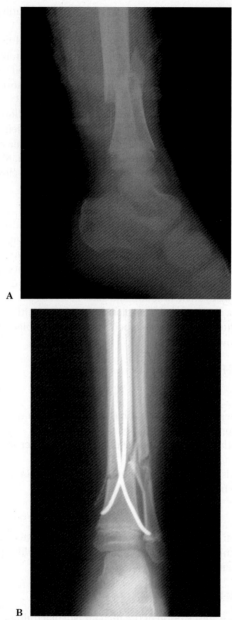

FIGURE 50.2 An 8-year-old child who sustained an open distal tibial metaphyseal fracture **(A)**. Treated with EIN **(B)**.

producing a spiral fracture of the tibia with or without concomitant fibular fracture.

- This injury has also been reported as a result of a fall.

Clinical Evaluation

- Patients typically present irritable and nonambulatory or with an acute antalgic limp.
- The examination of a child refusing to ambulate without readily identifiable causes should include a careful history, with attention to temporal progression of symptoms and signs (e.g., fever), as well as a systematic evaluation of the hip, thigh, knee, leg, ankle, and foot, with attention to points of tenderness, swelling, or ecchymosis. This should be followed by radiographic evaluation as well as appropriate laboratory analysis if the diagnosis remains in doubt.
- In the case of a toddler's fracture, pain and swelling are variable on palpation of the tibia. These features are usually appreciated over the anteromedial aspect of the tibia, where its subcutaneous nature allows for minimal soft tissue protection.

Radiographic Evaluation

- See above.
- Occasionally, an incomplete fracture may not be appreciated on presentation radiographs but may become radiographically evident 7 to 10 days after the injury as periosteal new bone formation occurs.
- Technetium bone scans may aid in the diagnosis of toddler's fracture by visualization of diffusely increased uptake throughout the tibia. This may be differentiated from infection, which tends to produce a localized area of increased uptake.

Treatment

- A long leg cast for 2 to 3 weeks followed by conversion to a short leg walking cast for an additional 2 to 3 weeks is usually sufficient.
- Manipulation is generally not necessary because angulation and displacement are usually minimal and within acceptable limits.

Complications

- Complications of toddler's fractures are rare owing to the low-energy nature of the injury, the age of the patient, and the rapid and complete healing that typically accompanies this fracture pattern.

■ **Rotational deformity:** Toddler's fractures may result in clinically insignificant rotational deformity of the tibia as the fracture slides minimally along the spiral configuration. This is usually unnoticed by the patient but may be appreciated on comparison examination of the lower limbs.

STRESS FRACTURES

Epidemiology

■ Most tibia stress fractures occur in the proximal third.
■ The peak incidence of tibia stress fractures in children is between the ages of 10 and 15 years.
■ Most fibula stress fractures occur in the distal third, but may also occur in the proximal third.
■ The peak incidence of fibula stress fractures in children is between the ages of 2 and 8 years.
■ The tibia is more often affected than the fibula in children; the opposite is true in adults.

Mechanism of Injury

■ An acute fracture occurs when the force applied to a bone exceeds the bone's capacity to withstand it. A stress fracture occurs when a normal bone is subjected to an abnormal repeated strain.
■ With microtrauma, osteoclastic tunnel formation increases to re-model microcracks. New bone formation results in the production of immature, woven bone that lacks the strength of the mature bone it replaced, predisposing the area to fracture with continued trauma.
■ Stress fractures in older children and adolescents tend to be as a result of athletic participation.
■ Distal fibula stress fractures have been referred to as the "ice skater's fracture," because of the repeated skating motion that results in a characteristic fibular fracture approximately 4 cm prox-imal to the lateral malleolus.

Clinical Evaluation

■ Patients typically presents with an antalgic gait that is relieved by rest, although younger patients may refuse to ambulate.
■ The pain is usually described as insidious in onset, worse with activity, and improved at night.

- Swelling is generally not present, although the patient may complain of a vague ache over the site of fracture with tenderness to palpation.
- Knee and ankle range of motions are usually full and painless.
- Occasionally, the patient's symptoms and signs may be bilateral.
- Muscle sprains, infection, and osteosarcoma must be excluded. Exercise-induced compartment syndrome overlying the tibia may have a similar clinical presentation.

Radiographic Evaluation

- AP and lateral views of the leg should be obtained to rule out acute fracture or other injuries, although stress fractures are typically not evident on standard radiographs for 10 to 14 days after initial onset of symptoms.
- Radiographic evidence of fracture repair may be visualized as periosteal new bone formation, endosteal radiodensity, or the presence of "eggshell" callus at the site of fracture.
- Technetium bone scan reveals a localized area of increased tracer uptake at the site of fracture and may be performed within 1 to 2 days of injury.
- Computed tomography rarely demonstrates the fracture line, although it may delineate increased marrow density and endosteal/periosteal new bone formation and soft tissue edema.
- Magnetic resonance imaging may demonstrate a localized band of very low signal intensity continuous with the cortex.

Classification

- Stress fractures may be classified as complete versus incomplete or acute versus chronic or recurrent. They rarely are displaced or angulated.

Treatment

- The treatment of a child presenting with a tibia or fibula stress fracture begins with activity modification.
- The child may be placed in a long leg (tibia) or short leg (fibula) cast, initially non–weight bearing with a gradual increase in activity level. The cast should be maintained for 4 to 6 weeks until the fracture site is nontender and radiographic evidence of healing occurs.
- Nonunion may be addressed with open excision of the nonunion site with iliac crest bone grafting or electrical stimulation.

Complications

- **Recurrent stress fractures:** These may be the result of overzealous training regimens, such as for gymnastics or ice skating. Activity modification must be emphasized to prevent recurrence.
- **Nonunion:** Rare, occurring most commonly in the middle third of the tibia.

51

Pediatric Ankle

EPIDEMIOLOGY

- Ankle injuries account for up to 25% of all physeal injuries, third in frequency following phalangeal and distal radius physeal injuries.
  - Fifty-eight percent of ankle physeal injuries occur during athletic participation.
  - They represent 10% to 40% of all injuries in skeletally immature athletes.
  - Tibial physeal fractures are most common from 8 to 15 years of age.
  - Fibular physeal injuries are most common from 8 to 14 years of age.
- Ligamentous injuries are rare in children because their ligaments are stronger relative to the physis.
- After age 15 to 16 years, see adult fracture pattern.

ANATOMY

- The ankle is a modified hinge joint stabilized by medial and lateral ligamentous complexes. All ligaments attach distal to the physes of the tibia and fibula—important in the pathoanatomy of pediatric ankle fracture patterns.
- The distal tibial ossific nucleus appears between the ages of 6 and 24 months; it fuses with the tibial shaft at about age 15 years in girls and 17 years in boys. Over an 18-month period, the lateral portion of the distal tibial physis remains open while the medial part has closed.
- The distal fibular ossific nucleus appears at the age of 9 to 24 months and unites with the fibula shaft 12 to 24 months after tibial physis closure.
- Secondary ossification centers occur and can be confused with a fracture of either the medial or lateral malleolus; they are often bilateral.

MECHANISM OF INJURY

- **Direct:** Trauma to the ankle from a fall, motor vehicle accident, or pedestrian–motor vehicle accident.

- **Indirect:** Axial force transmission through the forefoot and hindfoot or rotational force of the body on a planted foot; it may be secondary to a fall or, more commonly, athletic participation.

CLINICAL EVALUATION

- Patients with displaced ankle fractures typically present with pain and gross deformity, as well as an inability to ambulate.
- Physical examination may demonstrate tenderness, swelling, and ecchymosis.
- Ligamentous instability may be present, but it is usually difficult to elicit on presentation owing to pain and swelling from the acute injury.
- Ankle sprains are a diagnosis of exclusion and should be differentiated from a nondisplaced fracture based on the location of tenderness.
- Neurovascular examination is essential, with documentation of dorsalis pedis and posterior tibial pulses, capillary refill, sensation to light touch and pinprick, and motor testing.
- Dressings and splints placed in the field should be removed and soft tissue conditions assessed, with attention to skin lacerations that may indicate open fracture or fracture blisters that may compromise wound healing.
- The ipsilateral foot, leg, and knee should be examined for concomitant injury.

RADIOGRAPHIC EVALUATION

- Anteroposterior (AP), lateral, and mortise views of the ankle should be obtained. Tenderness of the proximal fibula warrants appropriate views of the leg.
- Clinical examination will dictate the possible indication for obtaining views of the knee and foot.
- Stress views of the ankle may be obtained to determine possible undisplaced transphyseal fractures.
- The presence of secondary ossification centers (a medial os subtibiale in 20% of patients or a lateral os subfibulare in 1% of patients) should not be confused with fracture, although tenderness may indicate injury.
- A Tillaux fragment represents an osseous fragment from the lateral distal tibia that has been avulsed during injury.
- Computed tomography (CT) is often helpful for evaluation of complex intra-articular fractures, such as the juvenile Tillaux or triplane fracture.

■ Magnetic resonance imaging has been used to delineate osteo-chondral injuries in association with ankle fractures.

CLASSIFICATION

Dias and Tachdjian

■ Lauge-Hansen principles are followed, incorporating the Salter–Harris classification.
■ The typology is simplified by noting the direction of physeal displacement, Salter–Harris type, and location of the metaphyseal fragment.
■ The classification aids in determining the proper maneuver for closed reduction (Fig. 51.1).

Supination–External Rotation (SER)

Stage I: Salter–Harris type II fracture of the distal tibia with the metaphyseal fragment located posterolaterally; the distal fragment is displaced posteriorly, but the Thurston-Holland fragment is seen on the AP x-ray, which differentiates it from a supination–plantar flexion (SPF) injury.

Stage II: As external rotation force continues, a spiral fracture of the fibula occurs beginning medially and extending posterosuperiorly; it differs from an adult SER injury.

Pronation–Eversion–External Rotation (PEER)

■ This type comprises 15% to 20% of pediatric ankle fractures.
■ Marked valgus deformity occurs.
■ Tibial and fibular fractures occur simultaneously.

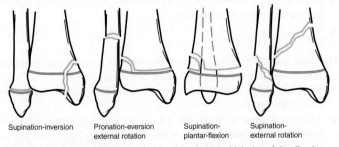

Supination-inversion   Pronation-eversion external rotation   Supination-plantar-flexion   Supination-external rotation

FIGURE 51.1 Dias–Tachdjian classification of physeal injuries of the distal tibia and fibula. (From Bucholz RW, Heckman JD, eds. *Rockwood and Green's Fractures in Adults.* 5th ed. Baltimore: Lippincott Williams & Wilkins; 2002.)

■ Salter–Harris type II fracture of the distal tibial physis is most commonly seen, but type I also occurs; the metaphyseal fragment is located laterally.

■ The short oblique distal fibular fracture occurs 4 to 7 cm proximal to the fibula tip.

Supination–Plantar Flexion (SPF)

■ Most commonly, this is a Salter–Harris type II fracture of the distal tibial physis with the metaphyseal fragment located posteriorly; type I Salter–Harris fractures are rare.

■ Fibula fracture is rare.

Supination–Inversion (SI)

■ This is the most common mechanism of fracture and has the highest incidence of complications.

Stage I: Salter–Harris type I or II fracture of the distal fibular physis is most common because the adduction or supination force avulses the epiphysis; pain is noted along the physis when x-rays are negative. This is the most common pediatric ankle fracture.

Stage II: Salter–Harris type III or IV fracture of the medial tibial physis occurs as the talus wedges into the medial tibial articular surface; rarely, this is a type I or II fracture. These are intra-articular fractures that exhibit the highest rate of growth disturbance (i.e., physeal bar formation).

Axial Compression

■ A Salter–Harris type V injury to the distal tibia (Fig 51.2).

■ A rare injury with poor prognosis secondary to physeal growth arrest.

■ Diagnosis is often delayed until premature physeal closure is found with a leg length discrepancy.

Juvenile Tillaux Fractures

■ These are Salter–Harris type III fractures of the anterolateral tibial epiphysis; they occur in 2.9% of ankle fractures (Fig 51.3).

■ External rotation force causes the anterior tibiofibular ligament to avulse the fragment.

■ These fractures occur in the 13- to 16-year age group when the central and medial portions of the distal tibial physis have already fused, and the lateral physis remains open (Fig. 51.4).

■ Patients with Tillaux fractures are generally older than those with triplane fractures.

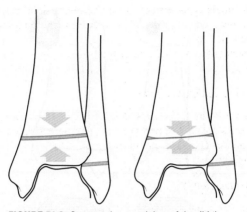

FIGURE 51.2 Compression-type injury of the tibial physis. Early physeal arrest can cause leg length discrepancy. (From Bucholz RW, Heckman JD, eds. *Rockwood and Green's Fractures in Adults.* 5th ed. Baltimore: Lippincott Williams & Wilkins; 2002.)

- CT scans or tomograms are helpful in distinguishing these injuries from triplane fractures.

Triplane Fractures

- **Occur in three planes:** transverse, coronal, and sagittal.
- Fractures are explained by fusion of tibial physis from central to anteromedial to posteromedial and finally to lateral.

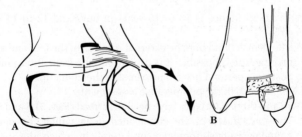

FIGURE 51.3 Juvenile Tillaux fracture. Mechanism of injury, the anteroinferior tibiofibular ligament avulses a fragment of the lateral epiphysis **(A)** corresponding to the portion of the physis that is still open **(B)**. (From Bucholz RW, Heckman JD, eds. *Rockwood and Green's Fractures in Adults.* 5th ed. Baltimore: Lippincott Williams & Wilkins; 2002.)

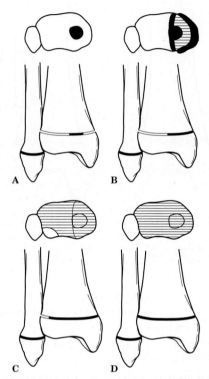

FIGURE 51.4 Closure of the distal tibial physis begins centrally **(A)** and extends medially **(B)** and then laterally **(C)** before final closure **(D)**. (From Bucholz RW, Heckman JD, eds. *Rockwood and Green's Fractures in Adults.* 5th ed. Baltimore: Lippincott Williams & Wilkins; 2002.)

- Peak age incidence is 13 to 15 years in boys and 12 to 14 years in girls.
- Mechanism is thought to be external rotation of the foot and ankle.
- Fibula fracture is possible; it is usually oblique from anteroinferior to posterosuperior 4 to 6 cm proximal to the fibula tip.
- CT is valuable in the preoperative assessment.
- Two- and three-part types have been described (Figs. 51.5 and 51.6):
  - □ Two-part fractures are either medial, in which the coronal fragment is posteromedial, or lateral, in which the coronal fragment is posterolateral.
  - □ Three-part fractures consist of (1) an anterolateral fragment that mimics the juvenile Tillaux fracture (Salter–Harris type III), (2) the remainder of the physis with a posterolateral spike of the tibial metaphysis, and (3) the remainder of the distal tibial metaphysis.

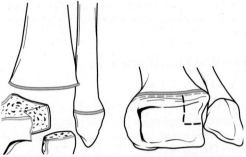

FIGURE 51.5 Anatomy of a two-part lateral triplane fracture (left ankle). Note the large posterolateral epiphyseal fragment with its posterior metaphyseal fragment. The anterior portion of the medial malleolus remains intact. (From Bucholz RW, Heckman JD, eds. *Rockwood and Green's Fractures in Adults.* 5th ed. Baltimore: Lippincott Williams & Wilkins; 2002.)

TREATMENT

Lateral Malleolar (Distal Fibula) Fracture

Salter–Harris Type I or II

- Closed reduction and casting with a short leg walking cast for 4 to 6 weeks is recommended.

Salter–Harris Type III or IV

- Closed reduction and percutaneous pinning with Kirschner wire fixation is followed by placement of a short leg cast.

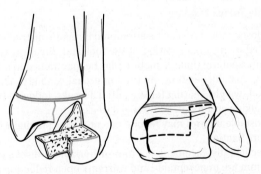

FIGURE 51.6 Anatomy of a three-part lateral triplane fracture (left ankle). Note the large epiphyseal fragment with its metaphyseal component and the smaller anterolateral epiphyseal fragment. (From Bucholz RW, Heckman JD, eds. *Rockwood and Green's Fractures in Adults.* 5th ed. Baltimore: Lippincott Williams & Wilkins; 2002.)

- Open reduction may be required for interposed periosteum, with fixation using an intramedullary Kirschner wire perpendicular to the physis.

Medial Malleolar (Distal Tibia) Fracture

Salter–Harris Type I or II

- Closed reduction is the treatment of choice; it is usually attainable unless soft tissue interposition prevents reduction.
- In children <10 years old, some residual angulation is acceptable because remodeling occurs.
- Open reduction may be necessary for interposed periosteum, with placement of a transmetaphyseal compression screw or Kirschner wire parallel and proximal to the physis.
- A long leg cast for 3 weeks is followed by a short leg walking cast for 3 weeks.

Salter–Harris Type III or IV

- Anatomic reduction is essential.
- Intra-articular displacement >2 mm is unacceptable; open reduction and internal fixation is indicated.
- Open reduction and internal fixation may be performed through an anteromedial approach with cancellous screw(s) placed parallel below and/or above the physis.
- Postoperative immobilization consists of short leg casting for 6 weeks.
- Weekly x-rays should be obtained for the first several weeks to ensure that the intra-articular fragment does not displace.

Juvenile Tillaux Fracture

- Closed reduction can be attempted by gentle distraction accompanied by internal rotation of the foot and direct pressure over the anterolateral tibia; reduction may be maintained in a short or long leg cast, depending on the rotational stability. The patient is non–weight bearing for the initial 3 weeks, followed by a short leg walking cast for an additional 3 weeks.
- Unstable injuries may require percutaneous pinning with Kirschner wire fixation.
- Vertical displacement >2 mm or horizontal displacement >3 to 5 mm are unacceptable and warrants open reduction and internal fixation.
- Open reduction and internal fixation may be achieved via an anterolateral approach with cancellous screw fixation.
- CT may be used to assess reduction.

Triplane Fracture

- Nondisplaced fractures may be treated in a long leg cast with the knee flexed to 30 degrees for 3 to 4 weeks, followed by an additional 3 weeks in a short leg walking cast.
- Articular displacement >2 mm warrants operative fixation, either by closed reduction and percutaneous pinning or by open reduction and internal fixation, using a combination of cancellous screws or Kirschner wires for fixation.
- CT may be used to assess the adequacy of reduction.
- Postoperative immobilization consists of a short or long leg cast (depending on stability of fixation) for 3 to 4 weeks followed by a short leg walking cast for an additional 3 weeks.

COMPLICATIONS

- **Angular deformity:** May occur secondary to premature physeal arrest, especially after Salter–Harris type III and IV injuries. Harris growth lines may be seen at 6 to 12 weeks after injury as an indication of growth arrest.
- Varus deformity is most common in SI injuries with premature arrest of the medial tibial physis.
- Valgus deformity is seen with distal fibula physeal arrest; it may result from poor reduction or interposed soft tissue.
- Rotational deformities may occur with inadequately reduced triplane fractures; extra-articular rotational deformities may be addressed with derotational osteotomies, but intra-articular fractures cannot.
- **Leg length discrepancy:** Complicates up to 10% to 30% of cases and is dependent on the age of the patient. Discrepancy of 2 to 5 cm may be treated by epiphysiodesis of the opposite extremity, although skeletally mature individuals may require osteotomy.
- **Posttraumatic arthritis:** May occur as a result of inadequate reduction of the articular surface in Salter–Harris type III and IV fractures.

52

Pediatric Foot

TALUS

Epidemiology

- Extremely rare in children (0.01% to 0.08% of all pediatric fractures)
- Most represent fractures through the talar neck

Anatomy

- The ossification center of the talus appears at 8 months in utero (Fig. 52.1).
- Two-thirds of the talus is covered with articular cartilage.
- The body of the talus is covered superiorly by the trochlear articular surface through which the body weight is transmitted. The anterior aspect is wider than the posterior aspect, which confers intrinsic stability to the ankle.
- Arterial supply to the talus is from two main sources:
  - **Artery to the tarsal canal:** This arises from the posterior tibial artery 1 cm proximal to the origin of the medial and lateral plantar arteries. It gives off a deltoid branch immediately after its origin that anastomoses with branches from the dorsalis pedis over the talar neck.
  - **Artery of the tarsal sinus:** This originates from the anastomotic loop of the perforating peroneal and lateral tarsal branches of the dorsalis pedis artery.
- An os trigonum is present in up to 50% of normal feet. It arises from a separate ossification center just posterior to the lateral tubercle of the posterior talar process.

Mechanism of Injury

- Forced dorsiflexion of the ankle from motor vehicle accident or fall represents the most common mechanism of injury in children. This typically results in a fracture of the talar neck.
- Isolated fractures of the talar dome and body have been described but are extremely rare.

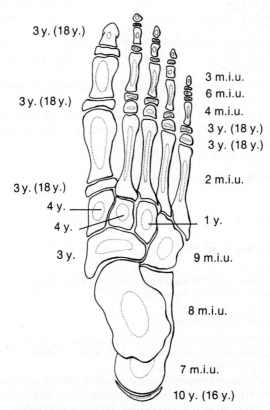

FIGURE 52.1 Time of appearance and fusion of ossification centers of the foot. Figures in parentheses indicate the time of fusion of primary and secondary ossification centers. *y.*, years; *m.i.u.*, months in utero. (Redrawn from Aitken JT, Joseph J, Causey G, et al. *A Manual of Human Anatomy.* Vol. 4. 2nd ed. London: E & S Livingstone; 1966:80.)

Clinical Evaluation

■ Patients typically present with pain on weight bearing on the affected extremity.

■ Ankle range of motion is typically painful, especially with dorsiflexion, and may elicit crepitus.

■ Diffuse swelling of the hindfoot may be present, with tenderness to palpation of the talus and subtalar joint.

■ A neurovascular examination should be performed.

Radiographic Evaluation

- Standard anteroposterior (AP), mortise, and lateral radiographs of the ankle should be obtained, as well as AP, lateral, and oblique views of the foot.
- Computed tomographic scanning may be useful for preoperative planning.
- Magnetic resonance imaging may be used to identify occult injuries in children <10 years old owing to limited ossification at this age.

Classification

Descriptive

- **Location:** Most talar fractures in children occur through the talar neck.
- Angulation.
- Displacement.
- **Dislocation:** Subtalar, talonavicular, or ankle joints.
- **Pattern:** Presence of comminution.

Hawkins Talar Neck Fractures

This classification is for adults, but it is often used for children.

Type I: Nondisplaced
Type II: Displaced with associated subtalar subluxation or dislocation
Type III: Displaced with associated subtalar and ankle dislocation
Type IV: Type III with associated talonavicular subluxation or dislocation

See Chapter 40 for figures.

Treatment

Nonoperative

- Nondisplaced fractures may be managed in a long leg cast with the knee flexed 30 degrees to prevent weight bearing. This is maintained for 6 to 8 weeks with serial radiographs to assess healing status. The patient may then be advanced to weight bearing in a short leg walking cast for an additional 2 to 3 weeks.

Operative

- Indicated for displaced fractures (defined as >5-mm displacement or >5-degree malalignment on the AP radiograph).

- Minimally displaced fractures can often be treated successfully with closed reduction with plantar flexion of the forefoot as well as hindfoot eversion or inversion, depending on the displacement.
  - □ A long leg cast is placed for 6 to 8 weeks; this may require plantar flexion of the foot to maintain reduction. If the reduction cannot be maintained by simple positioning, operative fixation is indicated.
- Displaced fractures are usually amenable to internal fixation using a posterolateral approach and 4.0-mm cannulated screws or Kirschner wires placed from a posterior to anterior direction. In this manner, dissection around the talar neck is avoided.
- Postoperatively, the patient is maintained in a short leg cast for 6 to 8 weeks, with removal of pins at 3 to 4 weeks.

Complications

- **Osteonecrosis:** May occur with disruption or thrombosis of the tenuous vascular supply to the talus. This is related to the initial degree of displacement and angulation and, theoretically, the time until fracture reduction. It tends to occur within 6 months of injury.
- Hawkins sign represents subchondral osteopenia in the vascularized, non–weight-bearing talus at 6 to 8 weeks; although this tends to indicate talar viability, the presence of this sign does not rule out osteonecrosis.

Type I fractures:	0% to 27% incidence of osteonecrosis reported
Type II fractures:	42% incidence
Type III, IV fractures:	>90% incidence

CALCANEUS

Epidemiology

- A rare injury (<2%), typically involving older children (>9 years) and adolescents.
- Most are extra-articular, involving the apophysis or tuberosity. Most occur secondary to a fall from height.
- Of these, 33% are associated with other injuries, including lumbar vertebral and ipsilateral lower extremity injuries.

Anatomy

- The primary ossification center appears at 7 months in utero; a secondary ossification center appears at age 10 years and fuses by age 16 years.

- The calcaneal fracture patterns in children differ from that of adults, primarily for three reasons:
  1. The lateral process, which is responsible for calcaneal impaction resulting in joint depression injury in adults, is diminutive in the immature calcaneus.
  2. The posterior facet is parallel to the ground, rather than inclined as it is in adults.
  3. In children, the calcaneus is composed of an ossific nucleus surrounded by cartilage.

These are responsible for the dissipation of the injurious forces that produce classic fracture patterns in adults.

Mechanism of Injury

- Most calcaneal fractures occur as a result of a fall or a jump from a height, although typically a lower-energy injury occurs than seen with adult fractures.
- Open fractures may result from lawnmower injuries.

Clinical Evaluation

- Patients typically are unable to walk secondary to hindfoot pain.
- On physical examination, pain, swelling, and tenderness can usually be appreciated at the site of injury.
- Examination of the ipsilateral lower extremity and lumbar spine is essential because associated injuries are common.
- A careful neurovascular examination should be performed.
- Injury is initially missed in 44% to 55% of cases.

Radiographic Evaluation

- Dorsoplantar, lateral, axial, and lateral oblique views should be obtained for evaluation of pediatric calcaneal fractures.
- **The Böhler tuber joint angle:** This is represented by the supplement (180-degree measured angle) of two lines: a line from the highest point of the anterior process of the calcaneus to the highest point of the posterior articular surface and a line drawn between the same point on the posterior articular surface and the most superior point of the tuberosity. Normally, this angle is between 25 and 40 degrees; flattening of this angle indicates collapse of the posterior facet (Fig. 52.2).
- Comparison views of the contralateral foot may help detect subtle changes in the Böhler angle.
- Technetium bone scanning may be utilized when calcaneal fracture is suspected but is not appreciated on standard radiographs.

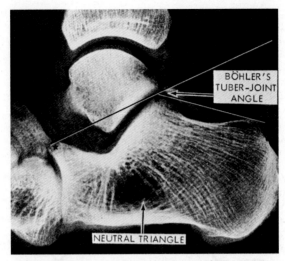

FIGURE 52.2 Bohler's Angle: The landmarks for measuring the Böhler angle are the anterior and posterior facets of the calcaneus and the superior border of the tuberosity. The neutral triangle, largely occupied by blood vessels, offers few supporting trabeculae directly beneath the lateral process of the talus. (From Harty MJ. Anatomic considerations in injuries of the calcaneus. *Orthop Clin North Am.* 1973;4:180.)

■ Computed tomography may aid in fracture definition, particularly in intra-articular fractures in which preoperative planning may be facilitated by three-dimensional characterization of fragments.

Classification

Schmidt and Weiner

Type I: A. Fracture of the tuberosity or apophysis
            B. Fracture of the sustentaculum
            C. Fracture of the anterior process
            D. Fracture of the anterior inferolateral process
            E. Avulsion fracture of the body (Fig. 52.3)
Type II: Fracture of the posterior and/or superior parts of the tuberosity (Fig. 52.3)
Type III: Fracture of the body not involving the subtalar joint (Fig. 52.3)
Type IV: Nondisplaced or minimally displaced fracture through the subtalar joint (Fig. 52.3)

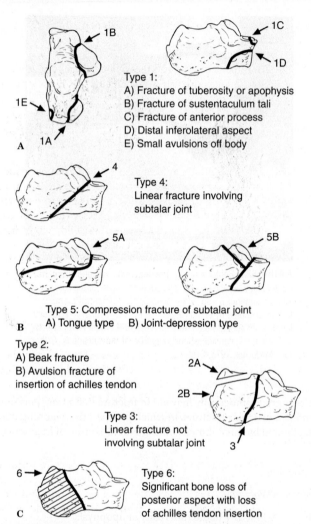

Type 1:
A) Fracture of tuberosity or apophysis
B) Fracture of sustentaculum tali
C) Fracture of anterior process
D) Distal inferolateral aspect
E) Small avulsions off body

A

Type 4:
Linear fracture involving subtalar joint

Type 5: Compression fracture of subtalar joint
B A) Tongue type   B) Joint-depression type

Type 2:
A) Beak fracture
B) Avulsion fracture of insertion of achilles tendon

Type 3:
Linear fracture not involving subtalar joint

Type 6:
Significant bone loss of posterior aspect with loss of achilles tendon insertion

C

FIGURE 52.3 Classification used to evaluate calcaneal fracture pattern in children. **(A)** Extra-articular fractures. **(B)** Intra-articular fractures. **(C)** Type VI injury with significant bone loss, soft tissue injury, and loss of insertion of Achilles tendon. (From Schmidt TL, Weiner DS. Calcaneus fractures in children: an evaluation of the nature of injury in 56 children. *Clin Orthop.* 1982;171:150.)

Type V: Displaced fracture through the subtalar joint
A. Tongue type
B. Joint depression type
Type VI: Either unclassified (Rasmussen and Schantz) or serious soft tissue injury, bone loss, and loss of the insertions of the Achilles tendon

Treatment

Nonoperative

- Cast immobilization is recommended for pediatric patients with extra-articular fractures as well as nondisplaced (<4 mm) intra-articular fractures of the calcaneus. Weight bearing is restricted for 6 weeks, although some authors have suggested that in the case of truly nondisplaced fractures in a very young child, weight bearing may be permitted with cast immobilization.
- Mild degrees of joint incongruity tend to remodel well, although severe joint depression is an indication for operative management.

Operative

- Operative treatment is indicated for displaced articular fractures, particularly in older children and adolescents.
- Displaced fractures of the anterior process of the calcaneus represent relative indications for open reduction and internal fixation because up to 30% may result in nonunion.
- Anatomic reconstitution of the articular surface is imperative, with lag screw technique for operative fixation.

Complications

- **Posttraumatic osteoarthritis:** This may be secondary to residual or unrecognized articular incongruity. Although younger children remodel very well, this emphasizes the need for anatomic reduction and reconstruction of the articular surface in older children and adolescents.
- **Heel widening:** This is not as significant a problem in children as it is in adults because the mechanisms of injury tend not to be as high energy (i.e., falls from lower heights with less explosive impact to the calcaneus) and remodeling can partially restore architectural integrity.
- **Nonunion:** This rare complication most commonly involves displaced anterior process fractures treated nonoperatively with cast immobilization. This is likely caused by the attachment of the bifurcate ligament that tends to produce a displacing force on

the anterior fragment with motions of plantar flexion and inversion of the foot.

■ **Compartment syndrome:** Up to 10% of patients with calcaneal fractures have elevated hydrostatic pressure in the foot; half of these patients (5%) will develop claw toes if surgical compartment release is not performed.

TARSOMETATARSAL (LISFRANC) INJURIES

Epidemiology

■ Extremely uncommon in children.
■ They tend to occur in older children and adolescents (>10 years of age).

Anatomy (Fig. 52.4)

■ The base of the second metatarsal is the "keystone" of an arch that is interconnected by tough, plantar ligaments.
■ The plantar ligaments tend to be much stronger than the dorsal ligamentous complex.
■ The ligamentous connection between the first and second metatarsal bases is weak relative to those between the second through fifth metatarsal bases.
■ Lisfranc ligament attaches the base of the second metatarsal to the medial cuneiform.

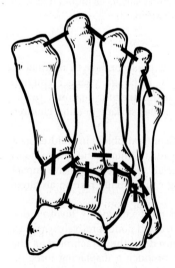

FIGURE 52.4 The ligamentous attachments at the tarsometatarsal joints. There is only a flimsy connection between the bases of the first and second metatarsals (not illustrated). The second metatarsal is recessed and firmly anchored. (From Wiley JJ. The mechanism of tarsometatarsal joint injuries. *J Bone Joint Surg Br.* 1971;53:474.)

Mechanism of Injury

- **Direct:** Secondary to a heavy object impacting the dorsum of the foot, causing plantar displacement of the metatarsals with compromise of the intermetatarsal ligaments.
- **Indirect:** More common and results from violent abduction, forced plantar flexion, or twisting of the forefoot.
    - ☐ Abduction tends to fracture the recessed base of the second metatarsal, with lateral displacement of the forefoot variably causing a "nutcracker" fracture of the cuboid.
    - ☐ Plantar flexion is often accompanied by fractures of the metatarsal shafts, as axial load is transmitted proximally.
    - ☐ Twisting may result in purely ligamentous injuries.

Clinical Evaluation

- Patients typically present with swelling over the dorsum of the foot with either an inability to ambulate or painful ambulation.
- Deformity is variable because spontaneous reduction of the ligamentous injury is common.
- Tenderness over the tarsometatarsal joint can usually be elicited; this may be exacerbated by maneuvers that stress the tarsometatarsal articulation.
- Of these injuries, 20% are missed initially.

Radiographic Evaluation

- AP, lateral, and oblique views of the foot should be obtained.
- AP radiograph
    - ☐ The medial border of the second metatarsal should be colinear with the medial border of the middle cuneiform.
    - ☐ A fracture of the base of the second metatarsal should alert the examiner to the likelihood of a tarsometatarsal dislocation because often the dislocation will have spontaneously reduced. One may only see a "fleck sign," indicating an avulsion of the Lisfranc ligament.
    - ☐ The combination of a fracture at the base of the second metatarsal with a cuboid fracture indicates severe ligamentous injury, with dislocation of the tarsometatarsal joint.
    - ☐ More than 2 to 3 mm of diastasis between the first and second metatarsal bases indicates ligamentous compromise.
- Lateral radiograph
    - ☐ Dorsal displacement of the metatarsals indicates ligamentous compromise.

□ Plantar displacement of the medial cuneiform relative to the fifth metatarsal on a weight-bearing lateral view may indicate subtle ligamentous injury.
■ Oblique radiograph
□ The medial border of the fourth metatarsal should be colinear with the medial border of the cuboid.

Classification

Quenu and Kuss

Type A: Incongruity of the entire tarsometatarsal joint
Type B: Partial instability, either medial or lateral
Type C: Divergent partial or total instability

Treatment

Nonoperative

■ Minimally displaced tarsometatarsal dislocations (<2 to 3 mm) may be managed with elevation and a compressive dressing until swelling subsides. This is followed by short leg casting for 5 to 6 weeks until symptomatic improvement. The patient may then be placed in a hard-soled shoe or cast boot until ambulation is tolerated well.
■ Displaced dislocations often respond well to closed reduction using general anesthesia.
□ This is typically accomplished with patient supine, finger traps on the toes, and 10 lb of traction.
□ If the reduction is determined to be stable, a short leg cast is placed for 4 to 6 weeks, followed by a hard-soled shoe or cast boot until ambulation is well tolerated.

Operative

■ Surgical management is indicated with displaced dislocations when reduction cannot be achieved or maintained.
■ Closed reduction may be attempted as described earlier, with placement of percutaneous Kirschner wires to maintain the reduction.
■ In the rare case when closed reduction cannot be obtained, open reduction using a dorsal incision may be performed. Kirschner wires are utilized to maintain reduction; these are typically left protruding through the skin to facilitate removal.
■ A short leg cast is placed postoperatively; this is maintained for 4 weeks, at which time the wires and cast may be discontinued and

the patient placed in a hard-soled shoe or cast boot until ambulation is well tolerated.

Complications

- **Persistent pain:** May result from unrecognized or untreated injuries to the tarsometatarsal joint caused by ligamentous compromise and residual instability.
- **Angular deformity:** May result despite treatment and emphasizes the need for reduction and immobilization by surgical intervention if indicated.

METATARSALS

Epidemiology

- Very common injury in children and accounts for up to 60% of pediatric foot fractures.
- The metatarsals are involved in only 2% of stress fractures in children; in adults, the metatarsals are involved in 14% of stress fractures.

Anatomy

- Ossification of the metatarsals is apparent by 2 months in utero.
- The metatarsals are interconnected by tough intermetatarsal ligaments at their bases.
- The configuration of the metatarsals in coronal section forms an arch, with the second metatarsal representing the "keystone" of the arch.
- Fractures through the metatarsal neck most frequently result from their relatively small diameter.
- Fractures at the base of the fifth metatarsal must be differentiated from an apophyseal growth center or an os vesalianum, a sesamoid proximal to the insertion of the peroneus brevis. The apophysis is not present before age 8 years and usually unites to the shaft by 12 years in girls and 15 years in boys.

Mechanism of Injury

- **Direct:** Trauma to the dorsum of the foot, mainly from heavy falling objects.
- **Indirect:** More common and results from axial loading with force transmission through the plantar flexed ankle or by torsional forces as the forefoot is twisted.

- Avulsion at the base of the fifth metatarsal may result from tension at the insertion of the peroneus brevis muscle, the tendinous portion of the abductor digiti minimi, or the insertion of the strong lateral cord of the plantar aponeurosis.
- **"Bunk-bed fracture"**: This fracture of the proximal first metatarsal is caused by jumping from a bunk bed landing on the plantar flexed foot.
- Stress fractures may occur with repetitive loading, such as long-distance running.

Clinical Evaluation

- Patients typically present with swelling, pain, and ecchymosis, and they may be unable to ambulate on the affected foot.
- Minimally displaced fractures may present with minimal swelling and tenderness to palpation.
- A careful neurovascular examination should be performed.
- The presence of compartment syndrome of the foot should be ruled out in cases of dramatic swelling, pain, venous congestion in the toes, or history of a crush mechanism of injury. The interossei and short plantar muscles are contained in closed fascial compartments.

Radiographic Evaluation

- AP, lateral, and oblique views of the foot should be obtained.
- Bone scans may be useful in identifying occult fractures in the appropriate clinical setting or stress fractures with apparently negative plain radiographs.
- With conventional radiographs of the foot, exposure sufficient for penetration of the tarsal bones typically results in overpenetration of the metatarsal bones and phalanges; therefore, when injuries to the forefoot are suspected, optimal exposure of this region may require underpenetration of the hindfoot.

Classification

Descriptive

- **Location:** Metatarsal number, proximal, midshaft, distal
- **Pattern:** Spiral, transverse, oblique
- Angulation
- Displacement
- Comminution
- Articular involvement

Treatment

Nonoperative

■ Most fractures of the metatarsals may be treated initially with splinting, followed by a short leg walking cast once swelling subsides. If severe swelling is present, the ankle should be splinted in slight equinus to minimize neurovascular compromise at the ankle. Care must be taken to ensure that circumferential dressings are not constrictive at the ankle, causing further congestion and possible neurovascular compromise.

■ Alternatively, in cases of truly nondisplaced fractures with no or minimal swelling, a cast may be placed initially. This is typically maintained for 3 to 6 weeks until radiographic evidence of union.

■ Fractures at the base of the fifth metatarsal may be treated with a short-leg walking cast for 3 to 6 weeks until radiographic evidence of union. Fractures occurring at the metaphyseal-diaphyseal junction have lower rates of healing and should be treated with a non–weight-bearing short leg cast for 6 weeks; open reduction and intramedullary screw fixation may be considered, especially if a history of pain was present for 3 months or more before injury, which indicates a chronic stress injury.

■ Stress fractures of the metatarsal shaft may be treated with a short leg walking cast for 2 weeks, at which time it may be discontinued if tenderness has subsided and walking is painless. Pain from excessive metatarsophalangeal motion may be minimized by the use of a metatarsal bar placed on the sole of the shoe.

Operative

■ If a compartment syndrome is identified, release of all nine fascial compartments of the foot should be performed.

■ Unstable fractures may require percutaneous pinning with Kirschner wires for fixation, particularly with fractures of the first and fifth metatarsals. Considerable lateral displacement and dorsal angulation may be accepted in younger patients, because remodeling will occur.

■ Open reduction and pinning are indicated when reduction cannot be achieved or maintained. The standard technique includes dorsal exposure, Kirschner wire placement in the distal fragment, fracture reduction, and intramedullary introduction of the wire in a retrograde fashion to achieve fracture fixation.

■ Postoperatively, the patient should be placed in a short leg, non–weight-bearing cast for 3 weeks, at which time the pins are removed and the patient is changed to a walking cast for an additional 2 to 4 weeks.

Complications

- **Malunion:** This typically does not result in functional disability because remodeling may achieve partial correction. Severe malunion resulting in disability may be treated with osteotomy and pinning.
- **Compartment syndrome:** This uncommon but devastating complication may result in fibrosis of the interossei and an intrinsic minus foot with claw toes. Clinical suspicion must be high in the appropriate clinical setting; workup should be aggressive and treatment expedient because the compartments of the foot are small in volume and are bounded by tight fascial structures.

PHALANGES

Epidemiology

- Uncommon; the true incidence is unknown because of underreporting.

Anatomy

- Ossification of the phalanges ranges from 3 months in utero for the distal phalanges of the lesser toes, 4 months in utero for the proximal phalanges, 6 months in utero for the middle phalanges, and up to age 3 years for the secondary ossification centers.

Mechanism of Injury

- Direct trauma accounts for nearly all these injuries, with force transmission typically on the dorsal aspect from heavy falling objects or axially when an unyielding structure is kicked.
- Indirect mechanisms are uncommon, with rotational forces from twisting responsible for most.

Clinical Evaluation

- Patients typically present ambulatory but guarding the affected forefoot.
- Ecchymosis, swelling, and tenderness to palpation may be appreciated.
- A neurovascular examination is important, with documentation of digital sensation on the medial and lateral aspects of the toe as well as an assessment of capillary refill.
- The entire toe should be exposed and examined for open fracture or puncture wounds.

Radiographic Evaluation

■ AP, lateral, and oblique films of the foot should be obtained.
■ The diagnosis is usually made on the AP or oblique films; lateral radiographs of lesser toe phalanges are usually of limited value.
■ Contralateral views may be obtained for comparison.

Classification

Descriptive

■ **Location:** Toe number, proximal, middle, distal
■ **Pattern:** Spiral, transverse, oblique
■ Angulation
■ Displacement
■ Comminution
■ Articular involvement

Treatment

Nonoperative

■ Nonoperative treatment is indicated for almost all pediatric phalangeal fractures unless there is severe articular incongruity or an unstable, displaced fracture of the first proximal phalanx.
■ Reduction maneuvers are rarely necessary; severe angulation or displacement may be addressed by simple longitudinal traction.
■ External immobilization typically consists of simple buddy taping with gauze between the toes to prevent maceration; a rigid-soled orthosis may provide additional comfort in limiting forefoot motion. This is maintained until the patient is pain free, typically between 2 and 4 weeks (Fig. 52.5).
■ Kicking and running sports should be limited for an additional 2 to 3 weeks.

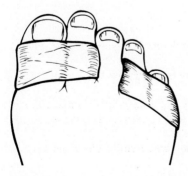

FIGURE 52.5 Method of taping to adjacent toe(s) for fractures or dislocations of the phalanges. Gauze is placed between the toes to prevent maceration. The nailbeds are exposed to ascertain that the injured toe is not malrotated. (From Weber BG, Brunner C, Freuler F. *Treatments of Fractures in Children and Adolescents.* New York: Springer-Verlag; 1980:392.)

Operative

- Surgical management is indicated when fracture reduction cannot be achieved or maintained, particularly for displaced or angulated fractures of the first proximal phalanx.
- Relative indications include rotational displacement that cannot be corrected by closed means and severe angular deformities that, if uncorrected, would lead to cock-up toe deformities or an abducted fifth toe.
- Fracture reduction is maintained via retrograde, intramedullary Kirschner wire fixation.
- Nailbed injuries should be repaired. Open reduction may be necessary to remove interposed soft tissue or to achieve adequate articular congruity.
- Postoperative immobilization consists of a rigid-soled orthosis or splint. Kirschner wires are typically removed at 3 weeks.

Complications

- Malunion uncommonly results in functional significance, usually a consequence of fractures of the first proximal phalanx that may lead to varus or valgus deformity. Cock-up toe deformities and fifth toe abduction may cause cosmetically undesirable results as well as poor shoe fitting or irritation.

Page numbers followed by *f* indicate figure; those followed by *t* indicate table.